Workbook for

Paramedic Practice Today: Above and Beyond

Volume 1

Revised Reprint

Workbook for

Paramedic Practice Today: Above and Beyond

Volume 1

Revised Reprint

Neil Coker
Robert Vroman, editor

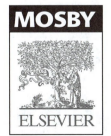

MOSBY

ELSEVIER

3251 Riverport Lane
St. Louis, Missouri 63043

WORKBOOK FOR PARAMEDIC PRACTICE TODAY:
ABOVE AND BEYOND, REVISED REPRINT
Volume 1   978-0-323-08536-6
Two-Volume Set   978-0-323-08540-3

Notices

Knowledge and best practice in this field are constantly changing. As new research and experience
broaden our understanding, changes in research methods, professional practices, or medical treatment may
become necessary.
Practitioners and researchers must always rely on their own experience and knowledge in evaluating and
using any information, methods, compounds, or experiments described herein. In using such information
or methods they should be mindful of their own safety and the safety of others, including parties for whom
they have a professional responsibility.
With respect to any drug or pharmaceutical products identified, readers are advised to check the most
current information provided (i) on procedures featured or (ii) by the manufacturer of each product to be
administered, to verify the recommended dose or formula, the method and duration of administration, and
contraindications. It is the responsibility of practitioners, relying on their own experience and knowledge
of their patients, to make diagnoses, to determine dosages and the best treatment for each individual
patient, and to take all appropriate safety precautions.
To the fullest extent of the law, neither the Publisher nor the authors, contributors, or editors, assume any
liability for any injury and/or damage to persons or property as a matter of products liability, negligence or
otherwise, or from any use or operation of any methods, products, instructions, or ideas contained in the
material herein.

ISBN: 978-0-323-08536-6

Managing Editor: Laura Bayless
Editorial Assistant: Kate O'Toole
Publishing Services Manager: Catherine Jackson
Senior Project Manager: Rachel E. McMullen
Cover Designer: Amy Buxton

Printed in the United States of America

Last digit is the print number: 9 8 7 6 5 4 3 2 1

Preface

The workbooks for *Paramedic Practice Today: Above and Beyond* have been developed to aid you in understanding and retaining material presented in the textbook.

There is a workbook chapter for each chapter of the textbook. Textbook objectives and summaries provide you with a quick overview of the key concepts presented in each chapter for convenient review. The workbooks use a variety of question types to aid comprehension, including matching, labeling, short-answer, multiple choice, and case study formats. Matching exercises reinforce key vocabulary and concepts. Labeling exercises provide you with a visual aid in learning core body systems. Short-answer exercises give you an opportunity to explain concepts in your own words and better test your understanding. Multiple-choice test items are established in an educationally sound format. Case studies are used frequently and aid you in putting your knowledge in context. Answers with rationales are provided for you at the back of the book to allow you to check your own work for instant feedback.

For best results, read the corresponding textbook chapter in *Paramedic Practice Today: Above and Beyond* before beginning the workbook chapter. If you have trouble completing these exercises, reread the text chapter and return here to try the workbook chapter again.

Acknowledgments

The editors would like to extend their appreciation to the reviewers who diligently worked on this book.

Jeffrey K. Benes, BS, NREMT-P
Aurora Medical Center
Kenosha, Wisconsin

Kristen Borchelt, NREMT-P
Cincinnati Children's Hospital
Cincinnati, Ohio

Michael Brewer, Med, NREMT-P
University of Mississippi Medical Center
Jackson, Mississippi

Robert Joseph Carter, Flight Paramedic
Center for Emergency Medicine
STAT MedEvac
Pittsburgh, Pennsylvania

Chief Thomas J. Cerbarano, BS, NREMT-P, PPS, CRS
Thomas County Fire Rescue Station 8
Ochlocknee, Georgia

Kevin Thomas Collopy, BA, NREMT-P, WEMT
Bell Ambulance, Inc.
Wilderness Medical Associates
Milwaukee, Wisconsin

Peter Connick, EMT-P
Chatham Fire–Rescue
Chatham, Massachusetts
Cape Cod Community College
Emergency Medical Teaching Services, Inc.
Dennis, Massachusetts

Jon Steven Cooper, NREMT-P
Baltimore City Fire and EMS Academy
Baltimore, Maryland

Elizabeth Criss, RN, Med, MS, CEN, CCRN
University Medical Center
Tucson, Arizona

Jeff Dietrich, BSAS, AAS, NREMT-P, CCP
Greenville Technical College
Greenville, South Carolina

Hunter Elliot, NREMT-P
The Center for Emergency Health Services
Williamsburg, Virginia

Jeffrey S. Force, BA, NREMT-P
Pikes Peak Community College
Penrose–St. Francis Health Services
Colorado Springs, Colorado

Fidel Garcia, EMT-P
Professional EMS Education, LLC
EMS Program
Mesa State College
Grand Junction, Colorado

Mark K. Goldstein, BSN, RN, EMT-P
William Beaumont Hospital
Royal Oak, Michigan
Oakland Community College
Auburn Hills, Michigan

Leslie Hernandez, BS, NREMT-P
Bulverde–Spring Branch EMS
LPMH and Associates
Spring Branch, Texas

Terry Horrocks, NREMT-P
Baltimore City Fire Department
Baltimore, Maryland

Robert L. Jackson, Jr., NREMT-P, CCEMTP, BA, MAPS, MAR
Paramedic
University of Missouri Health Care
Columbia, Missouri
Capital Regional Medical Center
Jefferson City, Missouri

Sean Kivlehan, BA, AAS, EMT-P, CIC
St. Vincent's Hospital
New York, New York

Robert Lamey, MSIT, NREMT-P
University of Baltimore (retired)
Baltimore, Maryland

Michael G. Miller, BS, RN, NREMT-P
EMS Education
Creighton University
Omaha, Nebraska

Kirk E. Mittelman, BS, NREMT-P
University of Utah
Salt Lake City, Utah
Mt. Nebo Training Association
Provo, Utah
Lone Peak Fire District
Alpine, Utah

Laraine Moody, MSN, RN, CP NP
Children's Hospital of Michigan
Detroit, Michigan

Greg Mullen, MS, NREMT-P
National EMS Academy
Lafayette, Louisiana

Timothy J. Perkins, BS, EMT-P
Virginia Department of Health
Office of Emergency Services
Richmond, Virginia

Gregg D. Ramirez, BS, EMT-P
Northwest Regional Training Center
Vancouver, Washington

Ken Reardon, Paramedic
Our Lady of Mercy Medical Center
New York, New York

Larry Richmond, AS, NREMT-P, CCEMT-P
Mountain Plains Health Consortium
Fort Meade, South Dakota

Maureen Shanahan, RN, BSN, MN
City College of San Francisco
San Francisco, California

G. Everett Stephens, MD, FAAEM
Department of Emergency Medicine
University of Louisville
Louisville, Kentucky

Contents

1 EMS Safety and Well-Being of the Paramedic

READING ASSIGNMENT

Chapter 1, pages 2-20, in *Paramedic Practice Today: Above and Beyond.*

OBJECTIVES

After completing this chapter, you will be able to:
1. List the components of wellness and discuss how paramedics can promote wellness.
2. Discuss the principles as well as personal and professional benefits of positive lifestyle choices that promote wellness related to nutrition, rest, exercise, weight control, and not smoking.
3. Discuss the ways cardiovascular endurance, muscle strength, and flexibility contribute to physical fitness.
4. Define circadian rhythm and discuss the impact it can have on those who work shifts and ways to manage that impact.
5. List risk factors and warning signs of cardiovascular disease and cancer and discuss the role of risk assessments.
6. Discuss proper lifting techniques and the safety factors related to lifting and moving patients during emergency and nonemergency situations.
7. Describe the steps that should be taken, and the equipment used, to protect yourself from airborne and bloodborne pathogens or other adverse conditions and situations.
8. Outline actions that would reduce infectious disease exposure as related to field scenarios.
9. Develop a decontamination plan for equipment exposed to body substances.
10. List and discuss the three phases of the stress response and factors that can trigger the response.
11. Identify causes (life and EMS), signs, and symptoms of stress and discuss positive and negative coping mechanisms.
12. Discuss the importance of dealing with stress.
13. When given a scenario involving a stressful situation, develop examples of positive coping responses and discuss how these could be used both on and off duty.
14. List and discuss the five stages of the grieving process.
15. Describe and discuss the needs that may arise when paramedics deal with stressed patients, families, death, and dying.

CHAPTER SUMMARY

- In EMS, "safety" includes mentally, emotionally, and physically preparing and protecting yourself. Physical preparation includes exercise as well as proper nutrition and ongoing risk assessments.
- In the world of EMS, eating wisely and well is difficult but can be done with preparation and planning.
- Maintaining a healthy weight contributes to lifelong health and decreases disease, but it also makes lifting easier by using appropriate body mechanics and decreases the chances of injury.
- Being physically fit decreases injury as well as disease and increases life span and an individual's ability to deal well with the physical, mental, and emotional demands found in EMS.
- Cardiovascular fitness, music strength, and flexibility should all be maintained; they enhance health and help and help provent disease.
- Regular medical check-ups and risk assessments increase longevity.
- Rest and sleep are phusical requirements and should not be considered luxuries.
- A wide variety of addictive behaviors is possible; identification is the first step to better health, and seeking assistance or treatment is the second.
- Stress management is an important component of remaining healthy in EMS; deal with emotions or they will deal with you; develop and practice positive coping mechanisms.
- One of the areas of self-protection that has become increasingly important is PPE; proper use can save your life.
- Paramedics work to save lives, but all have to deal with death and dying; be prepared through self-assessment of stress levels and by developing healthy coping strategies.

1

- Dealing with stressed individuals, those who are in pain, or those who have just experienced loss is challenging; keep your cool and remain professional and appropriate.
- Difficult calls and critical incidents bring special stress to the paramedic during and after the event; be alert and aware of your own emotions, feelings, and needs and deal with them in the most positive way possible; get professional help if needed.
- Be prepared for age-related differences found when death affects individuals of different ages, ethnicities, or cultural backgrounds; be supportive and nonjudgmental.

SHORT ANSWER

1. What are the three components of wellness?

   _____
   _____
   _____
   _____

2. Describe how cardiovascular endurance, muscle strength, and flexibility contribute to physical fitness.

   _____
   _____
   _____
   _____

3. What is the impact of shift work on circadian rhythms?

   _____
   _____
   _____
   _____

4. List four steps you can take to reduce the impact of shift work on circadian rhythms.

   _____
   _____
   _____
   _____

5. What is a risk assessment and why is risk assessment important in maintaining wellness?

   _____
   _____
   _____
   _____

6. List six steps that can reduce the risk of cardiovascular disease.

   _____
   _____
   _____
   _____

7. List seven warning signs of cancer.

   _____
   _____
   _____
   _____

8. Describe proper body mechanics for lifting and moving.

   _____
   _____
   _____
   _____

9. List factors that trigger the stress response.

   _____
   _____
   _____
   _____

10. List four specific physiologic effects of stress.

    _____
    _____
    _____
    _____

11. List four specific cognitive effects of stress.

    _____
    _____
    _____
    _____

12. Differentiate between positive and negative coping mechanisms for anxiety and stress.

    _____
    _____
    _____
    _____

13. Describe the stages of the grieving process (according to Kübler-Ross).

    _____
    _____
    _____
    _____

14. Describe methods of communicating death to survivors.

    _____
    _____
    _____
    _____

15. What is an exposure when referring to the spread of infectious diseases?

    _____
    _____
    _____
    _____

16. Describe procedures and equipment useful for minimizing exposure to air-borne pathogens.

    _____
    _____
    _____
    _____

17. Describe procedures and equipment useful in minimizing exposure to blood-borne pathogens.

_____

_____

_____

_____

18. What steps should you take if you are exposed to an infectious disease?

_____

_____

_____

_____

MULTIPLE CHOICE

1. Which of the following would be considered a significant communicable disease exposure?
   A. The blood of a patient with tuberculosis splashes on your shirt.
   B. The patient's blood contacts the intact skin of your forearm.
   C. You accidentally stick your finger with a clean, hollow-bore needle.
   D. Your patient's blood splashes into your eye.

2. Among the advantages of physical fitness for the paramedic is _____.
   A. physical fitness has little value to the paramedic
   B. physical fitness reduces the risk of injuries
   C. physical fitness will minimize the risk posed by violent patients
   D. the physically fit paramedic will not experience a back injury

3. Which of these activities during lifting and moving would be most likely to result in a back injury?
   A. Avoiding twisting and turning while carrying a load
   B. Enlisting help when lifting and moving a patient
   C. Exhaling during the lift rather than holding your breath
   D. Reaching over your head for a heavy box at the station supply room

4. Which of the following is the most appropriate respirator that the paramedic can use to provide protection from tuberculosis?
   A. Hospital-grade surgical face mask
   B. N-95 or HEPA face mask
   C. Organic vapor purifying respirator
   D. Self-contained breathing apparatus

5. The most important infection-control practice for healthcare workers is _____.
   A. avoiding contact with people who have infectious diseases
   B. constant use of protective equipment such as gloves
   C. ensuring immunizations are always up-to-date
   D. frequent hand-washing

6. For an EMS provider, the best method of minimizing his/her risk of disease transmission is to _____.
   A. always wear gloves
   B. ask the patient if he or she has any infectious diseases
   C. assume all body fluids and secretions are infectious
   D. assume all body fluids and secretions of the homeless are infectious

7. You are called to the home of a 38-year-old woman who is dying of lung cancer. Her children are concerned about her because she appears suicidal. She has been withdrawn and unwilling to communicate with others. You believe this behavior may also be due to the stage of grief referred to as _____.
   A. depression
   B. denial
   C. acceptance
   D. anger

8. When conveying the news of death to a family, which of the following would be the most appropriate statement?
   A. Your son has died, but he felt no pain.
   B. Your son has died. Can we call someone to come be with you?
   C. Your son has died. It was just his time to go.
   D. Your son has just passed away.

9. Steps you can take to help yourself sleep more easily after ending a shift include _____.
   A. attempting to maintain the same sleep schedule on and off duty
   B. drinking caffeine to relax yourself
   C. exercising hard before bed so you are tired
   D. going to bed immediately to maximize your sleep time

10. Which statement about patient responses to death and dying is most correct?
   A. A person's age affects how they respond to death and dying.
   B. After a stage in the process of dealing with death and dying is completed, it is not repeated.
   C. All persons will pass through the stages of dealing with death in the same order and at the same rate.
   D. Responses to death and dying are not affected by ethnicity or culture.

2 Paramedic Roles and Responsibilities

READING ASSIGNMENT

Chapter 2, pages 21-41, in *Paramedic Practice Today: Above and Beyond*.

OBJECTIVES

After completing this chapter, you will be able to:
1. Define the following terms:
   - EMS systems
   - Licensure
   - Certification
   - Profession
   - Professionalism
   - Health care professional
   - Ethics
   - Medical direction
   - Protocols
2. Describe key historical events that influenced the development of national EMS systems.
3. Discuss the role of a national registry and how national groups are important to the development, education, and implementation of EMS.
4. Identify the standards (components) of an EMS system, as defined by the National Highway Traffic Safety Administration.
5. Distinguish between the local and nationally recognized levels of EMS training and education, leading to licensure, certification, and/or registration.
6. Explain paramedic licensure and/or certification, recertification, and reciprocity requirements.
7. Evaluate the importance of maintaining your license and/or certification.
8. Describe the benefits of continuing education for paramedics.
9. Describe how professionalism applies to paramedics while on and off duty.
10. Describe the attributes of a paramedic as a healthcare professional.
11. Give examples of professional behavior in the areas of integrity, empathy, self-motivation, appearance and personal hygiene, self-confidence, communication, time management, teamwork and diplomacy, respect, patient advocacy, and careful delivery of service.
12. List the primary and additional responsibilities of paramedics.
13. Discuss the benefits of paramedics teaching in their community.
14. Analyze how the paramedic can benefit the healthcare system by providing primary care to patients in the prehospital setting.
15. Discuss citizen involvement in the EMS system.
16. Describe the role of the EMS physician, and discuss the benefits of on line and off line medical direction.
17. Describe the process for the development of local policies and protocols.
18. Describe the components of continuous quality improvement and its role regarding continuing medical education and research.
19. Explain the basic principles of research, the EMS provider's role in data collection, and the process of evaluating and interpreting research.
20. Describe the importance of quality EMS research to the future of EMS.

CHAPTER SUMMARY

- EMS is a dynamic field with a young but proud history and exciting future.
- EMS systems are an integral part of the medical community.
- Primary education is the beginning of a paramedic's education. Paramedics need to be committed to lifelong learning.
- Paramedics need to be licensed or certified to practice. If their credentials expire, they will be unable to practice.
- National, state, and local EMS organizations work to build EMS. Paramedics should participate in these organizations.
- Professionalism is a daily commitment for the paramedic, both on and off duty.
- Medical directors function as the medical conscience for EMS systems. They should be consulted in all aspects of an EMS system's development and growth.
- Research is critical if EMS is to grow and expand.

SHORT ANSWER

1. What is an EMS system?

   _____
   _____
   _____
   _____

2. Compare and contrast licensure, certification, and registration.

_____

_____

_____

_____

3. What is a profession?

_____

_____

_____

_____

4. What is professionalism?

_____

_____

_____

5. Why must paramedics practice professionalism both on and off duty?

_____

_____

_____

_____

6. How would you define medical direction?

_____

_____

_____

_____

7. What is prospective medical direction?

_____

_____

_____

_____

8. What is on-line medical direction?

_____

_____

_____

_____

9. What is retrospective medical direction?

_____

_____

_____

_____

10. What is the difference between a "protocol" and a "standing order"?

_____

_____

_____

_____

11. What is the role of the National Registry of Emergency Medical Technicians?

_____

_____

_____

_____

12. What are the titles of the four levels of EMS professionals defined by the *National EMS Scope of Practice Model*?

_____

_____

_____

13. What common name is used to refer to the 1966 publication *Accidental Death and Disability: The Neglected Disease of Modern Society*?

_____

_____

_____

_____

14. What did the National Highway Safety Act of 1966 require states to accomplish?

_____

_____

_____

_____

15. List the 15 specific EMS system components identified in the 1973 EMS Systems Act.

_____

_____

_____

_____

16. What was the date of development of the first EMT-Basic curriculum in the United States?

_____

_____

_____

_____

17. What was the date of development for the first paramedic curriculum in the United States?

_____

_____

_____

_____

18. List at least two specific EMS system elements added to the 1973 list by the 1988 Statewide EMS Technical Assessment Program.

_____

_____

_____

_____

19. What are the essential attributes of an EMS system as defined by the *EMS Agenda for the Future*?

_____
_____
_____
_____

20. What are the primary responsibilities of a paramedic?

_____
_____
_____
_____

21. Why are appearance and personal hygiene critical professional attributes of a paramedic?

_____
_____
_____
_____

22. Describe the benefits of paramedic continuing education.

_____
_____
_____
_____

23. List at least four examples of expanding/emerging roles for paramedics.

_____
_____
_____
_____

24. Describe how EMS personnel can support primary care for patients in the prehospital setting.

_____
_____
_____
_____

25. What are the benefits of having paramedics teach in their communities?

_____
_____
_____
_____

26. Why is citizen involvement important to the development of an EMS system?

_____
_____
_____
_____

27. What is the importance of quality EMS research to the future of EMS?

_____
_____
_____
_____

MULTIPLE CHOICE

1. The creation of "modern EMS" systems is often associated with the _____.
   A. creation of cardiopulmonary resuscitation at Johns Hopkins Medical Center in Baltimore, Maryland
   B. federal appropriation of $9 million for EMS demonstration projects.
   C. passage of the Emergency Medical Services Systems Act in 1973
   D. passage of the National Highway Safety Act in 1966

2. Standing orders, training programs, and case reviews are examples of _____.
   A. off-line medical control and direction
   B. on-line medical control and direction
   C. quality assurance procedures
   D. standard operating procedures

3. Of the following, the *most significant advantage* to the paramedic who reads professional journals is the ability to _____.
   A. find new employment opportunities
   B. learn about new ambulance designs
   C. learn from clinical research
   D. network with other EMS personnel

4. The National Highway Safety Act of 1966 required states to _____.
   A. create a formalized paramedic training program
   B. develop effective EMS systems or risk losing federal highway construction funds
   C. establish regional EMS projects and communications systems
   D. establish various levels of trauma centers

5. Which of the following statements best describes the role of a paramedic in prehospital care?
   A. A paramedic must surrender control of a scene to any physician with proper identification.
   B. A registered nurse who is not a paramedic may direct on-scene actions by paramedics.
   C. Paramedics are directed in the field by any healthcare provider with more than 1000 clock hours of training.
   D. The paramedic is the on-scene authority in prehospital care.

6. What is the difference between a "protocol" and a "standing order"?
   A. A protocol applies to management of patients in-hospital; standing orders are used to manage patients in out-of-hospital settings.
   B. A protocol applies to out-of-hospital care; standing orders are used only by personnel in hospitals.
   C. A protocol provides uniform guidelines for management of patients; standing orders are portions of protocols that may be used without direct radio contact with a physician.
   D. There is no difference. Both protocols and standing orders are sets of instructions that can be carried out before making radio contact with a physician.

7

7. Two elements that were not included in the components of an EMS system under the Emergency Medical Services Systems Act of 1973 were _____.
   A. consumer participation and critical care units
   B. patient transfer and access to care
   C. system financing and medical direction
   D. training and coordinated record keeping

8. The process by which an EMS professional who is approved to practice in one state obtains approval to practice in another state is _____.
   A. mutual recognition
   B. national registration
   C. reciprocity
   D. transfer of certification

9. Doing the right thing, even when no one is looking, is _____.
   A. advocacy
   B. diplomacy
   C. integrity
   D. respect

10. Completing tasks without constant supervision is an example of _____.
    A. empathy
    B. respect
    C. self-confidence
    D. self-motivation

11. Referring to patients as "frequent flyers" or "turkeys" demonstrates lack of the professional attribute of _____.
    A. empathy
    B. integrity
    C. respect
    D. self-confidence

12. Always placing the needs of your patients above your own self-interests is an example of _____.
    A. advocacy
    B. diplomacy
    C. integrity
    D. respect

13. What is the difference between empathy and sympathy?
    A. Empathy is sharing the feelings of another; sympathy is showing compassion to another and an appreciation of his or her situation without feeling the same emotions.
    B. Empathy is the process by which a professional demonstrates compassion while sympathy refers to showing compassion and sharing feelings by laypeople.
    C. Sympathy is sharing the feelings of another; empathy is showing compassion to another and an appreciation of his or her situation without feeling the same emotions.
    D. Sympathy is the process by which a professional demonstrates compassion whereas *empathy* refers to showing of compassion and sharing of feelings by laypeople.

14. A paramedic's first priority when arriving at the scene of a call is always to _____.
    A. ensure that bystanders are not in danger
    B. identify and deal with any threats to his or her safety
    C. immediately access patients and begin treatment
    D. remove any patients from hazardous environments

15. What agency of the federal government establishes national guidelines for education and training of emergency medical services personnel?
    A. The Department of Health and Human Services
    B. The Department of Homeland Security
    C. The National Highway Traffic Safety Administration
    D. The Office of the Surgeon General of the U.S. Public Health Service

16. Under the National EMS Scope of Practice Model, the minimum level of training needed to provide transport of a patient to an acute care facility is _____.
    A. advanced emergency medical technician
    B. emergency medical responder
    C. emergency medical technician
    D. paramedic

17. A paramedic's primary responsibilities include _____.
    A. documentation
    B. encouraging citizen involvement in EMS
    C. personal professional development
    D. supporting primary care efforts

18. The role of the National Registry of Emergency Medical Technicians is to _____.
    A. develop standards and guidelines for EMS education programs on a national level
    B. provide a nationwide certification for EMS personnel that all states must recognize
    C. provide a uniform testing process to ensure that graduates of EMS training programs have met minimum standards for competent practice
    D. provide a unified voice for EMS personnel and promote the advancement of EMS as a healthcare profession

3 Illness and Injury Prevention

READING ASSIGNMENT

Chapter 3, pages 42-61, in *Paramedic Practice Today: Above and Beyond.*

OBJECTIVES

After completing this chapter, you will be able to:
1. Describe the incidence, morbidity, and mortality of unintentional and alleged unintentional events.
2. Identify the human, environmental, and socioeconomic impact of unintentional and alleged unintentional events.
3. Identify the role of EMS in local municipal and community prevention programs.
4. Identify situations in which you can intervene in a preventive manner.
5. Document primary and secondary injury prevention opportunities.
6. Recognize the ways in which culture plays a role in injury patterns.
7. Identify national resources available for injury prevention data, strategies, and activities.

CHAPTER SUMMARY

- Paramedics are in a perfect position to decrease injuries and make a difference in communities.
- Primary injury prevention, or keeping an injury from occurring, is an essential activity. It must be undertaken by the leaders, decision makers, and providers of every EMS system. Traditionally, EMS providers have focused on secondary injury prevention, or preventing further injury from an event that has already occurred.
- In the United States, unintentional injuries are the leading cause of death for individuals aged 1 to 44 years.
- An injury is defined as intentional or unintentional damage to a person that results from acute exposure to thermal, mechanical, electrical, or chemical energy or the absence of essentials such as heat or oxygen.
- Unintentional injuries occur without intent to harm. In contrast, intentional injuries include all injuries and deaths that are self-inflicted or perpetrated by another person, usually involving some type of violence.
- Some people are more prone to injuries as a result of their actions or the actions of those around them. An injury risk is defined as a real or potentially hazardous situation that puts individuals at risk for sustaining an injury.

- Injury surveillance is the ongoing systematic collection, analysis, and interpretation of injury data essential to the planning, implementation, and evaluation of public health practice. Your run reports contribute to this collection of data.
- Measuring death (mortality) rates is much easier than measuring nonfatal injury (morbidity) rates. Nearly all reported deaths involve some type of tracking, whereas nonfatal injuries are difficult to track because reporting systems generally exclude clinics, physicians' offices, school nurses' offices, and the home medicine cabinet.
- Unintentional injuries are predictable and therefore are preventable.
- EMS personnel are well suited to injury prevention education for the following reasons:
  - They are widely distributed among the population.
  - More than 600,000 are in the United States.
  - They are high-profile role models.
  - They are welcome in schools and other environments.
  - They are champions of the healthcare consumer.
  - They reflect the composition of the community.
  - They may be the most medically educated individuals in a rural setting.
  - They are considered authorities on injury and prevention.
- If paramedics have the duty to respond to injuries and illness, then they have the duty to prevent injuries and illness.
- Because the job is physically demanding and inherently dangerous, both employer and employee should take responsibility for EMS provider safety.
- All employers are required to have policies and procedures in place that address workplace safety, including topics such as the use of personal protective equipment on calls and safe driving strategies.
- A teachable moment is the time immediately after an injury has occurred when the patient and observers remain acutely aware of what has happened and may be more receptive to learning how the event or illness could have been prevented. Speaking with patients or bystanders after they have experienced a crisis may be the best way to deliver effective injury prevention messages.
- KDF, SAFE, and EPIC Medics are examples of provider-driven community injury prevention programs.
- To start your own local injury prevention program, first evaluate the five *E*'s (*e*ducation, *e*nforcement, *e*ngineering, *e*nvironment, and *E*MS). Components of an injury prevention program include the five *P*'s (*p*roblem, *p*rogram, *p*artnership, *p*reparation, and *p*olicy).

9

SHORT ANSWER

1. Define *injury*.

_____

_____

_____

_____

2. Distinguish between primary and secondary injury prevention.

_____

_____

_____

_____

3. Why should EMS personnel be involved in injury and illness prevention activities?

_____

_____

_____

_____

4. What is a teachable moment?

_____

_____

_____

_____

5. Identify and describe each of the five *E*'s that are common aspects of successful injury prevention interventions.

_____

_____

_____

_____

6. Identify and describe the five *P*'s of community prevention programs.

_____

_____

_____

_____

7. Define *epidemiology*.

_____

_____

_____

_____

8. How can EMS personnel assist epidemiologists in identifying leading causes of injuries and strategies for correcting them?

_____

_____

_____

_____

9. Why are the narratives that are completed as part of EMS reports particularly important to injury prevention data collection efforts?

_____

_____

_____

_____

MULTIPLE CHOICE

1. The leading cause of death in persons from ages 1 to 44 is _____.
   A. cancer
   B. heart disease
   C. intentional injuries
   D. unintentional injuries

2. For all ages combined, where does injury (intentional and unintentional) rank as a cause of death?
   A. First
   B. Second
   C. Third
   D. Fourth

3. The leading cause of death among all age groups is

   _____.
   A. cancer
   B. cerebrovascular accident
   C. heart disease
   D. intentional and unintentional injuries

4. Applying a cervical collar, spine board, and head blocks to a patient involved in a motor vehicle collision is an example of what type of prevention?
   A. Primary
   B. Secondary
   C. Tertiary
   D. Environmental

5. Which of the following is an example of education as an injury prevention strategy?
   A. Doubling traffic fines for exceeding the posted speed limit in areas where maintenance crews are working on a highway
   B. Placing concrete barriers in the median of a highway to prevent vehicles from crossing into on-coming traffic
   C. Placing sand on overpasses before the arrival of an ice storm
   D. Presenting a program to preschoolers on identifying poisons in their homes

6. Presenting a program designed to encourage seat belt use to students in the public school is an example of what type of injury prevention?
   A. Primary
   B. Secondary
   C. Tertiary
   D. Educational

7. Your EMS system has started a new program in which paramedics visit the homes of the elderly and provide suggestions for eliminating physical injury hazards in the home. This is an example of EMS system involvement in _____.
   A. primary prevention
   B. secondary prevention
   C. tertiary prevention
   D. EMS response reduction

8. Which of the following is the best example of taking advantage of a teachable moment to provide effective public health education?
   A. Asking a 72-year-old female being transported for a hip fracture whether she has received influenza and pneumococcal pneumonia immunizations
   B. Discussing child restraint devices with a 25-year-old female who was involved in a minor motor vehicle collision with her 3-year-old daughter in the vehicle
   C. Explaining to a 72-year-old male being transported for chest pain how having throw rugs in his home puts him at risk for falls
   D. Providing a presentation of the consequences of driving while intoxicated to a high school health class

9. Ongoing systematic collection, analysis, and interpretation of injury data for planning, implementing, and evaluating injury prevention efforts is _____.
   A. an injury data collection system
   B. an injury epidemiology program
   C. an injury surveillance program
   D. a trauma registry

10. A situation that puts people in danger of sustaining injury is _____.
    A. an epidemiologic trigger
    B. a prevention target
    C. an injury hazard
    D. an injury risk

4 Legal and Regulatory Issues

READING ASSIGNMENT

Chapter 4, pages 62-82, in *Paramedic Practice Today: Above and Beyond*.

OBJECTIVES

After completing this chapter, you will be able to:
1. Distinguish legal from ethical responsibilities.
2. Describe the basic structure of the legal system in the United States.
3. Distinguish administrative, civil, and criminal law as they pertain to the paramedic.
4. Identify and explain the importance of laws relevant to the paramedic.
5. Define the following terms:
   - Abandonment
   - Advance directives
   - Assault
   - Battery
   - Breach of duty
   - Causation
   - Confidentiality
   - Consent (expressed, implied, informed, involuntary)
   - Damages
   - Defamation
   - Do not resuscitate orders
   - Duty to act
   - Emancipated minor
   - False imprisonment
   - Immunity
   - Invasion of privacy
   - Liability
   - Libel
   - Medical Practice Act
   - Minor
   - Negligence
   - Scope of practice
   - Slander
   - Standard of care
   - Tort (intentional, unintentional)
6. Distinguish the scope of practice from the standard of care for paramedic practice.
7. Discuss the concept of medical direction, including offline and online medical direction, and its relation to the standard of care of a paramedic.
8. Distinguish licensure from certification as they apply to the paramedic.
9. Explain the concept of liability as applied to paramedic practice, including physicians providing medical direction and paramedics supervising other care providers.
10. List the specific problems or conditions that paramedics are required to report. Identify in each instance to whom the report is made.
11. Describe the four elements that must be present to prove negligence.
12. Given a scenario in which a patient is injured while a paramedic is providing care, determine whether the four components of negligence are present.
13. Given a scenario, identify patient care behaviors that would protect the paramedic from claims of negligence.
14. Discuss the legal concept of immunity, including Good Samaritan statutes and governmental immunity, as it applies to the paramedic.
15. Distinguish assault from battery and describe how to avoid each.
16. Describe the differences between expressed, informed, implied, and involuntary consent.
17. Given a scenario in which a paramedic is presented with a conscious patient in need of care, describe the process used to obtain consent.
18. Identify the steps to take if a patient refuses care.
19. Given a refusal of care scenario, demonstrate appropriate patient management and care techniques.
20. Describe what constitutes abandonment.
21. Identify the legal issues involved in the decision to reduce the level of care being provided during transportation.
22. Explain the importance and necessity of patient confidentiality and the standards for maintaining patient confidentiality that apply to the paramedic.
23. Describe the conditions under which the use of force, including restraint, is acceptable.
24. Identify the legal issues involved in the decision not to transport a patient.
25. Describe how hospitals are selected to receive patients based on patient need and hospital capability as well as the paramedic's role in such selection.
26. Explain the purpose of advance directives as they relate to patient care and how paramedics should care for a patient who is covered by an advance directive.
27. Discuss your responsibilities regarding resuscitation efforts for patients who are potential organ donors.

28. Describe the actions you should take to preserve evidence at a crime or accident scene.
29. Describe the importance of providing accurate documentation (oral and written) in substantiating an incident.
30. Describe the required characteristics of a prehospital care report for it to be considered an effective legal document.
31. Given a scenario, prepare a prehospital care report, including an appropriately detailed narrative.

CHAPTER SUMMARY

- Paramedics have legal duties and ethical responsibilities.
- Paramedics are subject to operational policies, clinical protocols, and other state and local requirements.
- EMS law comes from the three branches of government: legislative, judicial, and executive.
- A scope of practice is a predefined set of skills, interventions, or other activities that paramedics are authorized to perform.
- Standard of care is the conduct expected of a reasonably prudent paramedic.
- Medical direction or physician oversight of paramedic practice includes the development of clinical practice standards, such as training curricula and protocols.
- Concurrent medical direction occurs when a paramedic consults a physician by phone, radio, or other electronic means on the scene or during transport.
- Retrospective medical direction occurs after the fact. It includes quality improvement programs and case reviews.
- Licensure through state or local levels is thought of as recognition of minimal competency and completion of prescribed training.
- Certification through state or local levels is thought of as evidence of competency in certain skills or tasks.
- Liability is the legal responsibility of a person for the consequences of his or her acts or omissions.
- Negligence is the failure to act as a reasonably prudent or careful person.
- The following are four elements of a paramedic's malpractice case:
  - Legal duty (or duty to act): the obligation of the paramedic to act with due regard for the patient and to uphold an applicable standard of care
  - Breach of duty: the paramedic violated the standard of care applicable to the circumstances
  - Damages: compensable harm or other losses suffered because of negligence
  - Causation: proof that negligence by the paramedic caused or created the harm sustained by the plaintiff
- Many states recognize immunity provisions or Good Samaritan laws to protect paramedics.
- Paramedics may also be subject to intentional torts, which encompass battery, assault, false imprisonment, invasion of privacy, defamation, libel, and slander.
- Consent is the informed permission (expressed or implied) given by a patient or another person legally responsible for decision making for the care and transportation provided by EMS providers.
- Refusal of care occurs when a competent patient, after being properly informed of risks and benefits, refuses medical care and/or transportation.
- HIPAA requires that all individually identifiable health information be safeguarded and used only for purposes specifically permitted by the regulation.
- EMTALA requires a hospital to provide medical screening examinations and stabilizing treatment to anyone who comes to that hospital.
- Advance directives document instructions for care in case a person becomes incapacitated or unable to make decisions.
- DNR patients direct healthcare professionals to withhold cardiac compressions, intubation, artificial ventilation, resuscitative drugs, defibrillation, and other invasive resuscitative measures.
- Paramedics play a vital role in organ donation by maintaining viability until organs can be harvested.
- Providing care is the paramedic's first priority regardless of crime or accident scene responsibilities.
- Accurate documentation from incident to transport is a crucial step for any paramedic.

SHORT ANSWER

1. What are the three sources of law that affect the practice of EMS personnel?

_____
_____
_____
_____

2. What is a tort?

_____
_____
_____
_____

3. What is the difference between battery and assault?

_____
_____
_____
_____

4. What is the difference between libel and slander?

_____
_____
_____
_____

5. Who may grant consent to medical care?

_____
_____
_____
_____

6. Who is considered a minor for purposes of consenting to medical care?

_____
_____
_____
_____

7. What is consent?

_____
_____
_____
_____

8. What is involuntary consent?

_____
_____
_____
_____

9. When can involuntary consent be used to treat a patient?

_____
_____
_____
_____

10. What is implied consent?

_____
_____
_____
_____

11. What conditions are necessary to treat an adult using implied consent?

_____
_____
_____
_____

12. What are the four elements that must be proved to obtain a judgment for negligence?

_____
_____
_____
_____

13. What determines the standard of care to which a paramedic is held?

_____
_____
_____
_____

14. Will the Good Samaritan Act provide a defense for an act of gross negligence?

_____
_____
_____
_____

15. You are transporting a patient in end-stage congestive heart failure who has DNR orders. The patient is awake and alert and is having extreme difficulty breathing. Is it appropriate to administer oxygen to this patient? Why or why not?

_____
_____
_____
_____

16. A 24-year-old male is in police custody for DWI following a motor vehicle crash (MVC). He has a fracture of the left humerus and a deep scalp laceration. He refuses treatment. The police officer that made the arrest tells you to treat the patient and take him to the hospital. Can you treat and transport this patient? Why or why not?

_____
_____
_____
_____

17. A 68-year-old male is conscious but is unable to speak coherently or understand what you are saying. He also has left hemiplegia. His wife tells you to "leave him alone." Can you treat and transport this patient? Why or why not?

_____
_____
_____
_____

18. You arrive at the hospital on a Friday evening with a 22-year-old male who has been stabbed in the right upper quadrant of his abdomen. The emergency department is very busy, and none of the nurses are immediately available to receive the patient. What should you do?

_____
_____
_____

19. At the scene of an MVC, you find a 23-year-old male with a deep scalp laceration. The patient is awake and alert. He refuses treatment and transportation. What should you do?

_____
_____
_____

20. You respond to a small hospital to transfer a patient who is suffering from *Pneumocystis carinii* pneumonia (PCP). Since you know that PCP is the most common life-threatening opportunistic infection in HIV-positive patients, you document in your report that the patient "probably has AIDS." Subsequently, you learn that the patient acquired

PCP secondary to immunosuppression produced by medications administered to prevent rejection of a kidney transplant. Your comments in the run report place you at risk for being sued for which tort?

_____

_____

_____

_____

MULTIPLE CHOICE

1. The recognition of minimal competency and the completion of prescribed education or training in a prescribed process or occupation is called _____.
   A. authorization to practice
   B. certification
   C. licensure
   D. reciprocity

2. You are called to a residence for an "ill man." You arrive to find an 18-year-old girl who states she has been unable to awaken her father this morning. Your initial evaluation of the patient reveals he is unresponsive to verbal and painful stimuli. He is sweating profusely. Treatment of this patient is initiated using which form of consent?
   A. Expressed consent
   B. Implied consent
   C. Informed consent
   D. Informed consent from the daughter

3. You are transporting an adult male patient. During your partner's casual conversation with the man, your partner states that her neighbor was permanently harmed by care she received from the patient's personal physician. If this statement is false, your partner may be guilty of _____.
   A. making libelous statements regarding the physician
   B. malpractice because your partner is not qualified to assess the degree of harm done to her neighbor
   C. simple negligence because the physician was not physically harmed
   D. slandering the physician

4. The conduct that would be expected of a reasonable, prudent individual with similar training and experience under similar circumstances is called _____.
   A. professional ethics
   B. scope of care
   C. scope of practice
   D. standard of care

5. A car struck an 8-year-old female as she was crossing the street. The child has moderate bleeding from an open femur fracture. She is crying and says she does not want you to take her to the hospital. The child's parents have not yet been located. Your best course of action will be to _____.

A. assume consent for treatment is implied and proceed with all appropriate emergency medical treatment
B. load the patient in the ambulance and transport rapidly to the closest appropriate hospital but withhold any invasive treatments until the parents are located
C. obtain consent to treat from the nearest police officer on the scene
D. withhold treatment until the police can locate the patient's parents

6. You and your partner are attempting to deal with a patient who is obviously intoxicated. The patient is belligerent and refuses to be treated. He repeatedly tells your partner to leave him alone. Your partner calmly, but firmly, insists on performing a brief physical examination. Which statement best describes your partner's liability in this situation?
   A. He is not liable because the patient is not competent to give consent.
   B. He is not liable because the patient's consent is implied.
   C. He is liable for assault for touching the patient without consent.
   D. He is liable for battery for touching the patient without consent.

7. You are unable to defibrillate a patient because the defibrillator did not charge. The patient later dies, and the family learns you failed to replace the battery the morning of the call, according to your service's standard operating procedures. The family most probably will sue you for _____.
   A. abandonment
   B. malpractice
   C. negligence
   D. tort violation

8. Your 20-year-old patient tells you that she may be pregnant. Upon arrival at the hospital, the patient's mother approaches you and asks you whether her daughter is pregnant. You respond by answering "yes." Your action is an example of _____.
   A. breach of confidentiality
   B. libel
   C. obtaining parental consent
   D. slander

9. A 90-year-old woman is in cardiac arrest. The patient's family says she has a DNR order, but they cannot produce evidence of any advance directive. You promise the family you will only perform basic life support measures and transport. By providing basic life support measures only, you and your partner are _____.
   A. complying with the patient's advance directive
   B. complying with the patient's DNR
   C. following the wishes of the family since they have the legal right to consent for the patient
   D. not following the standard of care for paramedics

10. A 60-year-old woman reportedly has a DNR order. While the family is searching for it, you feel obligated to begin resuscitation efforts. You are ventilating the patient, administering IV medications, and performing CPR. The family now presents the DNR order, which they have just found. You should _____.
    A. ask the family what they want you to do
    B. continue your efforts and ignore the DNR order
    C. stop all resuscitative efforts and honor the DNR order
    D. stop giving medications and just perform CPR until you arrive at the hospital

11. A home healthcare worker calls you to see your next patient. This patient is a 19-year-old male who has a history of brain cancer. There are no family members present; however, a woman arrives shortly after you. She presents a durable power of attorney for healthcare document. The patient is unresponsive and in respiratory distress but has an adequate pulse rate and blood pressure. The woman states she does not want any medical care for this patient, apologizes for the inconvenience, and asks that you leave. You should _____.
    A. call the police since this woman is endangering the patient
    B. ignore the woman and begin appropriate therapies for the patient
    C. leave immediately since this person has the ability to direct healthcare for the patient
    D. offer assistance, document the names of the parties involved, write a refusal document, and have the woman sign the refusal

12. A state court renders a decision that paramedics have a responsibility to show their license or certificate to the patient when asked. A state appellate court upholds the lower court's decision. This decision by the court is an example of _____.
    A. administrative law
    B. case law
    C. constitutional law
    D. legislative law

13. You and your partner transport a well-known celebrity to the hospital. After returning to the station, your co-workers want to know what was wrong with the celebrity patient. Which of the following statements would not disclose medically confidential patient information?
    A. The patient appeared to have pneumonia.
    B. The patient was fine and was only going to the hospital for a pregnancy test.
    C. The patient was hallucinating possibly because of a nervous breakdown.
    D. The patient was ill.

14. In which of the following situations would releasing information be a breach of confidentiality?
    A. Insurance companies that must have specific information about patients to pay claims
    B. Legal subpoenas to disclose the information
    C. Other EMS personnel who did not participate in the patient's care
    D. Other healthcare providers who need the information to continue patient care

15. Which of the following actions could result in a lawsuit against a paramedic for battery?
    A. Caring for an adult who has suffered a humerus fracture and is awake, alert, and refusing treatment
    B. Caring for an unconscious patient
    C. Treating a child for a femur fracture whose parents are not present to give consent
    D. Treating a patient in police custody who is refusing treatment when the arresting officer tells you to treat him

16. A paramedic's "standard of care" is judged by comparing his or her actions to _____.
    A. the actions expected of a paramedic in the same situation
    B. the actions expected of a physician in the same situation
    C. the care provided in the hospital emergency department
    D. the medical director's standards for how the paramedic should have performed

17. Your best protection from liability when a patient refuses treatment or transportation is a _____.
    A. detailed written report that documents all attempts made to obtain consent
    B. good attorney who understands EMS and the law of consent
    C. "release from liability" form signed by the patient
    D. report documenting that your more experienced partner agreed the patient did not need transport

18. Release of information about a patient to which of the following groups of persons would be a breach of confidentiality?
    A. Insurance companies that must have specific information about patients to pay claims
    B. Law enforcement officers who are attempting to determine whether a patient was using drugs
    C. Legal subpoenas or other orders from a court of law to disclose the information
    D. Other healthcare providers who need the information to continue patient care

19. For the purpose of consenting to medical treatment, a child becomes an adult at _____.
    A. 17 years of age for females and 18 years of age for males
    B. 17 years of age for males and 18 years of age for females
    C. 18 years of age whether the patient is male or female
    D. 21 years of age unless he or she already is married

20. A 32-year-old mentally incompetent patient has fallen and fractured his femur. His court-appointed guardian is present. You should _____.
    A. begin treatment using implied consent since a femur fracture is a life-threatening injury
    B. obtain an order from the court that originally declared the patient incompetent
    C. obtain consent from the guardian because he is authorized to consent for the patient
    D. obtain consent from the patient because he is an adult

21. A 10-year-old male fell from his bicycle and hit his head. He is conscious, but has a 2-inch laceration to the right temporal area of his scalp. While you are examining the patient, you hear radio traffic regarding a major auto collision with multiple casualties five blocks away. You ask the child's parents to transport him to the hospital in the family car so you can respond to the collision. In route to the hospital, the child has a seizure, vomits, and asphyxiates on the aspirate. You probably will be sued for _____.
    A. abandonment
    B. assault
    C. battery
    D. dereliction of duty

22. A 73-year-old male with a history of lung cancer lost consciousness approximately 5 minutes ago. He is pulseless and apneic. The family tells you the patient has a DNR order. However, they cannot find it. What should you do?
    A. Act like the DNR order was available and do not start CPR.
    B. Contact on-line medical control for advice on how to proceed before starting CPR.
    C. Start CPR, go to the ambulance, and then discontinue resuscitation once you are in route.
    D. Start CPR and then contact on-line medical control for advice on how to proceed.

23. Your patient is a 70-year-old retired federal judge who exhibits confusion, slurred speech, and a staggering gait. The odor of alcohol is present on his breath. As you are taking him to the ambulance, a neighbor asks what is wrong, and you reply, "He's just drunk." The patient is subsequently diagnosed as having a cerebrovascular accident (a stroke). Your comment to the neighbor could result in you being sued for _____.
    A. invasion of privacy
    B. slander
    C. libel
    D. negligence

Case one

A 20-year-old college junior who is home on spring break complains of severe abdominal pain, nausea, and vomiting. She wants to go to the hospital. However, her mother, who is a lay minister of the Central Unification Church of East Kalamazoo, says to leave the girl alone because you are an "agent of the devil."

1. Can you treat and transport this patient?

2. Why or why not?

3. What type of consent are you operating under in this situation?

Case two

You respond to a report of a child having seizures. The patient is a 13-year-old male with a history of epilepsy who is having a tonic-clonic seizure when you arrive. The patient's parents are not available. The patient's 18-year-old sister is present. She tells you to treat and transport her brother. However, the patient's 72-year-old grandmother tells you to leave the boy alone.

1. Can you treat and transport this patient?

2. Why or why not?

3. What type of consent are you operating under in this situation?

Case three

You respond to a report of an overdose. A 47-year-old male tells you his 42-year-old wife ingested the contents of a bottle of Seconal. You find the patient sitting in bed, awake and alert. She tells you she is fine and orders you out of the house.

1. Can you treat and transport this patient at this time?

2. What should you do?

3. What type of consent are you operating under in this situation?

Case four

You respond to a report of a child struck by a motor vehicle. The patient is a 10-year-old female who was hit by a car and thrown at least 30 feet. She is unresponsive. Respirations are shallow and gasping. Radial pulses are absent. Her skin is cool and moist, and her abdomen is distended. As you prepare to transport, a man approaches. He identifies himself as the girl's father and tells you not to treat the patient.

1. Can you treat and transport this patient at this time?

2. Why or why not?

3. What should you do?

4. What type of consent are you operating under in this situation?

5. What individuals can provide you with this type of consent?

Case five

At 0730 hours on a Tuesday morning, you respond to the First Baptist Church, where the custodian has found a middle-aged male unconscious in the flowerbeds. The patient is unresponsive. He is exuding a number of strong aromas, including that of cheap wine.

1. Can you treat and transport this patient at this time?

2. Why or why not?

3. What type of consent are you operating under in this situation?

Case six

A 14-year-old male was struck in the throat by a line drive during baseball practice. He is hoarse and slightly dyspneic, and he has ecchymosis and edema of the anterior aspect of his neck. He does not want to go to the hospital. His parents cannot be reached. His coach tells you to leave the patient alone because the pain "will make a man of him."

1. Can you treat and transport this patient?

2. Why or why not?

3. What type of consent are you operating under in this situation?

    _____

4. What are the elements of this form of consent?

    _____
    _____
    _____
    _____

Case seven

You are on the scene of a motor vehicle crash. As you are preparing to apply a cervical collar and extricate the patient to a long-board, a man approaches. He tells you he is a physician and states that he is "in charge here now." He then directs you to, "Stop all that TV stuff, drag the patient out of there, and rush him to the hospital where professionals can care for him." Recall what you learned in chapter 2 about on scene physicians. Combining that knowledge with the legal principles of this chapter, please answer the following questions.

1. What should you do?

    _____
    _____
    _____
    _____

2. What is your relationship to your medical director relative to a physician who intervenes on a scene?

    _____
    _____
    _____
    _____

Case eight

A truck ran down a 12-year-old male who was crossing the street. He is unconscious and unresponsive with unequal pupils. He also has a fractured pelvis and right femur. Present are his 17-year-old sister and 22-year-old first cousin.

1. Can his sister give you consent?

    _____

2. Why or why not?

    _____
    _____
    _____
    _____

3. Can his cousin give you consent?

    _____

4. Why or why not?

    _____
    _____
    _____
    _____

5. Can you treat this patient?

    _____

6. Why or why not?

_____
_____
_____
_____

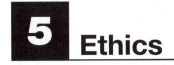

5 Ethics

READING ASSIGNMENT

Chapter 5, pages 83-94, in *Paramedic Practice Today: Above and Beyond.*

OBJECTIVES

After completing this chapter, you will be able to:
1. Define the terms *ethics, morals, unethical,* and *medical ethics.*
2. Distinguish ethical from moral decisions.
3. Identify the premise that should underlie the paramedic's ethical decisions in prehospital care.
4. Discuss the kinds of ethical dilemmas that paramedics typically en-counter in the field.
5. Analyze the relation between the law and ethics in EMS.
6. Discuss the rights of patients.
7. Compare the criteria that may be used in allocating scarce EMS resources.
8. Identify the issues surrounding the use of advance directives in making a prehospital resuscitation decision.
9. Discuss the basic virtues that are most essential in EMS professionals.

CHAPTER SUMMARY

- Ethics are societal principles of conduct that people or groups of people adopt as guidelines for personal behavior.
- Morals are values that help a person define right (what a persion ought to do) versus wrong (what a person ought not to do). Morals are derived from teachings from parents, grandparents, mentors, and religious beliefs.
- *Unethical* refers to conduct that does not conform to approved standards of social or professional behavior.
- Protection of patient privacy is paramount.
- Honesty and respect for humanity are essential traits for the paramedic.
- Medical codes of ethics throughout history and in modern times focus on first doing no harm and the responsibilities of healthcare professionals to the patient.
- Patients' rights are based on their intrinsic autonomy and dignity.
- Professional accountability includes staying current with certificates and maintaining healthy relationships with oneself and colleagues while always placing the patient's best interests foremost.

- Basic virtues exemplify the basis of ethical behavior and are evident in how paramedics treat each other as well as their patients.

SHORT ANSWER

1. Define *ethics.*

_____
_____
_____
_____

2. Integrating what you learned about legal issues in chapter 4, and what you learned in this chapter, how would you answer the following question: How do ethical standards differ from legal requirements?

_____
_____
_____
_____

3. If you are faced with an ethical dilemma when you are caring for a patient. What do you believe to be the "guiding principle" that will help you determine the appropriate response?

_____
_____
_____
_____

4. Define *beneficence.*

_____
_____
_____
_____

5. Define *autonomy.*

_____
_____
_____
_____

6. Define *justice.*

_____
_____
_____
_____

7. Explain the meaning of the Latin phrase *primum non nocere*.

_____

_____

_____

_____

8. Integrating your prior knowledge of the legal issues of EMS, and the information in this chapter, how would you answer the following question? What conditions must exist for a patient to exercise autonomy in making decisions relating to his or her healthcare?

_____

_____

_____

_____

9. Integrating your prior knowledge of the legal issues of EMS, and the information in this chapter, how would you answer the following question? Ethically, why is maintaining patient confidentiality important?

_____

_____

_____

_____

MULTIPLE CHOICE

1. The term *ethics* is best described as _____.
   A. legal standards of conduct for a profession
   B. one's personal choices of standards for conduct and behavior
   C. painstaking attention, caring, and management of patients
   D. standards of conduct and behavior defined by society

2. Your adult, mentally competent patient refuses all medical care. He realizes the potential consequences of his actions. By complying with this patient's wishes, the paramedic recognizes the patient's right to _____.
   A. autonomy
   B. beneficence
   C. justice
   D. nonmaleficence

3. Applying the principles you learned in this chapter, how would you answer the following question: A paramedic student has been riding with you and your partner for 10 shifts. The student is performing at or near the level of competence expected of an entry-level paramedic. You have been called to see a 36-year-old female who has had vomiting and diarrhea for 2 days. She is complaining of weakness and dizziness when she attempts to stand. The student is preparing to start an IV with Ringer's lactate. How should you explain the student's status and role to the patient?
   A. Do not bring up the issue of who the student is unless the patient asks.

B. Introduce the student to the patient, explain that you are supervising the student and will take over if there are any problems, and ask for the patient's permission for the student to start the IV.
   C. Tell the patient that the student is fully qualified and competent to perform an IV.
   D. Tell the patient that the student is a member of your crew and is competent to start the IV.

4. Your patient is a 34-year-old male with a history of narcotic abuse. You have been called to see him a number of times for a variety of vague painful complaints. Today the patient is complaining of substernal chest pain that radiates to his left shoulder, nausea, and shortness of breath. He says the pain is the worst he ever has felt and that he needs a shot of morphine "right now." What should you do?
   A. Treat the patient according to his signs and symptoms, following appropriate treatment for chest pain, including the administration of morphine if indicated.
   B. Treat the patient according to his signs and symptoms. However, withold morphine, if indicated, due to his history of narcotic abuse.
   C. Due to the patient's history of narcotic abuse, withhold all ALS treatment and treat him with BLS interventions only.
   D. Tell the patient you are not going to treat him for his chest pain because he is a "drug seeker."

5. If you would treat a physician with chest pain by giving morphine but would withhold morphine from a homeless person with a history of drug abuse, what principle of ethics would you be violating?
   A. Autonomy
   B. Beneficence
   C. Justice
   D. Nonmaleficence

6. A 22-year-old female, who was driving while intoxicated, fractured her right ankle and nose and lacerated her forehead during a frontal collision with a tree. She is conscious and highly agitated. She curses continuously at you and your partner while you extricate her from her vehicle and prepare her for transport. She has no evidence of chest or abdominal trauma. Her vital signs are, P—124 beats/min strong, regular; R—18 breaths/min regular; BP—136/100 mm Hg. Capillary refill time is less than 2 seconds. After moving her to the ambulance, you prepare to start a keep open IV as a precautionary measure. Your partner hands you a needle that is inappropriately large for the patient's condition. He winks at you, and says, "Here, use this one in the back of her hand." What fundamental principle of medical ethics is your partner violating?
   A. Autonomy
   B. Beneficence
   C. Justice
   D. *Primum non nocere*

7. Your patient is a 73-year-old male suffering from end-stage Alzheimer's disease. He is in respiratory distress after aspirating the contents of his feeding tube. His wife states she wants nothing done and produces her husband's advance directives that correspond to those wishes. By following the wishes of the patient as expressed in his advance directives, you are respecting the fundamental principle of medical ethics known as _____.
   A. autonomy
   B. beneficence
   C. justice
   D. nonmaleficence

8. If a physician asks you to perform an act that is illegal or unethical, what should you do?
   A. Perform the act as ordered because you could lose your certification from refusing a physician's orders.
   B. Perform the act as ordered but report the physician to the appropriate authorities.
   C. Refuse to perform the act.
   D. Refuse to perform the act and report the physician to the appropriate authorities.

READING ASSIGNMENT

Chapter 6, pages 95-107, in *Paramedic Practice Today: Above and Beyond*.

OBJECTIVES

After completing this chapter, you will be able to:
1. Explain why using correct medical terminology in medical setting is important.
2. Identify and describe the three word parts that make up medical terms.
3. State why understanding how each word part functions is important.
4. Pronounce various medical terms correctly by applying the appropriate pronunciation guidelines.
5. Correctly change various medical terms from their singular to plural form.
6. Define and give an example of a homonym, an antonym, and a synonym.
7. Describe the impact on patient care when paramedics have a solid grasp of the correct medical terminology.

CHAPTER SUMMARY

- Paramedics use medical terminology daily, so you must know how to determine the meaning of medical terms.
- The word parts used to build medical words are root words, prefixes, and suffixes.
- Understanding the function of the word parts can help you determine the meaning of unfamiliar medical terms.
- Practice makes perfect. Use flashcards, practice writing and saying the word parts and their meanings, and look up unfamiliar word parts in a medical dictionary if necessary.
- Practice pronouncing difficult medical terms.
- You may have to change a medical term from its singular to plural form to record it. Knowing the guidelines for changing English, Greek, and Latin words from singular to plural will help.
- A homonym is a word that has the same pronunciation as another word, but a different spelling and meaning.
- An antonym is a word that has the opposite meaning of another word.
- A synonym is a root word, suffix, or prefix that has the same or almost the same meaning as another root word, suffix, or prefix.
- The correct use of medical terminology correctly creates a good impression and builds credibility with your patients and their families.

MATCHING

1. Match each prefix to its meaning.

_____a-, an-	A. backward, behind
_____aden-	B. difficult, bad, painful
_____bi-	C. excessive, above
_____contra-	D. half
_____derma-	E. large
_____dia-	F. many, much, excessive
_____dys-	G. opposed, against
_____edem-	H. pertaining to gland
_____erythro-	I. pertaining to muscle
_____hemi-	J. red
_____hyper-	K. skin
_____hypo-	L. small
_____macro-	M. swelling
_____micro-	N. through, completely
_____my-	O. two, double, twice
_____poly-	P. under, deficient
_____retro-	Q. without, from

2. Match each root word to its meaning.

_____arthr-	A. arm
_____brachi-	B. bladder
_____bucc-	C. brain
_____cardi-	D. cartilage
_____carp-	E. cell
_____cephal-	F. cheek
_____chondr-	G. face
_____cost-	H. fibers
_____cyst-	I. head
_____cyt-	J. heart
_____encephal-	K. intestine
_____enter-	L. jaw
_____faci-	M. joint
_____fibr-	N. rib
_____gastr-	O. stomach
_____gloss-	P. tissue
_____gnath-	Q. tongue
_____hist-	R. wrist

3. Match each suffix to its meaning.

____-algia	A. blood
____-cyte	B. breathing
____-dipsia	C. causing
____-ectomy	D. cell
____-emia	E. condition of
____-esthesia	F. creation of an opening
____-genic	G. cutting out
____-gram	H. eating
____-itis	I. fear
____-logy	J. flow or discharge
____-ostomy	K. inflammation
____-oma	L. order, arrangement of
____-osis	M. pain
____-paresis	N. paralysis
____-phagia	O. record
____-plegia	P. rhythm
____-pnea	Q. science, study of
____-phasia	R. sensation
____-phobia	S. speech
____-rhythmia	T. thirst
____-rrhea	U. to do with urine
____-taxia	V. tumor
____-uria	W. weakness

SHORT ANSWER

1. Explain why it is important to use correct medical terminology in medical settings.

_____

_____

_____

_____

2. List the three word parts that make up medical terms.

_____

_____

_____

_____

3. Understanding how each word part functions can:

_____

_____

_____

_____

TRUE/FALSE

1. *Chromosome* begins with a hard *k* sound.
   A. True
   B. False

2. *Genitourinary* begins with a hard *g* sound.
   A. True
   B. False

MULTIPLE CHOICE

1. *Ad-* and *ab-* are examples of _____.
   A. antonyms
   B. eponyms
   C. homonyms
   D. synonyms

2. *Hemi-* and *semi-* are examples of _____.
   A. antonyms
   B. eponyms
   C. homonyms
   D. synonyms

3. The plural of *myopathy* is _____.
   A. myopathes
   B. myopathies
   C. myopathyes
   D. myopathys

4. Words that sound alike but are spelled differently and have different meanings are _____.
   A. antonyms
   B. eponyms
   C. homonyms
   D. synonyms

5. Words that derive their names from a specific person, place, or thing are called _____.
   A. antonyms
   B. eponyms
   C. homonyms
   D. synonyms

6. An example of an eponym is _____.
   A. carpal
   B. cystic fibrosis
   C. pinkeye
   D. postpartum

7. A word that begins with the prefix *my-* is referring to _____.
   A. glands
   B. muscles
   C. red blood cells
   D. speech

8. *Pulmon/o-* and *pneumo-* are examples of _____.
   A. antonyms
   B. eponyms
   C. homonyms
   D. synonyms

9. *Every day* is abbreviated _____.
   A. qd
   B. qh
   C. qid
   D. qn

10. *After* is abbreviated _____.
    A. ā
    B. p̄
    C. q̄
    D. s̄

7 Body Systems: Anatomy and Physiology

READING ASSIGNMENT

Chapter 7, pages 108-204, in *Paramedic Practice Today: Above and Beyond*.

OBJECTIVES

After completing this chapter, you will be able to:

1. Define *anatomy, physiology*, and *pathophysiology* and discuss the importance of human anatomy and physiology to the paramedic profession.
2. Define *homeostasis*.
3. Describe the anatomic position.
4. Describe the sagittal, midsagittal, transverse, and frontal planes.
5. List the structures that comprise the axial and appendicular regions of the body.
6. Name the body cavities, membranes, and some organs within each cavity.
7. Define the function of cellular structures.
8. Describe the cytoplasm.
9. Describe the function of the cell organelles.
10. State the function of the nucleus.
11. Describe how cells reproduce.
12. Discuss input and output of aerobic and anaerobic cellular metabolism.
13. Discuss mechanisms that move substances across cell membranes, including diffusion, facilitated diffusion, osmosis, and active transport.
14. Describe the function of epithelial tissue and how it can be classified on the basis of shape or arrangement.
15. Describe the functions of connective tissue and relate them to the function of the body or an organ system.
16. Explain the basic differences in skeletal, smooth, and cardiac muscle.
17. Describe nervous tissue.
18. Define the 11 major organ systems of the human body. Be prepared to label a diagram listing their major anatomic features, function, and interrelations to the other body systems.
19. State the functions of the integumentary system.
20. Name the two layers of the skin.
21. Describe the function of hair and nails.
22. Describe the functions of the sebaceous and sweat glands.
23. Describe the function of the skeleton.
24. List the parts of the axial and appendicular skeleton.
25. Describe the bones of the upper and lower extremities.
26. Explain how joints are classified. Give an example of each and describe the possible movements.
27. Describe the purpose of the muscular system.
28. List and describe the four basic properties of muscles.
29. State the three primary functions of muscles.
30. Describe the process of muscle movement.
31. Name the three main functions of the nervous system.
32. Name the divisions of the nervous system and state their general functions.
33. List and describe the three layers of the meninges.
34. State the locations and functions of the cerebrospinal fluid.
35. List and describe the three divisions of the brainstem.
36. Describe the diencephalons of the brain.
37. Describe the cerebrum, cerebellum, and spinal cord.
38. Describe the peripheral nervous system.
39. List the groups of cranial nerves and describe them.
40. List and describe the two branches of the autonomic nervous system.
41. Identify the primary endocrine glands and list the major hormones they secrete.
42. List the two parts of the circulatory system.
43. List the parts of the cardiovascular system.
44. Describe the parts of the blood.
45. Describe the location of the heart.
46. State the Frank-Starling law and explain why increased preload will increase myocardial contractility and cardiac output.
47. Discuss the relations among blood pressure, peripheral vascular resistance, cardiac output, stroke volume, and heart rate.
48. Name the great vessels and their functions.
49. Name and describe the chambers and valves of the heart.
50. Trace the pathway of blood flow through the heart and pulmonary circulation.
51. Describe the coronary circulation.
52. Describe the coronary conduction system and cardiac action potential.
53. Describe the systemic circulation.
54. Describe the structure and function of arteries, veins, and capillaries.
55. Describe the functions of the lymphatic system.
56. List the parts of the respiratory system.
57. Describe the pathway of the respiratory system, including nasal cavities, pharynx, and larynx.
58. Describe the structure and function of the larynx.
59. Describe the lower airway structures.
60. State the roles of the visceral and parietal pleura in respiration.
61. Describe the general function of the digestive system and name its major divisions.

62. Describe the structure and function of the parts of the gastrointestinal tract.
63. Describe the essential functions of the urinary system.
64. Describe the location and general function of each organ in the urinary system.
65. Name the parts of a nephron.
66. List the essential and accessory organs of the male and female reproductive systems and give the general function of each.
67. Describe the sense of smell.
68. Describe the sense of taste.
69. Name the parts of the eye and explain their functions in sight.
70. Name the parts of the ear and explain their functions in hearing.
71. Define *isotonic*, *hypotonic*, and *hypertonic*.
72. Describe the mechanisms that affect distribution of body water between the intracellular and extracellular spaces.
73. Define *ion, electrolyte, anion*, and *cation*.
74. Identify the principal intracellular and extracellular anions and cations.
75. Describe the physiologic mechanisms used to maintain acid-base balance.
76. Given values for pH and $PaCO_2$, determine the acid-base imbalance present.

SUMMARY

■ The paramedic must understand human anatomy. This understanding will help the paramedic organize a patient assessment by body regions. Mastering the anatomy of the human body also will help the paramedic communicate illness and injury information for the continuity of care for the patients he or she encounters.

■ Having an understanding of physiology will help the paramedic predict injury and illness patterns.

■ The anatomic position refers to a patient who is standing erect with his or her palms facing the examiner.

■ Directional terms are used to discuss the body. Such terms include *superior, inferior, anterior*, and *posterior*. These terms are used to give direction to findings during assessments.

■ The appendicular skeleton is composed of the extremities, including the arms, pelvic bones, and legs. The *axial skeleton* refers to the head, neck, thorax, and, abdomen.

■ The abdomen is divided into four quadrants: upper right, lower right, upper left, and lower left.

■ The major cavities of the human body are the ventral and dorsal cavities. These are further divided into subcavities including the thoracic cavity, the abdominopelvic cavity, the cranial cavity, and the spinal cavity.

■ The thoracic cavity contains the trachea, esophagus, thymus, heart, great vessels, lungs, and the cavities and membranes surrounded by them. The abdominopelvic cavity is surrounded by membranes and contains organs and blood vessels.

■ The cytoplasm lies between the cytoplasmic membrane and the nucleus. Specialized structures in the cell (organelles) are located in the cytoplasm. These organelles perform jobs that are key to the survival of the cell. The nucleus controls all other organelles in the cytoplasm.

■ All human cells reproduce by a process known as *mitosis*. In this process, cells divide to multiply.

■ Four types of tissue comprise the many organs of the body: epithelial, connective, muscle, and nervous. Epithelial tissue covers surfaces and forms structures. Connective tissue is composed of cells separated from each other by intercellular material known as the extracellular matrix. Muscle tissue is contractile tissue and is responsible for movement. The nervous tissue has the ability to conduct electrical signals know as action potentials.

■ A system is a group of organs arranged to perform a more complex function than any one organ can perform alone. The 10 major organ systems in the body are the integumentary, skeletal, muscular, nervous, endocrine, circulatory (cardiovascular and lymphatic/immune), respiratory, digestive, urinary, and reproductive.

■ The integumentary system consists of the skin and accessory structures such as hair, nails, and a variety of glands. It protects the body against injury and dehydration, defends the body against infection, and regulates the body's temperature.

■ The skeletal system consists of bone and associated connective tissue, including cartilage, tendons, and ligaments. The skeletal system provides a rigid framework for support and protection. It also provides a system of levers on which muscles act to produce body movements.

■ The three primary functions of the muscular system are movement, the maintenance of posture, and the production of heat.

■ The nervous and the endocrine systems are the major regulatory and coordinating systems of the body. The nervous system rapidly sends information by means of nerve impulses conducted from one area of the body to another. The endocrine system sends information more slowly by means of chemicals secreted by ductless glands into the bloodstream.

■ The heart and cardiovascular system are responsible for circulating blood throughout the body. Blood carries carbon dioxide and waste products away from tissues as well as hormones produced in endocrine glands to their target tissues. Blood regulates temperature, balances fluid, and protects the body from bacteria and foreign substances.

■ The lymphatic system is composed of lymph, lymphocytes, lymph nodes, the tonsils, the spleen, and the thymus gland. The lymphatic system has three basic functions: helping maintain fluid balance in tissues, absorb fats and other substances from the digestive tract, and assist the immune defense system of the body.

- The organs of the respiratory system and the cardiovascular system move oxygen to cells. They move carbon dioxide from cells to where it is released into the air. The respiratory system begins at the nasal cavity, with the nasopharynx, oropharynx, laryngopharynx, and larynx. The glottis is located at the lower airway, which leads to the lungs and consists of the trachea, the bronchial tree, the alveoli, and the lungs.
- The digestive system provides the body with water, electrolytes, and other nutrients needed to ensure the best use of the body's cells. Associated accessory organs (mainly glands) secrete fluid into the digestive tract.
- The urinary system works with other body systems to maintain homeostasis. It does this by removing waste products from the blood and helping maintain a constant body fluid volume and composition. The structures of the urinary system include two kidneys, two ureters, the urinary bladder, and the urethra.
- The purpose of the male reproductive system is to make and transfer spermatozoa to the female. The purpose of the female reproductive system is to make oocytes and receive the spermatozoa for fertilization, conception, gestation, and birth.
- The male reproductive system consists of the testes, epididymis, ductus deferens, urethra, seminal vesicles, prostate gland, bulbourethral glands, scrotum, and penis. The female reproductive organs consist of the ovaries, uterine/fallopian tubes, uterus, vagina, external genital organs, and mammary glands.
- The senses provide the brain with information about the outside world. Four senses are recognized as special senses: smell, taste, sight, and hearing and balance.

LABELING

1. Label the figure with the directional terms and planes listed below:

Anterior	Posterior
Coronal plane	Sagittal plane
Inferior	Superior
Lateral	Transverse, horizontal,
Medial	or axial plane

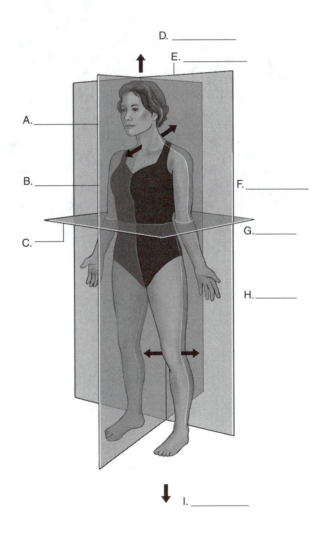

D. _____
E. _____
A. _____
B. _____
C. _____
F. _____
G. _____
H. _____
I. _____

2. Label the figure with the parts of the skin listed below:

Arrector pili muscle
Cutaneous nerve
Dermis
Epidermis
Hair follicle
Hair shaft

Papilla of hair
Sebaceous (oil) gland
Subcutaneous layer
Sweat gland
Sweat gland opening

A. _____

H. _____

B. _____

I. _____

C. _____

D. _____

E. _____

F. _____

G. _____

J. _____

K. _____

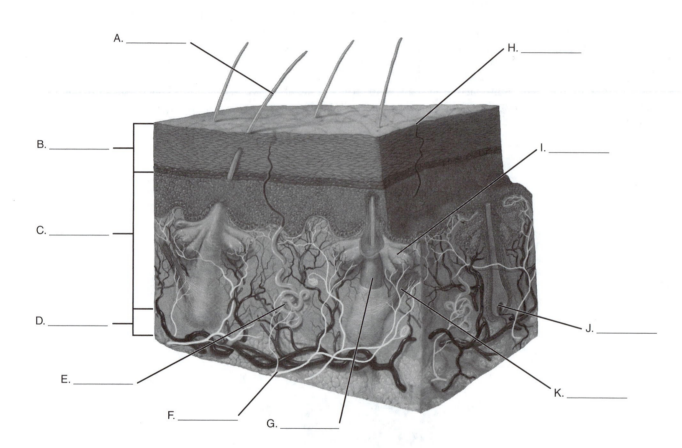

3. Label the figure with the terms for each bone listed below. One term will be used twice.

Carpals	Fibula	Patella	Sternum
Clavicle	Hip bone	Phalanges	Tarsals
Costal cartilage	Humerus	Radius	Tibia
Cranium	Mandible	Ribs	Ulna
Facial bones	Metacarpals	Sacrum	Vertebral column
Femur	Metatarsals	Scapula	

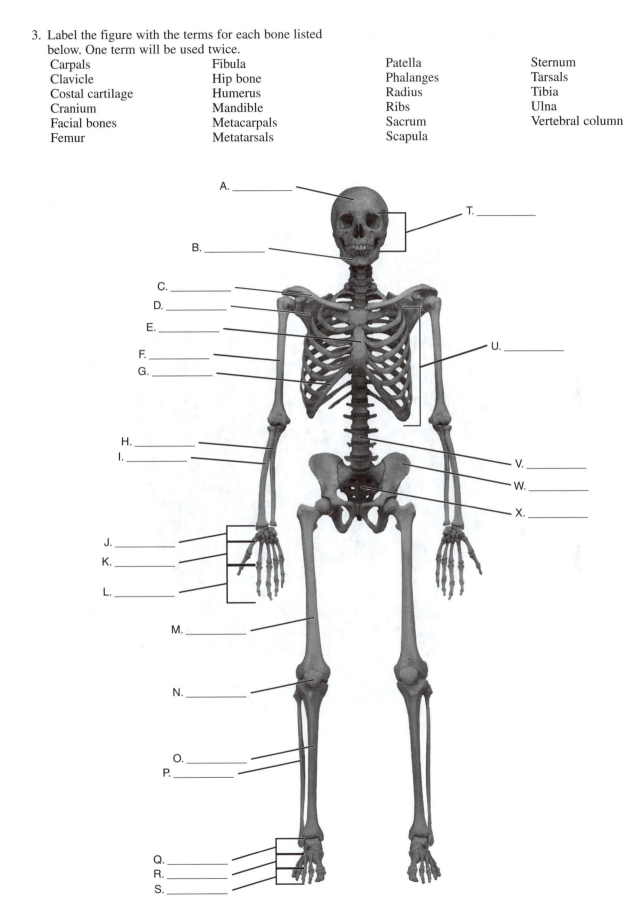

A. _____

T. _____

B. _____

C. _____
D. _____
E. _____
F. _____
G. _____

U. _____

H. _____
I. _____

V. _____
W. _____
X. _____

J. _____
K. _____
L. _____

M. _____

N. _____

O. _____
P. _____

Q. _____
R. _____
S. _____

4. Label the figure with the parts of the skull listed below:

Frontal bone

Lacrimal bone

Mandible

Mastoid process

Maxilla

Nasal bone

Nasal conchae

Parietal bone

Sphenoid bone

Temporal bone

Vomer

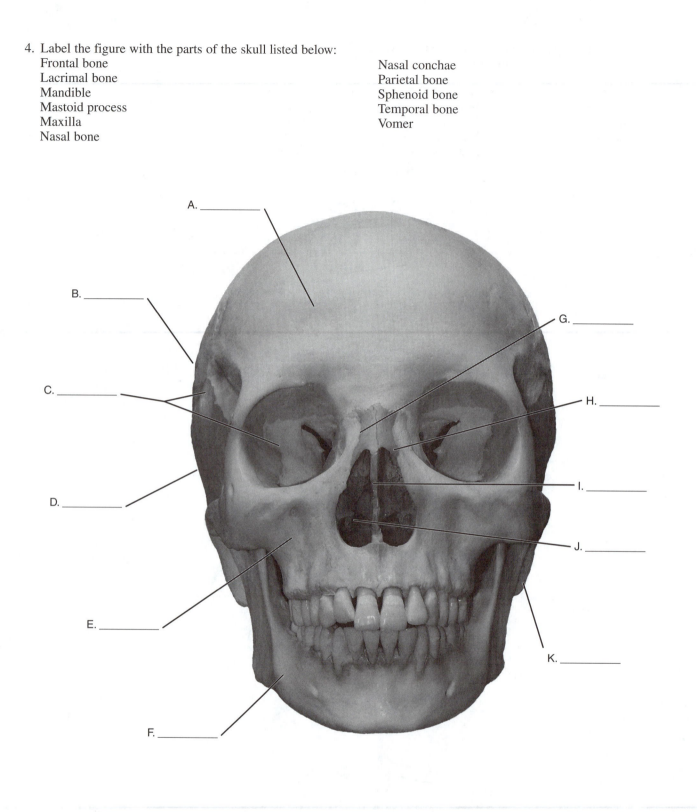

A. _____

B. _____

C. _____

D. _____

E. _____

F. _____

G. _____

H. _____

I. _____

J. _____

K. _____

5. Label the figure with the parts of the spine listed below:
   C1; atlas
   C2; axis
   Cervical curve
   Cervical vertebrae
   Coccyx (tailbone)
   Lumbar curve

   Lumbar vertebrae
   Sacral curve
   Sacrum vertebrae
   Thoracic curve
   Thoracic vertebrae

A. _____

B. _____

C. _____

D. _____

E. _____

F. _____

G. _____

H. _____

I. _____

J. _____

K. _____

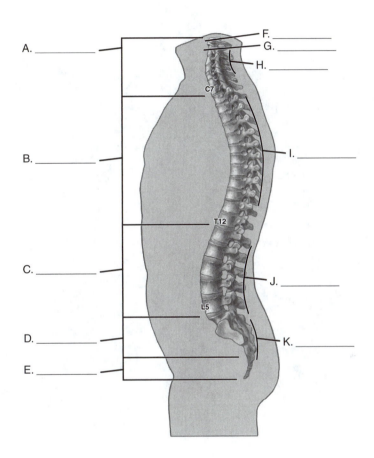

6. Label the figure with the parts listed below:

Body

Clavicle

Costal cartilage

False ribs

Floating ribs

L1 vertebra

Manubrium

Sternum

True ribs

Xiphoid process

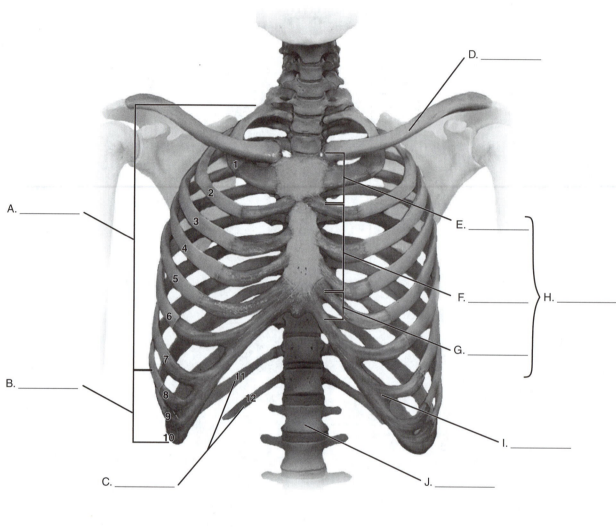

D. _____

A. _____

B. _____

C. _____

E. _____

F. _____

G. _____

H. _____

I. _____

J. _____

7. Label the figure with the parts of the pelvis listed below:

Coccyx

Coxal bone

Obturator foramen

Sacrum

Symphysis pubis

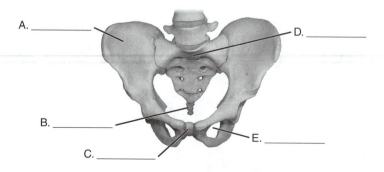

A. _____

B. _____

C. _____

D. _____

E. _____

8. Label the figure with the names of the muscles listed below:

Adductor longus
Adductor magnus
Biceps brachii
Brachialis
Brachioradialis
Buccinator
Deltoid

External oblique
Frontalis
Iliopsoas
Internal oblique
Linea alba
Masseter
Orbicularis oculi

Orbicularis oris
Pectoralis major
Peroneus longus
Rectus abdominis
Rectus femoris
Sartorius
Serratus anterior

Sternocleidomastoid
Temporalis
Tibialis anterior
Transversus abdominis
Vastus lateralis
Vastus medialis
Zygomaticus

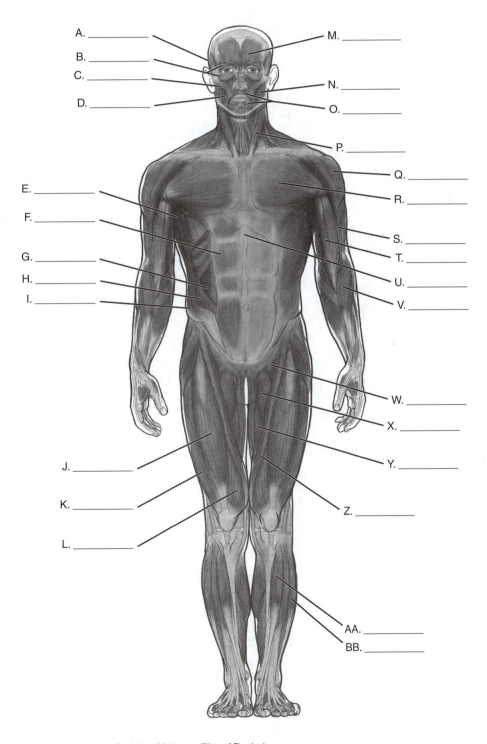

A. _____
B. _____
C. _____
D. _____
E. _____
F. _____
G. _____
H. _____
I. _____
J. _____
K. _____
L. _____
M. _____
N. _____
O. _____
P. _____
Q. _____
R. _____
S. _____
T. _____
U. _____
V. _____
W. _____
X. _____
Y. _____
Z. _____
AA. _____
BB. _____

9. Label the figure with the names of the muscles listed below:

Adductor magnus
Biceps femoris
Calcaneal (Achilles) tendon
Deltoid
Gastrocnemius
Gluteus maximus
Gluteus medius
Gracilis

Hamstring group
Latissimus dorsi
Semimembranosus
Semitendinosus
Soleus
Trapezius
Triceps brachii

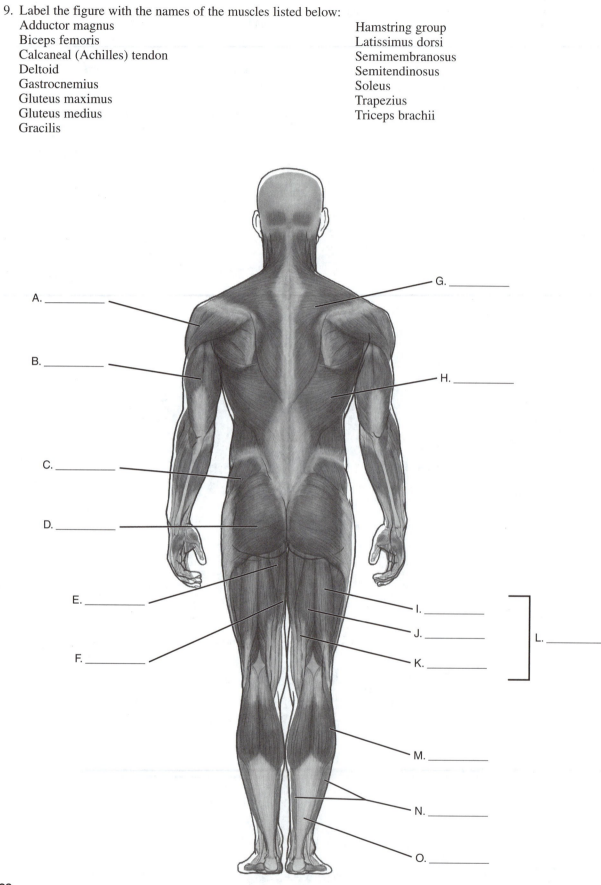

A. _____

B. _____

C. _____

D. _____

E. _____

F. _____

G. _____

H. _____

I. _____

J. _____

K. _____

L. _____

M. _____

N. _____

O. _____

10. Label the figure with the parts of the brain listed below:

Brainstem
Cerebellum
Cerebrum
Diencephalon
Hypothalamus
Medulla

Midbrain
Pituitary gland
Pons
Spinal cord
Thalamus

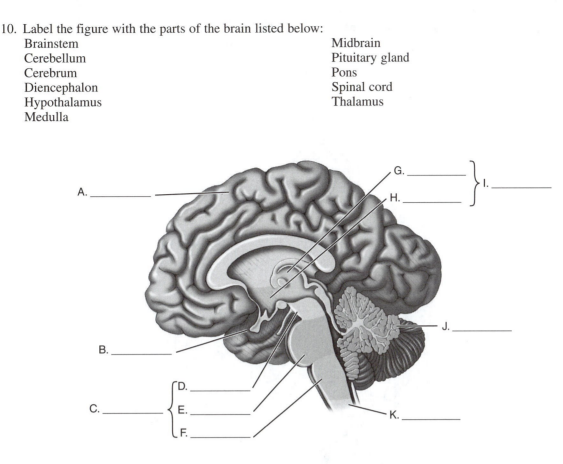

A. _____ _____

G. _____ ⎫
H. _____ ⎬ I. _____

J. _____

B. _____

C. _____ ⎰ D. _____
⎱ E. _____
⎱ F. _____

K. _____

11. Label the figure with the elements of the endocrine system listed below:

Adrenals   Pituitary
Ovaries (female)   Testes (male)
Pancreas   Thyroid
Parathyroids

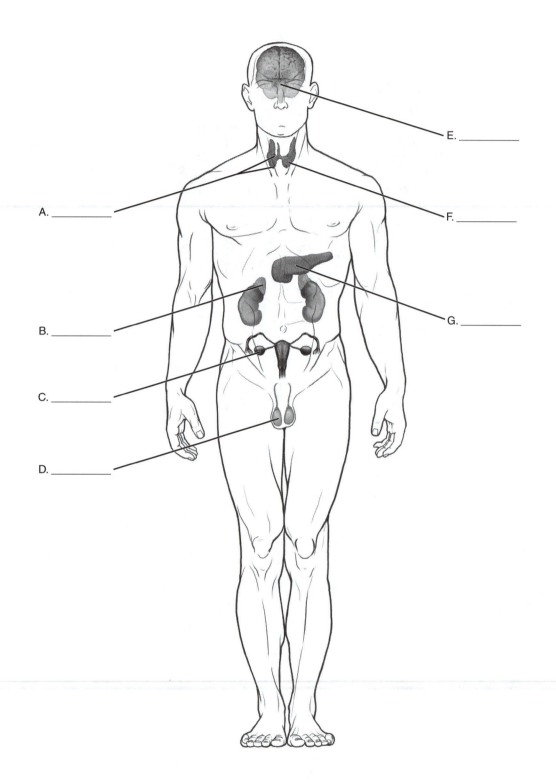

E. _____

A. _____

F. _____

B. _____

G. _____

C. _____

D. _____

12. Label the figure with the parts of the heart listed below:

Aortic valve   Pulmonic valve
Atrioventricular valves   Right atrium
Bicuspid (mitral) valve   Right ventricle
Chordae tendineae   Semilunar valves
Left atrium   Tricuspid valve
Left ventricle

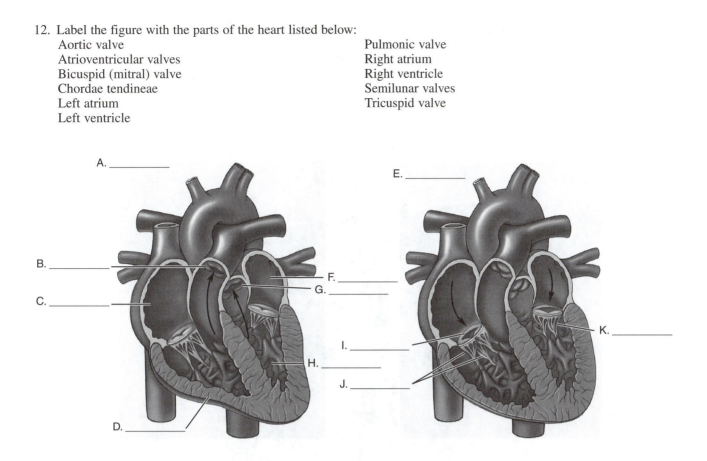

A. _____

B. _____
C. _____
D. _____

E. _____

F. _____
G. _____
I. _____
H. _____
J. _____
K. _____

13. Label the figure with the parts of the heart listed below:

Atrial conduction fibers   Purkinje fibers
Atrioventricular (AV) node   Right and left bundle branches
Bundle of His   Sinoatrial (SA) node or pacemaker

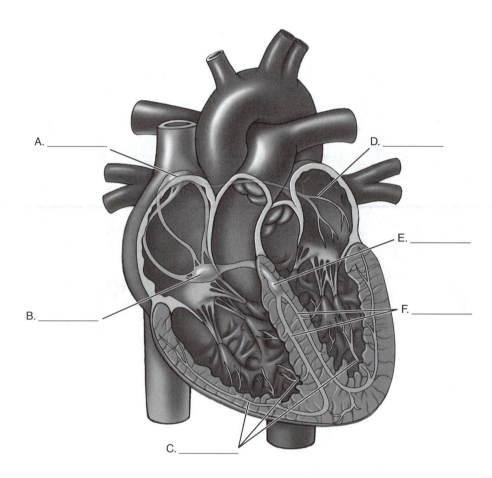

A. _____

D. _____

E. _____

B. _____

F. _____

C. _____

14. Label the figure with the names of the parts of the lymphatic system listed below:

Axillary nodes   Pharyngeal tonsil
Cervical nodes   Spleen
Lingual nodes   Subclavian vein
Lingual tonsil   Thymus gland
Palatine tonsil   Tonsils

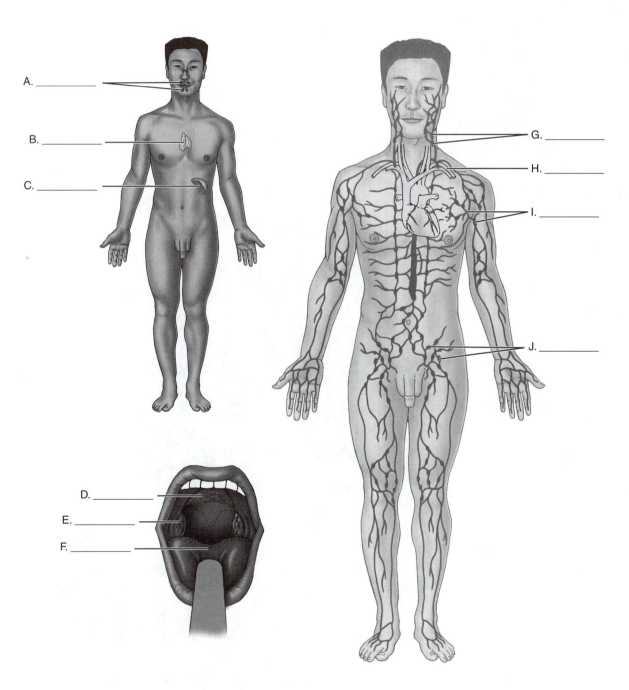

A. _____

B. _____

C. _____

D. _____

E. _____

F. _____

G. _____

H. _____

I. _____

J. _____

15. Label the figure with the names of the parts of the respiratory system listed below. Some terms may be used twice.

Alveolar ducts	Bronchiole	Middle lobe	Tertiary bronchi
Alveolar sacs	Capillaries	Primary bronchi	Trachea
Alveoli	Cartilaginous rings	Secondary bronchi	
Apex	Hilus	Superior lobe	
Base	Inferior lobe	Terminal bronchiole	

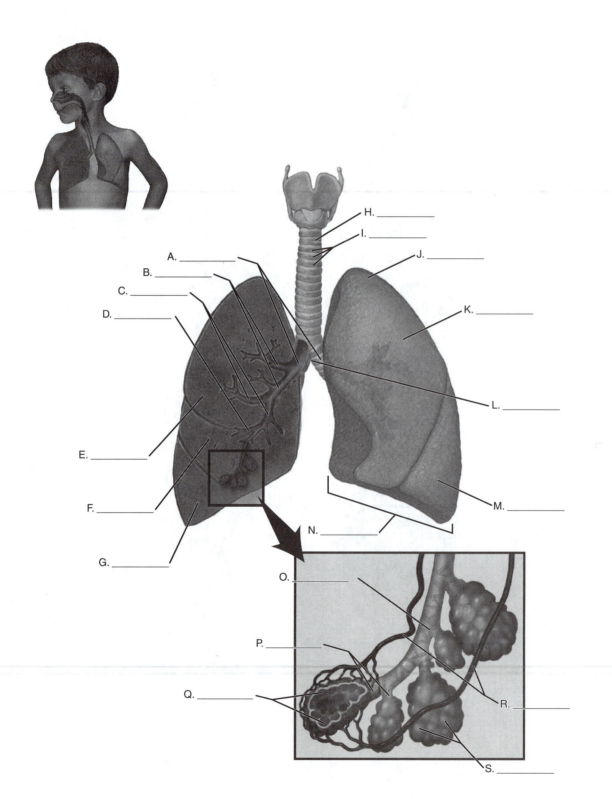

A. _____
B. _____
C. _____
D. _____
E. _____
F. _____
G. _____
H. _____
I. _____
J. _____
K. _____
L. _____
M. _____
N. _____
O. _____
P. _____
Q. _____
R. _____
S. _____

16. Label the figure with the names of the parts of the gastrointestinal system listed below. Some terms may be used twice.

Anal canal	Ileum
Cecum	Liver
Colon	Pancreas
Cystic duct	Rectum
Duodenum	Spleen
Esophagus	Stomach
Gallbladder	Tongue
Hepatic bile duct	

A. _____

B. _____

C. _____

D. _____

E. _____

F. _____

G. _____

H. _____

I. _____

J. _____

K. _____

L. _____

M. _____

N. _____

O. _____

P. _____

17. Label the figure with the names of the parts of the genitourinary system listed below.
    Some terms may be used twice.

    Bladder   Ureter
    Kidney   Urethra
    Penis   Urinary meatus
    Pubic symphysis   Vagina
    Rectum

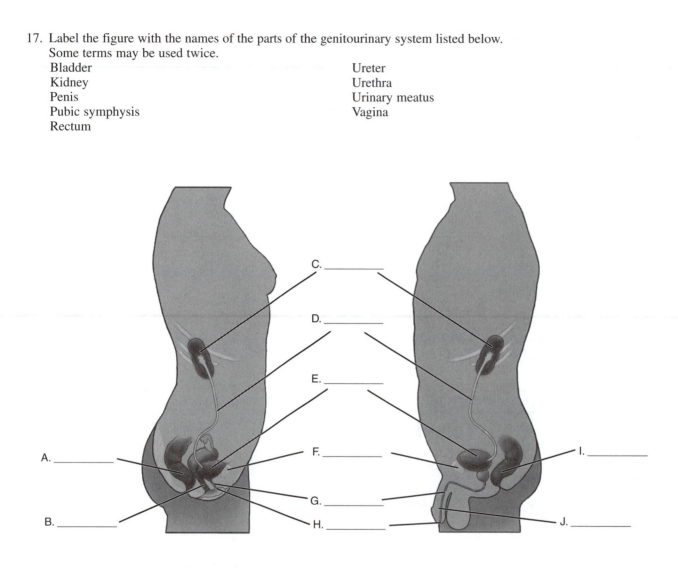

C. _____

D. _____

E. _____

A. _____   F. _____   I. _____

                       G. _____

B. _____   H. _____   J. _____

SHORT ANSWER

1. Describe the effects of sympathetic stimulation on each of the four adrenergic receptors.

   Alpha   **Beta**

   1 _____

   2 _____

2. Using the concept of Starling's law of the heart, explain why increasing cardiac preload increases contractility only up to a point.

   _____

   _____

   _____

   _____

3. List all of the cranial nerves, in order and with their number, and describe the function of each nerve.

   Nerve **Name**   **Function**

   I   _____

   II   _____

   III _____

   IV   _____

   V   _____

   VI   _____

   VII _____

   VIII _____

   IX   _____

   X   _____

   XI   _____

   XII _____

4. Describe the steps involved in pulmonary ventilation, including the factors affecting thoracic dimensions, pressures, pressure gradients, and direction of air flow.

   _____

   _____

   _____

   _____

5. Describe the steps involved in gas exchange at the pulmonary and systemic capillary beds. Include partial pressures of both oxygen and carbon dioxide.

   _____

   _____

   _____

   _____

6. Discuss the five phases of the electrical cardiac cycle (action potential) of cardiac muscle cells, including the direction of ion flow at phases 0 through 4.

   _____

   _____

   _____

   _____

7. Trace the circulation of blood through the heart and lungs. Begin with the return of blood to the heart through the vena cava and end with the blood exiting the heart through the aorta. Name all chambers, valves, and blood vessels.

   _____

   _____

   _____

   _____

8. Indicate whether the following structures contain high or low oxygen concentrations in the blood they carry.

   _____ aortic arch

   _____ pulmonary vein

   _____ inferior vena cava

   _____ right ventricle

   _____ renal artery

   _____ left atrium

   _____ pulmonary artery

   _____ carotid artery

9. Trace the path of a normal excitation impulse through the conduction system of the heart.

   _____

   _____

   _____

   _____

10. Indicate whether each of the following valves is open or closed during ventricular systole.

    _____ aortic

    _____ tricuspid

    _____ mitral

    _____ pulmonic

11. Complete the following equation:

    Stroke volume × Heart rate = _____

12. Complete the following equation:

    Cardiac output × Peripheral vascular resistance =

    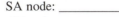

13. What is the intrinsic rate of firing of each of the following cardiac pacemaker sites?

    SA node: _____

    AV node: _____

    Purkinje system: _____

14. What effect will a decreased heart rate have on the cardiac output and blood pressure if the stroke volume and peripheral resistance do not change?

    _____

    _____

    _____

    _____

15. What effect does increasing the heart rate have on the length of systole and diastole?

_____

_____

_____

_____

16. What effect will increasing the peripheral vascular resistance have on blood pressure if cardiac output remains constant?

_____

_____

_____

_____

17. Applying what you have learned about the heart, please construct an answer for the following question: Why will a severe tachycardia decrease the cardiac output? (HINT: When does the heart fill with blood?)

_____

_____

_____

_____

18. What effect will stimulation of the sympathetic nervous system have on the heart rate?

_____

_____

_____

_____

19. What effect will stimulation of the parasympathetic nervous system have on the heart rate?

_____

_____

_____

_____

20. Applying what you learned about cellular respiration, please predict the effect on this process when the cells become hypoxic.

_____

_____

_____

_____

21. Compare and contrast diffusion, osmosis, and active transport mechanisms.

_____

_____

_____

_____

22. List at least three functions of the integumentary system.

_____

_____

_____

23. List the seven general cell functions.

_____

_____

_____

_____

_____

_____

_____

24. List the organelles of the cell and their functions.

_____

_____

_____

_____

25. Define isotonic, hypotonic, and hypertonic solutions.

_____

_____

_____

_____

26. Describe how hormones work.

_____

_____

_____

_____

27. What is the role of adenosine triphosphate in cellular function?

_____

_____

_____

_____

28. Name two nucleic acids.

_____

_____

_____

29. What is the role of nucleic acids in cell function?

_____

_____

_____

_____

30. What is a phospholipid bilayer?

_____

_____

_____

_____

31. What is the fluid that fills the interior of the cell?

_____

_____

_____

_____

32. What term is used to describe the phase of metabolism during which large molecules are broken down into smaller molecules?

_____

_____

_____

_____

33. What term is used to describe the phase of metabolism during which smaller molecules are put together to form larger molecules?

_____

_____

_____

_____

34. Applying the principles you learned about feedback loops, please answer the following question: When the blood glucose level rises, the pancreas normally releases insulin, which promotes uptake of glucose by the cells and storage of excess glucose as glycogen in the liver, thus decreasing the blood glucose level. What type of feedback loop does this represent?

_____

_____

_____

_____

35. Applying the principles you learned about feedback loops, please answer the following question: When blood is lost from the cardiovascular system and the blood pressure falls, the sympathetic nervous system releases norepinephrine. Norepinephrine causes an increased heart rate and peripheral vasoconstriction, raising the blood pressure. In response to the increase in blood pressure, more blood is lost from the cardiovascular system. What type of feedback loop does this represent?

_____

_____

_____

_____

36. Which part of the autonomic nervous system arises primarily from the thoracic and lumbar portions of the spinal cord?

_____

_____

_____

_____

37. What cation does the sodium-potassium pump move into the cells?

_____

_____

_____

_____

38. What cation does the sodium-potassium pump move out of the cells?

_____

_____

_____

_____

39. Which division of the autonomic nervous system mediates the body's response to physiologic stress?

_____

_____

_____

_____

40. What is cardiac output?

_____

_____

_____

41. How is cardiac output calculated?

_____

_____

_____

_____

42. What are the two variables that contribute to blood pressure?

_____

_____

_____

_____

43. If preload is increased, what happens to the contractility of the myocardium? What is this effect called?

_____

_____

_____

_____

49

TRUE/FALSE

1. The most important component of the lymphocyte is the iron-containing protein called *hemoglobin*.
   A. True
   B. False

2. An isotonic solution has an osmotic pressure greater than that of normal body fluids.
   A. True
   B. False

3. Surfactant serves to promote collapse of the alveoli.
   A. True
   B. False

MULTIPLE CHOICE

1. At the *end* of a normal expiration _____.
   A. the diaphragm contracts, decreasing the volume of air in the thoracic cavity
   B. air pressure inside the lungs exceeds atmospheric pressure
   C. the diaphragm contracts, increasing the volume of air in the thoracic cavity
   D. air pressure inside the lungs is equal to atmospheric pressure

2. Small hairlike processes on the outer surface of some cells that produce motion or current in a fluid are called _____.
   A. conchae
   B. cilia
   C. pleura
   D. turbinates

3. What effect does sympathetic nervous system stimulation have on cardiac output?
   A. Heart rate slows and blood vessels constrict, decreasing cardiac output.
   B. Heart rate increases and blood vessels dilate, increasing cardiac output.
   C. Heart rate and force of contraction increase, increasing cardiac output.
   D. Blood vessels dilate and bronchial smooth muscle relaxes, decreasing cardiac output.

4. Parasympathetic stimulation of the heart causes _____.
   A. an increase in the rate of conduction through the AV node
   B. an increase in heart rate
   C. a decrease in the rate of discharge of the SA node
   D. a decrease in the force of myocardial contraction

5. The process that occurs when the cell membrane actively pumps sodium out of the cell and potassium into the cell is called _____.
   A. repolarization
   B. plateau
   C. depolarization
   D. hypersensitization

6. Select the correct statement about pH.
   A. pH is used to express the sodium-ion concentration of a solution.
   B. The normal pH range for human blood is 7.0 to 7.35.
   C. A solution with a pH below 7 is an alkaline solution.
   D. H^+ concentration changes by a factor of 10 for each unit change in pH.

7. Which heart valves are open during ventricular diastole?
   A. Aortic and mitral
   B. Tricuspid and pulmonic
   C. Mitral and tricuspid
   D. Pulmonic and aortic

8. Bile is produced by the _____.
   A. gallbladder and stored in the liver
   B. pancreas and stored in the gallbladder
   C. liver and stored in the pancreas
   D. liver and stored in the gallbladder

9. The right and left nasal cavities are separated by the _____.
   A. nasal septum
   B. frontal sinus
   C. nasal turbinate
   D. olfactory membranes

10. Applying what you learned about acid base balance, what does a pH of 7.70 and a $P\text{CO}_2$ of 20 indicate?
    A. Respiratory acidosis
    B. Metabolic acidosis
    C. Respiratory alkalosis
    D. Metabolic alkalosis

11. Movement of particles from an area of higher concentration to an area of lower concentration, resulting in an even distribution, is _____.
    A. diffusion
    B. osmosis
    C. active transport
    D. dialysis

12. Which of the following sequences correctly describes the flow of air during inhalation?
    A. Nose, nasopharynx, laryngopharynx, oropharynx, larynx, trachea
    B. Nose, nasopharynx, larynx, laryngopharynx, oropharynx, trachea
    C. Nose, nasal cavities, laryngopharynx, nasopharynx, oropharynx, larynx, trachea
    D. Nose, nasal cavities, nasopharynx, oropharynx, laryngopharynx, larynx, trachea

13. The most numerous formed elements of blood are the _____.
    A. neutrophils
    B. erythrocytes
    C. platelets
    D. eosinophils

14. Which compounds combine to form carbonic acid (H_2CO_3)?
    A. Bicarbonate and water
    B. Water, bicarbonate, and carbon dioxide
    C. Carbon dioxide and bicarbonate
    D. Water and carbon dioxide, or bicarbonate and hydrogen ions

15. Applying what you learned about acid base balance, what dose a pH of 7.58 and a P_{CO_2} of 36 indicate?
    A. Respiratory acidosis
    B. Metabolic acidosis
    C. Respiratory alkalosis
    D. Metabolic alkalosis

16. Carbon dioxide is transported in the body primarily _____.
    A. as bicarbonate
    B. dissolved in plasma
    C. as carbaminohemoglobin
    D. bound to hemoglobin

17. The thyroid gland secretes _____.
    A. calcitonin
    B. oxytocin
    C. antidiuretic hormone
    D. epinephrine and norepinephrine

18. The islets of Langerhans secrete _____.
    A. insulin from beta cells, which decreases the blood glucose level
    B. insulin from alpha cells, which increases the blood glucose level
    C. glucagon from alpha cells, which decreases the blood glucose level
    D. glucagon from beta cells, which increases the blood glucose level

19. The major electrolytes that influence cardiac function are _____.
    A. magnesium, sodium, and chloride
    B. calcium, bicarbonate, and magnesium
    C. potassium, sodium, and calcium
    D. phosphate, bicarbonate, and chloride

20. The abdominal cavity extends from the _____.
    A. spinal cord to the scapula
    B. base of the neck to the pelvic bones
    C. base of the neck to the diaphragm
    D. diaphragm to the pelvic bones

21. The semilunar valves of the heart are the _____.
    A. tricuspid and mitral
    B. aortic and pulmonic
    C. mitral and aortic
    D. pulmonic and tricuspid

22. A person in the anatomic position would be _____.
    A. lying on his or her left side
    B. lying with the face and abdomen downward
    C. standing erect, facing forward, palms and feet facing forward
    D. standing erect, facing forward, palms and feet facing backward

23. The part of a neuron that carries impulses away from the cell body is the _____.
    A. axon
    B. nucleus
    C. dendrite
    D. myelin sheath

24. Applying what you learned about acid base balance, how you answer the following question? (Hint, think of what bradypnea would do to carbon dioxide elimination). A teenager has overdosed on diazepam. She is breathing shallowly at 2 to 4 breaths/min. This patient's P_{CO_2} should to be _____ than normal, and her pH should be _____ than normal, resulting in an acid-base disorder called _____.
    A. lower, higher, respiratory alkalosis
    B. higher, higher, respiratory alkalosis
    C. higher, lower, respiratory acidosis
    D. lower, lower, respiratory acidosis

25. Capillaries are _____
    A. the resistance vessels of the cardiovascular system, constricting and dilating as needed. They are thin-walled vessels that are just large enough to allow RBCs to pass single-file through them.
    B. thin-walled vessels that permit the flow of glucose, oxygen, fluid, carbon dioxide, and other substances through their walls.
    C. the resistance vessels of the cardiovascular system, constricting and dilating as needed to function as exchange vessels. They permit the flow of glucose, oxygen, fluid, carbon dioxide, and other substances through their walls.
    D. the resistance vessels of the cardiovascular system, constricting and dilating as needed. They are thin-walled vessels that are just large enough to allow RBCs to pass single-file through them. They permit the flow of glucose, oxygen, fluid, carbon dioxide, and other substances through their walls.

26. Acid-base balance is the regulation of which ion's concentration in body fluids?
    A. Nitrogen
    B. Hydrogen
    C. Sodium
    D. Potassium

27. Tidal volume is the amount of gas _____.
    A. moved in and out of the respiratory tract per minute
    B. contained in the lungs at the end of a maximal inspiration
    C. inhaled or exhaled during a normal breath
    D. that remains in the respiratory system after forced expiration

28. The meningeal layer that lies closest to the brain's surface is the _____.
    A. pia mater
    B. dura mater
    C. epidural layer
    D. arachnoid layer

29. Blood pressure is influenced by _____.
    A. stroke volume and peripheral vascular resistance
    B. stroke volume and heart rate
    C. heart rate and cardiac output
    D. cardiac output and peripheral vascular resistance

30. What is the principal intracellular cation?
    A. Sodium
    B. Potassium
    C. Calcium
    D. Magnesium

31. What is the principal extracellular cation?
    A. Sodium
    B. Potassium
    C. Calcium
    D. Magnesium

32. The coronary arteries fill during _____.
    A. atrial systole
    B. ventricular systole
    C. atrial diastole
    D. ventricular diastole

33. The point at which the trachea divides into the right and left mainstem bronchi is the _____.
    A. pleura
    B. xiphoid process
    C. carina
    D. sternal angle

34. The thickest part of the myocardium is located in the _____.
    A. right ventricle
    B. right atrium
    C. left atrium
    D. left ventricle

35. Substances whose molecules dissociate into electrically charged components when placed in water are called _____.
    A. proteins
    B. buffers
    C. minerals
    D. electrolytes

36. The outer boundary of the human cell is formed by the _____.
    A. nucleus
    B. cytoplasm
    C. organelles
    D. plasma membrane

37. Which type of tissue can conduct electrical signals called *action potentials*?
    A. Nervous
    B. Connective
    C. Epithelial
    D. Hemopoietic

38. The lungs are covered by a smooth, moist epithelial layer called the _____.
    A. visceral pleura
    B. parietal pleura
    C. visceral peritoneum
    D. parietal peritoneum

39. The three main components of a nerve cell are the _____.
    A. dendrite, neuron terminal, myelin sheath
    B. axon, synapse, ganglion
    C. myelin sheath, ganglion, cell body
    D. axon, dendrite, cell body

40. Epinephrine is produced naturally, or may be administered. Because this substance has alpha 1 and 2, and beta 1 and 2 effects, why might it be used to treat some patients who are in respiratory distress?
    A. Decrease bronchial secretions
    B. Increase blood pressure
    C. Relax bronchial smooth muscle
    D. Decrease myocardial contractility

41. Effects of alpha$_1$-adrenergic receptor stimulation include _____.
    A. renal vessel dilation
    B. increased heart rate
    C. peripheral vasoconstriction
    D. bronchial smooth muscle relaxation

42. The atrioventricular valves of the heart are the _____.
    A. mitral and aortic
    B. mitral and tricuspid
    C. aortic and pulmonic
    D. tricuspid and pulmonic

43. The heart is enclosed in a fibrous sac called the _____.
    A. pericardium
    B. myocardium
    C. endocardium
    D. adventitia

44. Which of the following statements best describes insulin?
    A. Insulin raises blood glucose levels by stimulating the liver to release glucose stores.
    B. Insulin is responsible for decreasing glucose metabolism by cells.
    C. Insulin is released by pancreatic cells when blood glucose levels fall.
    D. Insulin lowers blood glucose levels by increasing glucose transport into the cells.

45. Minute volume is the amount of gas _____.
    A. moved in and out of the respiratory system per minute
    B. contained in the lungs at the end of a maximal inspiration
    C. inhaled or exhaled during a normal breath
    D. that remains in the respiratory system after forced expiration

46. The larynx is _____ to the esophagus.
    A. inferior
    B. posterior
    C. distal
    D. anterior

47. Cardiac output is equal to _____.
    A. blood pressure × heart rate
    B. stroke volume × blood pressure
    C. heart rate × stroke volume
    D. systolic pressure + diastolic pressure

48. Applying what you learned about acid base balance, what does pH of 7.55 and a P_{CO_2} of 40 indicate?
    A. Respiratory acidosis
    B. Metabolic acidosis
    C. Respiratory alkalosis
    D. Metabolic alkalosis

49. The vessels that empty into the right atrium are the superior vena cava, the inferior vena cava, and the _____.
    A. pulmonary artery
    B. coronary sinus
    C. aorta
    D. right coronary artery

50. The thin strands of fibrous tissue connecting the AV valves to the papillary muscles are the _____.
    A. fibrous pericardium
    B. Purkinje fibers
    C. chordae tendineae
    D. trabeculae carneae

51. When the heart rate increases, ventricular filling time _____, resulting in _____ stroke volume.
    A. increases, decreased
    B. decreases, decreased
    C. decreases, increased
    D. increases, increased

52. Applying what you learned about acid base balance what does a pH of 7.30 and a P_{CO_2} of 50 indicate?
    A. Metabolic acidosis
    B. Respiratory acidosis
    C. Respiratory alkalosis
    D. Metabolic alkalosis

53. The junction between two neurons is called _____.
    A. an axon
    B. a synapse
    C. a ganglion
    D. a dendrite

54. Afterload is the _____.

    A. amount of blood ejected by the ventricle during a contraction
    B. volume of blood expelled per minute by the ventricles of the heart
    C. resistance against which the left ventricle must eject blood volume
    D. pressure exerted by the blood on the walls of the arteries

55. The sinoatrial (SA) node normally depolarizes at a rate of _____.
    A. 20 to 40 per minute
    B. 40 to 60 per minute
    C. 60 to 100 per minute
    D. 100 to 150 per minute

56. The part of the brain responsible for balance and coordination is the _____.
    A. cerebrum
    B. hypothalamus
    C. cerebellum
    D. occipital lobe

57. Which of the following structures serves as a passageway for both the respiratory and digestive systems?
    A. Trachea
    B. Pharynx
    C. Esophagus
    D. Cricoid cartilage

58. What is the minute volume if the respiratory rate is 12 breaths/min and the tidal volume is 800 mL/breath?
    A. 67 mL
    B. 788 mL
    C. 812 mL
    D. 9600 mL

59. The lymphatic system consists of lymph nodes, lymph vessels, and the _____.
    A. liver, spleen, and gallbladder
    B. thymus, spleen, and tonsils
    C. genitalia, thyroid, and liver
    D. brain, thymus, and pancreas

60. The ability of cardiac cells to spontaneously depolarize is _____.
    A. conductivity
    B. automaticity
    C. contractility
    D. excitability

61. Which statement best describes the cerebrum?
    A. The cerebrum is the largest part of the brain.
    B. The cerebrum controls respiration, heart rate, and blood pressure.
    C. The cerebrum includes the diencephalon, midbrain, pons, and medulla.
    D. The cerebrum coordinates muscle activity and maintains posture and equilibrium.

62. Which of the following statements best describes expiration?
    A. The chest wall expands, decreasing the size of the thoracic cavity.
    B. The chest wall relaxes, increasing the size of the thoracic cavity.
    C. The diaphragm and intercostal muscles contract, reducing the thoracic cavity's volume.
    D. The diaphragm and intercostal muscles relax, reducing the thoracic cavity's volume.

63. The only complete cartilaginous ring in the larynx is the _____.
    A. corniculate cartilage
    B. thyroid cartilage
    C. cricoid cartilage
    D. arytenoid cartilage

64. The process that occurs when an electrical stimulus causes sodium to rush into a resting cell is called _____.
    A. plateau
    B. repolarization
    C. depolarization
    D. hypersensitization

65. Applying what you learned about acid base balance, what does blood gas results of a pH of 7.26 and a P_{CO_2} of 40 reflect?
    A. Respiratory acidosis
    B. Metabolic acidosis
    C. Respiratory alkalosis
    D. Metabolic alkalosis

66. The primary neurotransmitter of the parasympathetic nervous system is _____.
    A. acetylcholine
    B. dopamine
    C. epinephrine
    D. norepinephrine

67. A type of extracellular fluid located outside the vascular bed and between the cells of the body is called _____ fluid.
    A. interstitial
    B. intracellular
    C. intravascular
    D. intracerebral

68. The digestive organs are surrounded by a connective tissue membrane called the _____.
    A. perineum
    B. pericardium
    C. pleura
    D. peritoneum

69. Which of the following statements best describes the brainstem?
    A. The brainstem connects the spinal cord to the remainder of the brain.
    B. The brainstem incompletely separates the right and left cerebral hemispheres.
    C. The brainstem is responsible for visual reception and visual association.
    D. The brainstem is responsible for personality, judgment, thought, and logic.

70. The medulla's functions include which of the following?
    A. Maintenance of posture and balance
    B. Regulation of temperature, sleep, and appetite
    C. Coordination of fine voluntary muscle movements
    D. Regulation of heart rate and blood vessel diameter

71. When the right ventricle contracts, blood is pumped into the _____.
    A. aorta
    B. pulmonary arteries
    C. pulmonary veins
    D. inferior vena cava

72. Effects of beta$_2$-adrenergic receptor stimulation include _____.
    A. bronchial smooth muscle relaxation
    B. increased heart rate
    C. renal vessel dilation
    D. peripheral vasoconstriction

73. Total body water makes up approximately _____ of body weight in adults. It is divided into two fluid-containing compartments: _____ fluid and _____ fluid.
    A. 50%, interstitial, plasma
    B. 60%, intracellular, extracellular
    C. 40%, plasma, transcellular
    D. 90%, intracellular, interstitial

74. What is the primary neurotransmitter of the sympathetic nervous system?
    A. Dopamine
    B. Acetylcholine
    C. Muscarine
    D. Norepinephrine

75. What is cardiac output?
    A. Amount of blood ejected by the ventricle during a ventricle contraction
    B. Pressure exerted by the blood on the walls of the arteries
    C. Volume of blood expelled by the ventricles per minute
    D. Resistance against which the left ventricle must eject blood

76. Which of the following contain thin epithelial linings and dense capillary networks and are responsible for oxygen and carbon dioxide exchange?
    A. Bronchioles
    B. Alveoli
    C. Secondary bronchi
    D. Right and left mainstem bronchi

77. Which blood component surrounds and digests infectious organisms (phagocytosis)?
    A. Thrombocytes
    B. Erythrocytes
    C. Neutrophils
    D. Basophils

78. Components of the integumentary system include the _____.
    A. skin, nails, hair, sweat, and oil glands
    B. heart, blood, and blood vessels
    C. trachea, bronchi, bronchioles, and alveoli
    D. brain, spinal cord, and peripheral nerves

79. Blood consists of three formed elements, which are the _____.
    A. plasma, lymph, and erythrocytes
    B. platelets, leukocytes, and erythrocytes
    C. lymph, erythrocytes, and leukocytes
    D. leukocytes, plasma, and platelets

80. Which of the following hormones is secreted by the adrenal cortex?
    A. Acetylcholine
    B. Norepinephrine
    C. Vasopressin
    D. Cortisol

81. Norepinephrine is an _____.
    A. alpha-adrenergic receptor stimulator
    B. alkalinizing agent
    C. antianginal and vasodilator
    D. antiinflammatory agent

82. The portion of the action potential in which a stronger than normal electrical stimulus is needed to cause the cardiac cells to respond is called the _____.
    A. plateau phase
    B. diastolic phase
    C. absolute refractory period
    D. relative refractory period

83. The movement of water through a semipermeable membrane from a solution that has a lower solute concentration to one that has a higher solute concentration is _____.
    A. active transport
    B. osmosis
    C. diffusion
    D. facilitated diffusion

84. Inspiratory reserve volume is the amount of _____.
    A. additional air that can be inhaled at the end of a normal inspiration
    B. air that is inhaled or exhaled during normal breathing
    C. air that can be inhaled after a normal exhalation
    D. air that can be forcefully exhaled after a maximum inspiration

85. The thoracic and abdominal cavities are separated by _____.
    A. the diaphragm
    B. the right lung
    C. the mediastinum
    D. an imaginary line called the *thoracoabdominal boundary*

86. Which blood component participates in blood clotting and helps to seal leaks in injured blood vessels?
    A. Neutrophils
    B. Thrombocytes
    C. Erythrocytes
    D. Basophils

87. Conditions that reduce alveolar ventilation can result in the retention of carbon dioxide. Knowing carbon dioxide is an acid, what can this result in?
    A. Respiratory acidosis
    B. Metabolic acidosis
    C. Respiratory alkalosis
    D. Metabolic alkalosis

88. The ability of cardiac cells to propagate an impulse from cell to cell is called _____.
    A. automaticity
    B. conductivity
    C. contractility
    D. excitability

89. Where is the sinoatrial (SA) node located?
    A. Near the aortic valve, just above the ventricular septum
    B. Near the bicuspid (mitral) valve, just above the ventricular septum
    C. At the junction of the right ventricle and pulmonary artery
    D. At the junction of the superior vena cava and the right atrium

90. An ion with a negative charge is called _____.
    A. an anion
    B. a protein
    C. a cation
    D. a nonelectrolyte

91. Which blood component is made up of water and dissolved molecules?
    A. Plasma
    B. Leukocytes
    C. Platelets
    D. Erythrocytes

92. Which statement best describes the trachea?
    A. The trachea prevents aspiration of material into the lungs.
    B. The trachea prevents collapse of the esophagus.
    C. The trachea is the only cartilage of the larynx that is a complete ring.
    D. The trachea has a ciliated inner lining.

93. What is the force that causes water to move from an area of low particle concentration to an area of higher concentration?
    A. Pulse pressure
    B. Hydrostatic pressure
    C. Osmotic pressure
    D. Isotonic pressure

94. Which of the following statements best describes the functional differences between the right and left sides of the heart?
    A. The right atrium and right ventricle make up a low-pressure pump whose purpose is to pump blood to the pulmonary circulation.
    B. The right atrium and right ventricle make up a high-pressure pump whose purpose is to pump blood to the systemic circulation.
    C. The left atrium and left ventricle make up a high-pressure pump whose purpose is to pump blood to the pulmonary circulation.
    D. The left atrium and left ventricle make up a low-pressure pump whose purpose is to pump blood to the systemic circulation.

95. The spinal cord passes through which of the following structures?
    A. Vertebral body
    B. Spinous process
    C. Vertebral foramen
    D. Transverse process

96. What substance prevents the collapse of the alveoli when little or no air is in them?
    A. Carbon dioxide
    B. Cartilage
    C. Interstitial fluid
    D. Surfactant

97. The most inferior cartilage of the larynx is the _____.
    A. thyroid cartilage
    B. hyoid cartilage
    C. cricoid cartilage
    D. pharyngeal cartilage

98. The middle layer of an artery is the _____.
    A. tunica adventitia
    B. tunica media
    C. tunica ligamentum
    D. tunica intima

99. The inner membranous surface of the heart wall that lines the heart valves and chambers is called the _____.
    A. epicardium
    B. endocardium
    C. myocardium
    D. pericardium

100. Which of the following is an effect of beta$_1$-adrenergic receptor stimulation?
    A. Peripheral vasoconstriction
    B. Bronchial smooth muscle relaxation
    C. Renal vessel dilation
    D. Increased heart rate

101. A solution with the same solute concentration as normal extracellular fluid is _____.
    A. isotonic
    B. hypotonic
    C. hypertonic
    D. hydrostatic

102. Which cranial nerve is responsible for slowing the heart rate and accelerating peristalsis?
    A. IV—trochlear
    B. IX —glossopharyngeal
    C. XII—hypoglossal
    D. X—vagus

103. Which of the following structures are found in the lower airway?
    A. Esophagus, trachea, and bronchioles
    B. Hard palate, bronchi, and alveoli
    C. Mouth, nose, larynx, and trachea
    D. Trachea, bronchi, bronchioles, and alveoli

104. Which statement best describes the movements of the diaphragm and intercostal muscles during inspiration?
    A. Diaphragm contracts and the intercostal muscles relax.
    B. Diaphragm relaxes and the intercostal muscles relax.
    C. Diaphragm relaxes and the intercostal muscles contract.
    D. Diaphragm contracts and the intercostal muscles contract.

105. What structure normally is the dominant pacemaker of the heart?
    A. SA node
    B. Bundle of His
    C. AV junction
    D. Purkinje fibers

106. What structure connects the right and left cerebral hemispheres?
    A. Diencephalon
    B. Corpus callosum
    C. Glia limitans
    D. Aqueduct of Sylvius

107. Which of the following events causes the "plateau" phase of the cardiac cycle?
    A. Na^+ influx
    B. K^+ efflux
    C. Ca^{2+} influx
    D. Na^+ efflux

108. Applying what you learned about types of fluids, what type of solution will cause water to move from the cells and interstitial space into the vascular space?
    A. Hypotonic
    B. Isotonic
    C. Hypertonic
    D. Crystalloid

109. What is the anatomic difference between the right and left mainstem bronchi?
    A. Right bronchus is shorter and straighter than left.
    B. Right bronchus is much smaller than left.
    C. Left bronchus is much smaller than right.
    D. Left bronchus is shorter and straighter than right.

110. Which of the following systems responds most rapidly to changes in pH?
    A. The liver and spleen
    B. The buffer system
    C. The renal system
    D. The respiratory system

111. The normal arterial CO_2 pressure (Pa_{CO_2}) is _____.
    A. 20 to 30 mm Hg
    B. 35 to 45 mm Hg
    C. 40 to 50 mm Hg
    D. 50 to 60 mm Hg

112. The Frank-Starling law states that when cardiac muscle is stretched, it contracts _____.
    A. with greater force
    B. with less force
    C. more frequently to handle the extra stroke volume
    D. less frequently to handle the extra preload

113. A membrane that allows certain substances to pass from one side to another but does not allow others to pass is _____.
    A. dissociated
    B. permeable
    C. semipermeable
    D. filterizable

114. The lymphatic system includes the _____.
    A. heart
    B. kidneys
    C. spleen
    D. pituitary gland

115. Building up and breaking down of biochemical substances collectively is called _____.
    A. cannibalism
    B. anabolism
    C. metabolism
    D. catabolism

116. A process that works to reverse or compensate for a physiologic change is called _____.
    A. a negative feedback loop
    B. a positive feedback loop
    C. homeostasis
    D. hemostasis

117. The constructive phase of metabolism is _____.
    A. anabolism
    B. catabolism
    C. apoptosis
    D. necrosis

118. Approximately 75% of all body water is _____.
    A. intracellular
    B. interstitial
    C. extracellular
    D. intravascular
    D. improving tissue oxygenation

8 Pathophysiology

READING ASSIGNMENT

Chapter 8, pages 205-274, in *Paramedic Practice Today: Above and Beyond*.

OBJECTIVES

After completing this chapter, you will be able to:
1. Discuss cellular adaptation.
2. Describe cellular injury and cellular death.
3. Describe the factors that lead to disease in the human body.
4. Describe the systemic manifestations that result from cellular injury.
5. Describe the cellular environment.
6. Discuss familial diseases and the associated risk factors.
7. Describe environmental risk factors.
8. Describe aging as a risk factor for disease.
9. Discuss the process of analyzing disease risk.
10. Discuss the combined effects of risk factors and the interactions among risk factors.
11. Discuss hypoperfusion.
12. Define *cardiogenic, hypovolemic, neurogenic, anaphylactic*, and *septic shock*.
13. Describe multiple organ dysfunction syndrome.
14. Define the characteristics of the immune response.
15. Discuss activation of the immune system.
16. Discuss fetal and neonatal immune function.
17. Discuss aging and the immune function in the elderly.
18. Describe the inflammation response.
19. Discuss the role of mast cells as part of the inflammation response.
20. Describe the plasma protein system.
21. Discuss the cellular components of inflammation.
22. Describe the systemic manifestations of the inflammation response.
23. Describe the resolution and repair from inflammation.
24. Discuss the effect of aging on the mechanisms of self-defense.
25. Discuss hypersensitivity.
26. Describe deficiencies in immunity and inflammation.
27. Discuss the interrelations between stress, coping, and illness.
28. Describe neuroendocrine regulation.

CHAPTER SUMMARY

- The human body is a fascinating and complex organism.
- The cell is the basic unit of life.
- Tissues are groupings of similar cells that perform a common function.
- Organs are composed of tissues that work together to accomplish specific functions.
- All the organs of the body work to maintain the homeostasis of the organism.
- Changes in the structure and function of cells can be helpful or harmful to the host. These changes occur as a result of a stimulus. The most common forms of adaptation include atrophy, hypertrophy, hyperplasia, dysplasia, and metaplasia.
- The most common forms of cellular injury are hypoxia, chemical injury, infectious injury, immunologic and inflammatory injury, genetic factors, nutritional imbalances, and physical agents.
- Cellular death can occur as a result of spreading irreversible injury, called *necrosis*, or it can be a preprogrammed response for tissue regeneration, called *apoptosis*.
- Viruses are the most common cause of infections in the human organism.
- Water in the body is distributed between intracellular and extracellular compartments. The proper distribution of fluid between these compartments is essential for proper function.
- The movement of water and other substances between the various compartments of the body occurs by osmosis, diffusion, and mediated transport.
- Water balance is greatly affected by the distribution and concentration of electrolytes.
- The proper electrolyte balance is essential for the body systems to function.
- Upsetting the proper balance of electrolytes generates signs and symptoms, primarily in the central nervous system, peripheral nervous system, and the heart.
- The body strives to maintain a constant concentration of hydrogen ions. This concentration is known as pH. he pH should be between 7.35 and 7.45. Anything greater than 7.45 is known as *alkalosis*, and anything less than 7.35 is called *acidosis*.
- Acid-base derangements can be respiratory or metabolic in nature. The body attempts to compensate for any change through the carbonic acid–bicarbonate buffer system, protein buffering, and renal mechanisms.
- Hypoperfusion is a state of inadequate tissue perfusion. To maintain adequate perfusion, the body must

be able to deliver oxygen and remove cellular waste products from the tissues. The most important determinant of adequate blood flow is cardiac output.

■ MODS is the progressive impairment of two or more organ systems. This usually is the result of an uncontrolled inflammatory response from severe illness or injury, such as sepsis, trauma, or severe burn injuries. The cause of this condition is largely unknown. However, clinicians' ability to identify patients at high risk is improving.

■ The human immune system has multiple mechanisms to defend the body against foreign invaders. The first of these are the anatomic barriers, such as the skin. The second line of defense includes certain chemical attacks and the inflammatory response. The third line includes the adaptive mechanism.

■ When the immune system produces an exaggerated response to a stimulus, it can be harmful to the body. This type of response is known as a *hypersensitivity reaction.*

■ Research is ongoing into the effects of stress on the body and its link to disease. The communication between the immune system, the nervous system, and the endocrine system is believed to play a role in the progression of disease as it relates to the stress response.

■ You should understand the way in which cells interact in the various tissues in the body. This knowledge will assist you in understanding the physiologic basis of the condition of your patient as well as the best approach for treatment.

MATCHING

1. Integrating what you learned in Chapter 7 and in this chapter, match the term with its definition.

____ Negatively-charged ions	A. Anions
____ Positively-charged ions	B. Cations
____ Substances forming ions in water	C. Electrolytes
	D. Extracellular fluid
	E. Intracellular fluid
____ Water inside blood vessels	F. Intravascular fluid
____ Water contained inside cells	
____ Water outside cells	

2. Based on the knowledge you gained from the chapter, match the type of solution with its behavior.

____ Hypertonic solution	A. Rapidly leaves the vascular space
____ Hypotonic solution	B. Remains in the vascular space and pulls in extra fluid
____ Isotonic solution	C. Remains in the vascular space without pulling in extra fluid

3. Based on what you learned about hypoperfusion, match the description of the patient with the most likely type of shock they are experiencing.

____ 23 y.o. h/o vomiting and diarrhea × 4 days; BP—98/76 mm Hg, P—120 beats/min, R—22 breaths/min	A. Cardiogenic B. Hypovolemic C. Neurogenic D. Septic
____ 27 y.o. c/o abdominal pain following an incomplete abortion 3 days ago; skin warm, flushed; BP—96/56 mm Hg, P—136 beats/min, R—26/min, shallow	
____ 30 y.o. c/o loss of lower extremity motor function following an MVC; BP—96/40 mm Hg, P—72 beats/min, R—24/min, shallow	
____ 77 y.o. c/o substernal chest pain and SOB; BP—70/56 mm Hg, P—130 beats/min, irregular, R—36 breaths/min	

4. Match the type of necrosis with the disease process in which it tends to occur or where it tends to occur.

____ Caseous necrosis	A. Kidneys, adrenal glands, heart
____ Coagulative necrosis	B. Pancreatic infarctions
____ Fatty necrosis	C. Tuberculosis
____ Liquefactive necrosis	D. Neural tissue

SHORT ANSWER

1. What is the difference between hypertrophy and hyperplasia?

2. What is the most common cause of injury to cells?

3. What type of necrosis typically is associated with tuberculosis?

4. When extensive liquefactive necrosis occurs, what happens to the cells?

5. When extensive coagulative necrosis occurs, what happens to the cells?

6. Define *osmosis*.

7. What is the principal intracellular cation?

8. What is the principal extracellular cation?

9. List in order of their speed of action the three mechanisms used by the body to maintain acid-base balance.

10. Integrating what you learned in Chapter 7, and this chapter, what change in pH will be caused by an increase in hydrogen ion concentration?

11. Integrating what you learned in Chapter 7 and this chapter, what change in pH will be caused by a decrease in hydrogen ion concentration?

12. What is the normal range of pH in the human body?

13. Applying what you learned in Chapters 7 and 8, how would you answer the following question? Since large protein molecules in the plasma hold water molecules within the vascular space, what will tend to happen to patients with problems such as liver disease or renal disease who tend to develop lowered plasma protein levels, and therefore a decreased plasma osmotic pressure?

14. If a patient is hyperventilating as a result of anxiety, what change will occur in the pH? What acid-base imbalance will the patient develop?

15. A diabetic patient who is in distress after not taking his insulin for several days and has developed diabetic ketoacidosis. What change will take place in his pH?

16. A diabetic patient who has not taken insulin for several days will create energy by breaking fat down into fatty acids and triglycerides. With this knowledge, what acid base disorder do you think would be present?

17. A patient with depressed ventilations secondary to a drug overdose will have what change in his pH?

_____
_____
_____
_____

18. What acid-base imbalance will be present in a patient with depressed respirations?

_____
_____
_____
_____

19. A patient who has received excessive amounts of sodium bicarbonate will have what change in his pH? What acid-base imbalance will be present?

_____
_____
_____
_____

20. Based on the principles you learned in this chapter, what type of fluid (hypotonic, isotonic, hypertonic) do you think should be used if a patient is in hypovolemic shock? Applying the principle of osmosis, explain why you think this fluid is used.

_____
_____
_____
_____

21. What type of fluid (hypotonic, isotonic, hypertonic) should be used if a patient is in neurogenic shock? Applying the principle of osmosis, explain why this fluid is used.

_____
_____
_____
_____

22. Define *shock*.

_____
_____
_____
_____

23. What are the three elements of the Fick principle that must be present for adequate tissue perfusion to occur?

_____
_____
_____
_____

24. What happens to cellular metabolism as a result of hypoperfusion?

_____
_____
_____

25. What substance is produced by the cells as a result of anaerobic glycolysis (anaerobic metabolism)?

_____
_____
_____
_____

26. Explain how the renin-angiotensin system supports blood pressure.

_____
_____
_____
_____

27. ACE inhibitors are medications that block the effect of angiotensin converting enzyme (ACE). Applying what you have learned about the renin-angiotensin system in this chapter, what effect will this class of medication have on a patient's blood pressure? Why?

_____
_____
_____

28. Angiotensin receptor blockers (ARBs) are medications that block the receptor sites for angiotensin II. Applying what you have learned in this chapter, what effect do you think this class of medication will have on a patient's blood pressure? Why?

_____
_____
_____

29. Based on what you have learned in this chapter, what do you believe is the most important thing that can be administered in the prehospital setting to a patient in shock?

_____
_____
_____
_____

30. Integrating what you learned in this chapter, describe the physiologic mechanism that produces neurogenic shock.

_____
_____
_____

31. As discussed in this chapter, neurogenic shock is the result of the loss of neurovascular control, and the inability to release catecholamines. Integrating this knowledge with what you learned about the autonomic nervous system in Chapter 7, explain why patients in neurogenic shock present with dry skin and bradycardia.

_____
_____
_____
_____

32. Based on the principles you learned in this chapter, what type of fluid (hypotonic, isotonic, hypertonic) should be used if a patient is in anaphylactic shock? Applying the principle of osmosis, explain why this fluid is used.

_____
_____
_____
_____

33. As you learned in this chapter, cardiogenic shock is the result of inadequate myocardial function. This results in hypoperfusion to the tissues and organs, including the myocardium itself. Part of the body's response to this is to retain fluid in an attempt to increase volume, even though it is not a hypovolmemic problem. Based on this knowledge, and your knowledge of anatomy and physiology, what complication could result if the paramedic rapidly infused fluid into a patient with inadequate cardiac function in an attempt to raise the blood pressure?

_____
_____
_____
_____

34. What effect will a prolonged state of hypoperfusion have on the kidneys?

_____
_____
_____

35. What effect will a prolonged state of hypoperfusion have on the liver?

_____
_____
_____

36. What is disseminated intravascular coagulation (DIC)? Why can a period of prolonged hypoperfusion cause DIC?

_____
_____
_____
_____

37. Integrating what you learned about the immune system, allergic reactions, and anaphylaxis, what substance released by the body is primarily responsible for causing anaphylactic shock?

_____
_____
_____
_____

38. What are the effects of this substance on the peripheral vascular resistance, on capillary permeability, and on extravascular smooth muscle (bronchioles, gastrointestinal tract)?

_____
_____
_____

39. What three drugs can be given to counteract the effects of this substance?

_____
_____
_____

40. What is the difference between immunity and inflammation?

_____
_____
_____
_____

41. A pathogen is anything capable of producing disease or infectious injury in the human body. Name four general classes of pathogens.

_____
_____
_____
_____

42. What are the four classic indicators that an inflammatory reaction is taking place?

_____
_____
_____
_____

43. What is the role of the helper T-cell in the functioning of the immune system?

_____
_____
_____
_____

44. What is the function of the macrophage in the functioning of the immune system?

_____
_____
_____
_____

45. What is systemic lupus erythematosis?

_____
_____
_____
_____

46. What is the principal role of the B-lymphocyte in the immune response?

_____
_____
_____
_____

47. What is the role of the cytotoxic ("killer") T-cell in the immune response?

_____
_____
_____
_____

48. Describe the process by which the immune system is able to generate B-cell precursors for antigens that will respond to every possible antigen.

_____
_____
_____
_____

49. What organ is responsible for promoting the development of T-cells?

_____
_____
_____
_____

50. Explain how autoimmunity is responsible for producing type 1 diabetes.

_____
_____
_____
_____

51. Which type of immune globulin is responsible for most (but not all) allergic reactions?

_____
_____
_____
_____

52. How is acquired immunity developed?

_____
_____
_____
_____

53. What is the difference between active and passive acquired immunity?

_____
_____
_____
_____

54. What is a cytokine?

_____
_____
_____
_____

55. What is the first antibody produced during the primary immune response?

_____
_____
_____
_____

MULTIPLE CHOICE

1. A decrease in cell size resulting from a decreased workload is called _____.
   A. atrophy
   B. dysplasia
   C. hyperplasia
   D. mitosis

2. An increase in the number of cells resulting from an increased workload is known as _____.
   A. atrophy
   B. dysplasia
   C. hyperplasia
   D. hypertrophy

3. An increased workload gradually causes what change in the skeletal muscle and myocardium?
   A. Atrophy
   B. Dilation
   C. Hyperplasia
   D. Hypertrophy

4. The most common cause of cellular injury is _____.
   A. acidosis
   B. alkalosis
   C. hypoxia
   D. inflammation

5. *Necrosis* means _____.
   A. a buildup of cell waste products
   B. an injured cell destroying itself
   C. cell death
   D. oxygen deficiency

6. The most prevalent extracellular cation is _____.
   A. calcium
   B. nitrogen
   C. potassium
   D. sodium

7. The principal buffer of the body is _____.
   A. bicarbonate
   B. chloride
   C. diphosphate
   D. sodium

8. The difference in concentration between solutions on opposite sides of a semipermeable membrane is called _____.
   A. diffusion
   B. osmosis
   C. the electrical gradient
   D. the osmotic gradient

9. When a solution on one side of a semipermeable membrane is hypotonic, it _____.
   A. has a greater concentration of solute molecules
   B. has a lesser concentration of solute molecules
   C. is equal in concentration of solute molecules
   D. will not move through the membrane

10. The pressure exerted by the concentration of solutes on one side of a membrane that, if hypertonic, tends to "pull" water from the other side of the membrane is called _____.
    A. hydrostatic pressure
    B. net filtration
    C. oncotic force
    D. osmotic pressure

11. The total amount of water lost from blood plasma across the capillary membrane into the interstitial space is called _____.
    A. net filtration
    B. oncotic force
    C. osmolarity
    D. osmotic pressure

12. Edema is caused by _____.
    A. excessive osmotic pressure
    B. imbalance between hydrostatic and oncotic pressures
    C. inadequate hydrostatic pressure
    D. inadequate intracellular fluid volume

13. Ringer's lactate is what type of solution?
    A. Hypertonic
    B. Hypotonic
    C. Isotonic
    D. Normotonic

14. A high concentration of hydrogen ions is known as _____.
    A. acidosis
    B. alkalosis
    C. base
    D. carbonosis

15. The fastest mechanism the body has for removing hydrogen ions is _____.
    A. kidney function
    B. the potassium buffer system
    C. respirations
    D. the bicarbonate buffer system

16. Impaired ventilation is the cause of which acid-base imbalance?
    A. Metabolic acidosis
    B. Metabolic alkalosis
    C. Respiratory acidosis
    D. Respiratory alkalosis

17. Vomiting, diarrhea, or diabetes can cause which acid-base imbalance?
    A. Metabolic acidosis
    B. Metabolic alkalosis
    C. Respiratory acidosis
    D. Respiratory alkalosis

18. Which of the following statements describes the relationship between hydrogen ion concentration and pH?
    A. As $[H^+]$ decreases, pH decreases.
    B. As $[H^+]$ increases, pH decreases.
    C. As $[H^+]$ increases, pH increases.
    D. There is no relationship between $[H^+]$ and pH.

19. pH is the _____.
    A. inverse logarithm of $[CO_2]$
    B. logarithm of $[H^+]$
    C. negative logarithm of $[H^+]$
    D. percent of hydrogen in solution

20. Normal pH is _____.
    A. 7.00
    B. 7.20
    C. 7.40
    D. 7.60

21. Normal P_{CO_2} is _____ mm Hg.
    A. 25 to 35
    B. 35 to 45
    C. 45 to 55
    D. 55 to 65

22. Given a pH of 7.00, a P_{CO_2} of 60, and an HCO_3^- of 24, you would suspect which acid-base imbalance?
    A. Metabolic acidosis
    B. Metabolic alkalosis
    C. Respiratory acidosis
    D. Respiratory alkalosis

23. Given a pH of 7.50, a P_{CO_2} of 20, and an HCO_3^- of 26, you would suspect which acid-base imbalance?
    A. Metabolic acidosis
    B. Metabolic alkalosis
    C. Respiratory acidosis
    D. Respiratory alkalosis

24. Given a pH of 7.20, a P_{CO_2} of 40, and an HCO_3^- of 12, you would suspect which acid-base imbalance?
    A. Metabolic acidosis
    B. Metabolic alkalosis
    C. Respiratory acidosis
    D. Respiratory alkalosis

25. Given a pH of 7.50 and a P_{CO_2} of 60, you would suspect which acid-base imbalance?
    A. Metabolic acidosis
    B. Metabolic alkalosis
    C. Respiratory acidosis
    D. Respiratory alkalosis

26. The clotting factor deficiency caused by an X-linked recessive gene is _____.
    A. anemia
    B. encephalitis
    C. hemochromatosis
    D. hemophilia

27. Integrating the knowledge you gained from Chapter 7 and this chapter, how do you believe the respiratory center will respond when blood [H⁺] concentrations rise above normal?
    A. Decreasing rate and decreasing tidal volume
    B. Decreasing rate and increasing tidal volume
    C. Increasing rate and decreasing tidal volume
    D. Increasing rate and increasing tidal volume

28. Integrating and applying what you learned in Chapter 7 and this chapter, what do you believe is released by the sympathetic nervous system when the baroreceptors detect a drop in blood pressure?
    A. Acetylcholine
    B. Dopamine
    C. Histamine
    D. Norepinephrine

29. Integrating what you learned in Chapter 7 and this chapter, what is produced by the cells in the setting of inadequate tissue perfusion?
    A. ATP and glucose
    B. Glucose and pyruvic acid
    C. Lactic acid and glucose
    D. Lactic acid and pyruvic acid

30. According to Fick's principle, which of the following best describes the factors affecting tissue perfusion?
    A. Hemoglobin levels, circulation of erythrocytes
    B. Hemoglobin levels, circulation of erythrocytes, ability to onload and offload oxygen
    C. Hemoglobin levels, circulation of erythrocytes, pH
    D. Hemoglobin levels, circulation of erythrocytes, pH, body temperature

31. Anaerobic metabolism is _____.
    A. 18 times less efficient than aerobic metabolism
    B. 50% as efficient as aerobic metabolism, but uses less oxygen
    C. a normal compensatory response that can be maintained for several hours without damage
    D. able to provide sufficient energy for vital body functions

32. Aldosterone acts on the kidneys to _____.
    A. conserve potassium and water
    B. conserve sodium and water
    C. eliminate potassium and water
    D. eliminate sodium and water

33. Angiotensin II produces _____.
    A. increased heart rate and vasoconstriction
    B. increased norepinephrine and vasoconstriction

C. vasoconstriction and decreased rate of urine production
    D. vasodilation and increased urine production

34. Disseminated intravascular coagulation initially begins with _____.
    A. activation of fibrinolysis
    B. uncontrolled severe hemorrhage
    C. uncontrolled, widespread clot formation
    D. vasodilation that triggers widespread clot formation

35. The primary cause of anaphylaxis is the release of which of these chemicals?
    A. Glucagon
    B. Histamine
    C. Norepinephrine
    D. Prednisone

36. You learned neurogenic shock is the result of loss of control of the sympathetic nervous system. Integrating this knowledge with what you learned about the sympathetic nervous in Chapter 7, why are pallor, diaphoresis, and tachycardia absent in neurogenic shock?
    A. In neurogenic shock there is no blood loss.
    B. Neurogenic shock is not as severe as hypovolemic shock.
    C. Norepinephrine is not released because of decreased sympathetic tone.
    D. These symptoms are due to vasoconstriction and this does not occur in neurogenic shock.

37. Protection from infection or disease that is developed by the body after exposure to an antigen is called _____.
    A. acquired immunity
    B. natural immunity
    C. primary immune response
    D. synthetic immunity

38. The type of leukocyte responsible for recognizing foreign antigens, producing antibodies, and developing memory is the _____.
    A. cytoplast
    B. erythrocyte
    C. lymphocyte
    D. thrombocyte

39. The type of leukocyte that does not produce antibodies but directly attacks antigens is _____.
    A. B-cells
    B. T_C-cells
    C. T_H-cells
    D. T_S-cells

40. A universal donor has which blood type?
    A. A
    B. AB
    C. C
    D. O

41. The development by B-cell precursors in the bone marrow of receptors that allow for the development of millions of single antigen responses from only several hundred to a few thousand genes is called clonal _____.
    A. application
    B. diversity
    C. integration
    D. selection

42. The first antibody produced during the primary immune response is _____.
    A. IgA
    B. IgE
    C. IgG
    D. IgM

43. The cells that transfer delayed hypersensitivity and secrete proteins that activate other cells are called _____.
    A. T_C-cells
    B. T_D-cells
    C. T_H-cells
    D. T_S-cells

44. Proteins produced by white blood cells, known as the "messengers" of the immune response, are _____.
    A. autokines
    B. cytokines
    C. monokines
    D. prokines

45. The organ responsible for T-cell development is the _____.
    A. hypothalamus
    B. thymus
    C. thyroid
    D. tonsils

46. One of the functions of the inflammatory response is _____.
    A. attacking foreign substances
    B. causing allergic reactions to specific antigens
    C. developing memory for antigens
    D. "walling off" the infected area

Life Span Development

READING ASSIGNMENT

Chapter 9, pages 275-294, in *Paramedic Practice Today: Above and Beyond*.

OBJECTIVES

After completing this chapter, you will be able to:

1. Describe the body system developmental milestones, characteristics, and vital signs of infants, toddlers and preschoolers, school-age children, adolescents, early adults, middle adults, and late adults.
2. Distinguish the unique psychosocial characteristics of infants, toddlers and preschoolers, school-age children, adolescents, early adults, middle adults, and late adults.
3. Explain the psychosocial development of children and adolescents that results from parenting styles, sibling and peer relationships, and environmental factors.
4. Explain the physiologic characteristics and emotional challenges faced when treating older adults.

SUMMARY

- The newborn is a baby in the first few hours of life, and a neonate is younger than 28 days old.
- The typical newborn weighs 3 to 3.5 kg at birth but should triple its weight by the end of a year. Twenty-five percent of the weight is the infant's head.
- The infant is born with several circulatory structures necessary for a fetus that should change shortly after birth.
- Nervous system functions in an infant are primarily reflex actions.
- Toddlers are children aged 1 to 3 years, and preschoolers are aged 3 to 5 years.
- Toddlers and preschoolers grow rapidly and undergo an increase in muscle and bone mass.
- Walking generally occurs by 14 to 15 months of age but may start earlier.
- Parenting styles can have a significant impact on the development of children and adolescents.
- School-age children are from 6 to 12 years old. Brain function increases rapidly, and these children are likely to begin puberty.
- Adolescents are 13 to 19 years old. They have nearly completed their growth, and their form has changed to that of an adult. Adolescents reach sexual maturity.
- Early adulthood is from 20 to 40 years of age. Body systems are at their peak performance. This is the age when love relationships occur and parenting takes place.

- Age 41 to 60 years is considered middle adulthood. This is when menopause occurs and when systems begin to show signs of aging.
- Late adulthood encompasses those older than 60 years. Body system deterioration becomes more apparent at different times for different people in this age group on the basis of genetics, health, and lifestyle.

MATCHING

1. Match the age group with the typical characteristics of that group.

   _____ Become assertive, take initiative, and assert their independence

   _____ Develop a unique personality and a strong set of likes and dislikes

   _____ Master environment through information; develop self-discipline; self-esteem issues may develop; begin to develop morals

   _____ Seeking self-determination; fragile self-esteem; very acute body image; establish identity and autonomy

   A. Toddlers
   B. Preschoolers
   C. School-age children
   D. Adolescents

2. Match the infant reflex response to its name.

   _____ Fanning of the toes outward when the sole of the foot is stroked

   _____ Flinging of the arms up and out in response to being startled

   _____ Grasping when an object is placed in the hand

   _____ Lifting one foot after another when the feet are held flat on a surface

   _____ Turning of the head toward anything that brushes the face

   A. Babinski reflex
   B. Moro reflex
   C. Palmar reflex
   D. Rooting reflex
   E. Stepping reflex

SHORT ANSWER

1. Applying what you learned in this chapter, what is the normal weight in kilograms of a 1-year-old child?

_____
_____
_____
_____

2. If an infant or small child is placed in a supine position, what happens to the airway? Why? How can this problem be prevented?

_____
_____
_____
_____

3. What are the fontanels? When does the anterior fontanel close? How can the fontanel be useful in assessment?

_____
_____
_____
_____

4. Applying what you learned in the chapter, why will gastric distention have a more significant impact on ability to ventilate adequately in an infant rather than in an adult?

_____
_____
_____
_____

5. Applying what you have learned in Chapters 7, 8, and 9, please answer the following question. Although infants younger than 6 months of age have a lower incidence of infection than older children, why are they more susceptible to severe and unusual infections if they are exposed to an infectious organism?

_____
_____
_____
_____

6. What response can you anticipate if you try to take an infant older than approximately 9 months away from his or her parents to do a physical examination?

_____
_____
_____
_____

7. How should you modify the physical examination of an older infant to accommodate the expected responses?

_____
_____
_____
_____

8. Applying the principles learned in this chapter, how would you modify your approach to the assessment of a pediatric patient who does not have a life threatening condition?

_____
_____
_____
_____

9. How does the pulse rate of a pediatric patient normally compare to that of an adult?

_____
_____
_____
_____

10. How will a typical toddler respond to your attempt to perform an examination on him or her?

_____
_____
_____
_____

11. What should you do to accommodate the expected responses of a toddler to a physical examination?

_____
_____
_____
_____

12. For children aged 1-10 years, how can the minimum acceptable blood pressure be estimated?

_____
_____
_____
_____

13. Applying what you learned in the chapter, how do you think adolescents are likely to respond to the need to undress in order to undergo a physical examination?

_____
_____
_____
_____

14. Based on what you learned in the chapter, how can you accommodate the likely response of an adolescent to being undressed for a physical examination?

_____
_____
_____
_____

15. What changes occur in the kidneys of older adults?

_____
_____
_____
_____

16. What is the "terminal drop" hypothesis of aging?

_____
_____
_____
_____

MULTIPLE CHOICE

1. Applying the principles you have learned in this chapter, please answer the following question. An 80-year-old female who is a resident of a local nursing home has severe pedal edema. However, her neck veins are flat, her lung fields are clear, and there is no apparent abdominal distention. A nursing home staff members tells you that she spends 12 to 16 hours a day sitting in her wheelchair in front of the TV in the lobby. The edema probably is the result of _____.
   A. kidney failure
   B. left-sided congestive heart failure
   C. prolonged immobility and dependent position of the feet
   D. right-sided congestive heart failure

2. Treating pediatric patients is different from treating adults because children _____.
   A. are less fearful than adults
   B. are more trusting than adults
   C. like riding in the ambulance
   D. may have difficulty communicating

3. When a pediatric patient is suffering from a problem that is not life-threatening, what should you do?
   A. Do not waste time doing an assessment.
   B. Perform the examination the same way it would be performed on an adult.
   C. Take a little more time to perform the examination.
   D. Think of the pediatric patient as a small adult.

4. When treating a sick or injured child, you should _____.
   A. allow only one parent to be present at any time
   B. allow parents to be present only if absolutely necessary
   C. never allow parents to be present
   D. use the parents to assist you when appropriate

5. The pulse rate of a pediatric patient is normally _____.
   A. faster than an adult's pulse rate
   B. slower than an adult's pulse rate
   C. the same as an adult's pulse rate
   D. weak and thready

6. The fontanelle of an infant _____.
   A. is only beneficial in the assessment of children up to 4 months old
   B. may be sunken if an infant is dehydrated
   C. should be checked with the infant lying flat
   D. will be sunken if there is an increase in intracranial pressure

7. In children younger than school age, how should the detailed physical examination be performed?
   A. From toe to head
   B. In the same manner as in the adult
   C. Rapidly to avoid agitating or upsetting the patient
   D. Very slowly to avoid agitation

8. When examining older infants and toddlers, you should _____.
   A. ask the parents to leave the room
   B. examine the child quickly to avoid creating distress
   C. hold the child in your lap
   D. leave the child on the parent's lap

9. Differences in airway anatomy between children and adults include _____.
   A. the child's tongue is larger in relation to the other structures in the airway
   B. the glottic opening is lower in the airway in children than in adults
   C. the mandible is relatively larger and the head is relatively smaller than in adults
   D. the tongue is set further forward in the airway than in adults

10. Which of the following groups of pediatric patients generally would be expected to be uncooperative?
    A. 2 to 3 year olds
    B. 4 to 5 year olds
    C. 6 to 10 year olds
    D. 10 to 14 year olds

11. Applying the principles you learned in the chapter, what do you believe the ideal initial approach for assessment of the conscious, non–acutely ill child is?
    A. Conduct the initial assessment and the detailed history and physical before talking to the child.
    B. Continue with your assessment, even with an uncooperative child, to avoid missing any important signs.
    C. Gain as much information as possible through history and observation before touching the child.
    D. Immediately perform a head to toe physical examination as your partner obtains the history.

12. Applying the principles you learned in the chapter, which of the following assessment techniques would you incorporate into your assessment of a patient in late adulthood?
    A. Call the patient "dear" or "honey" to let the patient know that you care.
    B. Separate the patient from friends and family as soon as possible to reduce anxiety.
    C. Talk louder than normal since most of the elderly have difficulty hearing.
    D. Use physical contact to compensate for loss of sight or hearing.

13. Which of these statements about specific age groups of pediatric patients is *correct*?
    A. Two to 3 year olds are usually cooperative and like to be touched.
    B. Six-12 year olds are usually cooperative and like to "help out" the paramedic.
    C. Adolescents usually have high self-esteem and are not concerned about lasting effects of injury or illness.
    D. School-aged children usually are frightened by information and do not like to be told what is being done to them.

CASE STUDY

Your patient is a 16-year-old female who is complaining of weakness, dizziness, and pain in the left lower quadrant of her abdomen. Her skin is pale, cool, and moist. Vital signs are P–114 beats/min, weak, regular; R–24 breaths/min shallow, regular; BP–98/68 mm Hg. Her mother is present on the scene.

1. Describe how you would take a history from this patient.

   _____
   _____
   _____
   _____

2. Discuss any modifications that might be necessary when performing a physical examination on this patient.

   _____
   _____
   _____
   _____

10 Public Health and EMS

READING ASSIGNMENT

Chapter 10, pages 295-304, in *Paramedic Practice Today: Above and Beyond.*

OBJECTIVES

After completing this chapter, you will be able to:
1. Define the term *public health*.
2. Identify the potential public health roles of EMS providers.
3. Describe opportunities for EMS to enhance access to care.
4. Define the public health role of EMS in emergency preparedness.
5. Explain opportunities to reduce medical costs through the appropriate use of emergency medical services.

CHAPTER SUMMARY

- Health is a state of complete physical, mental, and social well-being and not merely the absence of disease or infirmity.
- Public health can be defined as the science and practice of protecting and improving the health of a community.
- In the United States, public health services are provided through various means. At the federal level, public health services are a core function of the Department of Health and Human Services. This agency serves the public health community.
- The role of a public health agency is to prevent and control communicable disease and promote health.
- One of the most visible ways in which EMS professionals have interacted with public health agencies is through the provision of immunizations. EMS personnel also are well positioned to screen the population for the presence or absence of disease, recognize evidence of abuse or addiction, and educate the public on matters of public health and safety.
- EMS professionals are ideally suited to reach at-risk populations because of the credibility of EMS in the community as well as their inherent mobility. EMS stations often are located in areas of ready community access.
- Public health services are not obligated to provide individual healthcare; however, a strong desire exists to ensure that all people have access to care. Expanded EMS scopes of care can help accomplish this goal.

- EMS personnel have the opportunity to enhance access to care by using EMS stations as community health resources. Examples include providing medication compliance checks, blood pressure and blood sugar measurements, and chronic wound care on site.
- EMS agencies also may participate in home health visits, providing wound care, assessing the status of home intravenous or injection therapy, and performing well-being checks on those identified by their physicians as at particularly high risk.
- Prehospital personnel may also serve as a cost-effective supplement to hospital emergency department or nursing care staff.
- The EMS, law enforcement, and public health communities must work more closely together than ever before to be prepared for all-hazard emergencies.
- EMS systems generally view preparedness as responding to transient and time-limited situations that temporarily stress the medical care system but have minimal aftereffects on capabilities or infrastructure. In contrast, public health agencies adopt a longer term view of preparedness, focusing on the prolonged incident (such as the multiple waves of pandemic influenza) and prolonged recovery periods (as seen in the 2005 hurricanes). Because of these differences, EMS and public health must work together to enhance understanding and promote working relationships well in advance of when an actual emergency arises.
- Many jurisdictions in the United States use an emergency management model that designates service realms as an ESF.
- Epidemiology is the study of the prevalence and spread of disease in a community. In the context of preparedness, it is the ability to interpret incidence and prevalence data to determine the cause, geographic source, and nature of an imminent threat to public health. The earlier a potential biohazard can be detected, the sooner it can be traced to its source and those likely to be at risk can be identified and treated.
- Public healthcare agencies use the tools of isolation and quarantine to help prevent the spread of disease. Isolation refers to the seclusion of individuals with an illness to prevent transmission to others. Quarantine pertains to the seclusion of entire groups of exposed but asymptomatic individuals for monitoring.
- EMS systems may be able to address cost containment by revising the traditional paradigm of "triage, treatment, and transport." Some services are experimenting

with the idea of triaging callers. With this concept, those who call EMS dispatch centers may be referred to alternate, less-costly forms of care rather than summon EMS response and hospital transport. In Nova Scotia, primary care paramedics treat patients on site when possible, reducing the need for transport and hospitalization.

■ EMS personnel must take care that the requirements for reimbursement and the desire for cost containment do not jeopardize the core public service mission of prehospital care.

MATCHING

_____ A state of complete physical, mental, and social well-being, not merely the absence of disease or infirmity

_____ Comparison of number and nature of medical cases to expected number at a given time and place to identify disease outbreaks

_____ Evaluating a population for the presence or absence of disease

_____ Study of prevalence and spread of disease in a community

_____ The science and practice of protecting and improving a community's health

A. Epidemiology
B. Health
C. Screening
D. Syndromic surveillance
E. Public health

SHORT ANSWER

1. How does the practice of public health professionals differ from the practice of most healthcare professionals?

_____
_____
_____

2. List three reasons why EMS is well suited to provide immunizations as a public health service.

_____
_____
_____
_____

3. Identify at least three issues that must be addressed before an EMS organization initiates an immunization program.

_____
_____
_____
_____

4. Discuss strategies an EMS organization can use to recover the costs of providing an immunization program.

_____
_____
_____
_____

5. Applying the principles you learned in this chapter, should the concept of "screening" in public health be limited to simply evaluating a population for the presence or absence of disease? Why or why not?

_____
_____
_____

6. Why does EMS have an advantage in performing public health screening activities?

_____
_____
_____
_____

7. List five problems that can be routinely screened by EMS personnel when a patient's health history is being taken.

_____
_____
_____
_____
_____

8. What is a "teachable moment"?

_____
_____
_____
_____

9. Why does EMS have an advantage in using teachable moments to provide effective public health education?

_____
_____
_____

10. What is advocacy?

_____
_____
_____
_____

11. List five issues related to public health in which EMS organizations and personnel can act as effective advocates.

_____
_____
_____
_____
_____

12. Applying the principles learned in this chapter, and aside from the importance to their personal health and safety, why should EMS personnel practice behaviors such as seat belt use, tobacco avoidance, and good eating habits both on and off duty?

_____

_____

_____

_____

13. How does the public health view of emergency preparedness and response differ from the typical EMS organization's view of these functions? Why is this difference an important consideration during planning for significant incidents?

_____

_____

_____

_____

14. Why is healthcare cost containment considered a public health issue?

_____

_____

_____

_____

MULTIPLE CHOICE

1. Which of the following statements about the organization of public health services in the federal government of the United States is correct?
   A. Activities impacting public health take place in a variety of agencies including the Department of Agriculture and the Environmental Protection Agency.
   B. All functions related to public health are performed by the Department of Health and Human Services.
   C. The Environmental Protection Agency is a component of the Department of Health and Human Services.
   D. The Office of the Surgeon General is an agency of the Department of Homeland Security.

2. Which of the following statements about the structure of public health at the state and local levels is correct?
   A. Every state has a designated State Health Official.
   B. Federal law determines the relationship between state and local health departments.
   C. Public health at the local level always is a function of municipal government.
   D. The State Health Official always is the executive head of an independent state department of health.

3. Which of the following statements about EMS personnel performing public health screening is correct?
   A. EMS agencies that implement screening programs are legally obligated to develop and fund a system for ensuring follow-up action.

   B. EMS personnel generally do not have the time while responding to a call to screen patients and their environments for risks and hazards.
   C. For screening by EMS to be effective, patients must be given information on community resources and resource agencies must be notified of potential referrals.
   D. Studies have indicated that EMS personnel receive adequate initial education in recognizing situations that place patients or populations at risk.

4. What does taking an "all hazards" approach to emergency preparedness mean?
   A. Emergencies resulting from all hazards present in the community are managed from a single plan that provides common terminology and structure.
   B. The community assesses the hazards that could result in a disaster (e.g., tornado, flood, earthquake) and develops a comprehensive plan for each of them.
   C. The local emergency management director designates one agency to be in command for each hazard likely to impact a community.
   D. The local public health agency provides guidance to other government agencies on the health problems likely to result from all hazards identified in the community.

5. Which of the following statements best distinguishes between *isolation* and *quarantine*?
   A. Isolation is seclusion of asymptomatic individuals exposed to a disease for monitoring; quarantine is seclusion of persons with an illness to prevent transmission.
   B. Isolation is seclusion of persons with an illness to prevent transmission; quarantine is seclusion of asymptomatic individuals exposed to a disease for monitoring.
   C. Quarantine takes place in hospitals; isolation takes place in the residences of persons who are sick or have been exposed to a disease.
   D. Quarantine takes place in the residences of persons who are sick or have been exposed to a disease; isolation takes place in hospitals.

6. Which of the following statements about cost containment in EMS is correct?
   A. Actions and attitudes of EMS personnel can be adversely affected by mandating aggressive cost containment or revenue generation strategies.
   B. Efforts to contain costs by EMS organizations are unlikely to have a significant impact on the rest of the healthcare system.
   C. Having EMS dispatchers triage callers to less costly forms of care or transport has been shown to be a safe, effective cost containment strategy.
   D. Requiring patients to be billed for EMS services does not have an adverse effect on willingness to seek care or on patient outcomes.

7. In an emergency management model that groups agencies by emergency services functions (ESFs), EMS is most likely to function as part of the _____.

A. health and medical care ESF headed by the fire chief
B. health and medical care ESF headed by the local health officer
C. public safety ESF headed by the fire chief
D. public safety ESF headed by the police chief

8. Which of the following is the best example of taking advantage of a teachable moment to provide effective public health education?

A. Asking a 67-year-old male being transported for chest pain whether he has received influenza and pneumococcal pneumonia immunizations
B. Discussing child restraint devices with a 26-year-old female who was involved in a minor motor vehicle collision with her 2-year-old daughter in the vehicle
C. Explaining to a 72-year-old female being transported for shortness of breath and a productive cough how having throw rugs in her home puts her at risk for falls
D. Providing a presentation of the consequences of driving while intoxicated to a high school health class

CASE STUDIES

Case one

You are the director of a municipal third-service EMS organization serving a city of approximately 500,000 people located in the Southwestern United States. The community is located along an interstate highway, is served by an international airport, and is home to several large companies that operate internationally in Europe and Asia. For the last week you have been hearing news reports of syndrome X, a new viral respiratory tract infection that recently emerged in East Asia. The disease presents initially with a sore throat and nasal congestion and rapidly progresses to a flulike syndrome characterized by high fever, productive cough, and severe respiratory distress. More than 300 deaths have occurred in China, South Korea, and Japan both as a result of the primary disease process and from secondary bacterial infections, primarily pneumococcal pneumonia. The disease is airborne, has an incubation period of 96 hours, and is highly transmissible. Children younger than age 6, the elderly, and persons with chronic pulmonary disease are at greatest risk.

You have just received a call from the county public health director. She tells you that the Centers for Disease Control and Prevention has informed her that 10 cases of syndrome X have been identified in Los Angeles and San Francisco among persons who recently traveled to South Korea on business. One death has been documented.

A meeting is scheduled this afternoon to discuss strategies for rapidly identifying an outbreak of syndrome X in the community and controlling its spread.

1. Discuss the role EMS could play in this effort.

_____
_____
_____
_____
_____
_____

Case two

You are the director of a hospital-based EMS organization serving a city of approximately 70,000 people located in the South Central United States 200 miles inland from the Gulf of Mexico. A hurricane formed in the eastern Gulf of Mexico 3 days ago and began moving toward the northwest. The storm now is predicted to make landfall in 48 hours near a coastal city of 2,000,000 located 180 miles away. The storm is expected to be at category 4 strength when it makes landfall. Forecasters are predicting category 1 strength at your location. The governor has declared a state of emergency and ordered an evacuation of the areas of the coast likely to be affected. During a conference call with the local emergency management coordinator and the county public health director 20 minutes ago, you were advised that shelters for evacuees are being opened at five locations in the community. You just received a call from the State Health Department to stand-by to support the evacuation effort and respond to the storm's aftermath.

1. What types of activities should you anticipate?

   _____
   _____
   _____
   _____
   _____
   _____

11 Basic Principles of Pharmacology

READING ASSIGNMENT

Chapter 11, pages 306-347, in *Paramedic Practice Today: Above and Beyond.*

OBJECTIVES

After completing this chapter, you will be able to:
1. Describe historic trends in pharmacology.
2. Differentiate the chemical, generic, and trade names of a drug.
3. List the main sources of drug products.
4. Describe how drugs are classified.
5. List the authoritative sources for drug information.
6. List legislative acts controlling drug use and abuse in the United States.
7. Differentiate Schedule I, II, III, IV, and V substances and list examples of each.
8. Discuss standardization of drugs.
9. Discuss investigational drugs, including the Food and Drug Administration approval process and classifications for newly approved drugs.
10. Discuss the paramedic's responsibilities and scope of management pertinent to the administration of medications.
11. Review the specific anatomy and physiology pertinent to pharmacology with additional attention to autonomic pharmacology.
12. List and describe general properties of drugs.
13. List and describe liquid and solid drug forms.
14. List and differentiate routes of drug administration, including the enteral and parenteral routes.
15. Describe mechanisms of drug action.
16. List and differentiate the phases of drug activity, including the pharmaceutical, pharmacokinetic, and pharmacodynamic phases.
17. Describe the processes of pharmacokinetics and pharmacodynamics, including theories of drug action, drug-response relation, factors altering drug responses, predictable drug responses, iatrogenic drug responses, and unpredictable adverse drug responses.
18. Discuss special considerations in drug treatment regarding pregnant, pediatric, and geriatric patients.
19. Differentiate drug interactions.
20. Discuss considerations for storing and securing medications.
21. List the components of a drug profile by classification.

CHAPTER SUMMARY

- A drug's trade name is also called its *brand name.* The generic name often is a simplified form of the chemical name. The chemical name represents the chemical structure of the compound.
- Orphan drugs are products used to treat rare diseases or conditions.
- Sources of drugs include plants, animal/human products, minerals, synthetic chemicals, and recombinant DNA technology.
- Three drug classification systems are used in healthcare: body system, class of agent, and mechanism of action.
- Sources of information for drugs include the *Physicians' Desk Reference,* hospital formularies, people (such as physicians, nurses, and pharmacists), pocket references, and package inserts.
- The 1970 Comprehensive Drug Abuse Prevention and Control Act established the schedule of controlled substances.
- The *United States Pharmacopoeia* is the official public standards–setting authority for all prescription and over-the-counter medicines, dietary supplements, and other healthcare products manufactured and sold in the United States.
- The FDA has an approval process for investigational drugs that totals four phases.
- Safe and effective drug administration is the responsibility of the paramedic. Obtaining a history is crucial for proper administration of medications.
- The nervous system contains the central and the peripheral nervous system. The CNS contains the brain and the spinal cord. The peripheral nervous system contains all the nerves outside the CNS. The somatic nervous system includes nerves under voluntary control. The ANS is automatic and a division of the peripheral nervous system. Two divisions of the ANS have been classified: the sympathetic and parasympathetic.

79

- The sympathetic division also is called the *adrenergic division* and is responsible for the fight-or-flight response. Neurotransmitters in the sympathetic division include epinephrine and norepinephrine. Receptors in the sympathetic division include alpha$_1$, alpha$_2$, beta$_1$, beta$_2$, and dopaminergic receptors. The parasympathetic division also is called the *cholinergic system* and referred to as the "feed and breed" or "resting and digesting" response of the ANS. The neurotransmitter in the parasympathetic division is acetylcholine. Two receptors are present in the parasympathetic division: muscarinic and nicotinic.
- Synaptic transmission occurs at the synaptic junction. The preganglionic and postganglionic nerves are connected at the ganglion.
- Drugs come in liquid, solid, or gaseous forms.
- The route of drug administration affects the type of effect and onset of action. Enteral drugs enter the systemic circulation by the GI tract. Parenteral drugs enter the systemic circulation by bypassing the digestive tract.
- Medications typically alter a normal body response; they do not generate a new function or response.
- Pharmacokinetics is the process of how drugs are processed in the body. Drugs are absorbed, distributed, metabolized, and finally excreted. Absorption is highly dependent on the route of administration. Distribution depends on a number of physiologic factors, including blood supply, pH, and body temperature. Metabolism may render a drug active, inactive, or ready for excretion. Excretion and elimination are the body's mechanisms for removing the drug or its metabolites from circulation.
- An agonist stimulates a receptor, causing a physiologic response. A partial agonist or antagonist may cause a physiologic response but not to the extent of an agonist. An antagonist binds with a receptor but does not elicit a response.
- The biologic half-life is the time required to eliminate half of a substance from the bloodstream.
- Drugs have been rated for their safety in pregnancy by the FDA. Pediatric patients have different physiologic functions and thus their response to medications is different from adults. Geriatric patients also have different physiologic characteristics, compounded by multiple medical problems and medications. Their response to medications also is affected.
- A side effect is an effect of a drug other than the one for which it was given. Side effects may or may not be harmful.
- An iatrogenic drug response is an unintentional disease or drug effect produced by a physician's prescribed therapy.
- Many factors may affect drug action, including intestinal absorption, drug metabolism, excretion, electrolytes, drug-drug interactions, and incompatibilities.
- Drug storage is important because certain medications require special storage instructions. Drug storage for controlled substances is important and is the responsibility of the paramedic.
- A drug profile is a complete description of a drug and its characteristics.

MATCHING

1. Match the terms used to describe drug forms with their definitions.
   - _____ A medication consisting of an extract in an alcohol solution
   - _____ A drug dissolved in water with sugar, flavorings, and alcohol added
   - _____ Gelatin containers enclosing a dose of a drug
   - _____ Drug mixed in a firm base that melts at body temperature
   - _____ Medication suspended in a liquid, such as an oral antibiotic
   - _____ One liquid suspended in another; usually oil in water
   - _____ Powdered drugs molded or compressed into disks
   - _____ Volatile substance dissolved in alcohol

   A. Capsule
   B. Elixir
   C. Emulsion
   D. Spirits
   E. Suppository
   F. Suspension
   G. Tablet
   H. Tincture

2. Match the terms used to describe drug actions with their definitions.
   - _____ A condition or situation in which a drug is not given
   - _____ A condition that is a reason to give a drug action
   - _____ A predictable effect of a drug other than its therapeutic action
   - _____ Decreased intensity of drug effect after several doses
   - _____ Enhancement of one drug's effects by those of a related drug with similar effects
   - _____ A prolongation or increase in the effect of a drug by another drug
   - _____ Increased intensity of drug effect after several doses

   A. Additive effects
   B. Antagonism
   C. Contraindication
   D. Cumulative action
   E. Idiosyncrasy
   F. Indication
   G. Potentiation
   H. Side effect
   I. Synergism
   J. Desired action
   K. Tolerance

_____ Joint action of two drugs when combined
    exceeds the sum of their individual effects
_____ Opposing action between drugs
_____ Response to a drug that is peculiar to an individual
_____ The beneficial effect of a drug

3. Match the type of drug name with its definition.
    _____ Description of a drug's exact molecular composition
    _____ Name given to a drug by a specific manufacturer
    _____ Name given to a drug by first manufacturer before
        approval by government
    _____ Name listed in the _United States Pharmacopoeia_

    A. Chemical
    B. Generic
    C. Official
    D. Trade

4. Match the federal agency with its function in drug regulation.
    _____ Establishes drug effectiveness, safety. Approves new
        drugs for use.
    _____ Enforces controlled substance laws and monitors the
        need for changing schedules of abused drugs.
    _____ Suppresses misleading drug advertising.

    A. Drug Enforcement Administration
    B. Federal Trade Commission
    C. Food and Drug Administration

5. Match the drug legislation with its function.
    _____ Authorized government to determine drug safety/
        effectiveness
    _____ Authorized "scheduling" of drugs based on use and
        abuse potential
    _____ Controlled import, manufacture, and sale of opium,
        cocaine, and their derivatives; required physicians,
        pharmacists, and manufacturers to register with
        government
    _____ Required accurate labeling of products; established
        United States Pharmacopoeia as official information
        source
    _____ Required prescriptions for dangerous drugs; created
        over-the-counter medications

    A. Controlled Substances Act (1970)
    B. Durham-Humphrey Amendment (1951)
    C. Federal Food, Drug, and Cosmetic Act
       (1938)
    D. Harrison Narcotic Act (1914)
    E. Pure Food and Drug Act (1906)

6. Using Appendix B (compilation of drug profiles) in the text, please mach the proprietary name of each drug with
    its generic name.
    _____ albuterol
    _____ diazepam
    _____ diphenhydramine
    _____ epinephrine
    _____ furosemide
    _____ lidocaine
    _____ naloxone
    _____ procainamide
    _____ propranolol

    A. Adrenalin
    B. Benadryl
    C. Inderal
    D. Lasix
    E. Narcan
    F. Pronestyl
    G. Proventil
    H. Valium
    I. Xylocaine

SHORT ANSWER

1. How would a controlled substance with an accepted
    medical use and high abuse potential be scheduled?
    _____
    _____
    _____
    _____

2. How would a controlled substance with no accepted
    medical use and high abuse potential be scheduled?
    _____
    _____
    _____
    _____

3. From what source was insulin originally obtained?
    _____
    _____
    _____
    _____

4. From what source are digitalis and morphine obtained?
    _____
    _____
    _____
    _____

5. From what source are calcium chloride, sodium bicarbonate, and magnesium sulfate obtained?

_____

_____

_____

_____

6. What is a synthetic drug?

_____

_____

_____

_____

7. Applying the principles you learned in this chapter, if a patient has liver disease, what prediction can you make about the duration of the effects of drugs administered to the patient? Why?

_____

_____

_____

_____

8. Applying the principles you learned in this chapter, if a patient has renal disease, what prediction can you make about the duration of the effects of drugs administered to the patient? Why?

_____

_____

_____

_____

9. Naloxone (Narcan) is a narcotic antagonist. What does the term *antagonist* mean?

_____

_____

_____

_____

10. A patient who is receiving narcotics to control pain requires increasing doses of the drugs to relieve the pain. This is due to what drug effect?

_____

_____

_____

_____

11. In addition to its beneficial action, Benadryl produces drowsiness and a dry mouth. What would such actions be called?

_____

_____

_____

_____

12. List the components of pharmacokinetics.

_____

_____

_____

_____

13. Describe facilitated transport, including direction of movement relative to relevant gradients and use of proteins and energy, if applicable.

_____

_____

_____

_____

14. Describe active transport, including direction of movement relative to relevant gradients and use of proteins and energy, if applicable.

_____

_____

_____

_____

15. Applying what you have learned in prior chapters and in this chapter, compare and contrast osmosis and diffusion.

_____

_____

_____

_____

MULTIPLE CHOICE

1. Which of the following is one of the four types of drug names?
   A. Biologic
   B. Proper
   C. Sales
   D. Trade

2. The four main sources for drugs include _____.
   A. animals
   B. minerals and animals
   C. plants and minerals
   D. plants, minerals, and animals

3. For many years, the primary source of insulin was the extract of _____.
   A. feline pancreas
   B. equine pancreas
   C. porcine pancreas
   D. primate pancreas

4. Which publication is a commercially published compilation of information for more than 4000 medications including indications, interactions, mechanism of action, side effects, adverse effects, and other information?
   A. *AMA Drug Evaluation*
   B. *Monthly Prescribing Reference*
   C. *Physicians' Desk Reference*
   D. *United States Pharmacopoeia*

5. Name, classification, mechanism of action, and indications are examples of information found in a drug's _____.
   A. overview
   B. profile
   C. review
   D. synopsis

6. According to the Controlled Substances Act of 1970, a Schedule I drug _____.
   A. has a low abuse potential
   B. has a low physical, but high psychologic, dependence potential
   C. may lead to limited psychologic and/or physical dependence
   D. has no accepted medical indications

7. Drug legislation passed in the United States to protect the public from adulterated or mislabeled drugs was the _____.
   A. Comprehensive Drug Abuse Prevention and Control Act
   B. Federal Food, Drug, and Cosmetic Act
   C. Harrison Narcotic Act
   D. Pure Food and Drug Act

8. Which test determines the amount and purity of a given chemical in a pharmaceutical preparation?
   A. Assay
   B. Bioassay
   C. Bioequivalence
   D. Pharmacokinetics

9. The process by which a drug is absorbed, distributed, metabolized, and eliminated is called _____.
   A. bioequivalence
   B. pharmacokinetics
   C. pharmacodynamics
   D. pharmacology

10. A medication that may deform or kill a fetus is called a _____.
    A. category A drug
    B. fetal risk drug
    C. fundalgenic drug
    D. teratogenic drug (teratogen)

11. A drug's mechanism of action is described by its _____.
    A. bioequivalence
    B. pharmacodynamics
    C. pharmacokinetics
    D. pharmacology

12. The liver's partial or complete breakdown of a drug before it reaches the systemic circulation is called the _____.
    A. antidrug effect
    B. first-pass effect
    C. hepatic filtration effect
    D. liver-blood barrier

13. Certain barriers hamper the distribution of some drugs. An example of this is the _____.
    A. arterial-venous barrier
    B. blood-brain barrier
    C. endothelial barrier
    D. uterine-fetal barrier

14. A liquid form of a drug prepared using an alcohol extraction process is called a(n) _____.
    A. emulsion
    B. solution
    C. spirit
    D. tincture

15. The force of attraction between a drug and a receptor is _____.
    A. affinity
    B. binding
    C. combining
    D. efficacy

16. An agonist is a drug that binds to a receptor _____.
    A. and causes a deformity on the binding site
    B. and causes a physiologic response
    C. and stimulates some of its effects but blocks others
    D. but does not cause it to initiate the expected response

17. By developing a tolerance for morphine sulfate, a patient may also develop tolerance for other opioid agents. This effect is an example of _____.
    A. addiction
    B. cross tolerance
    C. idiosyncrasy
    D. tachyphylaxis

18. An antagonist agent binds to a receptor _____.
    A. and causes a deformity on the binding site
    B. and causes it to initiate the expected response
    C. and stimulates some of its effects but blocks others
    D. but does not elicit a response

19. The "lock and key" and "induced fit" analogies of drug action describe drugs that _____.
    A. activate second messenger systems such as cAMP
    B. are specific for a certain receptor morphology
    C. cause the body to increase the production of a substance
    D. escort substances through cell membranes

12 Drug and Chemical Classes

READING ASSIGNMENT

Chapter 12, pages 348-402, in *Paramedic Practice Today: Above and Beyond.*

OBJECTIVES

After completing this chapter, you will be able to:
1. List and describe drugs that the paramedic may administer according to local protocol.
2. Integrate pathophysiologic principles of pharmacology with patient assessment.
3. Synthesize patient history information and assessment findings to form a field impression.
4. Discuss the analgesic class of medications, including prescription and nonprescription medications.
5. Discuss anesthetics, including types, routes of administration, and indications.
6. Discuss serums, vaccines, and antidotes.
7. Discuss antiinfective agents, including antibiotics, antivirals, antifungals, and antiparasitic agents.
8. Discuss antineoplastic drugs.
9. Discuss vitamins and minerals.
10. Discuss fluids and electrolytes.
11. Discuss and give examples of anxiolytics, antidepressants, mood stabilizers, and antipsychotics.
12. Discuss and give examples of anticonvulsant drugs.
13. Discuss and give examples of muscle relaxants.
14. Discuss central nervous stimulants.
15. Discuss drugs used for Parkinson's and Alzheimer's disease.
16. Discuss drugs affecting the parasympathetic division of the autonomic nervous system.
17. Discuss drugs affecting the sympathetic division of the autonomic nervous system.
18. Discuss drugs affecting the cardiovascular system, including antidysrhythmics, antihypertensives, and vasodilator agents.
19. Discuss anticoagulants, fibrinolytics, and blood components.
20. Discuss antihyperlipidemic drugs.
21. Discuss oxygen, mucokinetic, and bronchodilator drugs.
22. Discuss drugs affecting the renal system.
23. Discuss drugs affecting the gastrointestinal system.
24. Discuss drugs affecting the eyes and ears.
25. Discuss drugs affecting the endocrine system, including hormones.
26. Discuss uricosuric drugs.
27. Discuss drugs that affect the reproductive system.
28. Discuss drugs affecting the immunologic system.
29. Discuss dermatologic preparations.
30. Discuss drugs of abuse, including alcohols and amphetamines.
31. Discuss environmental chemicals, including herbicides, rodenticides, and insecticides.
32. Discuss toxic substances, including alcohols, heavy metals, household chemicals, and hazardous materials.

CHAPTER SUMMARY

- An indication is an appropriate use of a drug. A contraindication is an instance when a drug should not be used.
- Poison Control Centers can be accessed by phone for information on overdose and poisons.
- Gastric lavage is the cleansing of the stomach through a pump and irrigation with water.
- Activated charcoal is used to bind medications so they cannot be absorbed into the systemic circulation.
- Acetaminophen toxicity can affect the liver. Acetaminophen is used as an analgesic and for fever.
- Salicylates can be used as an antiplatelet or analgesic or for fever.
- NSAIDs are used for fever and analgesia.
- Morphine is an opioid. Opioids are narcotics. Some synthetic narcotics, such as fentanyl, do not have a profound effect on blood pressure. Opioid combinations are medications that combine two different types of analgesics. Aspirin or acetaminophen often is combined with a narcotic.
- Partial opioid agonists (agonist-antagonists) provide some effect but block the effect of a full agonist when given together.
- Opioid antagonists block the effects of the agonists.
- Anesthetics are used for deep sedation during procedures, including surgery and rapid-sequence intubation.
- Conscious sedation is a state in which a patient maintains the airway but is not aware of the procedure or pain.
- Benzodiazepines are used for anxiety and to induce sleep.
- Flumazenil (Romazicon) is an antidote for benzodiazepine overdose. It must be used cautiously because of a risk of seizures.
- Anticonvulsants are used to prevent seizure or treat seizure disorders.
- Antidepressants are used to treat both depression and bipolar disorder.

- Most antidepressants are very serious in overdose and can cause cardiac dysrhythmias.
- CNS stimulants include anorexiants and amphetamines.
- Antipsychotics are used to treat schizophrenia.
- Medications have been designed to treat Parkinson's and Alzheimer's diseases. They often alter acetylcholine or dopamine levels in the brain.
- Cholinergic drugs are rarely used therapeutically. These drugs include physostigmine, which is used to treat atropine overdose.
- Cholinergic drugs such as atropine are used in advanced cardiac life support.
- Sympathomimetics or catecholamines are used in advanced cardiac life support and in other medical conditions when the sympathetic nervous system needs to be stimulated.
- Antidysrhythmics are used to treat and prevent disorders of cardiac rhythm. Class I antidysrhythmics affect the sodium channel and work on slow conduction. Class II antidysrhythmics are beta-blockers, which block beta-receptors. They slow heart rate and conduction velocity and limit the force of contraction. Class III antiarrhythmics block the potassium channel. Included in this class is amiodarone. Class IV antiarrhythmics block the calcium channel. These are also used for blood pressure control. Adenosine is used to slow supraventricular tachycardias. It is in a class of its own.
- Digitalis is used for dysrhythmias and blocks ion pumps.
- Diuretics often are used to control pulmonary edema and blood pressure.
- Anticoagulants are used to inhibit clot formation. Thrombolytics (fibrinolytics) are used to break up an existing clot.
- Antihemophilic agents are used to treat bleeding after trauma in patients who are deficient in clotting cascade components.
- Bronchodilators are used to help stop bronchospasm and improve respiratory function.
- Mucokinetic drugs are used to loosen mucus so it can be expelled.
- Antihistamines are used to block the release of histamine, which helps reduce tissue edema.
- Antacids treat overproduction of acid and heartburn.
- Antiemetics are used for protracted vomiting and nausea.
- H_2-receptor antagonists are used to block histamine in the gastrointestinal tract.
- Ophthalmic agents are used for the diagnosis and treatment of diseases of the eye.
- Otic preparations are used for analgesia and treatment of diseases of the ear.
- Many hormones are used to treat various endocrine problems.
- Antibiotics are used to treat bacterial infections. Many different types are available.
- Antivirals are used to treat viral infections. Many types are used to treat HIV.

- Antifungals are used to treat fungal infections. Fungal infections can affect the skin as well as the entire systemic circulation.
- Gout is a painful type of arthritis treated with uricosuric drugs, including NSAIDs.
- Vitamins and minerals are necessary for normal body function.
- Crystalloids include normal saline, Ringer's lactate, D_5W, $D_5{}^{1/2}NS$, and D_5NS.
- Immunizations are designed to prevent infection.
- Immunoglobulins are used to treat infection; they are preformed antibodies.
- Antidotes are used to treat poisons or toxins.
- Drugs of abuse include stimulants, benzodiazepines, narcotics, hallucinogens, and sedative/hypnotics.
- Ethanol is a common drug of abuse that can cause respiratory depression.
- Herbicides, rodenticides, and insecticides can be highly toxic to human beings.
- Isopropyl alcohol, ethylene glycol, and methanol are in the alcohol family and can be highly toxic if ingested or absorbed.
- Hazardous materials can cause significant toxicity to human beings.

MATCHING

1. Match each drug with the classification to which it belongs.

____ Alpha with some beta effects	A. Atropine
____ Beta-blocker	B. Epinephrine
____ Beta with some alpha effects	C. Isoproterenol (Isuprel)
____ Parasympathetic blocker	D. Norepinephrine (Levophed)
____ Pure alpha	E. Phenylephrine (Neo-Synephrine)
____ Pure beta	F. Propranolol (Inderal)

SHORT ANSWER

1. List the classes and subclasses of antidysrhythmic drugs and give an example of a drug in each class.

_____

_____

_____

_____

2. Why do angiotensin-converting enzyme (ACE) inhibitors reduce blood pressure?

_____

_____

_____

_____

3. What condition are antihyperlipidemic agents used to treat?

_____

_____

_____

_____

4. What are thrombolytic agents?

_____

_____

_____

_____

5. In what type of tissue are "fast potentials" found?

_____

_____

_____

_____

6. In what type of tissue are "slow potentials" found?

_____

_____

_____

_____

7. Blocking calcium influx by giving a calcium channel blocker will have what effect on cardiac automaticity?

_____

_____

_____

_____

8. List the phases and indicate the direction of ion flow during each phase of a "fast potential."

_____

_____

_____

_____

9. What is the mnemonic for remembering the effects of atropine toxicity?

_____

_____

_____

_____

10. What are the components of the central nervous system?

_____

_____

_____

_____

11. What effect would a drug that is an opioid agonist-antagonist have on the pain response? On respirations?

_____

_____

_____

_____

12. Benzodiazepines and barbiturates are members of which functional class of medications?

_____

_____

_____

_____

13. What condition is methylphenidate (Ritalin) used to treat?

_____

_____

_____

_____

14. Taken over an extended time, antipsychotic medications may produce side effects that include tremors, shuffling gait, muscle spasms, and repetitive motions that are called *extrapyramidal symptoms (or extrapyramidal reactions)*. What medication may be given to treat these effects?

_____

_____

_____

_____

15. List the names of three selective serotonin reuptake inhibitors (SSRIs).

_____

_____

_____

_____

16. What condition are SSRIs used to treat?

_____

_____

_____

_____

17. List the names of three monoamine oxidase inhibitors (MAOIs).

_____

_____

_____

_____

18. What condition is treated with MAOIs?

_____

_____

_____

_____

19. Describe the action of MAOIs.

_____

_____

_____

_____

20. What effect will parasympathetic stimulation have on:

Heart rate:_____

GI tract gland secretions:_____

Pupils:_____

Muscle tone in the lower airway:_____

21. What are the two types of acetylcholine receptors?

_____

_____

22. Where is each of the acetylcholine (ACh) receptor types found?

_____

_____

_____

23. Which type of ACh receptor site is blocked by atropine?

_____

_____

_____

_____

24. Define the acronym SLUDGE.

_____

_____

_____

_____

25. SLUDGE suggests toxicity with what kind of drug?

_____

_____

_____

_____

26. What is the effect of stimulation of the sympathetic nervous system on each of the following?

Blood flow to the abdominal organs:_____

Peristalsis in the GI tract:_____

Muscle tone in the urinary bladder wall:_____

Glycogen stores in the liver:_____

27. What effect is produced by stimulation of the dopaminergic receptors?

_____

_____

_____

_____

28. Complete the following chart:

	Alpha Effect	Beta Effect
Heart	_____	_____
Lungs (bronchioles)	_____	_____
Blood vessels	_____	_____

29. What division of the ANS mediates the body's response to stress?

_____

_____

_____

_____

30. What division of the ANS mediates day-to-day vegetative functions?

_____

_____

_____

_____

31. What division of the ANS produces its effects by release of norepinephrine?

_____

_____

_____

_____

32. What division of the ANS produces its effects by release of ACh?

_____

_____

_____

_____

33. What division of the ANS functions primarily through the vagus nerve (cranial nerve X)?

_____

_____

_____

_____

34. What division of the ANS functions primarily through nerves arising from the thoracolumbar spine?

_____

_____

_____

_____

35. A $beta_1$ agent acts primarily on what organ? What are the effects of a $beta_1$ agent?

_____

_____

_____

_____

36. A $beta_2$ agent acts primarily on what anatomic structures? What are the effects of a $beta_2$ agent?

_____

_____

_____

_____

37. Stimulation of which division of the ANS will produce pupillary constriction, salivation, increased gastrointestinal motility and secretion, slight bronchoconstriction, decreased heart rate, and increased urine production?

_____

_____

_____

_____

38. Stimulation of which division of the ANS will produce pupillary dilation, decreased salivation, decreased gastrointestinal motility, bronchodilation, increased heart rate and myocardial irritability, and urinary retention?

_____

_____

_____

_____

39. If you wanted to give a drug to a patient that would increase the rate and contractility of the patient's heart without causing peripheral vasoconstriction, what combination of alpha and beta effects would you select?

_____

_____

_____

40. If you wanted to give a drug to a patient that would constrict blood vessels in the skin and digestive tract without directly affecting the heart rate, rhythm, and contractility, what combination of alpha and beta effects would you select?

_____

_____

_____

_____

41. What effect would a nonselective beta-blocker be expected to have on each of the following?
    a. Heart rate:_____
    b. Blood vessels:_____
    c. Bronchi:_____
    d. Cardiac automaticity:_____

42. If increasing dopamine levels in the brain is the goal of drugs that treat Parkinson's disease, why is levodopa used rather than dopamine itself?

_____

_____

_____

_____

43. How does an H_2 receptor antagonist decrease acid secretion?

_____

_____

_____

_____

44. What effect does ACh have on gastric acid secretion? What is the effect of blocking these receptors?

_____

_____

_____

_____

45. What are the two areas of the brain that control emesis?

_____

_____

_____

_____

46. What stimulates emesis?

_____

_____

_____

_____

47. What are the four major ways to prevent emesis?

_____

_____

_____

_____

48. A release of insulin causes what change in blood glucose levels?

_____

_____

_____

_____

49. A release of glucagon causes what change in blood glucose levels?

_____

_____

_____

_____

50. How do glucocorticoids help an asthmatic?

_____

_____

_____

51. What effect will glucocorticoids have on an acute asthmatic attack?

_____

_____

_____

_____

52. H₁ blockers will cause what effects?

_____

_____

_____

_____

53. Define the term *antitussive* and give an example.

_____

_____

_____

_____

54. Define the term *expectorant* and give an example.

_____

_____

_____

_____

55. Define the term *mucolytic* and give an example.

_____

_____

_____

_____

MULTIPLE CHOICE

1. The drug that best demonstrates the common properties of opioid agonists and illustrates their particular characteristics is _____.
   A. chloroform
   B. heroin
   C. morphine
   D. nalbuphine

2. Which of the following is an opioid antagonist?
   A. Midazolam
   B. Naloxone
   C. Nalbuphine
   D. Opium

3. Which of the following statements about opioid agonist-antagonists drugs is true?
   A. Respiratory depression is a common side effect in therapeutic doses.
   B. They are often given in conjunction with other agents to enhance their effects.
   C. They cause decreased sensation of pain with amnesia.
   D. They decrease pain response and have few respiratory depressant effects.

4. Benzodiazepines and barbiturates are the two main pharmacologic classes in the functional class of _____.
   A. analgesics
   B. anesthetics
   C. antidepressants
   D. sedative-hypnotics

5. Xanthines include _____.
   A. amphetamine sulfate
   B. methylphenidate
   C. pseudoephedrine
   D. theophylline

6. Methylphenidate is the most commonly prescribed drug for _____.
   A. asthma
   B. attention deficit–hyperactivity disorder
   C. congestive heart failure
   D. motion sickness

7. Which of the following is a phenothiazine?
   A. Chlorpromazine
   B. Diphenhydramine
   C. Haloperidol
   D. Methylphenidate

8. Which of the following is true regarding the intended therapeutic effects of phenothiazines and butyrophenones?
   A. They selectively block alpha₂ receptors in the CNS.
   B. They nonselectively block both alpha₁ and alpha₂ receptors in the CNS.
   C. They selectively block dopamine₂ receptors in the CNS.
   D. They selectively block norepinephrine receptors in the CNS.

9. Acute dystonic reactions are treated with _____.
   A. atropine
   B. diphenhydramine
   C. epinephrine
   D. phenytoin

10. SSRIs are use primarily to treat _____.
    A. bipolar disorder
    B. depression
    C. Parkinson's disease
    D. seizures

11. Which of the following is an MAOI?
    A. Nardil
    B. Paxil
    C. Prozac
    D. Zoloft

12. Stimulation of the parasympathetic nervous system results in _____.
    A. bronchodilation
    B. increase in heart rate and cardiac contractile force
    C. pupillary dilation
    D. secretion by digestive glands

13. The two main types of cholinergic receptors are _____.
    A. alpha and beta
    B. dopaminergic and adrenergic
    C. GABA and BZ
    D. nicotinic and muscarinic

14. SLUDGE is an acronym used to remember the effects of overdose of _____.
    A. adrenergics
    B. benzodiazepines
    C. butyrophenones
    D. cholinergics

15. Stimulation of the nerves in the sympathetic collateral ganglia of the abdominal cavity causes _____.
    A. increased blood flow to the abdominal organs
    B. increased digestive activity
    C. relaxation of the smooth muscle in the wall of the urinary bladder
    D. retention of glucose stores in the liver

16. Dopaminergic receptors are believed to cause _____.
    A. an increase in respiration and blood flow to the respiratory system
    B. constriction of the peripheral arteries
    C. constriction of the hepatic arteries
    D. dilation of the renal and mesenteric arteries

17. Terbutaline specifically targets _____.
    A. alpha$_1$ receptors
    B. alpha$_2$ receptors
    C. beta$_1$ receptors
    D. beta$_2$ receptors

18. Lidocaine and phenytoin belong to the class of _____.
    A. beta-blockers
    B. calcium channel blockers
    C. potassium channel blockers
    D. sodium channel blockers

19. Which class of drugs acts to decrease blood pressure by blocking the effects of a complex "cascade" system responsible for regulating fluid balance?
    A. ACE inhibitors
    B. Calcium channel blockers
    C. Direct vasodilators
    D. Ganglionic blockers

20. Drugs used to treat high blood cholesterol are called _____.
    A. ACE inhibitors
    B. antihyperlipidemics
    C. LDLs
    D. vasculotensives

21. Fibrinolytics are used to _____.
    A. break down thrombi
    B. decrease the formation of platelet plugs
    C. dilate blood vessels to reduce blood pressure
    D. interrupt the clotting cascade

22. Which of the following is a beta$_2$-specific agonist?
    A. Ipratropium
    B. Methylprednisolone
    C. Proventil
    D. Theophylline

23. Drugs that suppress the CNS stimulus to cough are _____.
    A. antihistamines
    B. antitussives
    C. expectorants
    D. mucolytics

24. The hormone oxytocin is released by the _____.
    A. anterior pituitary
    B. hypothalamus
    C. posterior pituitary
    D. thalamus

25. The pancreatic hormone that increases blood glucose level when released is _____.
    A. glucagon
    B. glycogen
    C. insulin
    D. somatostatin

26. A solution containing a modified pathogen that does not actually cause disease but still stimulates the development of antibodies specific to a disease is _____.
    A. an antibiotic
    B. an immunoglobulin
    C. a serum
    D. a vaccine

27. The antidote for organophosphate poisoning is _____.
    A. atropine
    B. diphenhydramine
    C. epinephrine
    D. lidocaine

Case one

While you are watering your lawn on your day off, your next-door neighbor wanders over to seek your "expert medical advice." He tells you his doctor just put him on a new "blood pressure" medicine, and he is "peeing like crazy." When you look at the bottle, you see that the medication is Captopril.

1. Why is this medication useful in the treatment of hypertension?

   _____
   _____
   _____
   _____

2. What effect of this medication is causing your neighbor's diuresis?

   _____
   _____
   _____
   _____

Case two

A 76-year-old man found an unknown plant growing in his yard and decided to see whether it was edible. He exhibits the following symptoms: he is restless, confused, and anxious; his skin is warm, flushed, and dry; his pupils are dilated and unreactive. The patient's wife tells you he was complaining of thirst and of blurry vision before his level of consciousness decreased. Vital signs are BP—146/100 mm Hg; P—138 beats/min strong, regular; R—24 breaths/min shallow, regular.

1. Based on the patient's clinical presentation, what type of substance has he ingested?

   _____
   _____
   _____
   _____

2. Explain why the substance is producing tachycardia, dilated pupils, and thirst. Be specific.

   _____
   _____
   _____
   _____

Case three

A patient is taking a monoamine oxidase inhibitor (MAOI). The patient has been instructed to avoid a variety of foods, including cheese, liver, wine, coffee, tea, and chocolate.

1. What disease processes are MAOI inhibitors used to treat?

   _____
   _____
   _____
   _____

2. Why are MAOI inhibitors useful in treating this disease process?

   _____
   _____
   _____
   _____

3. Why are patients taking MAOI inhibitors cautioned against consuming cheese, liver, and wine?

_____

_____

_____

_____

4. Why are patients taking MAOI inhibitors told not to consume coffee, tea, and chocolate?

_____

_____

_____

_____

5. What significant problem can occur if a patient taking an MAOI inhibitor consumes one of these foods?

_____

_____

_____

_____

Case four

A patient is requesting "pain medication" for a variety of nonspecific aches and pains. He tells you that he can take morphine and Demerol, but he is allergic to pentazocine (Talwin), butorphanol (Stadol), and nalbuphine (Nubain).

1. From what problem should you suspect this patient is actually suffering?

_____

_____

_____

_____

2. Why do patients with this problem want to avoid Talwin, Stadol, and Nubain?

_____

_____

_____

_____

Case five

A patient receiving a continuous infusion of lidocaine to control ventricular irritability complains of numbness of the lips, decreased hearing acuity, and depression.

1. Of what class of cardiac antidysrhythmics is lidocaine a member?

_____

_____

_____

_____

2. What is the common pharmacologic action of all members of this drug class?

_____

_____

_____

_____

3. How does this drug action account for the side effects being experienced by this patient?

_____

_____

_____

_____

4. How does this drug action account for lidocaine's ability to function as a local anesthetic?

_____

_____

_____

_____

Case six

A patient taking sildenafil citrate (Viagra) attained the desired effect. Unfortunately, the increase in myocardial oxygen demand associated with the accompanying activities produced an episode of angina pectoris. To relieve his chest discomfort, he took a dose of nitroglycerin.

1. What is the pharmacologic action by which Viagra produces its effects?

_____

_____

_____

_____

2. What complication can result from taking nitroglycerin following a dose of Viagra?

_____

_____

_____

_____

3. Why does nitroglycerin produce this effect when taken following Viagra?

_____

_____

_____

_____

4. How can the effects of combining nitroglycerin and Viagra be managed?

_____

_____

_____

_____

Case seven

You respond to a small community hospital to transport a 22-year-old female who is experiencing preterm labor. Before transport, the physician gives the patient a subcutaneous injection of terbutaline (Brethine).

1. What type of drug is terbutaline?

_____

_____

_____

_____

2. Why is terbutaline useful in treating preterm labor?

_____

_____

_____

_____

Case eight

A 22-year-old female with a 10-month history of severe clinical depression was found unconscious at her home. An empty bottle of amitriptyline (Elavil) was found nearby. The patient is unresponsive to painful stimuli. Radial pulses are rapid and weak. The patient's skin is warm, flushed, and dry. The pupils are dilated and react sluggishly. The patient's ECG showed sinus tachycardia with prolongation of the PR, QRS, and QT intervals. Vital signs are P—126 beats/min weak, regular; R—22 breaths/min shallow, regular; BP—86/42 mm Hg.

1. What type of agent is Elavil?

2. Why does Elavil toxicity produce tachycardia, dilated pupils, and dry, flushed skin?

3. Why does Elavil toxicity produce hypotension?

4. Why does Elavil toxicity produce slowed cardiac conduction with prolongation of ECG intervals?

5. What drug is given to antagonize the cardiotoxic effects of Elavil and related drugs?

6. Why is this drug effective against Elavil's cardiotoxic effects?

Case nine

A 58-year-old male with a history of alcohol abuse is unresponsive. The patient's blood glucose level is 30 mg/dL. Repeated attempts to establish an IV are unsuccessful. Your partner suggests that glucagon given IM might be useful in treating this patient's problem.

1. Where is glucagon produced?

2. What effect does glucagon have on blood glucose levels?

_____

_____

_____

_____

3. Could glucagon possibly be ineffective with this patient? Why?

_____

_____

_____

_____

Case ten

You are called to see an unconscious person at a large commercial greenhouse. Your patient is a 23-year-old female who lost consciousness while she was disinfecting the tropical plants. She is unconscious and unresponsive. She is salivating and sweating heavily. Auscultation of her chest reveals rales, wheezes, and rhonchi. She has lost continence of her bladder and bowels. Her pupils are pinpoint.

1. What division of the ANS is responsible for these effects?

_____

_____

_____

_____

2. What drug should be administered to reverse these effects?

_____

_____

_____

_____

13 Medication Administration

READING ASSIGNMENT

Chapter 13, pages 403-464, in *Paramedic Practice Today: Above and Beyond.*

OBJECTIVES

After completing this chapter, you will be able to:
1. List basic mathematic principles.
2. Review mathematic equivalents.
3. Differentiate temperature readings between the Celsius and Fahrenheit scales.
4. Discuss formulas as a basis for performing drug calculations.
5. Discuss applying basic principles of mathematics to the calculation of problems associated with medication dosages.
6. Discuss legal aspects affecting medication administration.
7. Discuss the "six rights" of drug administration.
8. Discuss medical asepsis and the differences between clean and sterile techniques.
9. Describe the use of standard precautions when giving a medication.
10. Describe the use of antiseptics and disinfectants.
11. Describe disposal of contaminated items and sharps.
12. Describe the different oral dosage forms and general principles of giving oral medications.
13. Describe the technique and general principles of rectal medication administration.
14. Describe the technique and general principles of giving medications are through a gastric tube.
15. Describe the technique and general principles of giving medications topically.
16. Describe the technique and general principles of giving medications by the inhalation route.
17. Describe the technique for withdrawing medication from an ampule.
18. Describe the technique for withdrawing medication from a vial.
19. Describe the technique and general principles of giving medications by the subcutaneous route.
20. Describe the technique and general principles of giving medications by the intramuscular route.
21. Describe the indications, equipment needed, technique used, precautions, and general principles of peripheral venous access.
22. Describe the indications, equipment needed, technique used, precautions, and general principles of intraosseous needle placement and infusion.
23. Describe the purpose, equipment needed, techniques used, complications, and general principles for obtaining a blood sample.

CHAPTER SUMMARY

Because the administration of drugs by the paramedic can be life saving but equally life threatening (or even lethal), this chapter addresses the critical areas of medication administration.

- Drugs were originally measured according to the apothecary system, which was based on the weight of a grain of wheat.
- The household system uses the dropper, teaspoon, tablespoon, cup, glass, pint, quart, and gallon for measuring. Household measures are expressed in Arabic numbers and fractions. Decimals are not used.
- The metric system is currently used for drug calculations. It is a logical system, organized and based on the basic unit of 10.
- The basic units of measurement in the metric system are the following:
  - Weight (solids, or mass): gram (g)
  - Length: meter (m)
  - Volume (liquid or fluid): liter (L)
- The four commonly used units in drug calculations today are centi, milli, micro, and kilo. The prefix *centi* (c) represents 1/100 of a basic unit. The prefix *milli* (m) represents 1/1000 of a basic unit. The prefix *micro* (mc or sometimes the Greek letter μ) represents 1/1,000,000 of a basic unit. *Kilo* means 1000 times a unit.
- When calculating drug dosages, you must be able to convert milligrams to grams, grams to milligrams, milligrams to micrograms, and micrograms to milligrams.
- Body temperature is measured by two scales: Celsius (centigrade) and Fahrenheit.
- Only four basic formulas are necessary to calculate any dosage for patient medications.
  - Formula 1: Single Dose Calculations

$$\frac{DD \times V}{DH}$$

  - Formula 2: Drip (Infusion) Calculations

$$\frac{\text{Total volume to be infused}}{\text{Total time of infusion in minutes}} \times \frac{\text{Drops (administration set)}}{mL}$$

  - Formula 3: Drip Not Based on Weight

$$\frac{DD \times V}{\text{Dose on hand}} \times \frac{gtt}{mL} \quad \text{(IV administration set)}$$

  - Formula 4: Drip Based on Weight
    Step 1: Calculate the patient's weight in kilograms by dividing the weight in pounds by 2.2.

97

Step 2: Multiply the patient's weight in kilograms by the desired dose per kilogram (cross out like terms).

Step 3: Prepare the infusion and calculate the dose on hand (concentration on hand).

Step 4: Cross out like terms that appear in the numerator and denominator, one for one. Determine the drip rate by a microdrip IV infusion set, such as one that delivers 60 gtt/mL.

- A paramedic is authorized to give specific medications for specific conditions under the direction of a physician. Federal, state, and local laws govern the purchasing, distribution, dispensing, and administration of drugs in the United States. The organization for which a paramedic works also has policies and procedures pertaining to medication administration. Every paramedic must know what those laws and regulations are in his or her area of employment.

- Protocols are a written form of medical direction and must be signed by the medical director. Medical direction may be given by radio or cell phone when a paramedic is on the scene (online medical direction). However, if communication fails, or in instances in which the paramedic has been given permission to function without radio communication, the written protocol must be followed (offline medical direction). If an event occurs that is not covered by protocol, the paramedic must communicate with medical direction before proceeding.

- Follow common safety protocols and procedures when giving medications.
  - Be sure you are familiar with the drug you are giving.
  - Be sure to convey important information about the patient to the online physician, including the patient's age, chief complaint, vital signs, signs and symptoms, allergies, current medications, and pertinent medical history.
  - Verify the physician's order. Repeat the order, including the name and dosage of the drug, back to the physician. Be certain to document the order received.
  - Concentrate on the task at hand.
  - Make sure the patient is properly positioned before giving a medication.
  - Assemble and use the correct supplies and equipment.
  - Handle all drugs carefully to avoid dropping or breaking.
  - Always use aseptic technique.
  - Carefully calculate drug dosages.
  - Monitor for signs of overdose.
  - Carefully document the drug given, dose, time, route, and the patient's response to the medication.

- The "six rights" of drug administration are the following:
  - Right drug
  - Right patient
  - Right dose
  - Right time
  - Right route

- Right documentation

- *Standard precautions* refers to the actions required by personnel every time they are in contact with a patient to prevent exposure to infectious substances from body fluids.

- Disinfection involves the process of cleaning the emergency vehicle, stretcher, and equipment. The substances used are called disinfectants. They are toxic to body tissues.

- Antisepsis is the process used to cleanse local skin areas before needle puncture. Alcohol-based or iodine-based products are used for antisepsis.

- Sterilization is the process that makes an object free of all forms of life by using extreme heat or certain chemicals.

- Observe proper precautions when handling sharps.

- Medications may be given orally, rectally (very rare in the prehospital setting), by gastric tube, topically, by an inhaled route, by injection, through vascular access, and by intraosseous infusion.

- A blood sample should be obtained before starting any IV lines or giving medications to provide the hospital team with accurate results.

SHORT ANSWER

1. State the two reasons why IV lines are started in the prehospital setting.

   _____

   _____

2. An IV catheter should never be withdrawn without first removing the needle. Why?

   _____

   _____

   _____

3. You establish an IV line and discover that bright red blood is moving up the line in pulsations. What has happened? What should you do?

   _____

   _____

   _____

   _____

4. Your patient is a 76-year-old male who is volume depleted. You have started an IV with Ringer's lactate. About 30 minutes after the IV is established, the patient begins to complain of backache and nausea. He is experiencing chills and is shivering. What has happened? What should you do? How can this complication of IV therapy be prevented?

   _____

   _____

   _____

   _____

5. While receiving an IV infusion, your patient suddenly develops cyanosis, hypotension, tachycardia, and extreme restlessness. Examination of the IV line reveals large numbers of air bubbles. What problem do you suspect? What should you do?

_____

_____

_____

_____

6. How many drops per milliliter does a microdrip administration set deliver?

_____

_____

_____

7. When you are starting an IV, what should the constricting band do to the arterial flow to the extremity? How does the constricting band affect the venous flow?

_____

_____

_____

_____

8. What will increasing the diameter (increasing the gauge) of an IV catheter do to the fluid flow through the catheter?

_____

_____

_____

_____

9. What will decreasing the length of an IV catheter do to the fluid flow through the catheter?

_____

_____

_____

_____

10. Rank the following administration routes from the one with the fastest absorption rate (1) to the one having the slowest (5).
    ____Subcutaneous
    ____Oral
    ____Intramuscular
    ____Intravenous
    ____Endotracheal

11. Which route for drug administration is the fastest and most dangerous?

_____

_____

_____

12. Why is air injected into a vial before attempting to withdraw a drug with a syringe?

_____

_____

_____

_____

13. Why is the top of a glass ampule tapped before it is broken off to withdraw a drug?

_____

_____

_____

_____

14. Why are the IM and subcutaneous (Sub-Q) routes not used to administer drugs to patients who are in shock?

_____

_____

_____

_____

15. If a physician gives you a radio order for a drug that is inappropriate, what should you do first?

_____

_____

_____

_____

16. When you are giving a drug by IM or Sub-Q injection, you should always aspirate by pulling back on the plunger before administering the drug. What is the purpose of this procedure?

_____

_____

_____

_____

17. Why is the IV tubing pinched off above the injection site when performing an IV push?

_____

_____

_____

_____

18. Contrast the procedures for IM and Sub-Q injection in each of the following areas:
    A. Angle at which the needle is inserted

_____

_____

    B. Whether the skin is pulled into a fold or held taut

_____

_____

19. What is the most important question you should ask before giving any patient a medication?

20. List four drugs other than oxygen that can be administered via the endotracheal route.

21. What is the most common cause of a needle stick among healthcare providers?

22. What does the term *parenteral* mean?

23. What does the term *enteral* mean?

24. You are giving a drug by IM injection. As you push the medication, the patient begins to complain of pain that radiates down the arm. What probably has happened? What should you do?

25. List two medications that can be administered by the rectal (pr) route.

26. By what route is nitroglycerin (Nitrostat) given?

27. What are the indications that an intraosseous line has been placed successfully?

28. What medications and fluids can be administered safely through an intraosseous line?

29. What are the "six rights" of drug administration?

DRUG DOSE CALCULATIONS

1. You are told to add 0.5 g of lidocaine to 250 mL of D_5W. Lidocaine is supplied in a concentration of 50 mg/mL. How many mL of this solution would you put in the bag?

2. You have an ampule containing a drug in a concentration of 500 mg/10 mL. You are to give 400 mg. How much of the solution will you give?

3. You are instructed to give 30 mg of a drug supplied in a concentration of 10 mg per 0.5 mL. How many mL will you administer?

4. You are instructed to administer 250 mg of a drug that is supplied as 1 g in 10 mL. How many mL will you administer?

5. You have a solution prepared by placing 1 g of lidocaine in 250 mL of D_5W. What is the concentration of this solution in mg/mL?

6. You have a solution that was prepared by placing 200 mg of dopamine in 250 mL of D_5W. What is the concentration of this solution in micrograms (mcg)/mL?

7. You have a solution that was prepared by placing 2 g of lidocaine in 500 mL of D_5W. You are asked to infuse 2 mg of lidocaine per minute by piggyback drip. What volume of lidocaine solution should you administer per minute?

8. Your patient is a 63-year-old male who weighs 220 pounds. You are told to administer 0.01 mg/kg of atropine. Atropine is supplied as 1 mg/10 mL. What volume of atropine solution should you administer?

9. You have a solution that was prepared by placing 1 g of lidocaine in 250 mL of D_5W. How fast will the infusion have to run in drops per minute using a microdrip infusion set to give the patient:
   a. 1 mg/min of lidocaine _____
   b. 2 mg/min of lidocaine _____
   c. 3 mg/min of lidocaine _____
   d. 4 mg/min of lidocaine _____

10. You are told to give a patient 0.04 g of a medication that is dispensed in tablets of 5 mg each. How many tablets should the patient receive?

   _____

11. A patient has taken two 7.5-g tablets. How many milligrams has the patient taken?

   _____

12. How many cubic centimeters are in 1 mL?

   _____

13. You are ordered to administer dopamine at 2 mcg/kg/min to a patient who weighs 220 pounds. You have a 250-mL bag of D_5W to which 200 mg of dopamine has been added. How many milliliters per minute should you infuse?

   _____

14. If your administration set gives 60 gtt/mL, how many gtt/min should you infuse to give the number of mL/min required in the previous question?

   _____

15. You are transporting a patient 135 miles. The patient is receiving Ringer's lactate at a rate of 10 gtt/min through a set that delivers 10 gtt/mL. During the first 120 miles of the trip, you are able to maintain an average speed of 60 miles/hr. However, once you reach the city to which the patient is being transferred, your average speed falls to 30 miles/hr. How many 1000-mL bags of Ringer's lactate will you need to complete the trip?

   _____

16. A 220-pound patient is receiving 30 gtt/min of dopamine solution through a 60 gtt/mL administration set. The dopamine infusion was mixed by placing 400 mg in a 500-mL bag. How many mcg/kg/min of dopamine is the patient receiving?

   _____

17. Your patient becomes nauseated. You administer 12.5 mg of promethazine. Promethazine is supplied in 25 mg/1 mL vials. How many milliliters should you administer?

   _____

18. Your patient is having a myocardial infarction and you need to administer aspirin. Aspirin is supplied in 80-mg tablets. You want to give 320 mg of aspirin. How many tablets do you give?

   _____

19. Morphine is supplied in 10 mg/1 mL vials. How many milliliters do you administer if you want to give 4 mg?

   _____

20. You hit a bump while you were giving the morphine and pushed too much. Your patient's respiratory rate is now 2 per minute and you give naloxone. Your protocols indicate you should give 2 mg of naloxone IV push. Naloxone is supplied as 5 mg/5 mL vial. How many milliliters do you give?

   _____

21. You have decided to give 7.5 mL of naloxone. If naloxone is supplied as 5 mg/5 mL vial, how many milligrams will you be giving?

   _____

22. Epinephrine 1:10,000 is supplied as 1 mg/10 mL prefilled syringe. You want to give 0.01 mg/kg of epinephrine to a 220-pound patient. How many milliliters will you administer?

   _____

23. Lidocaine is supplied as a 100 mg/5 mL vial. You want to give 1.5 mg/kg of lidocaine to a 220-pound patient. How many milliliters do you give?

   _____

24. The lidocaine (from question 23) seems to have worked. You now follow up with a lidocaine infusion. You have a premixed solution containing 1 g of lidocaine in 250 mL. You want to infuse 2 mg/min. Using a 60 gtt/mL set, what is your drip rate?

   _____

25. A 22-year-old patient is complaining of shortness of breath and hives. You decide to administer epinephrine 1:1000. Epinephrine 1:1000 is supplied as a 1 mg/1 mL vial. You want to give 0.3 mg Sub-Q. How many mL will you give?

   _____

26. You also decide to give diphenhydramine. Diphenhydramine is supplied as a 50 mg/1 mL vial. You want to give 25 mg IM. How many milliliters do you give?

   _____

14 Airway Management

READING ASSIGNMENT

Chapter 14, pages 466-555, in *Paramedic Practice Today: Above and Beyond.*

OBJECTIVES

After completing this chapter, you will be able to:
1. Explain the primary objective of airway maintenance.
2. Identify commonly neglected prehospital skills related to airway.
3. Identify the anatomy of the upper and lower airway.
4. Describe the functions of the upper and lower airway.
5. Define *gag reflex.*
6. Define atelectasis.
7. Explain the differences between adult and pediatric airway anatomy.
8. Explain the relation between pulmonary circulation and respiration.
9. List the concentrations of gases that comprise atmospheric air.
10. Describe the measurement of oxygen in the blood.
11. Describe the measurement of carbon dioxide in the blood.
12. List factors that cause decreased oxygen concentrations in the blood.
13. List the factors that increase and decrease carbon dioxide production in the body.
14. Describe peak expiratory flow.
15. Define FiO_2.
16. Describe the voluntary and involuntary regulation of respiration.
17. List the factors that affect respiratory rate and depth.
18. Define and differentiate hypoxia and hypoxemia.
19. Define normal respiratory rates and tidal volumes for the adult, child, and infant.
20. Describe causes of respiratory distress.
21. Describe the modified forms of respiration.
22. Identify types of oxygen cylinders and pressure regulators (including a high-pressure regulator and a therapy regulator).
23. List the steps for delivering oxygen from a cylinder and a regulator.
24. Explain safety considerations of oxygen storage and delivery.
25. Describe the indications, contraindications, advantages, disadvantages, complications, liter flow range, and concentration of delivered oxygen for supplemental oxygen delivery devices.
26. Describe the use of an oxygen humidifier.
27. Define and explain the implications of partial airway obstruction with good and poor air exchange.
28. Define *complete airway obstruction.*
29. Describe causes of upper airway obstruction.
30. Describe complete airway obstruction maneuvers.
31. Describe manual airway maneuvers.
32. Explain the purpose for suctioning the upper airway.
33. Identify types of suction equipment.
34. Describe the indications for suctioning the upper airway.
35. Identify types of suction catheters, including hard or rigid catheters and soft catheters.
36. Identify techniques of suctioning the upper airway.
37. Identify special considerations of suctioning the upper airway.
38. Describe the indications, contraindications, advantages, disadvantages, complications, equipment, and technique of tracheobronchial suctioning in the intubated patient.
39. Identify special considerations of tracheobronchial suctioning in the intubated patient.
40. Describe the use of an oral and nasal airway.
41. Describe the indications, contraindications, advantages, disadvantages, complications, and technique for inserting an oropharyngeal and nasopharyngeal airway.
42. Define *gastric distention.*
43. Describe the indications, contraindications, advantages, disadvantages, complications, and technique for ventilating a patient by the following resuscitation methods:
   - Mouth to mouth
   - Mouth to nose
   - Mouth to mask
   - One-person bag-mask
   - Two-person bag-mask
   - Three-person bag-mask
   - Flow-restricted, oxygen-powered ventilation device

103

44. Compare the ventilation techniques used for adult patients with those used for pediatric patients.
45. Explain the advantage of the two-person method when ventilating with the bag-mask.
46. Describe the Sellick (cricoid pressure) maneuver.
47. Describe indications, contraindications, advantages, disadvantages, complications, and technique for ventilating a patient with an automatic transport ventilator.
48. Define, identify, and describe tracheostomy, stoma, and tracheostomy tube.
49. Define, identify, and describe a laryngectomy.
50. Define how to ventilate a patient with a stoma, including mouth-to-stoma and bag-mask–to-stoma ventilation.
51. Describe the indications, contraindications, advantages, disadvantages, complications, equipment, and technique for inserting a nasogastric tube and orogastric tube.
52. Identify special considerations of gastric decompression.
53. Describe the special considerations in airway management and ventilation for patients with facial injuries.
54. Describe the special considerations in airway management and ventilation for the pediatric patient.
55. Differentiate endotracheal intubation from other methods of advanced airway management.
56. Describe the indications, contraindications, advantages, disadvantages, complications, equipment, and technique for using a dual-lumen airway.
57. Describe the indications, contraindications, advantages, disadvantages, and complications of endotracheal intubation.
58. Explain the risk of infection to EMS providers that is associated with ventilation.
59. Describe laryngoscopy for the removal of a foreign body airway obstruction.
60. Describe the indications, contraindications, advantages, disadvantages, complications, equipment, and technique for direct laryngoscopy.
61. Describe visual landmarks for direct laryngoscopy.
62. Describe methods of assessment for confirming correct placement of an endotracheal tube.
63. Describe methods for securing an endotracheal tube.
64. Describe methods of endotracheal intubation in the pediatric patient.
65. Describe the indications, contraindications, advantages, disadvantages, complications, equipment, and technique for nasotracheal intubation.
66. Describe indications, contraindications, advantages, disadvantages, complications, equipment, and technique for digital endotracheal intubation.
67. Describe the indications, contraindications, advantages, disadvantages, complications, and equipment for rapid-sequence intubation with neuromuscular blockade.
68. Identify neuromuscular blocking drugs and other agents used in rapid-sequence intubation.
69. Describe the indications, contraindications, advantages, disadvantages, complications, and equipment for sedation during intubation.
70. Identify sedative agents used in airway management.
71. Describe the indications, contraindications, advantages, disadvantages, complications, equipment, and technique for needle cricothyrotomy.
72. Describe the indications, contraindications, advantages, disadvantages, and complications for performing a surgical cricothyrotomy.
73. Describe the equipment and technique for performing a surgical cricothyrotomy.

CHAPTER SUMMARY

- The upper airway consists of structures located outside the chest cavity, including the nose and nasal cavities, pharynx, and larynx. The upper airway functions to filter, warm, and humidify the air, protecting the surfaces of the lower respiratory tract. The lower airway consists of the trachea, bronchial tree (primary bronchi, secondary bronchi, and bronchioles), alveoli, and the lungs. The lower airway is where gas exchange occurs. Functionally, oxygen diffuses from the alveoli into the pulmonary capillaries while carbon dioxide diffuses in the opposite direction.

- Ventilation is the mechanical process of moving air into and out of the lungs in two separate phases: inspiration and expiration. Respiration is the exchange of gases between a living organism and its environment. The bodies of human beings provide oxygen while removing carbon dioxide, one of the chief metabolic pollutants within our system.

- You must be able to identify respiratory problems quickly so you can provide appropriate and timely intervention. Assessment of age-appropriate respiratory rate, regularity, and work of breathing are essential parameters to evaluate early (and repeatedly) on every patient. When possible, use topographic landmarks of the chest to describe physical examination findings. These markers include the clavicles, nipples, angle of Louis, suprasternal notch, and costal angle.

- Auscultating lung sounds is essential for every patient with any type of respiratory symptom. The primary goal of auscultation is to determine if lung sounds are present and equal bilaterally. Compare sounds from side to side by listening to one lung and then the other in the same place. With each stethoscope placement, listen to at least one full inhalation and exhalation.

- Many supplemental oxygen delivery methods are available. You must choose the correct option for your patient's circumstances. When you administer supplemental oxygen to a patient, an adequate rate and depth (minute volume) of ventilation is necessary. If any doubt exists regarding the adequacy of ventilation in addition to oxygenation, you must support the patient with both supplemental oxygen and positive-pressure ventilation.

- Many devices exist for delivering supplemental oxygen to patients. Devices have various capabilities relating to percentage of oxygen delivery. Your patient's condition determines the method of delivery as well as the liter per minute flow rate.
- Airway obstruction can have many causes. Even a partial blockage of the airway may impair gas exchange to a degree that the patient's life is in jeopardy without quick corrective action. Classifications of airway obstruction include complete obstruction, partial obstruction with poor air exchange, and partial obstruction with good air exchange. Common causes leading to obstruction include the tongue, foreign bodies, laryngeal spasm and edema, trauma, and aspiration.
- Basic to any type of airway management procedure is the ability to manually open a patient's airway. Manual maneuvers require no special equipment and are noninvasive. The purpose of a manual maneuver is to position the anatomic structures of the patient's airway so that the airway passages are open to the flow of air.
- In an unresponsive patient, secretions, blood, and vomitus require removal with a suction device before ventilating. Ill patients often have nausea and many airway procedures may stimulate vomiting. You must anticipate such situations and have suction within arm's reach to minimize the potential risk of aspiration.
- Several devices can help keep the airway open. Two adjuncts specifically designed to prevent the tongue from falling back into the airway and blocking the flow of air are oral and nasal airways.
- Patients who are apneic or those with inadequate ventilation require artificial ventilation. Forcing air into the lungs is called *positive-pressure ventilation*. Methods by which positive-pressure ventilation may be accomplished include mouth-to-mouth, mouth-to-nose, mouth-to–barrier device, and mouth-to-mask ventilation; one-person, two-person, or three-person bag-mask ventilation; ventilation with an automatic transport ventilator (ATV); and ventilation using a flow-restricted, oxygen-powered ventilation device (FROPVD).
- Advanced airways include the Combitube, the laryngeal mask airway (LMA), and the endotracheal (ET) tube. Insertion of a Combitube or LMA does not require visualization of the vocal cords. In contrast, insertion of an ET tube through a patient's mouth and into the trachea (orotracheal intubation) does require direct visualization of the vocal cords. Nasotracheal intubation is an alternative approach for intubating the trachea. It is considered a blind procedure because the vocal cords are not visualized. Rapid-sequence intubation (RSI) is the use of medications to sedate and paralyze a patient to achieve rapid ET intubation. Capnography, or capnometry, at least, should be used with all endotracheal intubations.
- Pulse oximetry is a noninvasive measurement of the oxygen saturation of hemoglobin in peripheral tissues.
- Continuous positive airway pressure (CPAP) is the delivery of slight positive pressure to prevent airway collapse, reduce the work of breathing, and improve alveolar ventilation.
- Cricothyrotomy is an emergency procedure performed to allow rapid entrance to the airway for temporary oxygenation and ventilation. It can be accomplished by inserting a needle into the cricothyroid membrane (needle cricothyrotomy) or creating an opening into the cricothyroid membrane with a scalpel (surgical cricothyrotomy).

MATCHING

1. Match each of the following structures with its anatomic name.

_____ Air sacs in which gas exchange occurs	A. Epiglottis
_____ Double membrane covering lungs	B. Larynx
_____ Flap covering windpipe's opening	C. Trachea
_____ Point where mainstem bronchi branch	D. Alveoli
_____ Smaller airways without cartilage in their walls	E. Carina
_____ Space between base of tongue and epiglottis	F. Vallecula
_____ Throat	G. Bronchioles
_____ Voice box	H. Pharynx
_____ Windpipe	I. Pleura

2. Match the abnormal respiratory sound with its name.

_____ Fine bubbling sounds caused by fluid in small airways	A. Crackles (rales)
_____ High-pitched crowing sounds on inspiration resulting from a tight upper airway	B. Rhonchi
_____ Rattling sounds from mucus obstruction of large airways	C. Snoring
_____ Sound produced by partial obstruction of upper airway by tongue	D. Stridor
_____ Whistling sounds on exhalation caused by narrow or tight lower airways	E. Wheezing

3. Match each word or statement with the type of laryngoscope blade it describes.

_____ Curved	A. Miller
_____ Placed into vallecula	B. Macintosh
_____ Placed under epiglottis	
_____ Straight	

105

4. Match each respiratory volume or capacity with its definition.

____	Volume in lungs at end of maximum inspiration	A.	Minute volume
____	Volume inhaled or exhaled in 1 minute	B.	Vital capacity
		C.	Functional residual capacity
____	Volume inhaled or exhaled in one respiratory cycle	D.	Tidal volume
		E.	Residual volume
____	Volume left in lungs after maximum expiration	F.	Forced expiratory volume
		G.	Expiratory reserve volume
____	Volume remaining in lungs at end of normal expiration	H.	Inspiratory reserve volume
____	Volume that can be maximally exhaled after a normal expiration		
____	Volume that can be maximally expired after a maximum inspiration		
____	Volume that can be maximally inhaled after a normal inspiration		

SHORT ANSWER

1. Where in the central nervous system is the center controlling respirations located?

_____
_____
_____
_____

2. What is the name of the nerve that stimulates the diaphragm? Where does it originate?

_____
_____
_____
_____

3. What are the nerves that control the intercostal muscles? Where do they originate?

_____
_____
_____
_____

4. Respirations normally are stimulated by what change in the arterial blood gases?

_____
_____
_____
_____

5. What is the backup system for controlling respirations? What change in the arterial blood gases triggers this backup system?

_____
_____
_____
_____

6. Patients with long-standing chronic obstructive pulmonary disease (COPD) have what change in their arterial carbon dioxide levels?

_____
_____
_____
_____

7. What effect can administration of high concentration oxygen have on a COPD patient's breathing? Why does this happen? Is this a reason for withholding oxygen from a COPD patient? Why or why not?

_____
_____
_____
_____

8. Which phase of the respiratory cycle normally requires contraction of the intercostal muscles and diaphragm?

_____
_____
_____
_____

9. Which phase of the respiratory cycle does not require contraction of the intercostal muscles and diaphragm?

_____
_____
_____
_____

10. During respiration, what effect does contraction of the diaphragm have on the volume of air in the lungs?

_____
_____
_____
_____

11. What are the principal anatomic differences between the right and left mainstem bronchi? Why is this of practical importance in performing endotracheal intubation?

_____
_____
_____
_____

12. What is tidal volume? What is the normal tidal volume of a 70-kg male?

_____

_____

_____

_____

13. What is the minute volume of a patient who has a tidal volume of 500 mL and respirations of 20/minute?

_____

_____

_____

_____

14. What is anatomic dead space?

_____

_____

_____

_____

15. What is physiologic dead space?

_____

_____

_____

_____

16. What is atelectasis?

_____

_____

_____

_____

17. What is the normal $PaCO_2$?

_____

_____

_____

_____

18. What is the normal PaO_2?

_____

_____

_____

_____

19. If a patient's respiratory rate and tidal volume are decreased, what change would you expect to see in the patient's $PaCO_2$? What is this condition called?

_____

_____

_____

20. If a patient's respiratory rate increases and tidal volume decreases, what change would you expect to see in the patient's $PaCO_2$? What is this condition called?

_____

_____

_____

_____

21. Is cyanosis a late or early sign of hypoxia? Why?

_____

_____

_____

_____

22. What is usually the earliest sign that a patient is hypoxic?

_____

_____

_____

23. What is the most common cause of an obstructed airway in an unconscious person? If you attempt to ventilate an unconscious person and the chest does not rise, what should be your first action?

_____

_____

_____

24. If a patient reacts to placement of an oral airway by coughing and gagging, what should be done?

_____

_____

_____

25. If a patient will not tolerate an oral airway, but is not alert enough to manage his or her own airway unassisted, what device should be used?

_____

_____

_____

_____

26. How do you distinguish between a partial airway obstruction with poor air exchange and a partial airway obstruction with good air exchange? How do you manage a partial obstruction with good air exchange? How do you manage a partial obstruction with poor air exchange?

_____

_____

_____

_____

27. What oxygen mask should be used with a young adult who is having an acute asthma attack? Why?

_____

_____

_____

_____

Chapter **14**

28. Why is the Venturi mask the preferred oxygen administration device for a COPD patient who presents in mild to moderate respiratory distress? (Explain in terms of how the Venturi mask controls the patient's FiO_2.)

_____

_____

_____

_____

29. If a COPD patient who is receiving oxygen experiences depressed respirations, what should you do?

_____

_____

_____

_____

30. Should a person who has ingested a caustic agent be intubated with a dual-lumen airway? Why?

_____

_____

_____

_____

31. Should a person with a history of cirrhosis of the liver or chronic alcohol abuse be intubated with a dual-lumen airway? Why?

_____

_____

_____

_____

32. What is the maximum period of time that should elapse during an intubation attempt before ventilating?

_____

_____

_____

33. Since it is difficult to keep track of time during an intubation attempt, what method is used to determine when the patient needs to be ventilated?

_____

_____

_____

34. How can you estimate the correct endotracheal tube size to use when intubating a pediatric patient?

_____

_____

_____

35. After intubating a patient endotracheally, you auscultate the chest and discover absent breath sounds on the left. What is the most likely cause of this problem, and how do you solve it?

_____

_____

_____

_____

36. How do you determine the correct amount of air to place in the cuff of the endotracheal tube?

_____

_____

_____

37. When you are intubating a patient endotracheally, how do you know that the tube is in the trachea?

_____

_____

_____

_____

38. What is the most common complication of endotracheal suctioning? How can it be prevented?

_____

_____

_____

_____

39. What is the maximum time for which a patient's trachea should be suctioned without oxygenating?

_____

_____

_____

_____

40. What is the correct position in which to place a patient's head during an endotracheal intubation attempt?

_____

_____

_____

41. Why should an unconscious patient be intubated endotracheally before placing a gastric tube?

_____

_____

_____

42. Why should instrumentation of the nose be avoided in patients with mid-face trauma or signs of a possible basilar skull fracture (CSF otorrhea, CSF rhinorrhea, Battle's sign, and periorbital ecchymosis)?

_____

_____

_____

_____

43. What percentage of oxygen is delivered by a bag-mask and reservoir with oxygen flowing at 15 L/min?

_____
_____
_____
_____

44. What is the only reliable indicator that rescue breathing is inflating the lungs?

_____
_____
_____
_____

45. What term is used to describe dyspnea that is more severe when the patient is lying down, or inversely is relieved when the patient sits or stands?

_____
_____
_____
_____

46. List four signs of respiratory distress (increased work of breathing).

_____
_____
_____
_____

47. Why is a rigid (Yankauer) catheter the preferred device for suctioning the secretions of a patient whose upper airway is obstructed with blood or vomitus?

_____
_____
_____
_____

48. What term describes a crackling sensation under the skin of the chest wall or neck caused by leakage of air into the soft tissues?

_____
_____
_____
_____

49. A blood gas report shows a patient's $PaCO_2$ to be elevated. What is the most common reason that a patient will develop increased arterial CO_2 concentration? How can this problem be corrected?

_____
_____
_____
_____

50. A patient is receiving oxygenation and ventilation via a bag-mask device and an endotracheal tube. The blood gas report shows a PaO_2 of 120 mm Hg and a $PaCO_2$ of 50 mm Hg. What do these findings indicate about the patient's oxygenation and ventilation?

_____
_____
_____
_____

51. You respond to a report of a "man down" to find a 62-year-old male who is unconscious and unresponsive. Your initial assessment reveals that he is apneic and deeply cyanotic, but a pulse is present. Should you intubate him immediately or ventilate and oxygenate him first? Why?

_____
_____
_____
_____

52. What is the difference between the mechanism of action of a depolarizing and a nondepolarizing neuromuscular blocker?

_____
_____
_____
_____

53. What effect do neuromuscular blockers have on level of consciousness?

_____
_____
_____

54. What is the implication of the effect of neuromuscular blockers on level of consciousness when these agents are used to facilitate intubation?

_____
_____
_____
_____

MULTIPLE CHOICE

1. Which of the following is the most appropriate depth of insertion for an endotracheal tube in an adult male?
   A. 16 mm at the teeth
   B. 18 mm at the teeth
   C. 22 cm at the teeth
   D. 25 cm at the teeth

2. During a single-vehicle rollover, the driver has been ejected. He is unconscious and unresponsive. What technique should you use to open his airway?
   A. Head tilt/chin lift with extreme hyperextension of the neck
   B. Head tilt/neck lift with slight hyperextension of the neck
   C. Jaw thrust or chin lift with the head and neck in a neutral position
   D. Triple airway maneuver (head tilt/jaw thrust/mouth opened)

3. A 5-year-old female received an electrical shock. She is not breathing, but a pulse is present. This patient's lungs should be ventilated once every _____.
   A. 3 seconds
   B. 4 seconds
   C. 5 seconds
   D. 6 seconds

4. A 72-year-old male with a possible cerebrovascular accident presents unresponsive with snoring respirations. The most probable cause for the snoring is _____.
   A. fluid or edema partially obstructing the upper airway
   B. hypersecretion of mucus into the lower airway as a result of brain injury
   C. partial obstruction of the upper airway by the tongue
   D. spasms of the lower airway secondary to brain injury

5. A 26-year-old female was found unconscious in an alleyway. Her arms are covered with needle tracks and her pupils are constricted. Her respiratory rate is 6 breaths/min. The most probable values for her blood gases would be _____.
   A. elevated oxygen, low carbon dioxide
   B. high oxygen, high carbon dioxide
   C. low oxygen, high carbon dioxide
   D. low oxygen, low carbon dioxide

6. A patient is breathing 15 times a minute and has a tidal volume of 400 mL. What is the patient's minute volume (minute ventilation)?
   A. 400 mL
   B. 1500 mL
   C. 3750 mL
   D. 6000 mL

7. Which of the following poses the greatest risk to the paramedic when performing endotracheal intubation?
   A. The transmission of a bloodborne disease, such as HIV, by inhaling droplets from the airway of an infected person
   B. The transmission of an infectious disease, such as meningitis, by inhaling droplets from the airway of an infected person
   C. The transmission of hepatitis B by inhaling droplets from the airway of an infected person
   D. The transmission of tuberculosis by skin contact with droplets from the airway of an infected person

8. Which of the following most closely describes the normal tidal volume for a 70-kg adult?
   A. 150 mL
   B. 350 mL
   C. 500 mL
   D. 6000 mL

9. Rhonchi suggest which of the following problems?
   A. Fluid in the alveoli and small airways
   B. Mucus partially obstructing the larger airways
   C. Partial obstruction of the upper airway by edema or foreign body
   D. Partial obstruction of the upper airway by the tongue

10. Ventilations are normally stimulated by the _____.
    A. carbon dioxide content of arterial blood
    B. carbon dioxide content of venous blood
    C. oxygen content of arterial blood
    D. oxygen content of venous blood

11. In which part of the brain is the respiratory center located?
    A. Cerebellum
    B. Cerebrum
    C. Hypothalamus
    D. Medulla oblongata

12. Which statement best describes the purpose or objective of endotracheal intubation?
    A. To achieve complete control of the airway
    B. To permit chest compressions to be performed more rapidly during CPR
    C. To relieve gastric distention caused by artificial ventilation
    D. To relieve laryngospasm

13. When a stylet is used during endotracheal intubation, the tip of the stylet should _____.
    A. be even with the distal end of the endotracheal tube
    B. be moved in and out during the intubation attempt as needed
    C. be recessed approximately ½ inch from the distal end or Murphy eye of the endotracheal tube
    D. extend beyond the distal end of the endotracheal tube

14. The partial pressure of oxygen in arterial blood (systemic) is normally _____.
    A. 30 to 40 torr
    B. 50 to 60 torr
    C. 80 to 100 torr
    D. 120 to 140 torr

15. What is the anatomic difference between the right and left mainstem bronchi?
    A. The left bronchus is much smaller than the right.
    B. The left bronchus is shorter and straighter than the right.
    C. The right bronchus is much smaller than the left.
    D. The right bronchus is shorter and straighter than the left.

16. Your patient has a normal tidal volume and also has an arterial carbon dioxide pressure of 20 torr. This patient's ventilatory rate _____.
    A. cannot be evaluated from the information given
    B. is probably fast
    C. is probably normal
    D. is probably slow

17. Which of the following would be most likely to produce localized, unilateral wheezing in the lung fields?
    A. An acute asthma attack
    B. Aspiration of a foreign body into the lower airways
    C. Bronchospasms secondary to an allergic reaction
    D. Pulmonary edema secondary to congestive heart failure

18. Your patient is a 12-year-old who has a complete airway obstruction secondary to epiglottitis. Which of the following is the best course of action following two unsuccessful intubation attempts?
    A. Attempt the Heimlich maneuver.
    B. Continue to attempt intubation using direct laryngoscopy.
    C. Perform immediate needle cricothyrotomy.
    D. Perform immediate surgical cricothyrotomy.

19. Your patient is a 4-year-old girl who has been struck in the head with a baseball bat. She is not breathing. Which of the following is the best choice of endotracheal tube size for this patient?
    A. 3.5-mm tube
    B. 4.0-mm tube
    C. 5.0-mm tube
    D. 6.0-cm tube

20. For the 4-year-old patient in the previous question, what is the most appropriate depth of insertion for the endotracheal tube?
    A. 12 to 13 cm at the teeth
    B. 12 to 13 mm at the teeth
    C. 14 to 15 cm at the teeth
    D. 14 to 15 mm at the teeth

21. The most reliable indication that rescue breathing is adequately inflating the lungs is _____.
    A. constriction of the patient's pupils in response to light
    B. rise of the chest wall during ventilation
    C. the ease of air entry into the mouth during ventilation
    D. the absence of cyanosis

22. Extensive atelectasis would be expected to cause which changes in the arterial blood gases?
    A. PaO_2 decreased, $PaCO_2$ decreased
    B. PaO_2 decreased, $PaCO_2$ increased
    C. PaO_2 increased, $PaCO_2$ decreased
    D. PaO_2 increased, $PaCO_2$ increased

23. How should a patient's head and neck be positioned before an endotracheal intubation attempt (assuming spinal injury is not suspected)?
    A. Hyperextended
    B. Hyperflexed
    C. Left in a neutral position
    D. Placed in a sniffing position

24. Which statement about administration of oxygen is correct?
    A. Administration of oxygen to COPD patients may stimulate their hypoxic drive.
    B. Administration of oxygen to some COPD patients may depress spontaneous ventilations.
    C. Emphysema patients need high levels of oxygen to stimulate their ventilatory drive.
    D. High concentration oxygen should never be administered to patients with COPD.

25. Oxygen cylinders are potentially dangerous because _____.
    A. oxygen is a flammable gas
    B. oxygen vigorously supports combustion
    C. oxygen vigorously supports combustion and the oxygen in cylinders is under pressure
    D. the oxygen in the cylinders is stored under pressure

26. After intubating your patient, you auscultate the chest for lung sounds. Lung sounds are absent on the left but present on the right. This could mean _____.
    A. either the tube is in the right mainstem bronchus or there is a pneumothorax on the left
    B. the endotracheal tube is in the esophagus
    C. the endotracheal tube is in the right mainstem bronchus
    D. there is a pneumothorax on the left

27. The nasal cavity performs which of the following functions?
    A. Reduces the carbon dioxide content of the air, filters the air, humidifies the air
    B. Warms the air, filters the air, humidifies the air
    C. Warms the air, humidifies the air
    D. Warms the air, reduces the carbon dioxide content of the air

28. In which of the following patients would the assessment of peak expiratory flow be most useful?
    A. Asthma
    B. Congestive heart failure
    C. Pneumonia
    D. Tension pneumothorax

29. The preferred airway for use in the patient with severe facial injuries is _____.
    A. nasotracheal intubation
    B. orotracheal intubation
    C. the Combitude
    D. the laryngeal mask airway

30. After intubating a 50-year-old COPD patient with a 7.5-mm endotracheal tube, you assess the depth of the endotracheal tube insertion. Which of the following is the most correct depth for this patient?
    A. 18 cm at the teeth
    B. 21 cm at the teeth
    C. 25 cm at the teeth
    D. 27 cm at the teeth

31. You have just delivered a baby 10 weeks premature. Which of the following is the most appropriate size endotracheal tube for this neonate?
    A. 2.5 mm
    B. 3.5 mm
    C. 4.0 mm
    D. 4.5 mm

32. A 68-year-old male complains of shortness of breath and a productive cough of yellow-green sputum. He has a barrel chest and hypertrophied neck muscles. He purses his lips when he exhales. He reports smoking three packs of cigarettes per day for 45 years. He has a history of COPD. Because of this patient's history and physical findings, you should consider the possibility that this patient's ventilations are being stimulated by the _____.
    A. carbon dioxide content of his arterial blood
    B. carbon dioxide content of his venous blood
    C. oxygen content of his arterial blood
    D. oxygen content of his venous blood

33. You respond to a report of a "man down" at a cafeteria in the local mall. You find a 35-year-old man unconscious on the floor of the dining room. When you tilt his head back and check for breathing, you discover he is not breathing. Bystanders report that he stood up, grasped his throat, and tried to run to the men's bathroom before collapsing. When you attempt to ventilate him with the bag-mask, air will not go in. Your next step should be to _____.
    A. begin chest compressions at a rate of 100 compressions per minute
    B. intubate the trachea
    C. perform a surgical cricothyrotomy
    D. reposition the head and try again to ventilate

34. A 16-year-old male has overdosed on a CNS depressant drug. When you attempt to insert an oral airway, the patient gags. However, when you remove your hands from the patient's head, his neck flexes and he begins to snore. The best device for maintaining this patient's airway *initially* would be the _____.
    A. Combitude
    B. endotracheal tube
    C. nasopharyngeal airway
    D. oropharyngeal airway

35. A 12-year-old female has ingested 20 Darvocet, 10 Valium, 20 birth control pills, and 20 aspirin. She is unconscious and unresponsive to all stimuli. Her pupils are dilated and slow to react. Vital signs are: P—50 beats/min, weak, regular; BP—60/40 mm Hg; RR—6/min, shallow, regular; skin—pale, cool, dry. Which of the following is the best course of airway management before transport?
    A. Open airway, administer oxygen by nonrebreather mask, endotracheally intubate, and then transport.
    B. Open airway, administer oxygen by nonrebreather mask, insert a gastric tube to lavage the stomach, and then transport.
    C. Open airway, assist ventilations with bag-mask and oxygen, endotracheally intubate, and then insert an 18-French orogastric tube during transport.
    D. Open airway, assist ventilations with bag-mask and oxygen, nasotracheally intubate, and then insert an 18-French orogastric tube during transport.

36. What is the maximum amount of time in which the procedure of endotracheal intubation should be accomplished?
    A. 15 seconds
    B. 25 seconds
    C. 30 seconds
    D. 50 seconds

37. Which of the following is one of the most serious errors committed during endotracheal intubation?
    A. Attempting to intubate without first adequately oxygenating and ventilating
    B. Inadequately hyperextending the neck during the intubation attempt
    C. Selecting an endotracheal tube that is too small
    D. Using a Miller blade when a Macintosh blade is needed

38. The dual-lumen airway should be used only for _____.
    A. patients who are less than 5 feet or more than 6 feet 7 inches tall
    B. patients who have ingested substances such as acids or gasoline
    C. patients with a history of alcohol abuse or liver disease
    D. unconscious adults

39. Which of the following is the most appropriate initial method to remove a complete foreign body airway obstruction when basic life support techniques have failed?
    A. Insert the Magill forceps to remove the object but do not waste time using direct laryngoscopy.
    B. Perform a surgical cricothyrotomy to access the airway below the obstruction.
    C. Perform direct laryngoscopy and use the endotracheal tube to push the obstruction downward.
    D. Perform direct laryngoscopy and use the Magill forceps to remove the object if it is visualized.

40. Which patient is likely to be easiest to intubate?
    A. 3-year-old patient who is unconscious secondary to a motor vehicle collision
    B. 12-year-old patient who has experienced sudden cardiac arrest for an unknown reason
    C. 28-year-old, 300-pound offensive lineman for the local professional football team
    D. 32-year-old, 4 feet 10 inches tall, obese female who is unconscious secondary to a drug overdose

15 Therapeutic Communication

READING ASSIGNMENT

Chapter 15, pages 558-577, in *Paramedic Practice Today: Above and Beyond*.

OBJECTIVES

After completing this chapter, you will be able to:
1. Define *communication*.
2. Discuss the importance of developing effective communication skills.
3. Identify internal and external factors for effective communication.
4. Differentiate sympathetic and empathetic responses to facilitate the patient's history.
5. Understand the patient interview process, including the identification of verbal and nonverbal cues.
6. Discuss the importance of using open-ended versus direct questions.
7. Describe the use of facilitation, reflection, clarification, confrontation, and interpretation.
8. Identify various interviewing traps and pitfalls that can hinder effective communication.
9. Discuss ways to gather information from sources other than the patient.
10. Identify techniques to develop patient rapport and trust.
11. Discuss and overcome communication barriers between you and your patient.
12. Discuss special situations that require additional effort and diligence to obtain a comprehensive history.

CHAPTER SUMMARY

■ The ability to communicate effectively is an essential skill.
■ Internal and external factors affect your ability to communicate.
■ The interview process begins before actual contact with the patient and is a dynamic process in response to each individual situation.
■ Open-ended questions are usually the most effective and efficient means to gather information during the patient interview.
■ Nonverbal cues, from both the patient and the paramedic, have an impact on the communication process.

■ Building patient rapport, which can be done in several ways, is conducive to good patient communication and care.
■ Several traps of interviewing can negatively affect patient communication and care.
■ Paramedics must realize and take advantage of other sources of information regarding any call.
■ Special situations require adjusting your communication skills to maximize your chances of gathering information and promoting good care.

MATCHING

1. Match the feedback technique with its description.

_____ Asking the speaker to help you understand	A. Clarification
_____ Briefly reviewing the interview and your conclusions	B. Confrontation
_____ Echoing the patient's message using your own words	C. Empathy
	D. Explanation
	E. Facilitation
_____ Encouraging the patient to provide more information	F. Interpretation
_____ Focusing on a particular point made during the interview	G. Reflection
_____ Sharing objective information related to the message	H. Summarization
_____ Stating the conclusions you have drawn from the information	
_____ Using body language to show you understand and care	

SHORT ANSWER

1. Define *communication*.

_____

_____

_____

_____

115

2. List the external factors that affect a patient or bystander interview conducted by a paramedic.

_____

_____

_____

_____

3. List the internal factors that affect a patient or bystander interview conducted by a paramedic.

_____

_____

_____

_____

4. List seven strategies for building trust and rapport with patients.

_____

_____

_____

_____

_____

_____

5. Define *social distance*.

_____

_____

_____

6. Define *personal distance*.

_____

_____

_____

_____

7. Define *intimate distance*.

_____

_____

_____

_____

8. At what distance does most of the patient assessment take place?

_____

_____

_____

_____

9. What should you do before you enter a patient's personal or intimate spaces?

_____

_____

_____

_____

10. What message is communicated by placing yourself at the same eye level as a patient?

_____

_____

_____

_____

11. When might standing above or over a patient be appropriate?

_____

_____

_____

_____

12. What does dropping below eye level indicate?

_____

_____

_____

_____

13. Dropping below eye level might be most appropriate when dealing with which groups of patients?

_____

_____

_____

_____

14. What is an open-ended question?

_____

_____

_____

15. When is an open-ended question useful in history taking?

_____

_____

_____

16. What problems can open-ended questions cause during history taking?

_____

_____

_____

17. What is a direct (closed-ended) question?

_____

_____

_____

18. When is a direct (closed-ended) question useful in history taking?

_____

_____

_____

_____

19. What problems can direct (closed-ended) questions cause during history taking?

_____

_____

_____

_____

20. Discuss strategies a paramedic may use when interviewing a patient who is unmotivated to talk.

_____

_____

_____

_____

21. Discuss strategies a paramedic may use when interviewing a patient who is hostile or uncooperative.

_____

_____

_____

_____

22. Why do questions that begin with "why" often create problems during patient interviews?

_____

_____

_____

_____

23. Why should you be cautious about using phrases such as "I'm going to take your pulse" when you are talking to a child?

_____

_____

_____

_____

24. You are treating a patient with respiratory distress who is not responding to oxygen administration by nonrebreather mask. Your partner says, "I think we may need to bag her." What type of communication error has your partner made and what problem can it cause in dealing with the patient?

_____

_____

_____

_____

MULTIPLE CHOICE

1. In the United States, social distance—the acceptable distance between strangers—is _____.
   A. 0 to 1.5 feet
   B. 1.5 to 4 feet
   C. 4 to 12 feet
   D. 12 feet or more

2. In the United States, personal space—the distance from themselves that most people perceive as an extension of themselves—is _____.
   A. 0 to 1.5 feet
   B. 1.5 to 4 feet
   C. 4 to 12 feet
   D. 12 feet or more

3. Most of patient assessment takes place at what distance?
   A. Intimate distance
   B. Personal distance
   C. Public distance
   D. Social distance

4. Extended arms, open hands, relaxed large muscles, and a nodding head characterize _____.
   A. a closed stance, which sends a message of confidence and ease
   B. a closed stance, which suggests disinterest, discomfort, anger, or disgust
   C. an open stance, which communicates warmth and attentiveness
   D. an open stance, which sends negative signals to the patient

5. Flexed arms and clenched fists characterize _____.
   A. a closed stance, which communicates warmth and attentiveness
   B. a closed stance, which sends negative signals to the patient
   C. an open stance, which communicates disinterest, discomfort, or fear
   D. an open stance, which sends a message of confidence and ease

6. Positioning yourself below a patient's eye level indicates _____.
   A. willingness to let the patient have some control of the situation
   B. you are confident and in control of the situation
   C. you are in authority and have control of the encounter
   D. you consider yourself and the patient to be equals

7. When you are communicating with an elderly patient, you should _____.
   A. call the patient "dear" or "honey" to show the patient you care
   B. quickly separate the patient from friends and family to reduce anxiety
   C. talk louder than normal because most of the elderly have difficulty hearing
   D. use physical contact when necessary to compensate for decreased vision

117

8. Which statement about communicating with patients is correct?
   A. Interrupt the patient as soon as the patient says something that is unclear.
   B. Use medical terminology as much as possible to demonstrate you are an expert.
   C. Use nicknames for pediatric patients like "sonny" or "missy" to reinforce your authority.
   D. Use the patient's first name only after obtaining permission to do so.

9. A patient says, "My chest hurts." You respond to this by saying, "So, you are having chest pain." This is an example of the feedback technique called _____.
   A. clarification
   B. confrontation
   C. interpretation
   D. reflection

10. A question that guides the direction of a patient's answer is _____.
   A. a closed-ended question
   B. a direct question
   C. a leading question
   D. reflection

11. A question such as "Did you take your insulin today?" is referred to as _____.
   A. a clarification question.
   B. a closed-ended question.
   C. an open-ended question.
   D. a reflective question.

12. Which of the following questions is an example of an open-ended question?
   A. Are you having chest pain?
   B. Do you have a squeezing sensation in your chest?
   C. Have you eaten today?
   D. What would someone have to do to you to produce pain similar to what you are feeling?

13. While you are interviewing a patient you lean forward in your chair, nod your head, and occasionally say "Mm-hmm" or "go on." These are examples of feedback techniques called _____.
   A. confrontation
   B. empathy
   C. facilitation
   D. summarization

CASE STUDIES

Case one

You have been dispatched to an area of the community with a large population of refugees from the Balkans. Your patient is a 35-year-old female who is obviously pregnant and appears to be in pain. The only person present who speaks English is a 7-year-old boy.

1. Discuss points you would consider when using the boy as an interpreter.

   _____
   _____
   _____
   _____

Case two

You have responded to an area of your community with a large Cambodian population. When you attempt to determine the problem, you discover that the women will not talk to you and the men will not look you in the eye as they answer your questions.

1. How should you interpret these responses?

   _____
   _____
   _____
   _____

16 History Taking

READING ASSIGNMENT

Chapter 16, pages 578-587, in *Paramedic Practice Today: Above and Beyond*.

OBJECTIVES

After completing this chapter, you will be able to:
1. Describe the structure and purpose of a medical history.
2. List the components of a comprehensive history for adult patients.
3. Describe how to obtain a comprehensive health history.
4. List the unique components of a comprehensive history for pediatric patients.

CHAPTER SUMMARY

- The medical interview is designed to gather information about the patient's past and present medical conditions and establish rapport with the patient.
- The technique of active listening and knowledge of when to use open-ended versus direct questions allow you to obtain an accurate history from your patients efficiently.
- Understand that the components of a comprehensive medical history include the chief complaint, history of present illness, past medical history, current health status, and review of systems.
- Recognize that special challenges to obtaining the medical history require changing your standard approach to the medical interview to accommodate the issues facing the patient.

SHORT ANSWER

1. What is the importance of the history in the patient assessment process?

_____

_____

_____

_____

2. What are the components of a comprehensive health history?

_____

_____

_____

_____

3. What is the chief complaint?

_____

_____

_____

_____

4. Why is the chief complaint important in patient assessment and history taking?

_____

_____

_____

_____

5. What is an open-ended question?

_____

_____

_____

_____

6. When is an open-ended question useful in history taking?

_____

_____

_____

_____

7. What problems can open-ended questions cause during history taking?

_____

_____

_____

_____

8. What is a closed-ended question?

_____

_____

_____

_____

9. When is a closed-ended question useful in history taking?

_____

_____

_____

_____

10. What problems can closed-ended questions cause during history taking?

_____
_____
_____
_____

11. How does a patient's "chief complaint" differ from a patient's "primary problem"?

_____
_____
_____
_____

12. If a patient has difficulty describing his or her pain, what questions can you ask that may help?

_____
_____
_____
_____

13. Whenever you ask a patient to describe severity of pain on a scale of 0 to 10, what other questions should you always ask?

_____
_____
_____
_____

14. What is a differential diagnosis?

_____
_____
_____
_____

15. What role does the differential diagnosis play in the patient assessment process?

_____
_____
_____
_____

16. What do the letters in the memory aid OPQRST indicate?

_____
_____
_____
_____

17. A patient presents with a chief complaint of abdominal pain. Using the memory aid OPQRST, list questions you might ask as part of the history of the patient's present illness.

_____
_____
_____
_____

18. What is the purpose of the "review of systems" in a comprehensive health history?

_____
_____
_____
_____

19. List unique questions that should be asked when obtaining a history for a pediatric patient.

_____
_____
_____
_____

MULTIPLE CHOICE

1. A question such as "Are you having numbness in your left arm?" is referred to as _____.
   A. a clarified question
   B. a closed-ended question
   C. an open-ended question
   D. a reflective question

2. Which of the following statements about taking a history is correct?
   A. Ask the patient questions that can be answered "yes" or "no."
   B. Examine a body part or organ system before asking questions about it.
   C. If possible, question the patient before talking to relatives and bystanders.
   D. Suggest answers to the patient to speed the process.

3. Which of the following would be part of the history of the present illness of a patient complaining of abdominal pain?
   A. Allergies
   B. General health before onset of the pain
   C. Medications
   D. The duration of the pain

4. The first information you should obtain from a conscious patient is the _____.
   A. chief complaint
   B. history of the present illness
   C. medical history
   D. review of systems

5. Your patient is a 21-year-old male with a history of type 1 diabetes mellitus. He is complaining of a severe headache. In developing a history of the present illness, you will need to know _____.
   A. both the type of insulin he takes and the duration of his headache
   B. the amount of insulin he takes daily
   C. the duration of the headache
   D. the type of insulin he takes

17 Patient Assessment

READING ASSIGNMENT

Chapter 17, pages 588-634, in *Paramedic Practice Today: Above and Beyond.*

OBJECTIVES

After completing this chapter, you will be able to:
1. Explain the rationale for the use of an otoscope.
2. Explain the rationale for the use of an ophthalmoscope.
3. Define the terms *inspection, palpation, percussion,* and *auscultation.*
4. Describe the techniques of inspection, palpation, percussion, and auscultation.
5. Discuss medical identification devices and systems.
6. Describe trending of assessment components and explain the value of trending assessment components to other health professionals who assume care of the patient.
7. Describe the methods used to locate and assess a pulse.
8. Differentiate locating and assessing a pulse in an adult, child, and infant patient.
9. Distinguish among methods of assessing breathing in the adult, child, and infant patient.
10. Differentiate a patient with adequate and inadequate minute ventilation.
11. Discuss methods of assessing mental status and differentiate assessing altered mental status in the adult, child, and infant patient.
12. Categorize levels of consciousness in the adult, infant, and child.
13. Recognize hazards and potential hazards.
14. Determine and describe common hazards found at the scene of a traumatic event and at the scene of a medical patient.
15. Differentiate safe from unsafe scenes.
16. Describe methods for making an unsafe scene safe.
17. Discuss common mechanisms of injury and nature of illness.
18. Predict patterns of injury based on mechanism of injury.
19. Discuss the reason for identifying the total number of patients at the scene.
20. Organize the management of a scene after size-up.
21. Explain the reasons for identifying the need for additional help or assistance.
22. Summarize the reasons for forming a general impression of the patient.
23. Explain the value of performing an initial assessment.
24. State reasons for management of the cervical spine once the patient has been determined to be a trauma patient.
25. Discuss methods of assessing the airway in the adult, child, and infant patient.
26. Describe methods used for assessing whether a patient is breathing.
27. Discuss the need for assessing the patient for external bleeding.
28. Describe normal and abnormal findings when assessing skin color, temperature, and condition.
29. Describe the evaluation of a patient's perfusion status based on findings in the primary survey.
30. Discuss the reasons for reconsidering the mechanism of injury.
31. Analyze a scene to determine if spinal precautions are required.
32. Explain the reason for prioritizing a patient for care and transport.
33. Identify patients who require expeditious transport.
34. Differentiate the assessment performed for a patient who is unresponsive or has an altered mental status and other medical patients requiring assessment.
35. Apply the techniques of physical examination to the medical patient.
36. State the reasons for performing a rapid trauma assessment.
37. Cite examples and explain why patients should receive a rapid trauma assessment.
38. Apply the techniques of physical examination to the trauma patient.
39. Describe the areas included in the rapid trauma assessment and discuss what should be evaluated.
40. Discuss the reason for performing a focused history and physical examination.
41. Describe when and why a detailed physical examination is necessary.
42. Discuss the components of the detailed physical examination in relation to the techniques of examination.
43. State the areas of the body that are evaluated during the detailed physical examination.
44. Explain what additional care should be provided while performing the detailed physical examination.
45. Distinguish between the detailed physical examination performed on a trauma patient and that of the medical patient.
46. Differentiate patients requiring a detailed physical examination from those who do not.
47. Differentiate normal and abnormal findings of the assessment of the skin, hair, and nails.

121

48. Distinguish the importance of abnormal findings of the assessment of the skin.
49. Describe the examination of the head and neck.
50. Differentiate normal and abnormal findings of the scalp examination.
51. Describe the normal and abnormal assessment findings of the skull.
52. Describe the assessment of visual acuity.
53. Describe the examination of the eyes.
54. Distinguish between normal and abnormal assessment findings of the eyes.
55. Describe the examination of the ears.
56. Differentiate normal and abnormal assessment findings of the ears.
57. Describe the examination of the nose.
58. Differentiate normal and abnormal assessment findings of the nose.
59. Describe the examination of the mouth and pharynx.
60. Describe the examination of the neck.
61. Differentiate normal and abnormal assessment findings of the neck.
62. Describe the assessment of jugular venous pressure and pulsations.
63. Differentiate normal and abnormal assessment findings of the chest examination.
64. Describe the examination of the anterior and posterior chest.
65. Differentiate the characteristics of breath sounds.
66. Describe the examination of the heart and blood vessels.
67. Differentiate normal and abnormal assessment findings of the heart and blood vessels.
68. Describe the auscultation of the heart.
69. Differentiate the characteristics of normal and abnormal findings associated with the auscultation of the heart.
70. Describe special examination techniques of the cardiovascular examination.
71. Describe the examination of the abdomen.
72. Differentiate normal and abnormal assessment findings of the abdomen.
73. Describe auscultation of the abdomen.
74. Distinguish normal and abnormal findings of the auscultation of the abdomen.
75. Describe the examination of the female genitalia.
76. Differentiate normal and abnormal assessment findings of the female genitalia.
77. Describe the examination of the male genitalia.
78. Differentiate normal and abnormal findings of the male genitalia.
79. Describe the examination of the anus and rectum.
80. Distinguish between normal and abnormal findings of the anus and rectum.
81. Describe the examination of the musculoskeletal system.
82. Differentiate normal and abnormal findings of the musculoskeletal system.
83. Describe the examination of the nervous system.
84. Differentiate normal and abnormal findings of the nervous system.
85. Discuss the considerations of examination of an infant or child.
86. Discuss the reasons for repeating the primary survey as part of the ongoing assessment.
87. Describe the components of the ongoing assessment.
88. Describe the general guidelines of recording examination information.

CHAPTER SUMMARY

- A thorough and complete patient assessment is the paramedic's most important tool. To provide a thorough examination, the paramedic must have his or her equipment prepared and be familiar with how to use all the tools.
- A well-organized format to patient assessment is critical; it helps address higher priority problems earlier. First, identify and manage any scene-related problems. Second, identify and stabilize critical body system problems. Finally, perform a through examination to identify and manage all the patient's noncritical problems.
- Organize your physical examination in a logical pattern that makes sense for you. During the detailed examination, completely assess each anatomic region before moving on to another portion of the body.
- Remember, children are not small adults. Anytime a child is sick or injured, you have multiple patients—the child and his or her parents. Keep the immaturity of the child's organ systems in mind while performing an examination, and attempt to earn the patient's trust before trying to examine his or her body.
- As patients age, so do their organ systems. Anticipate multiple and more complicated problems in older adults. Also remember that older adults cannot compensate as well or as long as they once did. Intervene on seemingly minor problems early before they become life-threatening conditions.
- Never assume a patient is completely stable until you have the continued assessment evidence to back up your analysis. A single set of vital signs is only a place to start; two sets are merely interesting. Once you have three sets of vital signs you can begin to observe trends over time. These trends offer great insight into underlying conditions.
- Quite simply, if you do not write it down, you have not done it. Completely and thoroughly document all parts of your assessment. Do not simply document the interesting problems and conditions found; also remember to note normal findings and identify pertinent negatives. Select a documenting format that works for you and use it consistently to decrease your chances of forgetting to document that critical information.

MATCHING

1. Identify each of the following abnormal (adventitious) respiratory sounds.

   _____ Fine, popping sounds that indicate the presence of fluid in alveoli and small airways

   _____ Harsh, high-pitched crowing sound that indicates a narrow upper airway

   _____ Rattling sound produced by collections of mucus and other fluids in larger airways

   _____ High-pitched whistling sounds produced by air flowing through narrow lower airways

   A. Crackles
   B. Rhonchi
   C. Stridor
   D. Wheezes

SHORT ANSWER

1. When you arrive on the scene of an incident, what is the *first* action that you should always take?

   _____
   _____
   _____
   _____

2. What is the purpose of the initial assessment (primary survey) in patient assessment?

   _____
   _____
   _____
   _____

3. What are the elements of the initial assessment (primary survey)?

   _____
   _____
   _____
   _____

4. If a problem is discovered during the initial assessment (primary survey), what action should be taken?

   _____
   _____
   _____
   _____

5. What is the purpose of the focused or detailed history and physical (secondary survey) during patient assessment?

   _____
   _____
   _____
   _____

6. What is the most reliable indicator that a patient's brain is being perfused adequately?

   _____
   _____
   _____
   _____

7. What is normal capillary refill time?

   _____
   _____
   _____
   _____

8. What do the letters *AVPU* indicate?

   _____
   _____
   _____
   _____

9. When is the cervical spine controlled during the assessment of a trauma patient?

   _____
   _____
   _____
   _____

10. During what phase of the patient assessment is the pulse rate counted?

    _____
    _____
    _____
    _____

11. During what phase of the patient assessment is the respiratory rate counted?

    _____
    _____
    _____
    _____

12. During what phase of the patient assessment is the blood pressure taken by cuff?

    _____
    _____
    _____
    _____

13. List four possible causes of neck vein distention in a patient who is in a semisitting position.

    _____
    _____
    _____
    _____

14. What is the technical term used to describe ecchymosis over the mastoid process?

    _____
    _____
    _____
    _____

15. List four signs of increased work of breathing (respiratory distress).

_____

_____

_____

_____

16. What three pieces of information should be recorded and reported when a patient's pulse rate is taken?

_____

_____

_____

17. List the steps of the general approach to assessment of an emergency patient.

_____

_____

_____

_____

18. Define the terms *inspection, palpation, auscultation,* and *percussion.*

_____

_____

_____

_____

19. When should the diaphragm of the stethoscope be used?

_____

_____

_____

_____

20. When should the bell of the stethoscope be used?

_____

_____

_____

21. When should the fingertips be used for palpation?

_____

_____

_____

_____

22. What part of the hand should be used to palpate for vibrations or impulses?

_____

_____

_____

_____

23. Why should the back of the hand be used to check for skin moisture and temperature?

_____

_____

_____

_____

24. List the cranial nerves and describe how you would test the functions of each nerve.

_____

_____

_____

_____

_____

_____

_____

_____

_____

_____

_____

_____

25. Describe the methods used to assess for orthostatic hypotension. Include in your discussion specifics of the assessment process and the findings that would be considered abnormal.

_____

_____

_____

_____

26. A patient whose chest struck the steering wheel during a traffic collision complains of difficulty breathing and chest pain. When you auscultate the chest, breath sounds are absent on the right. Percussion of the right side of the chest produces a booming, hollow sound over the entire lung field. What problem do you suspect?

_____

_____

_____

_____

27. A patient whose chest struck the steering wheel during a traffic collision complains of difficulty breathing and chest pain. When you auscultate the chest, breath sounds are absent on the right. Percussion of the right side of the chest produces a dull sound in the inferior and posterior portions of the lung field. What problem do you suspect?

_____

_____

_____

_____

28. Why are terms such as *stuporous, obtunded, lethargic,* and *comatose* not useful in communicating a patient's mental status? What is a more appropriate way to describe a patient's mental status?

_____

_____

_____

_____

29. What change occurs in the fingertips of patients suffering from conditions that produce chronic hypoxia, such as emphysema or chronic bronchitis? Why does this change develop?

_____

_____

_____

_____

30. While transporting a patient from a nursing home, you notice that she has numerous transverse depressions on her nails, which appear to parallel the cuticle. The depressions give the nails a ridged appearance. What are these depressions called? What do they suggest about this patient's medical history?

_____

_____

_____

_____

31. Describe the use of a visual acuity wall chart and a visual acuity card for assessing visual acuity.

_____

_____

_____

_____

32. In the absence of a wall chart or visual acuity card, what techniques can be used to assess visual acuity in the field?

_____

_____

_____

_____

MULTIPLE CHOICE

1. A 32-year-old female says she was walking through her home when her arm bumped a door frame. She has an obvious hematoma on her forearm but no other obvious injuries. Considering this information, which of the following is the most appropriate examination for the paramedic to perform on this patient?
   A. A comprehensive physical examination, as would be performed in a physician's office
   B. A focused examination of the injured extremity
   C. A patient assessment including a head-to-toe examination, as would be performed on any trauma patient
   D. No physical examination is needed for this patient.

2. A 25-year-old male apparently was thrown from the vehicle during a collision. He is unconscious and unresponsive. His skin is pale, cool, and moist. Respirations are 36 breaths/min, shallow, and irregular. Radial pulses are absent. He has a large avulsion of his scalp with moderate bleeding. His abdomen is rigid and distended. He has an open fracture of his right tibia. Your *initial efforts* should be directed toward _____.
   A. immobilizing his open tibia fracture
   B. managing the scalp avulsion
   C. performing a secondary survey (detailed history and physical examination)
   D. supporting his respirations and beginning therapy for shock

3. Your patient is unconscious and does not respond to your voice. When you stimulate him with pain, his arms extend. Based upon this information, which of the following is the most descriptive and accurate assessment statement?
   A. Alert but responds to painful stimulus only
   B. Confused but responds to painful stimulus
   C. Responds to painful stimulus with decerebrate posturing
   D. Responsive to painful stimulus with posturing

4. The purpose of the primary survey (initial assessment) is to identify _____.
   A. any immediately life-threatening problems
   B. any threats to your safety or the safety of your patient
   C. clues at the scene that may help identify the cause of the problem
   D. the patient's most obvious injury

5. A patient's pupils react to light equally, are equal in size, and are round. The patient is able to follow your penlight in all directions making the shape of an **H**. When you place your penlight just in front of the patient's nose, the eyes move medially and the pupils constrict. The most accurate and complete way to document these findings is _____.
   A. pupils are equal and reactive to light (PERL)
   B. pupils are equal, round, and reactive to light (PERRL)
   C. pupils are equal, round, and reactive to light with absence of injury (PERRLA)
   D. pupils are equal, round, and reactive to light with accommodation intact (PERRLA)

6. A 24-year-old male fell from a ladder and suffered an open fracture of the right radius. He is awake and alert. There is no radial pulse on the side of the fracture, and blood is spurting from the injury. The patient has multiple small lacerations and abrasions on the right palm and both arms with blood flowing steadily from these injuries. What problem should be treated first?
   A. The abrasions
   B. The flowing hemorrhage
   C. The open fracture
   D. The spurting hemorrhage

125

7. The first step you should take when you arrive on the scene of a motor vehicle crash is to _____.
   A. begin disentanglement of any patients pinned in the vehicles
   B. immediately gain access to the patient and correct life threats
   C. immediately gain access to the patients and perform initial assessments
   D. survey for any special problems or hazards

8. Which of the following problems should be managed first?
   A. Femur fracture
   B. Forearm laceration with venous bleeding
   C. Partial airway obstruction with poor air exchange
   D. Penetrating abdominal trauma

9. The first step during the initial assessment (primary survey) always is to check for _____.
   A. adequate oxygenation and ventilation
   B. adequate perfusion
   C. an open airway
   D. cyanosis

10. Which of the following statements about assessment of vital signs is correct?
    A. Vital signs need to be reassessed only if the initial findings were abnormal.
    B. Vital signs only need to be assessed initially at the scene and again just before arrival at the hospital.
    C. Vital signs should be reassessed several times during transport.
    D. Vital signs should be reassessed several times if the blood pressure was palpated initially.

11. The purpose of the secondary survey (focused or detailed physical examination) is to detect _____.
    A. fractures and dislocations
    B. immediate life threats
    C. less obvious signs
    D. minor soft tissue injuries

12. The first information a paramedic should obtain from a conscious patient is the _____.
    A. blood pressure
    B. chief complaint
    C. history of the present illness
    D. medical history

13. Which of the following statements is the best description of a patient's mental status?
    A. The patient responded to pain by opening his eyes, moaning, and trying to push my hand away.
    B. The patient was oriented ×2.
    C. The patient was semiconscious.
    D. The patient was stuporous.

14. Which of the following pulses would be the last to vanish in a patient with decompensated shock?
    A. Brachial
    B. Carotid
    C. Femoral
    D. Radial

15. When you assess a patient with a chief complaint of abdominal pain, auscultation of the abdomen should _____.
    A. be performed with the bell of the stethoscope
    B. involve listening to each abdominal quadrant for at least 15 seconds
    C. be performed primarily to detect the presence or absence of bowel sounds
    D. only be performed after palpating the abdomen

16. A patient with a midshaft fracture of the left humerus complains of pain in her forearm and hand as well as at the fracture site. The hand and forearm are cold and pale. A radial pulse is absent. What is the most probable cause of these signs and symptoms?
    A. Compression of nerves resulting in vasoconstriction
    B. Occlusion of the extremity's arterial supply
    C. Occlusion of the extremity's venous supply
    D. Vasoconstriction in response to pain from the fracture

17. If a patient is unstable, an ongoing assessment should be performed every _____.
    A. 15 minutes
    B. 5 minutes
    C. 10 minutes
    D. 20 minutes

18. If a patient is stable, an ongoing assessment should be performed every _____.
    A. 15 minutes
    B. 5 minutes
    C. 10 minutes
    D. 20 minutes

19. Light popping, nonmusical lung sounds heard during inspiration are _____.
    A. crackles
    B. rhonchi
    C. stridor
    D. wheezes

20. Clubbing of the nailbeds is associated with _____.
    A. asthma
    B. diabetes or renal failure
    C. diseases causing chronic hypoxia
    D. liver disease or hypertension

21. The cranial nerve associated with the sense of smell is _____.
    A. cranial nerve I
    B. cranial nerve II
    C. cranial nerve III
    D. cranial nerve IV

22. Your patient is not awake. He does not respond to your voice. When you stimulate him with pain, his arms flex. Based upon this information, which of the following is the most descriptive and accurate assessment statement?
   A. Alert but responds to painful stimulus only
   B. Confused but responds to painful stimulus
   C. Responds to painful stimulus with decorticate posturing
   D. Responsive to painful stimulus with decerberate posturing

23. When viewed with an otoscope, a normal tympanic membrane would be _____.
   A. concave with a visible cone of light
   B. concave with no visible cone of light
   C. convex with a visible cone of light
   D. convex with no visible cone of light

24. A patient's left chest wall is hyporesonant to percussion. When you percuss the right chest wall, you hear normal sounds. Which of the following is most likely present and responsible for your specific findings?
   A. Hemothorax of the left chest
   B. Pneumothorax of the right chest
   C. Severe pneumonia of the left lung
   D. Tension pneumothorax of the left chest

25. Which of the following statements about heart sounds is correct?
   A. Closing of the aortic and pulmonic valves produces the S_1 sound.
   B. Closing of the mitral and tricuspid valves produces the S_1 sound.
   C. Closing of the mitral and tricuspid valves produces the S_2 sound.
   D. Closing of the semilunar valves produces the S_1 sound.

26. Jugular venous distention is best assessed while the patient is _____.
   A. in Trendelenburg's position
   B. sitting upright
   C. sitting upright and at a 45-degree incline
   D. supine

27. While assessing a patient with acute abdominal pain, your partner measures the vital signs while the patient is sitting. Her blood pressure in this position is 102/78 mm Hg and her pulse rate is 102 beats/min. Your partner now assesses the patient's vital signs while the patient is standing. Her blood pressure in this position is 122/84 mm Hg and her pulse rate is 82 beats/min. Which of the following is a correct evaluation of these data?
   A. The patient has negative orthostatic testing and may be experiencing a hypertensive event.
   B. The patient has positive orthostatic testing and may be hypovolemic.

C. The patient is taking some type of drug that is altering her vital signs.
   D. The vital sign data are not consistent with predictable changes that occur because of body position.

28. A 28-year-old man tripped while playing soccer. He complains only of his scraped elbow and knee. The patient correctly states his name, knows he is at the soccer field, cannot recall the day of the week, cannot recall the name of the current President of the United States, and thinks the year is 2005. Which of the following statements best describes this patient's mental status?
   A. He is alert and confused.
   B. He is alert and oriented to person and place only.
   C. He is alert and oriented to person, place, and time.
   D. He is alert and oriented ×3.

29. Which of the following cranial nerves has a function involving a structure other than the eye?
   A. Cranial nerve III
   B. Cranial nerve IV
   C. Cranial nerve V
   D. Cranial nerve VI

30. The "lub" of the heart sounds represents which event of the cardiac cycle?
   A. Closing of the aortic and pulmonic valves
   B. Closing of the mitral and tricuspid valves
   C. Ventricular contraction
   D. Ventricular filling

31. Wheezing is best described as _____.
   A. high-pitched sounds caused by asthma
   B. high-pitched sounds caused by constriction of the smaller airways
   C. high-pitched sounds caused by constriction of the upper airway
   D. high-pitched sounds caused by fluid in the alveoli

32. The S_3 heart sound is most commonly associated with _____.
   A. acute myocardial infarction
   B. cardiac tamponade
   C. congestive heart failure
   D. hypovolemia

33. The sounds of bruits are _____.
   A. associated with acute myocardial infarctions
   B. associated with turbulent blood flow in narrowed blood vessels
   C. only found in persons who have a shunt for hemodialysis
   D. present during high-output states as in a hypertensive crisis

34. When examining the interior of the eye, which of the following normally can be seen without increasing the depth of focus on the ophthalmoscope?
    A. Hyphema
    B. The optic blood vessels
    C. The optic disc
    D. The retina

35. You see retinal hemorrhages in the interior of your 40-year-old patient's eye. Which of the following must be added to your differential diagnosis?
    A. Cataracts
    B. Diabetes
    C. Increased intracranial pressure
    D. Papilledema

36. A patient is lying supine, and his neck veins are flat. Based on this observation, you might suspect that he has _____.
    A. cardiac tamponade
    B. hypovolemia
    C. right-sided heart failure
    D. tension pneumothorax

37. Battle's sign suggests the presence of _____.
    A. a basilar skull fracture
    B. a cervical spine injury
    C. a ruptured tympanic membrane
    D. an intracranial hematoma

38. Which of the following groups of findings would be consistent with the presence of pneumonia with pus and other fluid in the alveoli and small airways?
    A. Rales, increased fremitus, absence of egophony and bronchophony
    B. Rales, increased fremitus, presence of egophony and bronchophony
    C. Rhonchi, decreased fremitus, absence of egophony and bronchophony
    D. Rhonchi, decreased fremitus, presence of egophony and bronchophony

39. Bronchovesicular breath sounds are most easily heard _____.
    A. between the scapulae or at the second and third intercostal space lateral to the sternum
    B. in the periphery of the lung
    C. over the manubrium
    D. over the trachea

40. Which statement best describes vesicular sounds?
    A. Loud, high pitched, and hollow
    B. Soft, breezy, lower pitched
    C. Soft, swishy, lowest pitched
    D. Very loud, harsh

41. The sound of the aortic valve is best auscultated at which of the following locations?
    A. At the apex beat
    B. Over the sternum at the level of the fourth intercostal space
    C. The second intercostal space at the right of the sternum
    D. The second intercostal space at the left of the sternum

42. What is kyphosis?
    A. Exaggerated lumbar concavity
    B. Exaggerated lumbar convexity
    C. Exaggerated thoracic concavity
    D. Exaggerated thoracic convexity

43. What is scoliosis?
    A. Exaggerated lumbar concavity
    B. Exaggerated lumbar convexity
    C. Exaggerated thoracic concavity
    D. Lateral spinal curvature

44. Increased muscle tone when passive movement is applied, especially at the end of the range of motion, is _____.
    A. flaccidity
    B. paratonia
    C. rigidity
    D. spasticity

45. Increased resistance to active movement throughout the entire range of motion is _____.
    A. flaccidity
    B. paratonia
    C. rigidity
    D. spasticity

46. Loss of muscle tone, causing the limb to be loose, is _____.
    A. flaccidity
    B. paratonia
    C. rigidity
    D. spasticity

47. Sudden changes in muscle tone during passive movement, resulting in either increased or decreased resistance, are _____.
    A. flaccidity
    B. paratonia
    C. rigidity
    D. spasticity

Case one

A 23-year-old female's vehicle struck another vehicle at 55 mph. The patient was restrained with a lap belt and shoulder harness, and the airbag deployed. The patient is awake and alert. Radial pulses are present, rapid, and strong. The patient's skin is pale and cool. Her only complaint is pain in both arms and in her right ankle. There are abrasions on the anterior surfaces of both forearms. The right ankle is painful, swollen, and discolored.

1. Based on this information, should you perform a focused or a detailed examination?

   _____

2. Why?

   _____
   _____
   _____
   _____

Case two

On a summer day, a 25-year-old male was jogging when he tripped on an area of uneven pavement. As he fell, he attempted to catch himself with his right hand. The patient is awake and alert. Radial pulses are present, rapid, and strong. The skin is warm, moist, and flushed. He complains of pain in his right wrist, which is painful, swollen, and discolored. An abraded area is present on his right knee.

1. Based on this information, should you perform a focused or a detailed examination?

   _____

2. Why?

   _____
   _____
   _____
   _____

Case three

A 45-year-old male developed chest pain while he was sitting at home watching television. He states that the pain is "squeezing" in character and radiates to his left shoulder and left arm. He also is experiencing nausea and mild shortness of breath. He is awake, alert, and anxious. Radial pulses are present, rapid, weak, and irregular. His skin is pale, cool, and moist.

1. Based on this information, should you perform a focused or a detailed examination?

   _____

2. Why?

   _____
   _____
   _____
   _____

Case four

The police found a male, who appears to be in his late 50s, unconscious and unresponsive in an abandoned building. Radial pulses are present, strong, slow, and regular. Respirations are rapid, deep, and regular. The patient's skin is cool and dry. There is no immediately obvious trauma. The patient exudes a variety of aromas, including those of urine, feces, and cheap wine.

1. Based on this information, should you perform a focused or a detailed examination?

   _____

2. Why?

_____

_____

_____

_____

Case five

A patient with a mid-shaft fracture of the humerus complains of pain in the distal portions of the upper extremity as well as at the fracture site. Examination shows that the extremity is cold and cyanotic and that the radial pulses are absent.

1. What is the most probable cause of these signs and symptoms?

_____

_____

_____

_____

Case six

Your patient is a 30-year-old female who was thrown from the motorcycle. She is unconscious and unresponsive. Her skin is pale, cool, and moist. Her respirations are 28 breaths/min, shallow, and irregular. Radial pulses are absent. Her abdomen is rigid and distended. Breath sounds are absent on the left side of her chest. She has an open fracture of her right femur.

1. What are your priorities in managing this patient?

_____

_____

_____

_____

2. Why?

_____

_____

_____

_____

Case seven

A 32-year-old male complains of pain in the right lateral chest that worsens when he inhales. He also complains of a cough that is productive of yellow-green sputum. When you listen to his chest, you hear fine popping sounds in the right middle lobe of the lung as the patient inhales as well as a grating sound that is present both on inhalation and exhalation. You are able to hear his words clearly through the stethoscope when he speaks in a normal voice and in whispers. His body temperature is 101°F.

1. What is your field diagnosis for this patient?

_____

2. Explain how each of the observations made during the assessment supports this diagnosis.

_____

_____

_____

_____

Case eight

A 67-year-old female complains of shortness of breath that awakened her about 15 minutes ago. You find her sitting upright on the side of her bed. The patient is using her neck muscles to assist her respirations. Her neck veins are distended from the clavicles about halfway to the angle of the jaw. Auscultation of her chest reveals fine popping sounds on inhalation and high-pitched, whistling sounds on exhalation over the lower half of both lung fields. Radial pulses are present, rapid, and weak. When you auscultate the heart sounds, you hear "lub-dub-duh, lub-dub-duh." The patient's feet and ankles appear swollen. When you push on the swollen area, a depression of approximately ¾ inch forms and then slowly disappears.

1. What is your field diagnosis for this patient?

   _____

2. Explain how each of the observations made during the assessment supports this diagnosis.

   _____
   _____
   _____
   _____

Case nine

A 52-year-old male with a history of chronic alcohol abuse calls EMS because he "just doesn't feel well and is having a hard time breathing." Your examination reveals an emaciated male who appears significantly older than his stated age. His skin, eyes, and nailbeds have a yellowish color. His abdomen is grossly distended with enlarged veins radiating from the umbilicus. When you place the palm of your left hand against the left side of the patient's abdomen and slap the other side of the abdomen with your right hand, you can feel an impulse against your left hand. The abdomen is dull to percussion. There is a tender mass in the right upper abdominal quadrant.

1. What is your field diagnosis for this patient?

   _____

2. Explain how each of the observations made during the assessment supports this diagnosis.

   _____
   _____
   _____
   _____

Case ten

An 18-year-old female awakened this morning to find that she could not move the left side of her face. When she attempts to smile, the left side of her mouth will not move. When she tries to wrinkle her forehead, the portion left of the midline remains completely smooth. She has no impairment of speech or gait. She also reports that everything she tries to eat or drink "tastes funny."

1. From what problem is she suffering?

   _____

2. What cranial nerve is involved?

   _____

3. How does the involvement of this cranial nerve explain the alterations in motor function and sensation that are present?

   _____
   _____
   _____
   _____

Case eleven

A 38-year-old male with a history of diabetes mellitus experienced a sudden onset of severe pain in the distal portions of his left lower extremity about 10 minutes ago. The affected extremity rapidly became paralyzed and lost all sensation after passing through a period when the patient felt a "pins and needles" sensation in the limb. The patient's foot and distal calf are cool to the touch and very pale. The dorsal pedal and posterior tibial pulses are absent. Capillary refill time is so prolonged that it cannot be determined. The patient reports that he has been experiencing cramping and aching pain in the affected extremity for about 2 weeks when he climbs stairs or walks long distances. By comparison, the patient's right lower extremity is unremarkable.

1. What is your field diagnosis for this patient?

   _____

2. Explain how each of the observations made during the assessment supports this diagnosis.

   _____
   _____
   _____
   _____

Case twelve

A 68-year-old female has developed dull pain in the distal portion of her left lower extremity over about 2 days. The onset of the pain was preceded by a temperature of 100.6° F. Over the past hour the pain has become progressively more severe. The patient's foot and distal calf are warm to the touch and swollen, and have a purple-red appearance. The dorsal pedal and posterior tibial pulses are palpable, but are weak. Capillary refill is sluggish at about 4 seconds. When the patient attempts to dorsiflex her foot, she experiences pain in the posterior portion of the calf. A ropelike structure can be felt in the back of the calf.

1. What is your field diagnosis for this patient?

   _____

2. Explain how each of the observations made during the assessment supports this diagnosis.

   _____
   _____
   _____
   _____

Case thirteen

A 22-year-old male was involved in an altercation at a pool hall during which he was struck in the face repeatedly with a pool cue. He is awake and responds appropriately to questions. Bruising is present around both of his eyes, and blood is draining from his nose. When you check his eyes and pupil response, you find that his right pupil is fixed and dilated while the left pupil reacts briskly to light. Visual acuity in the right eye is unaffected. When you check extraocular muscle function, you discover that the left eye has a full range of movement. The right eye is able to look left and up-and-to-the left with difficulty. He is unable to move his right eye in any other direction.

1. What problem accounts for this patient's presentation?

   _____

2. Justify your answer based on your understanding of nerve anatomy and function.

   _____
   _____
   _____
   _____

Case fourteen

A 17-year-old female fell approximately 20 feet down an escalator in a department store. She is awake and alert, complaining of severe pain in her left arm. The patient's left humerus appears to have been fractured at mid-shaft and is severely angulated. The skin of the patient's hand and forearm are pale and cool. The patient's right forearm is warm and of normal color.

1. What problem do you suspect?

   _____

2. When you check for a radial pulse or check capillary refill in the patient's left arm, what findings would you anticipate?

   _____
   _____
   _____
   _____

18 Communication

READING ASSIGNMENT

Chapter 18, pages 635-647, in *Paramedic Practice Today: Above and Beyond*.

OBJECTIVES

After completing this chapter, you will be able to:
1. Identify why good communication skills are important when providing EMS.
2. Identify the roles of verbal, written, and electronic communication in providing EMS.
3. Identify why you should use the proper terminology when communicating during an EMS event.
4. Identify why you should use proper verbal communication during an EMS event.
5. List factors that enhance and hinder effective verbal communication.
6. Identify why you should use proper written communication during an EMS event.
7. List factors that enhance and hinder effective written communication.
8. Recognize the legal status of your written communication documenting an EMS event.
9. State why you should collect data during an EMS event.
10. Identify technology that you can use to collect and exchange patient and/or scene information electronically.
11. Recognize the legal status of any patient medical information that has been exchanged electronically.
12. Identify ways you use the following communication equipment:
    - Digital communications
    - Fax machine
    - Computer
13. Describe the phases of communication you will use to complete a typical EMS event.
14. Identify the various parts of a typical EMS communications system and describe their function and use.
15. Describe the functions and responsibilities of the Federal Communications Commission.
16. Identify and distinguish the following communications systems:
    - Simplex
    - Multiplex
    - Duplex
    - Half duplex
    - Trunked
17. Describe how an EMS dispatcher functions as an integral member of the EMS team.
18. Identify the role of emergency medical dispatch in a typical EMS event.
19. Identify the importance of prearrival instructions in a typical EMS event.
20. Describe the purpose or reason that you verbally communicate the patient's information to the hospital.
21. Describe any information that you should include in the patient assessment information that you verbally report to medical direction.

CHAPTER SUMMARY

- Each phase of an emergency requires good, effective communication.
- Accurate communication of every type—verbal, written, and electronic—is essential for the patient's health and documentation.
- Quality management is essential to the overall improvement of communication and patient care.
- A good knowledge of terminology helps eliminate communication problems.
- Radios are the backbone of the communication system in EMS.
- Repeater systems are essential to ensuring quality radio communication over extreme distances and rough terrain.
- Radio systems vary depending on the local EMS system and the type of equipment used.
- Computer-assisted dispatch systems send and receive numerous types of data quickly and accurately.

SHORT ANSWER

1. Define the following terms as they relate to radio communications systems:
   a. Simplex

   _____
   _____
   _____
   _____

   b. Duplex

   _____
   _____
   _____
   _____

c. Multiplex

_____

_____

_____

d. Trunked

_____

_____

_____

2. What are the three basic modes of communication used in EMS?

_____

_____

3. How are the basic modes of EMS communication used during a typical EMS call?

_____

_____

_____

_____

4. What is the function of a repeater in a communications system?

_____

_____

_____

_____

5. What is the function of an encoder in a communications system?

_____

_____

_____

_____

6. List three alternative technologies that can be used to supplement radio communications.

_____

_____

_____

7. Compare and contrast UHF and VHF frequencies including advantages and disadvantages of each.

_____

_____

_____

_____

8. What federal agency regulates the use of radio communication frequencies in the United States?

_____

_____

_____

_____

9. Describe methods used by the federal regulatory authorities to monitor compliance with rules and regulations.

_____

_____

_____

_____

10. Why should a radio frequency always be monitored for a few seconds before keying the microphone and beginning to transmit?

_____

_____

_____

11. Why should the microphone be keyed for about 2 seconds before beginning to transmit?

_____

_____

_____

_____

12. What are prearrival instructions? What is the advantage of providing prearrival instructions as part of an EMS communications system?

_____

_____

_____

_____

13. Diagram a basic EMS communications system. Include the following elements: portable radios, mobile radios, repeaters, base station, and remote console.

MULTIPLE CHOICE

1. Your EMS system uses a VHF simplex radio system with a repeater. Considering this type of system, which of the following statements is true?
   A. You are able to begin speaking into the radio microphone as soon as you depress the push-to-talk button.
   B. You are able to talk to medical control while also simultaneously transmitting ECG information.
   C. Your radio transmission range is increased by the fact that this radio system has a repeater.
   D. Your radio transmission range is limited by the fact that this is not a duplex system.

2. In Emergency Services Communications, *PSAP* refers to the _____.
   A. dispatch system in which the dispatcher is trained to provide prearrival aid instructions
   B. single location where 9-1-1 calls from a specific geographic area are routed for answering
   C. type of radio system that uses a computer to determine the frequency needed for talking
   D. type of radio system that uses a series of public repeater systems to access the emergency services radio system

3. The purpose of an encoder in an EMS communications system is to _____.
   A. allow base stations to share a frequency without having to listen to traffic not intended for them
   B. ensure privacy by keeping anyone other than the party to whom the message is directed from monitoring the system
   C. convert (encode) the patient's ECG into a signal that can be transmitted on the radio
   D. prevent interference from VHF frequencies arriving from distant areas caused by "skip"

4. Which statement best describes properties of a simplex radio system?
   A. One frequency is used; more than one unit can transmit at a time.
   B. One frequency is used; only one unit can transmit at a time.
   C. Two frequencies are used; more than one unit can transmit at a time.
   D. Two frequencies are used; only one unit can transmit at a time.

5. Which statement best describes a decision to be made by the EMS dispatcher?
   A. The code of travel on the way to the hospital
   B. The crew and vehicle that will respond to a call
   C. The equipment that should be taken on a call
   D. The route the ambulance will take to the scene

6. When a radio system has multiplex capability, it can _____.
   A. allow repeaters to use two or more frequencies simultaneously
   B. receive messages from two different mobile radios on the same frequency simultaneously
   C. receive signals on several frequencies simultaneously, but transmit on only one frequency at a time
   D. transmit two different signals (voice, ECG) on the same frequency simultaneously

7. Which of the following statements about radio frequency bands is correct?
   A. UHF has a greater range than VHF but is more susceptible to interference than VHF.
   B. UHF has better penetration in metropolitan areas.
   C. VHF has a greater range than UHF and is less susceptible to interference than UHF.
   D. VHF has better penetration in metropolitan areas since the signal "bounces" off of tall buildings.

8. What function do repeaters serve in an EMS communications system?
   A. They recycle radio traffic between mobile units and the base station at least five times to prevent the dispatcher from missing messages.
   B. They allow radio traffic to be heard only by the radio(s) intended to receive it.
   C. They extend the range of mobile radios by converting signals from VHF to UHF.
   D. They extend the range of mobile radios by receiving signals and retransmitting them at higher power on a different frequency.

9. The government agency that controls radio frequency allocations and regulates radio use is the _____.
   A. Federal Communications Commission
   B. United States Department of Health and Human Services
   C. United States Department of Homeland Security
   D. United States Department of Transportation

10. Radio reports to medical facilities always should follow a standard format because _____.
    A. hospital personnel may miss important details if the reporting format is unfamiliar
    B. significant information is less likely to be omitted and hospital personnel are less likely to miss significant details
    C. state and federal regulations require use of a standardized format
    D. this decreases the probability that significant information will be omitted

11. The principal transmitter and receiver of a communications system is the _____.
    A. base station
    B. mobile radio
    C. repeater
    D. satellite receiver

The following paragraph includes information about a patient you now are transporting to the hospital. Using the following information, write the specific details of your radio report to the receiving hospital. Include only those details that *should* be in your radio report. List the details of your radio report in the exact order in which you will be reporting the information to the receiving facility. What you write should be exactly what someone listening to your radio report would hear.

Hematoma to left forehead; bruising under both eyes; 24-year-old male; there is significant intrusion to the vehicle's passenger compartment; you establish IV access; you splinted the left arm during transport; you are dispatched to a vehicle versus concrete retaining wall; there are no other patients involved; vital signs are BP—118/70 mm Hg, P—144 beats/min, R—28 breaths/min; lung sounds are clear on the left and diminished with wheezes on the right; pupils are dilated, equal, and reactive; he is able to follow your penlight with his eyes; you transfer care to nurse Jones; patient is able to move his feet and hands; he complains of pain in his right chest and a headache; awake and responds appropriately to questions; he has a history of hypertension and thyroid disease; his abdomen is soft and nontender; he takes hydrochlorothiazide and L-thyroxine daily; he is able to open his mouth, stick out his tongue, and swallow; you provide spinal motion restriction using a back board, cervical collar, head blocks, tape, and spider straps; you provide oxygen before beginning your rapid trauma assessment; you transport the patient code 3 to the community level I trauma center.

_____
_____
_____
_____
_____
_____
_____
_____
_____
_____
_____
_____

19 Documentation

READING ASSIGNMENT

Chapter 19, pages 648-671, in *Paramedic Practice Today: Above and Beyond*.

OBJECTIVES

After completing this chapter, you will be able to:
1. Describe the potential consequences of illegible, incomplete, or inaccurate documentation.
2. Explain the role and importance of documentation as it pertains to the following:
   - Continuity of patient care
   - Quality management
   - Data collection
   - Research
   - Billing and reimbursement
3. Explain how to document information received from bystanders and other third-party sources.
4. Explain how to document scene assessment findings.
5. Discuss the importance of documenting pertinent positive and pertinent negative findings.
6. Explain the importance of using medical terminology appropriately.
7. Discuss the importance of using only locally approved medical abbreviations.
8. Discuss the importance of timely report writing and submission.
9. Be familiar with the different methods used to document, including the following:
   - Handwritten documentation
   - Electronic or computer-based documentation
   - Dictation
10. Discuss the importance of documenting with a consistent narrative style, as identified by local protocol.
11. Describe the differences between subjective and objective elements of documentation.
12. Identify irrelevant or unprofessional information.
13. Describe the special considerations for documenting a patient refusal of care or transport.
14. Describe the special considerations for documenting a multiple-casualty incident.
15. Evaluate a completed prehospital care report for the following:
    - Completeness
    - Thoroughness
    - Accuracy
    - Spelling
    - Grammar
    - Use of medical terminology
    - Use of approved abbreviations

CHAPTER SUMMARY

- Documentation is one of the most important parts of a paramedic's job.
- The report written by the paramedic commonly is the only documentation of the medical events on scene and during transport.
- Documentation can affect the following:
  - Patient care
  - Legal proceedings
  - Scope of practice
  - Education and training
  - Agency reimbursement
- The report written by the paramedic must be timely, complete, accurate, legible, objective, and free of errors.
- The report written by the paramedic should attempt to leave no questions in the reader's mind.
- The report written by the paramedic should leave no room for reader interpretation.
- Reports should be written in a set format, such as following the mnemonics CHART or SOAP or a narrative structure.
- Reports can be written by hand, entered in a computer-based system, or completed by dictation.
- All interactions with a patient should result in a written report.

SHORT ANSWER

1. List four uses of prehospital care reports (PCRs) in an EMS system.

   _____

   _____

   _____

   _____

2. If you make an error when filling out an EMS run report, how should you correct the error?

   _____

   _____

   _____

   _____

3. After you have filed an EMS run report, you discover you accidentally made an error while writing the report. What should you do?

   _____

   _____

   _____

   _____

4. What are the characteristics of a properly completed EMS run report?

_____
_____
_____
_____

5. State what is inappropriate about each of the following phrases from an EMS run report, and rephrase the statement so it would be more appropriate.
"The patient was drunk."

_____
_____
_____
_____

"The patient was shocky."

_____
_____
_____
_____

"Vital signs: pulse—normal; respirations—normal; BP—120/80"

_____
_____
_____
_____

6. What are the components of a report written in the SOAP format?

_____
_____
_____
_____

7. What are the components of a report written in the CHART format?

_____
_____
_____
_____

8. If a patient refuses care, what information should be included in the PCR?

_____
_____
_____
_____

9. What is the standard charting abbreviation for each of the following terms?
Chief complaint

_____

Date of birth

_____

History

_____

Signs and symptoms

_____

Vital signs

_____

Abdominal aortic aneurysm

_____

Left upper quadrant

_____

As needed

_____

Within normal limits

_____

10. What is the meaning of each of the following abbreviations?
PERRLA

_____

IDDM

_____

HPI

_____

EtOH

_____

CHF

_____

HTN

_____

CABG

_____

npo

_____

MULTIPLE CHOICE

1. Which of the following is an example of *correct* documentation on a medical record?
   A. A BP could not be obtained because of massive extremity trauma.
   B. The patient was drunk.
   C. The patient was shocky.
   D. Vital signs were normal.

2. Your patient states that she ingested six tablets of her prescription Prozac. She has a history of depression. You find an empty bottle of her prescription Prozac nearby. Which of the following statements regarding this information can be correctly included in the stated section of the PCR?
   A. In the assessment section state: "Possible OD and suicide attempt."
   B. In the objective section state: "The patient states she ingested six tablets of her prescription Prozac, which is supported by an empty prescription bottle found near the patient."
   C. In the subjective section state: "The patient states she ingested six tablets of her prescription Prozac. The patient reports she has a history of depression."
   D. In the subjective section state: "The patient states she ingested six Prozac tablets. She has a history of depression. An empty bottle of Prozac was found near the patient."

3. Which of the following is a *sign*?
   A. Dizziness
   B. Headache
   C. Jaundice
   D. Nausea

4. Which of the following is a *symptom*?
   A. Chest pain
   B. Cyanosis
   C. Diaphoresis
   D. Vomiting

5. Your patient is a woman experiencing pelvic pain. She states the pain comes and goes. During your assessment, she states the pain is beginning again. You measure the time that lapses until she states the pain has ended and determine it to be 2 minutes. This information should be included in which section of your patient care report?
   A. Either subjective or objective
   B. Objective
   C. Plan
   D. Subjective

6. If you make an error while writing a run report form, you should _____.
   A. carefully obliterate the error so its presence will not confuse future readers of the report
   B. carefully obliterate the error, write the word "error" over the obliteration, and then continue with the correct information
   C. draw a single line through the error, write in the correct information, and initial the change
   D. leave the error as is, and provide a note including the correct information at the end of the document

7. Writing on a PCR that a patient "probably has AIDS secondary to IV substance abuse" could place you at risk of being sued for _____.
   A. breach of confidence
   B. invasion of privacy
   C. libel
   D. slander

8. The prehospital care report becomes _____.
   A. a legal record of the care provided by the paramedics
   B. a source of information for research and quality improvement
   C. documentation of care, a legal record, and a source of research information
   D. documentation of the patient's initial condition, signs, and symptoms

9. If an error is discovered after a prehospital care report is submitted, you should _____.
   A. draw a single line through the error, write a note with the correct information at the end of the report, initial and date all changes, and distribute the corrected report to all appropriate personnel
   B. ignore it since there is no way to legally correct a report that has been submitted
   C. notify a supervisor to substitute a corrected report
   D. write an entirely new PCR, find and destroy the original form, and substitute the corrected form in its place

CASE STUDIES

Case one

Using any or all of the following information, write a SOAP report. You may reword any of this information. However, do not create new information or change the basic information presented. You will, however, need to create the assessment portion of the SOAP.

Hematoma to left forehead; bruising under both eyes; 24-year-old male; there is significant intrusion to the vehicle's passenger compartment; you establish IV access; you splinted the left arm during transport; you are dispatched to a vehicle vs. concrete retaining wall; there are no other patients involved; vital signs are BP—118/70 mm Hg, P—144 beats/min, RR—28/min; lung sounds are clear on the left and diminished with wheezes on the right; pupils are dilated, equal, and reactive; he is able to follow your penlight with his eyes; you transfer care to nurse Jones; patient is able to move his feet and hands; he complains of pain in his right chest and a headache; awake and responds appropriately to questions; he has a history of hypertension and thyroid disease; his abdomen is soft and nontender; he takes hydrochlorothiazide and

L-thyroxine daily; he is able to open his mouth, stick out his tongue, and swallow; you provide spinal motion restriction using a back board, cervical collar, head blocks, tape, and spider straps; you provide oxygen before beginning your rapid trauma assessment; you transport the patient code 3 to the community level I trauma center.

Case two

Write your CHART for the following patient using any or all of the information provided in the following paragraph. End your report with any further actions you might take if this was your patient.

You are dispatched to the parking lot of the local grocery store for a possible seizure patient. You arrive to find a 40-year-old man sitting on the curb. Initially, he is awake and alert but confused. Witnesses state the man was placing aluminum cans into a garbage bag. He regularly collects the cans along a nearby highway. The patient has alcohol on his breath. He denies pain of any type. He has no difficulty breathing. He has a history of seizures for which he takes Dilantin. He has been taking his Dilantin daily as prescribed. He denies recreational drug use today. His last meal was at noon today. In your examination, you find no obvious injuries other than the fact that he has bitten his tongue. He denies any other past medical history. He takes no other medications. During your examination, the patient's orientation improves and he is no longer confused. He is now aware of his present location, the day of the week, and his name. He refuses transportation to the hospital. You remind him that his medications make not be working well. You advise him that he should contact his physician and inform him of the seizure. You offer to transport the patient to the ER. Vital signs are BP—140/88 mm Hg, P—110 beats/min, RR—20/min; skin—warm and sweaty. The patient simply wants to go home. He lives only three blocks away.

---

20 Head, Ear, Eye, Nose, and Throat Disorders

READING ASSIGNMENT

Chapter 20, pages 674-689, in *Paramedic Practice Today: Above and Beyond.*

OBJECTIVES

After completing this chapter, you will be able to:
1. Describe the etiology, demographics, history, and physical findings for the following conditions:
   - Lice
   - Impetigo
   - Lesions
   - Headache
   - Bell's palsy
   - Ludwig's angina
2. By using the patient history and physical examination findings, develop a treatment plan for patients with the following conditions:
   - Lice
   - Impetigo
   - Lesions
   - Headache
   - Bell's palsy
   - Ludwig's angina
3. Describe the etiology, demographics, history, and physical findings for the following conditions:
   - Conjunctivitis
   - Inflammation of the eyelids
   - Glaucoma
   - Central retinal artery occlusion
   - Retinal detachment
4. By using the patient history and physical examination findings, develop a treatment plan for patients with the following conditions:
   - Conjunctivitis
   - Inflammation of the eyelids
   - Glaucoma
   - Central retinal artery occlusion
   - Retinal detachment
5. Describe the etiology, demographics, history, and physical findings for the following conditions:
   - Ear foreign bodies
   - Vertigo
   - Tinnitus
   - Otitis externa

6. By using the patient history and physical examination findings, develop a treatment plan for patients with the following conditions:
   - Ear foreign bodies
   - Vertigo
   - Tinnitus
   - Otitis externa
7. Describe the etiology, demographics, history, and physical findings for the following conditions:
   - Epistaxis
   - Nose foreign bodies
   - Piercing
   - Rhinitis
8. By using the patient history and physical examination findings, develop a treatment plan for patients with the following conditions:
   - Epistaxis
   - Nose foreign bodies
   - Piercing
   - Rhinitis
9. Describe the etiology, demographics, history, and physical findings for the following conditions:
   - Thrush
   - Broken, missing, or loose teeth
   - Sore throat
   - Epiglottitis
   - Peritonsillar abscess
10. By using the patient history and physical examination findings, develop a treatment plan for patients with the following conditions:
    - Thrush
    - Broken, missing, or loose teeth
    - Sore throat
    - Epiglottitis
    - Peritonsillar abscess

CHAPTER SUMMARY

HEAD

- Inspection and palpation are the primary ways to evaluate the structures of the head. Because of the vascular nature of this area, bleeding may be greater than the severity of the wound. Evaluate and reassure as needed. Both sides of the face should appear somewhat

143

symmetric on inspection. Gross deformities or a droop on one side should be further evaluated. Gross deformities of the face are typically the result of trauma. A droop on one side of the face, however, can be caused by several different illnesses. Illicit a good history to assist in the decision-making process.

EYES

■ The oval-shaped eyeballs sit in bony orbital cavities. The bones of the orbits are thin and susceptible to fracture from blunt force trauma. Assessment of the eye should primarily consist of inspection. Look for drainage, redness, movement through the fields of gaze, pupil size, and response to light. Whenever something being splashed into the eye is suspected, immediately begin flushing the eye and continue flushing the eye until instructed to stop by medical staff.

EARS

■ The external auditory canal should always be dry; any signs of drainage should be referred for further medical care. The tympanic membrane is located at the end of the auditory canal and serves as a barrier between the external and internal ear.

NOSE

■ The primary function of the nose is to filter, warm, and humidify incoming air before it gets to the lungs. The nose also houses the nerves that allow smell. Common problems with the nose usually involve foreign objects. Patient should be referred for removal and further medical care.

MOUTH

■ Assessment of the mouth requires visualization of the internal structures. Having the patient open the mouth should be adequate. Never put anything in the mouth.
■ Patients with hoarseness, stridor on inspiration or expiration, or drooling should be kept quiet and allowed to assume a position that facilitates breathing during transport. These signs suggest a possible life-threatening condition.

SHORT ANSWER

1. What differentiates the presence of louse eggs (nits) in the hair from dandruff?

2. Describe a patient who is suffering from otitis externa.

3. Describe a patient who is suffering from peritonsillar abscess.

4. What is the most immediate cause of concern for a patient with a peritonsillar abscess?

5. A 6-year-old male inserted a pea into his nasal cavity via the right nostril. How would you manage this patient?

6. What is vertigo?

7. What is thrush?

8. How should a tooth that has been knocked out of its socket be managed?

9. A patient with a history of severe osteoarthritis complains that she hears a constant buzzing sound. What is the medical term used for this sound and what question should you ask the patient that probably will identify the cause of the problem?

10. How should a patient with epistaxis be instructed to position his or her head? Why?

MULTIPLE CHOICE

1. A 30-year-old homeless man says he has lost the hearing in his left ear. He states his ear itches and is leaking fluid. You note a yellow-brown discharge from the left ear but not from the right ear. His ear is tender when you tug on it in order to look inside. You suspect this patient is suffering from _____.
   A. barotrauma
   B. otitis externa
   C. otitis media
   D. a ruptured eardrum

2. Your patient is a 65-year-old female with a history of chronic atrial fibrillation controlled with digoxin. She is complaining of severe pain in her right eye that radiates to her head and face. She also says she is nauseated and sees halos around lights. Her right eye is red with the pupil fixed and nonreactive in mid-position. The cornea appears "hazy." What problem should you suspect?
   A. Acute glaucoma
   B. Cerebrovascular accident
   C. Digitalis toxicity
   D. Retinal detachment

3. A 45-year-old male complains of loss of vision in his left eye. He says the vision in the affected eye "went gray" and then gradually disappeared completely. He denies any pain. The left eye is not red. The pupil does not react to light. The patient otherwise is neurologically intact. What problem should you suspect?
   A. Acute glaucoma
   B. Central retinal artery occlusion
   C. Cerebrovascular accident
   D. Retinal detachment

4. The patient is a 32-year-old female who awakened this morning to discover that she could not move the left side of her face or blink her left eye. She is awake and alert. Sensation over the affected side of her face is intact. She has no extremity motor or sensory deficits. There is no history of cardiopulmonary or neurologic disease. She takes no medications other than vitamins and birth control pills. Vital signs are: P—116 beats/min strong, regular; BP—136/90 mm Hg; R—16/min shallow, regular. What problem should you suspect?
   A. Bell's palsy
   B. Cerebrovascular accident
   C. Glossopharyngeal neuritis
   D. Trigeminal neuralgia

5. The problem being experienced by the patient in the previous question is due to inflammation of which cranial nerve?
   A. III
   B. V
   C. VII
   D. IX

6. Which statement about cluster headaches is correct?
   A. The pain is pulsating or throbbing.
   B. They begin during childhood.
   C. They occur more commonly in males than in females.
   D. They tend to be felt over the entire head.

7. Which statement about classic migraine headaches is correct?
   A. They are generalized and last for hours to days.
   B. They are generalized and last for only a short period of time.
   C. They involve one side of the head and last for hours to days.
   D. They involve one side of the head and last for only a short period of time.

8. Headaches associated with muscle tension _____.
   A. affect females more frequently than males
   B. affect males more frequently than females
   C. produce throbbing pain
   D. tend to be burning or stabbing in character

9. A 76-year-old male presents with redness and swelling on the left side of his face and neck. He says the swelling began near the base of his left ear and rapidly extended down his neck and up under his chin. The patient says he has had a toothache on the left side for about a week but cannot afford to go to the dentist. What problem should you suspect?
   A. Bell's palsy
   B. Ludwig's angina
   C. Peritonsillar abscess
   D. Retropharyngeal abscess

10. Which of the following statements best describes the severity of the disease for the patient in the previous question?
    A. This disease is immediately life-threatening because it can cause loss of the airway.
    B. This disease is immediately life-threatening because it can lead to meningitis.
    C. This disease is immediately life-threatening because it can spread to the mediastinum and cause pericarditis.
    D. This disease is not immediately life-threatening and can be treated easily with a tooth extraction and antibiotics.

11. An infection of the oil glands of the eyelid, commonly called a *stye*, also is known as a _____.
    A. chalazion
    B. hordeolum
    C. pengueculum
    D. pterygium

12. Which statement best describes the pattern of vision loss associated with chronic glaucoma?
   A. Gradual loss of eyesight near the central portion of the visual fields
   B. Gradual loss of peripheral vision, creating the sensation of looking down a tunnel
   C. Sudden, complete loss of eyesight associated with intense pain
   D. Sudden, painless loss of sight

13. A 6-year-old boy became ill about 4 hours ago and has been complaining of a severe sore throat. He will not eat or drink because he says it hurts too much to swallow. He is sitting up in bed, crying, and noticeably drooling. He appears very frightened. His axillary temperature is 104°F. Respirations are 30/min, shallow, regular. Nasal flaring is present on inhalation. The patient's chest is clear to auscultation. The life-threatening problem for which this patient is at greatest risk is _____.

A. airway obstruction
B. cardiac dysrhythmias
C. respiratory arrest
D. seizures

14. Which of the following statements about impetigo is correct?
   A. A honey-colored crust formed from the exudate released as the vesicles rupture characterizes impetigo.
   B. Impetigo can be distinguished from poison ivy because impetigo does not cause lesions on the face while poison ivy does.
   C. Impetigo produces fever, whereas chickenpox does not.
   D. The lesions of impetigo typically appear on the trunk and extremities.

CASE STUDY

You are called to see a 67-year-old female who is complaining of a severe headache radiating from her left eye. The patient also complains of seeing halos around lights. The affected eye is red. The cornea has a "steamy" appearance. The left pupil is midposition and nonreactive.

1. What problem do you suspect?

_____

_____

_____

_____

2. Describe the pathophysiology of this problem.

_____

_____

_____

_____

3. How would you manage this patient?

_____

_____

_____

_____

4. For long-term management of this patient's problem, her physician prescribes eye drops that contain timolol. Why would timolol be useful in preventing a reoccurrence of this problem?

_____

_____

_____

_____

21 Pulmonology

READING ASSIGNMENT

Chapter 21, pages 690-732, in *Paramedic Practice Today: Above and Beyond*.

OBJECTIVES

After completing this chapter, you will be able to:
1. Explain the importance of the respiratory tract and the prevalence of pulmonary disease.
2. Explain the basic role of pulmonary function testing in medical care.
3. Identify the anatomy of the upper airway.
4. Describe the etiology, epidemiology, history, and physical findings, and develop a treatment plan for a patient having any of the following upper airway disorders: upper respiratory tract infection, epiglottitis, croup, bacterial tracheitis, and peritonsillar abscess.
5. Describe the etiology, epidemiology, history, and physical findings, and develop a treatment plan for a patient having any of the following situations: upper airway obstruction, trauma, and tracheostomy.
6. Describe the etiology, epidemiology, history, and physical findings, and develop a treatment plan for a patient having any of the following disorders of the pleura, mediastinum, lung, and chest wall: costochondritis, pleurisy, pneumomediastinum, pneumothorax, pleural effusion, noncardiogenic pulmonary edema, and acute respiratory distress syndrome.
7. Identify the anatomy of the lower airway.
8. Describe the etiology, epidemiology, history, and physical findings, and develop a treatment plan for a patient having any of the following lower airway disorders: asthma, bronchiolitis, bronchopulmonary dysplasia, chronic obstructive pulmonary disease, cystic fibrosis, pneumonia, lung abscess, pulmonary thromboembolism, hyperventilation syndrome, atelectasis, and tumors.
9. Describe the etiology, epidemiology, history, and physical findings, and develop a treatment plan for a patient having a pulmonary infection such as pneumonia, tuberculosis, or aspiration pneumonia.
10. Describe the etiology, epidemiology, history, and physical findings, and develop a treatment plan for environmental and occupational exposure to inhaled agents and irritants, gases, fumes, and vapors.

CHAPTER SUMMARY

- Pulmonary dysfunction is generally the result of interference with ventilation, interference with diffusion, interference with perfusion, or combinations of any of these factors.
- Indicators of life-threatening respiratory distress include alterations in mental status, dyspnea at rest, severe cyanosis, absent breath sounds, audible stridor or other adventitious breath sounds, severe difficulty in speaking, tachycardia, pallor and diaphoresis, the presence of retractions, or the use of the accessory muscles.
- Hypoxia and/or hypercarbia can cause confusion, restlessness, irritability, lethargy, or coma.
- Indicators of respiratory compromise include the inability to complete sentences, the use of accessory muscles in the respiratory effort, or pursed lips on exhalation.
- Patients in respiratory distress are often tachycardic. However, bradycardia is associated with severe hypoxia and may indicate imminent cardiac arrest.
- Diagnostic tools available to the paramedic for evaluation of the patient in respiratory distress and the effectiveness of treatment include pulse oximetry, peak flow meters, and capnography.
- Respiratory diseases are categorized as two major varieties: upper respiratory conditions and lower respiratory conditions.
- Upper respiratory diseases tend to affect or limit inspired or expired air. An upper respiratory infection can cause a wide array of respiratory symptoms, including headache, nasal congestion, nasal drainage, nasal inflammation, sore throat, coughing, muscle aches, and mucus production with cough, fever, or chills.
- Epiglottitis is a potentially life-threatening infection of the supraglottic structures of the airway. It results in inflammation of the base of the tongue, aryepiglottic folds, arytenoids, tonsils, and the epiglottis itself. The patient with epiglottitis requires rapid transport and specialty care.
- Croup (laryngotracheobronchitis) affects young children and is manifested by infection of the upper airways. The area below the glottis is most commonly affected, resulting in swollen, inflamed mucosa.
- Bacterial tracheitis is a serious infection of the trachea, often requiring hospitalization.
- Peritonsillar abscess is a painful and frightening illness. The abscess begins when a bacterial infection forms on the back of the oropharynx, rooted in the richly vascular tissues of the adenoid tonsils. In rare instances it may compromise the upper airway.
- Foreign bodies in the airway can range from pins and needles to toys. Although the majority of patients are young children, some are adults.
- Penetrating and blunt trauma to the neck have the potential to generate life-threatening injuries.

147

- Most penetrating trauma to the neck is the result of knife or gunshot wounds. Blunt trauma is more frequently seen in motor vehicle crashes. Direct-force blunt trauma to the cricoid cartilage is capable of crushing the cartilage and creating an airway obstruction.
- In some chronic medical conditions, a tracheostomy must be surgically performed to support respiration.
- Costochondritis is inflammation of the cartilage in the anterior chest that causes chest pain.
- Pleurisy is painful rubbing of the pleural lining. The cause of the inflammation is often unknown.
- The presence of air in the mediastinum is called *pneumomediastinum*, which may occur spontaneously or as a result of trauma to the chest, mechanical ventilation, asthma, emphysema, lung or chest tumors, cocaine use, violent emesis or coughing, or childbirth, among other causes.
- Lower respiratory diseases limit the ability of the body to oxygenate the blood.
- A pneumothorax is a collection of air in the pleural space. Spontaneous pneumothorax is a pneumothorax that occurs in the absence of trauma. A primary spontaneous pneumothorax occurs in patients without underlying lung disease. A secondary spontaneous pneumothorax occurs in patients with an underlying lung disease.
- Fluid that collects in the pleural cavity is referred to as a *pleural effusion*. A pulmonary embolism is a common cause of pleural effusions in patients less than 40 years of age; therefore the presence of a coexisting embolus must be considered in these patients.
- Noncardiogenic pulmonary edema (NCPE) is a condition in which fluid accumulates in the alveoli in the absence of heart failure. NCPE has been noted in overdoses secondary to opioids, salicylates, cyclic antidepressants, and other medications.
- Acute respiratory distress syndrome is a clinical syndrome in which alveoli are damaged because of significant illness or injury. Some alveoli collapse and others fill with fluid, impairing the exchange of oxygen and carbon dioxide. As the syndrome progresses, more alveoli are affected, gas exchange is further impaired, and respiratory failure ensues, resulting in dyspnea, hypoxia, and pulmonary edema.
- Asthma is a type I allergic reaction associated with an inflammatory response that is expressed in the lower airways. Asthma is a reactive airway disease that many people underestimate.
- Bronchiolitis is an acute, infectious, inflammatory disease of the upper and lower respiratory tracts that results in obstruction of the small airways. Although it may occur in all age groups, the larger airways of older children and adults tolerate the respiratory syncytial virus infection better than infants.
- Bronchopulmonary dysplasia may occur in preterm infants as a result of prolonged treatment with positive-pressure ventilation and high oxygen concentrations.

- COPD may include varying degrees of bronchitis, emphysema, and asthma and is usually caused or worsened by tobacco abuse.
- Cystic fibrosis (CF) is a genetic disease in which glands create thicker-than-normal secretions. These thicker secretions cause chronic infections, resulting in the most common complication of the disease—pulmonary infections. Most fatalities from the disease result from progressive lung disease.
- Pneumonia is an infection in the alveoli and is particularly deadly in the elderly population. It can be caused by a wide variety of pathogens, ranging from bacteria to fungi to viruses. Pneumonia, regardless of cause, can prevent oxygenation. Thus it requires aggressive medical treatment.
- Pulmonary abscesses are collections of pus in the lung tissue itself. They are often the result of aspiration of gastric contents. It can take several weeks to develop clinical signs. Empyema is a collection of pus outside the lung in the pleural space.
- The inspiration of fluids not intended for the lungs is termed *aspiration*. Aspiration of gastric acid or food from the upper airway or stomach can cause an inflammatory response that can lead to hypoxia and respiratory failure. Aspiration pneumonitis is lung and bronchoalveolar irritation caused by aspirated stomach acid.
- Tuberculosis (TB) is a pulmonary disease caused by the bacterium *Mycobacterium tuberculosis*. It is transmitted by airborne droplets. Active TB is characterized by a productive cough, fever, and weight loss. Symptoms include hemoptysis, chest or chest wall pain, weight or appetite loss, fatigue, irritability, weakness, headache, chills, fever, and night sweats. TB requires respiratory isolation.
- A pulmonary embolus (PE) occurs when a thrombus (clot) becomes dislodged and travels (the clot is now an embolus), lodging in a pulmonary artery and obstructs blood flow to a portion of the lung. The clot may consist of blood, fat, or air. PE is often difficult to diagnose and can be a potentially fatal condition.
- Hyperventilation, strictly defined, is excess ventilation. This condition results in a respiratory alkalosis secondary to the increased elimination of carbon dioxide. Psychogenic hyperventilation is a diagnosis of exclusion and can be considered only after all other causes of respiratory distress have been ruled out.
- Partial or full physical collapse of the alveoli in parts of the lungs is called *atelectasis*. In atelectasis, the lung is fully expanded, but collections of alveoli are collapsed, inhibiting oxygenation.
- Pulmonary tumors have two varieties: benign (noncancerous) and malignant (cancerous). Malignant tumors may originate in the lung (called *primary tumors*) or may have spread from some other location, such as the liver, stomach, or pancreas (called *secondary tumors*).
- Environmental chemical exposures are often the result of mixing chemicals, usually cleaning products, or the use of solvent-based chemicals in enclosed spaces.

Respiratory symptoms include dyspnea, wheezing, tachypnea, anxiety, coughing, and sometimes coughing mucus, tearing, or drooling. Exposure to inhaled toxins is immediately managed by removal of the patient and medical team to a safe area.

- Continuous positive airway pressure (CPAP) is the delivery of slight positive pressure to prevent airway collapse and improve oxygenation and ventilation in spontaneously breathing patients. The patient wears a mask that covers the mouth and nose, providing continuous increased airway pressure throughout the respiratory cycle as the patient breathes. CPAP may be used to assist ventilation in patients with neuromuscular weakness, chronic pulmonary edema, or obstructive sleep apnea.
- Bilevel positive airway pressure (BiPAP) is delivered through a tight-fitting mask. In BiPAP therapy, two levels of positive pressure are delivered. One is delivered during inspiration to keep the airway open as the patient inhales, and the other (lower) pressure is delivered during expiration to reduce the work of exhalation.
- Care should be used when mechanically ventilating patients' lungs to avoid pneumothorax.

MATCHING

1. Match the structure with its anatomic name.
   - ____ Air sacs in which gas exchange occurs
   - ____ Double membrane covering lungs
   - ____ Flap covering the windpipe's opening
   - ____ Point where mainstem bronchi branch
   - ____ Smallest airways in respiratory tract
   - ____ Space between epiglottis and base of tongue
   - ____ Voice box
   - ____ Windpipe
   - ____ Throat

   A. Alveoli
   B. Bronchioles
   C. Carina
   D. Epiglottis
   E. Larynx
   F. Pharynx
   G. Pleura
   H. Trachea
   I. Vallecula

2. Match the disease with its description.
   - ____ 80% of cases begin before age 30 chitis
   - ____ Bronchospasm, excess mucus, bronchial edema
   - ____ Cyanosis present early in course of disease
   - ____ Cyanosis present only late in course of disease
   - ____ Excess bronchial mucus for at least

   A. Asthma
   B. Chronic bronchitis
   C. Emphysema

   - ____ 3 months for 2 successive years
   - ____ Progressive loss of alveolar wall elasticity
   - ____ Reversible obstructive airway disease

3. Match the sound with its description.
   - ____ Fine bubbling sounds caused by fluid in smaller airways and alveoli; do not change with coughing
   - ____ Harsh sound produced by partial obstruction of upper airway by base of tongue
   - ____ High-pitched, crowing sound on inspiration caused by narrowing of upper airway
   - ____ Rattling sound from mucus obstruction of larger airway; disappears or changes location and quality with coughing
   - ____ Sounds like two pieces of dry leather moving across each other; associated with inflammation of chest cavity's lining
   - ____ Whistling sound primarily on exhalation as air moves through narrow lower airways

   A. Crackles
   B. Friction rub
   C. Rhonchi
   D. Snoring
   E. Stridor
   F. Wheezing

SHORT ANSWER

1. Complete the following chart contrasting croup (laryngotracheobronchitis) and epiglottitis.

	Croup	Epiglottitis
Age group		
Type of organism		
Speed of onset		
Fever		
Drooling		
Sore throat		

2. What three beneficial actions does the nasal cavity have on inhaled air?

   _____

   _____

   _____

149

3. What is the name of the largest and most superior cartilage in the larynx?

_____

4. What is the name of the most inferior cartilage in the larynx?

_____

5. What is the only cartilage in the larynx that forms a complete ring?

_____

6. What is the thin, almost bloodless membrane that separates the thyroid and cricoid cartilages?

_____

7. Which of the mainstem bronchi is shorter and straighter? Why?

_____
_____
_____
_____

8. How many lobes does the right lung have? How many lobes does the left lung have? Why is there a difference?

_____
_____
_____
_____

9. What is the name of the double-walled membrane that encloses the lungs?

_____

10. What anatomic feature differentiates bronchioles from the larger airways?

_____
_____

11. What process is responsible for producing the exchange of oxygen and carbon dioxide between the alveolar air and the blood in the pulmonary capillaries?

_____

12. What nerve innervates the diaphragm?

_____

13. From what part of the central nervous system does this nerve arise?

_____

14. When a patient inhales, what does the diaphragm do? What do the intercostal muscles do?

_____
_____
_____
_____

15. What change do these movements produce in the intrathoracic volume? How do these movements affect the intrathoracic pressure?

_____
_____
_____
_____

16. Is inhalation an active or a passive process?

_____

17. When a patient exhales, what does the diaphragm do? What do the intercostal muscles do?

_____
_____
_____
_____

18. What change do these movements produce in the intrathoracic volume? How do these movements affect intrathoracic pressure?

_____
_____
_____
_____

19. Is exhalation an active or a passive process?

_____

20. Respirations normally are stimulated by what change in the arterial blood gases?

_____
_____
_____
_____

21. What is the drive that provides the backup to the respiratory drive?

_____
_____
_____

22. What change in the arterial blood gases triggers this drive?

_____
_____
_____

23. What change occurs in the arterial carbon dioxide levels of a patient with chronic obstructive pulmonary disease?

_____
_____
_____

150

24. Because of this change, patients with COPD may be breathing (theoretically) on what drive?

_____
_____
_____
_____

25. What effect can administration of high concentrations of oxygen have (theoretically) on the breathing of a COPD patient?

_____
_____
_____
_____

26. Is this potential problem ever a justification for withholding oxygen from a COPD patient? Why?

_____
_____
_____
_____

27. What is the minute volume of a patient who has a tidal volume of 500 mL and a respiratory rate of 20 breaths/minute?

_____

28. If a patient takes his deepest possible breath and then exhales the maximum amount of air possible, what is the volume of exhaled air called?

_____

29. What is the property of lung tissue that allows it to resume its resting shape after being stretched?

_____
_____
_____
_____

30. What happens to this property in the lungs of a patient with emphysema?

_____
_____
_____
_____

31. What is surfactant? What role does surfactant play in the mechanics of ventilation?

_____
_____
_____
_____

32. What is the anatomical dead air space?

_____
_____

33. What is the normal range for the $PaCO_2$?

_____

34. What is the normal range for the PaO_2?

_____

35. What is atelectasis?

_____
_____

36. What effect will extensive atelectasis have on the $PaCO_2$ and the PaO_2?

_____
_____

37. If a patient's respiratory rate and tidal volume are decreased, what change would you expect to see in the patient's $PaCO_2$?

_____
_____

38. If a patient's respiratory rate and tidal volume are increased, what change would you expect to see in the patient's $PaCO_2$?

_____
_____

39. In what form is most of the oxygen transported by the blood carried?

_____
_____

40. In what form is most of the carbon dioxide transported by the blood carried?

_____
_____

41. If the PaO_2 falls below 60 torr, what happens to the ability of hemoglobin to on-load and off-load oxygen? (HINT: Think oxyhemoglobin dissociation curve.)

_____
_____
_____
_____

42. When a patient becomes acidotic or hyperthermic, what happens to the affinity of hemoglobin for oxygen?

_____
_____
_____

43. When a patient becomes alkalotic or hypothermic, what happens to the affinity of hemoglobin for oxygen?

_____
_____
_____
_____

44. What effect would nebulized bronchodilators be expected to have on each of the following?
   a. Pulse rate: _____
   b. Skeletal muscles: _____
   c. Level of consciousness: _____

45. If a patient's respiratory rate and tidal volume are decreased:
   a. What change would you expect to see in the patient's arterial CO_2 level?

   _____

   b. What is this condition of decreased ventilation called?

   _____

   c. What change would you expect to see in the patient's pH?

   _____

   d. What would this acid-base imbalance be called?

   _____

46. If a patient's respiratory rate and tidal volume are increased:
   a. What change would you expect to see in the patient's arterial CO_2 level?

   _____

   b. What is this condition of increased ventilation called?

   _____

   c. What change would you expect to see in the patient's pH?

   _____

   d. What would this acid-base imbalance be called?

   _____

47. How is the acid-base imbalance that results from hyperventilation corrected?

   _____
   _____
   _____
   _____

48. If a patient has a partial airway obstruction with good air exchange and is coughing forcefully, how should the patient be managed?

   _____
   _____
   _____
   _____

49. If a patient has a partial airway obstruction with poor air exchange, how should the patient be managed?

   _____
   _____
   _____
   _____

50. Why is humidified oxygen administered during treatment of asthma?

   _____
   _____
   _____
   _____

51. What is the preferred oxygen administration device for a young adult who is having an acute asthma attack?

   _____

52. What is status asthmaticus? How is status asthmaticus managed?

   _____
   _____
   _____
   _____

53. Why is it important to obtain a medication history from a patient with asthma before giving any drugs?

   _____
   _____
   _____
   _____

54. Albuterol is what type of drug? Why are these drugs useful in the management of asthma attacks?

   _____
   _____
   _____
   _____

55. Racemic epinephrine is administered by what route to a child with croup?

   _____

56. Describe how racemic epinephrine is beneficial in a child with respiratory distress secondary to croup.

   _____
   _____
   _____
   _____

57. What is a normal SaO_2?

   _____

58. A patient presents with an SaO_2 of 90%. What action should you take?

_____
_____
_____
_____

59. A 16-year-old female was rescued from a house fire. The pulse oximeter reads 98%. What must be taken into consideration when interpreting this oximeter reading?

_____
_____
_____
_____

60. A patient is in cardiac arrest. Is there any value in placing a pulse oximeter on this patient as a means of evaluating oxygenation? Why or why not?

_____
_____
_____
_____

MULTIPLE CHOICE

1. You are called for a 24-year-old woman with a severe asthmatic attack. You find the patient sitting in a chair, alert, and anxious, but in obvious respiratory distress. Her family states she is now on her third nebulized Proventil treatment in the past 30 minutes with no relief. She has no other medical history. Her regular medications are Proventil, cromolyn, and Beclovent. Her vital signs are: BP—134/84 mm Hg, P—120 beats/min, R—28 breaths/min; lung sounds are difficult to hear but sound like wheezing in all fields; skin is warm, pink, clammy. She states her breathing is getting more difficult. Of the following, which is the most appropriate initial management of this patient after administering oxygen?
   A. 0.3 mg of epinephrine 1:1000 Sub-Q
   B. 0.5 mg of epinephrine 1:10,000 slow IV
   C. 2.5-mg unit-dose vial albuterol by SVN
   D. 125 mg of methylprednisolone IV

2. Epinephrine stimulates beta$_2$ receptors, which causes

   _____.
   A. an increased heart rate
   B. bronchial smooth muscle relaxation
   C. increased cardiac contractility
   D. cerebrospinal fluid

3. When blood bypasses alveoli without being oxygenated in the lungs because of malfunctioning alveoli (such as in pulmonary edema or atelectasis), the situation is referred to as a $\dot{V}/\dot{Q}$ mismatch or

   _____.
   A. intermittent ventilation
   B. perfusion
   C. shunting
   D. ventilation

4. You are called to a medical clinic for a 16-year-old girl who is hyperventilating. You arrive to find her sitting upright in a chair, appearing anxious. She is speaking in two- to three-word sentences. Auscultation of the chest reveals inspiratory and expiratory wheezes in all fields. According to the clinic nurse, the patient's pulse oximetry reading is 97% on room air. Her respiratory rate is 28 breaths/min, BP—122/78 mm Hg, P—110 beats/min. The nurse states the patient came into the office complaining of an upper respiratory tract infection and persistent cough, and the girl is accompanied by her mother. The 16-year-old was sitting in the waiting room when suddenly she felt short of breath. Your first impression of this patient leads you to suspect _____.
   A. an acute asthma attack
   B. chronic bronchitis
   C. hyperventilation syndrome
   D. pneumonia

5. A 65-year-old man is complaining of shortness of breath and chills. He states he has had a fever for 5 days and a productive cough with dark yellow sputum. Vital signs are BP—148/88 mm Hg, P—110 beats/min, R—24 breaths/min. Based on this information, your most likely diagnosis is _____.
   A. congestive heart failure
   B. pleuritis
   C. pneumonia
   D. sepsis

6. Which of the following conditions is characterized by the presence of a productive cough occurring on most days for at least 3 months of the year for at least 2 consecutive years?
   A. Asthma
   B. Chronic bronchitis
   C. Emphysema
   D. Pneumonia

7. While obtaining a history from your patient, you learn that she has difficulty sleeping. She states, "When I sleep flat, it becomes harder to breathe." This finding may be referred to as *orthopnea* or _____.
   A. aggravated dyspnea
   B. paroxysmal nocturnal dyspnea
   C. paroxysmal tachypnea
   D. spasmodic dyspnea

8. Clubbing of the fingers and peripheral cyanosis are associated with _____.
   A. atrial fibrillation
   B. chronic hypoxemia
   C. chronic pulmonary infections
   D. shock

153

9. You are called to see a 16-year-old female with respiratory difficulty. You arrive to find this patient with moderate respiratory difficulty. The girl's mother states that her daughter has a congenital condition that results in abnormal secretion of thick bronchial mucus. This condition is referred to as _____.
   A. cystic fibrosis
   B. Guillain-Barré syndrome
   C. myasthenia gravis
   D. pickwickian syndrome

10. You arrive at your local hospital to transport a 10-year-old asthmatic patient to a pediatric hospital. The receiving hospital physician has requested initiation of a terbutaline infusion at a specific rate. The physician's request is _____.
    A. correct because IV infusion is an acceptable route of administration for terbutaline
    B. correct because terbutaline can only be given by metered dose inhaler and IV infusion route
    C. incorrect because terbutaline cannot be given by the IV infusion route
    D. incorrect because terbutaline is only given by metered dose inhaler or subcutaneous injection

11. Neurologic initiation of ventilation begins in the _____.
    A. cerebellum
    B. cerebrum
    C. medulla
    D. pons

12. The *primary* control for ventilation relies on the _____.
    A. $PaCO_2$
    B. PaO_2
    C. pH of blood in the pulmonary artery
    D. pH of cerebrospinal fluid

13. Your unit is preparing to transfer a 50-year-old man from one hospital to another. You are told the patient is currently on CPAP. Based solely on this information, you correctly determine _____.
    A. the patient is breathing spontaneously
    B. the patient is definitely not on a ventilator
    C. the patient is on a ventilator
    D. the patient is intubated

14. Your patient has a history of asthma. You are seeing her today because she is having a mild asthma attack. She has not taken her Proventil inhaler because it is empty. At this early stage of her asthmatic episode, which of the following blood gas changes would you expect?
    A. Decreased $PaCO_2$, decreased PaO_2
    B. Decreased $PaCO_2$, increased PaO_2
    C. Increased $PaCO_2$, decreased PaO_2
    D. Increased $PaCO_2$, increased PaO_2

15. You respond to a group home to see a 17-year-old female experiencing difficulty breathing. She states she has a history of cystic fibrosis. Considering her disease, which of the following statements regarding her health history will most likely be a *correct* statement?
    A. Her breathing is best when she is in a warm environment.
    B. She has a history of pancreatic duct obstructions.
    C. She rarely experiences wheezing.
    D. She was just diagnosed with cystic fibrosis 2 years ago.

16. The signs and symptoms of hyperventilation syndrome result from _____.
    A. a metabolic acidosis secondary to anxiety
    B. a metabolic alkalosis secondary to some underlying pathology
    C. a respiratory acidosis resulting from poor peripheral perfusion
    D. a respiratory alkalosis without an underlying pathology

17. You are called to see a 2-year-old boy who is experiencing respiratory difficulty. He has been ill with a low-grade fever and cough for the past few days. Tonight, he awakened suddenly with stridor and difficulty breathing. His voice is hoarse and he has a strange sounding cough. You suspect this child is suffering from _____.
    A. bronchiolitis
    B. croup
    C. epiglottitis
    D. pneumonia

18. You are called to a residence where a 10-year-old girl is reportedly having a reaction to her medications. She has recently been diagnosed with asthma and used her own Ventolin inhaler for the first time today. Her mother believes the girl is having an allergic reaction to the medication because she is experiencing nausea, headache, and restlessness. Based on this information, you believe this patient _____.
    A. has overdosed on her medication
    B. is experiencing an allergic reaction to the Ventolin
    C. is experiencing typical side effects of this drug
    D. is having an anxiety reaction

19. The role of the Hering-Breuer reflex in pulmonary function is that it _____.
    A. initiates an inflammatory response when foreign substances enter the lungs
    B. initiates ventilation in response to increased $PaCO_2$.
    C. prevents overinflation of the lungs
    D. prevents use of the hypoxic drive

20. You are assessing a 78-year-old woman in her home. She has been resting in her bed in a semireclined position propped upright with four to five pillows. The patient's daughter believes her mother is retaining fluid. Where would you assess this patient for dependent edema?

A. Her ankles and lower legs
B. Her lungs
C. Her posterior legs, buttocks, and lower back
D. Her posterior trunk

21. You respond to a local high school to see a 15-year-old boy with difficulty breathing secondary to asthma. As you enter the room, the school nurse tells you that he is doing much better now. He came to her office 1 hour ago but did not have to use his inhaler. His respiratory rate was 40 breaths/min 1 hour ago but is now only 16 breaths/min. She does not believe you are needed and is ready to sign any form you have. Your next step is to _____.

A. assess the patient because this may be impending respiratory failure
B. assess the patient even though he seems to be breathing better now
C. have the nurse sign the refusal form
D. quickly look at the patient and ask if he wants your help

22. Your patient is a 50-year-old emphysema patient who is in severe respiratory distress. He has not responded to multiple inhaled beta-agonist treatments. Your partner is now assisting ventilations with a bag-mask. The patient has a history of severe episodes such as this one. He takes theophylline, prednisone, and albuterol daily. The patient has previously told his family he does not ever want to be intubated because he stays on the ventilator for too many weeks. Which of the following would be the next best course of action for you to initiate?

A. Administer another albuterol by nebulizer and drive quickly to the hospital.
B. Administer 0.3 mg of epinephrine 1:1000 Sub-Q.
C. Administer sedation and neuromuscular blockers in order to intubate the patient.
D. Administer 0.25 mg of terbutaline Sub-Q.

23. A 35-year-old man is complaining of shortness of breath. He states this began suddenly about 30 minutes ago. He had just left the airport after returning from a trip to Hawaii. He now complains of a sharp pain in his left chest. He has no significant medical history but has smoked cigarettes for the past 20 years. Lung sounds are clear bilaterally. Vital signs are: P—120 beats/min, BP—110/76 mm Hg, R—36/min, skin—pink, warm, dry. You suspect this patient is experiencing _____.

A. an acute myocardial infarction
B. an exacerbation of emphysema
C. a pulmonary embolism
D. a spontaneous pneumothorax

24. On arrival at a local medical clinic, the physician advises you this patient has a pleural effusion with an associated friction rub. He is referring to fluid within the patient's _____.

A. alveoli
B. chest soft tissue
C. interstitial space
D. pleural space

25. A 67-year-old male complains of severe dyspnea that awakened him approximately 20 minutes ago. He says he has been awakening in the night short of breath for several weeks. He had a myocardial infarction 1 year ago. He has a history of hypertension and has smoked two packs of cigarettes a day for 30 years. His respirations are noisy and labored, his lips and nailbeds are cyanotic, and he is coughing up pink, frothy sputum. When you listen to his chest, you hear wheezing and fine crackling noises throughout the lung fields. Vital signs: BP—140/86 mm Hg; P—100 beats/min weak, irregular; R—32/min labored, regular. What problem do you suspect?

A. Asthma
B. Congestive heart failure with pulmonary edema
C. Decompensated pulmonary emphysema
D. Lung cancer

26. A 16-year-old female complains of a sudden onset of dyspnea, dizziness, sharp chest pains, and tingling in her hands and feet that began after an argument with her boyfriend. She has no history of heart or lung disease. Vital signs are: BP—140/70 mm Hg; P—110 beats/min strong, regular; R—32 breaths/min deep, regular. How would you manage this patient?

A. Coach the patient to slow her breathing.
B. Give oxygen at 4 to 6 L/min by nasal cannula.
C. Give oxygen at 12 to 15 L/min by nonrebreather mask.
D. Transport immediately "code 3."

27. You are giving oxygen by nonrebreather mask at 12 L/min to a 57-year-old male with a history of pulmonary emphysema who is complaining of difficulty breathing and a productive cough. The patient suddenly becomes unconscious and stops breathing. A strong carotid pulse of 108 beats/min is present. What should you do?

A. Place the patient on oxygen by nasal cannula at 4 to 6 L/min.
B. Remove all oxygen and wait for the patient to resume breathing.
C. Ventilate the lungs using a bag-mask and oxygen at 4 to 6 L/min.
D. Ventilate the lungs using a bag-mask and oxygen at 12 to 15 L/min.

28. A 35-year-old male experienced sudden, sharp pain in his left chest followed by dyspnea while he was eating dinner. Breath sounds are decreased on the left side. His vital signs are: BP—144/96 mm Hg; P—110 beats/min strong, regular; R—26 breaths/min regular. What problem probably is present?
    A. Acute myocardial infarction
    B. Pulmonary embolism
    C. Spontaneous pneumothorax
    D. Tension pneumothorax

29. Which disease is characterized by excessive mucus production in the bronchial tree and a recurrent productive cough?
    A. Asthma
    B. Anaphylaxis
    C. Chronic bronchitis
    D. Emphysema

30. Which disease is characterized by loss of elasticity in the lung tissue and destructive changes in the alveolar walls?
    A. Anaphylaxis
    B. Asthma
    C. Chronic bronchitis
    D. Emphysema

31. Which statement *best* describes asthma?
    A. An inflammation of the bronchioles and alveolar walls caused by a viral infection that results in wheezing and shortness of breath
    B. An obstructive pulmonary disease characterized by distention of the pulmonary air spaces and destructive changes in their walls
    C. An obstructive pulmonary disease characterized by episodes of severe bronchospasm, bronchial edema, and hypersecretion of mucus in the lower airways
    D. An obstructive pulmonary disease characterized by excessive mucus production in the bronchial tree with a chronic productive cough

32. Which of the following statements about COPD is *correct*?
    A. Chronic bronchitis patients tend to purse their lips as they exhale.
    B. Cyanosis tends to occur early in the course of chronic bronchitis but late in the course of emphysema.
    C. Emphysema patients frequently cough up large amounts of mucus while chronic bronchitis patients seldom cough.
    D. COPD patients are usually females in rural areas who have no history of smoking.

33. Common signs and symptoms of an acute asthma attack include _____.
    A. a slow pulse rate and a lowered blood pressure
    B. squeezing chest pain
    C. wheezing heard primarily on expiration
    D. wheezing heard primarily on inspiration

34. Patients with COPD may breathe in response to _____.
    A. decreased carbon dioxide levels in the arterial blood
    B. decreased oxygen levels in the arterial blood
    C. increased carbon dioxide levels in the arterial blood
    D. increased oxygen levels in the arterial blood

35. Normally the body's stimulus to breathe is based on the level of _____.
    A. carbon dioxide in the arterial blood
    B. carbon dioxide in the venous blood
    C. either carbon dioxide or oxygen in the arterial blood
    D. oxygen in the arterial blood

CASE STUDIES

Case one

A 20-year-old female developed severe dyspnea approximately 20 minutes ago. She is conscious, but is agitated and confused. Her lips and nailbeds are cyanotic, and her neck veins are distended. She also complains of left-sided pleuritic chest pain. Breath sounds are present bilaterally with an area of localized wheezing on the left side. The patient has a history of recent surgery for damaged tendons in the right ankle. The right ankle is in a cast. The patient takes birth control pills and also is taking codeine for pain secondary to her ankle surgery. Vital signs: P—140 beats/min weak, regular; BP—88/50 mm Hg; R—34 breaths/min labored, regular.

1. From what problem is the patient suffering?

   _____

2. What is the most likely cause of this problem?

   _____

3. What other mechanisms can produce this problem?

_____

_____

4. What is Virchow's triad?

_____

_____

5. Why is this patient experiencing dyspnea?

_____

_____

6. Why are the patient's neck veins distended?

_____

_____

7. Why is the patient becoming hypotensive and developing a tachycardia?

_____

_____

_____

_____

8. Is the history of recent surgery significant? Why or why not?

_____

_____

_____

_____

9. Is the history of birth control pill use significant? Why or why not?

_____

_____

_____

_____

10. Is the use of codeine significant? Why or why not?

_____

_____

_____

_____

Case two

A 70-year-old retired fire captain complains of severe dyspnea that began suddenly about 45 minutes ago. The patient says that after he coughed forcefully, he experienced sharp pain in the right upper lung field that was followed by shortness of breath that rapidly increased in severity. His skin is flushed with some peripheral cyanosis. His chest has an increased anteroposterior (AP) diameter. The patient is thin and wasted. His fingertips are clubbed, and he purses his lips when he exhales. Distant breath sounds are present over the right lung field and the lower portion of the left lung field. However, breath sounds are absent over the upper portion of the right lung field.

1. From what underlying disease process is this patient suffering?

_____

2. What is the most common reason patients develop this disease?

_____

_____

3. What effect does this disease process have on a patient's $PaCO_2$ level? Why?

_____

_____

4. Why do patients with this disease process develop an increased thoracic AP diameter?

_____

_____

5. Why do patients with this disease process purse their lips when they exhale?

_____

_____

6. If you percussed this patient's chest, what would you expect to find?

_____

_____

7. Why do patients with this disease normally have distant breath sounds in their lung fields?

_____

_____

8. Do patients with this disease process normally have a productive cough?

_____

9. The presence of a recurrent cough productive of thick, white sputum would suggest the presence of what related disease process?

_____

10. The presence of a cough productive of yellow, green, rust-colored, or blood-streaked sputum would suggest what related disease process?

_____

11. What problem probably explains the sudden onset of dyspnea and the absent breath sounds over the upper right lung field?

_____

Case three

At 0400 hours, you are called to see "a child who can't breathe." You arrive at an apartment about 5 minutes from your station where two very anxious parents await you. They tell you that their 11-year-old son, who has a history of severe asthma, developed an attack the previous morning and "has just gotten worse and worse." He has been using his metered-dose inhaler without apparent benefit. You find a very sick-looking child who is sitting upright in bed and struggling to breathe. He is extremely agitated and restless and does not want to sit still for your examination. There are suprasternal and intercostal retractions on inhalation. The patient's skin is pale and dry. The mucous membranes are also dry. Pulse is 130 beats/min, weak, regular. Respirations are 30 breaths/min, shallow, regular. Auscultation of the chest reveals a few faint wheezes throughout the lung fields. The chest is hyperresonant to percussion.

1. What three events in a patient's lungs characterize an asthma attack?

_____

_____

_____

2. Why should oxygen given to patients suffering asthma attacks be humidified?

_____

_____

3. What term is used to describe an asthma attack that will not respond to beta-adrenergic agents?

_____

4. A patient with a prolonged asthma attack will tend to develop what acid-base abnormality?

_____

5. What impact does this acid-base abnormality have on the effectiveness of treatment with beta-adrenergic agents?

_____

_____

6. What is significant about the near absence of wheezing in the patient's lung fields?

_____

_____

7. Why is the dryness of the mucous membranes significant?

_____

_____

8. If you elect to give a beta-adrenergic agent to this patient, what problem should you anticipate?

_____

_____

_____

_____

9. Why could Atrovent be useful in the management of this patient?

_____

_____

_____

10. Why are steroids useful in the management of asthma?

_____

_____

_____

_____

11. What is the disadvantage of trying to use steroids in the acute management of an asthma attack?

_____

_____

_____

_____

Case four

An 23-year-old female with a history of asthma is complaining of difficulty breathing and is wheezing loudly. The patient's blood gases on oxygen by nonrebreather mask are PaO_2—350 mm Hg; $PaCO_2$—30 mm Hg; pH—7.48.

1. What acid-base imbalance is indicated by the blood gases?

_____

2. Is this what you would anticipate for this patient?

_____

_____

3. What physiologic process accounts for the acid-base imbalance?

_____

Thirty minutes later, the patient's blood gases are PaO_2—200 mm Hg; $PaCO_2$—40 mm Hg; pH—7.38. She continues to complain of difficulty breathing and is tachypneic.

4. What do the changes in the patient's blood gases indicate?

_____
_____
_____
_____

Case five

A 58-year-old male with a 30-pack-year smoking habit complains of difficulty breathing. He says that he has had a productive cough for "about 6 years" and that he has been "catching chest colds a lot lately." He reports that normally he coughs up "white stuff" but for the past couple of days "it's been yellow with blood in it." The patient is awake but appears to be very drowsy. His skin has a "bluish-red" appearance. Auscultation of the lung fields reveals distant breath sounds associated with diffuse wheezes and rhonchi. During the physical examination you discover that the patient has bilateral pitting edema of the lower extremities.

1. From what underlying disease process is this patient suffering?

_____

2. What is the most common reason patients develop this disease?

_____

3. What effect does this disease process have on a patient's $PaCO_2$ level? Why?

_____

4. Do patients with this disease process normally have a productive cough?

_____

5. When does cyanosis usually occur in the progression of this disease (early or late)?

_____

6. What problem is suggested by the changes occurring in this patient's sputum?

_____

7. Why does this patient have pitting edema of the lower extremities?

_____
_____

22 Cardiovascular Disorders

READING ASSIGNMENT

Chapter 22, pages 733-890, in *Paramedic Practice Today: Above and Beyond*. Questions in this chapter will require you to apply, integrate, and synthesize your prior knowledge of anatomy and physiology, pathophysiology, and pharmacology, as well as your new knowledge of cardiology.

OBJECTIVES

After completing this chapter, you will be able to:

1. Describe the epidemiology of cardiovascular disease.
2. Identify the risk factors most predisposing to coronary heart disease.
3. Discuss prevention strategies that may reduce the morbidity and mortality rates of coronary heart disease.
4. Identify the major structures of the vascular system.
5. Describe the anatomy of the heart, including the position in the thoracic cavity, layers of the heart, chambers of the heart, and location and function of cardiac valves.
6. Identify the normal characteristics of the point of maximal impulse.
7. Identify phases of the cardiac cycle.
8. Identify the arterial blood supply to any given area of the myocardium.
9. Compare the coronary arterial distribution with the major portions of the cardiac conduction system.
10. Identify the structures of the autonomic nervous system and their effects on heart rate, rhythm, and contractility.
11. Define and give examples of positive and negative inotropism, chronotropism, and dromotropism.
12. Identify and define the components of cardiac output and the factors affecting venous return.
13. Define *preload, afterload,* and *left ventricular end-diastolic* pressure and relate each to the pathophysiology of heart failure.
14. Describe the clinical significance of Starling's law.
15. Define the functional properties of cardiac muscle.
16. List the most important ions involved in the cardiac action potential and their primary functions in this process.
17. Describe the events involved in the steps from excitation to contraction of cardiac muscle fibers.
18. Define the events composing the cardiac action potential.
19. Correlate the electrophysiologic and hemodynamic events occurring throughout the entire cardiac cycle with the various ECG waveforms, segments, and intervals.
20. Identify the structure and course of all divisions and subdivisions of the cardiac conduction system.
21. Identify and describe how the heart's pacemaking control, rate, and rhythm are determined.
22. Explain the physiologic basis of conduction delay in the atrioventricular node.
23. Differentiate the primary mechanisms responsible for producing cardiac dysrhythmias.
24. Describe reentry.
25. Explain the purpose of ECG monitoring.
26. Identify the limitations of the ECG.
27. Relate the cardiac surfaces or areas represented by the ECG leads.
28. Describe correct anatomic placement of the chest leads.
29. Identify how heart rates, durations, and amplitudes may be determined from ECG recordings.
30. Describe how ECG waveforms are produced.
31. Recognize the changes on the ECG that may reflect evidence of myocardial ischemia and injury.
32. Describe a systematic approach to the analysis and interpretation of cardiac dysrhythmias.
33. Describe the ECG characteristics, possible causes, signs and symptoms, and initial emergency care for dysrhythmias originating in the sinus node.
34. Describe the ECG characteristics, possible causes, signs and symptoms, and initial emergency care for dysrhythmias originating in the atria.
35. Describe aberrant conduction.
36. Define *synchronized cardioversion* and discuss the indications and methods for this procedure.
37. Describe the significance of accessory pathways.
38. Describe the ECG characteristics, possible causes, signs and symptoms, and initial emergency care for dysrhythmias originating in the atrioventricular junction.
39. Describe the ECG characteristics, possible causes, signs and symptoms, and initial emergency care for dysrhythmias originating in the ventricles.
40. Describe the conditions of pulseless electrical activity.
41. Describe the process and pitfalls in the differentiation of wide QRS complex tachycardias.
42. Describe the dysrhythmias seen in cardiac arrest.
43. Define *defibrillation* and discuss the indications and methods for this procedure.
44. Describe the electrocardiographic characteristics, possible causes, signs and symptoms, and initial emergency care of atrioventricular blocks.
45. Describe the characteristics of an implanted pacemaking system.
46. List the causes and implications of pacemaker failure.

47. Recognize the complications of artificial pacemakers as evidenced on electrocardiogram.
48. Identify additional hazards that interfere with artificial pacemaker function.
49. Describe artifacts that may cause confusion when evaluating the electrocardiogram of a patient with a pacemaker.
50. Describe the components and the functions of a transcutaneous pacing system.
51. Identify the indications for transcutaneous cardiac pacing.
52. Describe the technique of applying a transcutaneous pacing system.
53. Explain what each setting and indicator on a transcutaneous pacing system represents and how the settings may be adjusted.
54. List the possible complications of transcutaneous pacing.
55. Based on the pathophysiology and clinical evaluation of the patient with a suspected acute myocardial infarction, list the anticipated clinical problems according to their life-threatening potential.
56. Identify the ECG changes characteristically seen during evolution of an acute myocardial infarction.
57. Recognize the limitations of the ECG in reflecting evidence of myocardial ischemia and injury.
58. Describe the abnormalities originating within the bundle branch system.
59. Identify the ECG changes characteristically produced by electrolyte imbalances.
60. Identify and describe the components of the focused history as it relates to the patient with cardiovascular compromise.
61. Identify what is meant by the OPQRST of chest pain assessment.
62. Explain the clinical significance of paroxysmal nocturnal dyspnea.
63. Identify patient situations for which ECG rhythm analysis is indicated.
64. Identify and describe the details of inspection, auscultation, and palpation specific to the cardiovascular system.
65. Identify and define the heart sounds.
66. Relate heart sounds to hemodynamic events in the cardiac cycle.
67. Describe the differences between normal and abnormal heart sounds.
68. Define pulse deficit, pulsus paradoxus, and pulsus alternans.
69. Describe how to determine if pulsus paradoxus, pulsus alternans, or electrical alternans is present.
70. Describe the clinical significance of unequal arterial blood pressure readings in the arms.
71. Describe the etiology, epidemiology, history, and physical findings of acute coronary syndromes.
72. Using the patient history, physical examination findings, and ECG analysis, develop a treatment plan for a patient with an acute coronary syndrome.

73. Describe the incidence of myocardial conduction defects.
74. List other clinical conditions that may mimic signs and symptoms of acute coronary syndromes.
75. Describe the etiology, epidemiology, history, and physical findings of heart failure.
76. Using the patient history, physical examination findings, and ECG analysis, develop a treatment plan for a patient in heart failure.
77. Describe the etiology, epidemiology, history, and physical findings of myocarditis.
78. Using the patient history, physical examination findings, and ECG analysis, develop a treatment plan for a patient with myocarditis.
79. Describe the etiology, epidemiology, history, and physical findings of cardiogenic shock.
80. Using the patient history, physical examination findings, and ECG analysis, develop a treatment plan for a patient in cardiogenic shock.
81. Describe the etiology, epidemiology, history, and physical findings of cardiac arrest.
82. Using the patient history, physical examination findings, and ECG analysis, develop a treatment plan for a patient in cardiac arrest.
83. Assess and manage an adult immediately after resuscitation from a cardiac arrest.
84. Identify and list the inclusion and exclusion criteria for termination of resuscitation efforts.
85. Identify communication and documentation protocols with medical direction and law enforcement used for termination of resuscitation efforts.
86. Describe the etiology, epidemiology, history, and physical findings of a hypertensive emergency.
87. Using the patient history, physical examination findings, and ECG analysis, develop a treatment plan for a patient with a hypertensive emergency.
88. Describe the etiology, epidemiology, history, and physical findings of endocarditis.
89. Using the patient history, physical examination findings, and ECG analysis, develop a treatment plan for a patient with endocarditis.
90. Describe the etiology, epidemiology, history, and physical findings of pericarditis.
91. Using the patient history, physical examination findings, and ECG analysis, develop a treatment plan for a patient with pericarditis.
92. Describe the etiology, epidemiology, history, and physical findings of pericardial tamponade.
93. Using the patient history, physical examination findings, and ECG analysis, develop a treatment plan for a patient with pericardial tamponade.
94. Describe the etiology, epidemiology, history, and physical findings of an aortic aneurysm.
95. Using the patient history, physical examination findings, and ECG analysis, develop a treatment plan for a patient with an aortic aneurysm.
96. Describe the etiology, epidemiology, history, and physical findings of vascular disorders.

97. Using the patient history, physical examination findings, and ECG analysis, develop a treatment plan for a patient with a vascular disorder.

CHAPTER SUMMARY

- Cardiovascular disorders are diseases and conditions that involve the heart and blood vessels. Heart disease refers to conditions affecting the heart. Heart disease is the leading cause of death in the United States. Coronary heart disease refers to disease of the coronary arteries and their resulting complications, such as angina pectoris or acute MI. Coronary artery disease affects the arteries that supply the heart muscle with blood.

- Risk factors are traits and lifestyle habits that may increase a person's chance of developing a disease. Some risk factors associated with coronary heart disease can be modified. Risk factors that cannot be modified are called *nonmodifiable* or *fixed risk factors*. Contributing risk factors are thought to lead to an increased risk of heart disease, but their exact role has not been defined.

- Arteries are conductance vessels that carry blood from the heart under high pressure. Arterioles are the smallest branches of the arteries. They are called *resistance vessels* because they have smooth muscle in their walls that allows the vessel to adjust its diameter, controlling the amount of blood flow to specific tissues. Capillaries are the smallest blood vessels. They connect arterioles and venules and function as exchange vessels. Venules connect capillaries and veins. Veins carry oxygen-poor blood from the body to the right side of the heart. Because most of the body's blood is located in them at any one time, veins are called *capacitance* (storage) *vessels*.

- The heart has four chambers that function as two functional pumps. The right atrium and right ventricle comprise one pump. The left atrium and left ventricle comprise the other. The right side of the heart is a low-pressure system (pulmonary circulation). The left side of the heart is a high-pressure pump (systemic circulation). The walls of the heart are composed of the endocardium, myocardium, and epicardium. Four valves in the heart (two atrioventricular [AV] valves and two semilunar [SL] valves) ensure blood flows in one direction through the heart's chambers and prevent the backflow of blood. The heart has three major coronary arteries: the left anterior descending (LAD), circumflex (CX), and right coronary artery (RCA).

- Parasympathetic stimulation of the heart slows the firing rate of the sinoatrial (SA) node, slows conduction through the AV node, decreases the strength of atrial contraction, and can cause a small decrease in the force of ventricular contraction. Sympathetic stimulation of the heart results in increased force of contraction, increased heart rate, and increased blood pressure.

- Cardiac output is the amount of blood pumped into the aorta each minute by the heart. It is defined as the stroke volume (amount of blood ejected from a ventricle with each heartbeat) multiplied by the heart rate. Stroke volume is determined by the degree of ventricular filling when the heart is relaxed (preload), the pressure against which the ventricle must pump (afterload), and the myocardium's contractile state (contracting or relaxing).

- The cardiac action potential is a five-phase cycle that reflects the difference in the concentration of charged particles across the cell membrane at any given time. The polarized state is the period after repolarization of a myocardial cell (also called the *resting state*) when the outside of the cell is positive and the interior of the cell is negative. Depolarization is movement of ions across a cell membrane, causing the inside of the cell to become more positive. It is an electrical event expected to result in contraction. Repolarization is movement of ions across a cell membrane in which the inside of the cell is restored to its negative charge.

- The SA node is the heart's normal pacemaker. The built-in (intrinsic) rate of the SA node is 60 to 100 beats/min. The AV junction is the AV node and the nonbranching portion of the bundle of His. The bundle of His has pacemaker cells capable of discharging at a rate of 40 to 60 beats/min. The Purkinje fibers have pacemaker cells capable of firing at a rate of 20 to 40 beats/min.

- The ECG records the electrical activity of a large mass of atrial and ventricular cells as specific waveforms and complexes. Three types of leads are used: standard limb leads, augmented limb leads, and chest (precordial) leads. The position of the positive electrode on the body determines which portion of the left ventricle is seen by each lead. Leads I, II, and III are the standard limb leads. Leads aVR, aVL, and aVF are augmented limb leads. The chest leads are identified as V_1, V_2, V_3, V_4, V_5, and V_6.

- ECG paper is graph paper composed of small and large boxes measured in millimeters. The horizontal axis of the paper corresponds with time. The vertical axis of the ECG paper measures the voltage or amplitude of a waveform. Voltage is measured in millivolts (mV).

- A waveform is movement away from the baseline in either a positive (upward) or a negative (downward) direction. Waveforms are named alphabetically, beginning with P, QRS, T, and U. A segment is a line between waveforms. It is named by the waveform that precedes or follows it. An interval is a waveform and a segment. A complex is several waveforms.

- The P wave represents atrial depolarization and the spread of the electrical impulse throughout the right and left atria. The QRS complex consists of the Q wave, R wave, and S wave. It represents the spread of the electrical impulse through the ventricles (ventricular depolarization). The T wave represents ventricular repolarization.

- The PR interval represents the interval between the onset of atrial depolarization and ventricular depolarization. The ST segment represents the early part of repolarization of the right and left ventricles. The point where the QRS complex and the ST segment meet is called the ST-junction, or J-point. The TP segment is the portion of the ECG tracing between the end of the T wave and the beginning of the next P wave.

- A rhythm that begins in the SA node has a positive (upright) P wave before each QRS complex, P waves that look alike, a constant PR interval, and (usually) a regular atrial and ventricular rhythm. A rhythm that begins in the atria has a positive P wave shaped differently than P waves that begin in the SA node.

- A rhythm that begins in the atria has a positive P wave shaped differently than P waves that begin in the SA node. This difference in P-wave configuration occurs because the impulse begins in the atria and follows a different conduction pathway to the AV node.

- If the AV junction paces the heart, the electrical impulse must travel in a backward (retrograde) direction to activate the atria. If a P wave is seen, it will be inverted in leads II, III, and aVF because the impulse is traveling away from the positive electrode. If the atria depolarize before the ventricles, an inverted P wave will be seen before the QRS complex. If the atria and ventricles depolarize at the same time, a P wave will not be visible because it will be hidden in the QRS complex. If the atria depolarize after the ventricles, an inverted P wave will appear after the QRS complex.

- When an ectopic site within a ventricle assumes responsibility for pacing the heart, the electrical impulse bypasses the normal intraventricular conduction pathway. This results in stimulation of the ventricles at slightly different times. As a result, ventricular beats and rhythms usually have QRS complexes that are abnormally shaped and longer than normal (measuring more than or equal to 0.12 second).

- In first-degree AV block, all components of the ECG tracing usually are within normal limits except the PR interval. This is because electrical impulses normally travel from the SA node through the atria, but a delay occurs in impulse conduction, usually at the level of the AV node. Second-degree AV blocks are types of incomplete blocks because the AV junction conducts at least some impulses to the ventricles. In third-degree AV block, impulses generated by the SA node are blocked before reaching the ventricles, so no P waves are conducted. Third-degree AV block also is called *complete AV block*. The block may occur at the AV node, bundle of His, or bundle branches.

- A pacemaker is an artificial pulse generator that delivers an electrical current to the heart to stimulate depolarization. Pacemaker systems usually are named according to where the electrodes are located and the route the electrical current takes to the heart.

- In right bundle branch block (BBB), the last portion of the QRS complex points up. In left BBB, the last portion of the QRS complex is directed downward. Patients with a temperature less than 32°C (89.6°F) may develop a unique ECG pattern called a *J wave* (also called an *Osborne wave*), which is seen at the J-point.

- A systematic approach to the assessment of the cardiac patient is important so that you do not overlook physical findings or important signs pertinent to the treatment plan for your patient.

- Acute coronary syndromes (ACSs) are conditions caused by a similar sequence of pathologic events—a temporary or permanent blockage of a coronary artery. This sequence of events results in conditions ranging from myocardial ischemia or injury to death (necrosis) of heart muscle. ACS include unstable angina, non–ST-segment elevation MI (NSTEMI), and ST-segment elevation MI (STEMI). Sudden cardiac death (SCD) can occur with any of these conditions.

- Heart failure is a condition in which the heart is unable to pump enough blood to meet the metabolic needs of the body. Heart failure is a syndrome, not a disease, that can result from disorders that impair the ability of the ventricle to fill with or eject blood. In acute heart failure, symptoms occur suddenly. In chronic heart failure, symptoms develop more slowly. Although failure of either ventricle can occur by itself, they often fail together. Right ventricular failure (RVF) often is a result of left ventricular failure (LVF).

- Shock is inadequate tissue perfusion that results from the failure of the cardiovascular system to deliver sufficient oxygen and nutrients to sustain vital organ function. The underlying cause must be recognized and treated promptly or cell and organ dysfunction and death may result.

- Cardiac arrest is the absence of cardiac pump function, confirmed by the absence of a detectable pulse, unresponsiveness, and apnea or agonal, gasping breathing. Cardiac arrest may be reversible but will lead to death without prompt emergency care. Sudden cardiac death (SCD) is an unexpected death from a cardiac cause that occurs either immediately or within 1 hour of the onset of symptoms. In some cases the patient in cardiac arrest will not respond despite appropriate basic and advanced life support care. Some EMS systems have developed protocols that allow field termination of resuscitation efforts in specific circumstances.

- Uncontrolled high blood pressure can lead to vision problems and increases the risk of serious health problems such as stroke, heart attack, heart failure, or kidney failure. Hypertensive urgencies are significant elevations in blood pressure with nonspecific symptoms that should be corrected within 24 hours. Hypertensive emergencies are situations that require rapid (within 1 hour) lowering of blood pressure to prevent or limit organ damage.

- Endocarditis occurs when bacteria in the bloodstream lodge and begin to multiply on a heart valve or other damaged tissue in the heart. If untreated, the bacteria can damage the heart valve, causing it to malfunction. Pericarditis is an inflammation of the double-walled sac (pericardium) that encloses the heart. A pericardial effusion is an increase in the volume and/or character of pericardial fluid that surrounds the heart. Cardiac tamponade occurs when the buildup of pericardial fluid compresses the heart and impairs contraction and ventricular filling.

- Congenital heart defects may obstruct blood flow in the heart or the vessels near it or cause an alteration in the normal pattern of blood flow through the heart.
- An aneurysm is a localized dilation or bulging of a blood vessel wall (or wall of a heart chamber). The dilated area may leak or rupture if it stretches too far. Dissection or rupture of the aorta is a medical emergency.
- An acute arterial occlusion is a sudden disruption of arterial blood flow that occurs because of a thrombus, embolus, tumor, direct trauma to an artery, or an unknown cause. Acute limb (extremity) ischemia results when an arterial occlusion suddenly reduces blood flow to an arm or leg. Intermittent claudication is pain, cramping, muscle tightness, fatigue, or weakness of the legs when walking or during exercise.
- Vasculitis is an inflammation of blood vessels. This disorder can affect vessels of any type in any organ. Thrombophlebitis is the development of a clot in a vein in which inflammation is present. Superficial thrombophlebitis occurs when a clot develops in a vein near the skin surface. If a clot develops in the deep veins of the extremities, deep venous thrombosis (DVT) is present. DVT is associated with an increased risk of pulmonary embolism.

SHORT ANSWER

1. What are the three layers that compose the walls of the heart?

2. What is the fibrous, double-walled sac that surrounds the heart?

3. What is the name of the inner layer of this sac that lies against the heart? What is the name of the outer layer of this sac that touches the diaphragm and the pleura?

4. What are the three layers that compose blood vessels?

5. What vessels carry blood away from the heart?

6. Integrating what you learned in Chapter 7 and this chapter, do these vessels always carry oxygenated blood? If there is an exception, what is it?

7. What vessels carry blood toward the heart?

8. Integrating what you learned in Chapter 7 and this chapter, do these vessels always carry unoxygenated blood? If there is an exception, what is it?

9. What type of blood vessel contains valves?

10. What is the purpose of these valves?

11. Based on your prior knowledge of cardiovascular anatomy and physiology (Chapter 7) and the information contained in this chapter, what type of blood vessel is primarily responsible for controlling the resistance to blood flow of the cardiovascular system?

12. Integrating your knowledge from Chapter 7 and the information in this chapter, what type of blood vessel is primarily responsible for controlling the capacitance (volume storage capacity) of the cardiovascular system?

13. What type of blood vessel provides the exchange surface between the cardiovascular system and the interstitial space?

_____
_____
_____

14. Applying your prior knowledge of anatomy and physiology and what you have learned in this chapter, what mechanism is responsible for the movement of blood on the arterial side of the cardiovascular system?

_____
_____
_____
_____

15. What is the function of the heart valves?

_____
_____
_____
_____

16. What valve separates the right atrium from the right ventricle? What valve separates the right ventricle from the pulmonary artery? What valve separates the left atrium from the left ventricle? What valve separates the left ventricle from the aorta?

_____
_____
_____
_____

17. Which valves are referred to collectively as the *atrioventricular (AV) valves*? What accounts for this name?

_____
_____
_____
_____

18. Which valves are referred to collectively as the *semilunar (SL) valves*? What accounts for this name?

_____
_____
_____
_____

19. Considering how blood flows through the heart, would the AV valves be open or closed during ventricular systole?

_____
_____
_____

20. Considering how blood flows through the heart, would the SL valves be open or closed during ventricular systole?

_____
_____
_____

21. Considering how blood flows through the heart, would the AV valves be open or closed during ventricular diastole?

_____
_____
_____

22. Considering how blood flows through the heart, would the SL valves be open or closed during ventricular diastole?

_____
_____
_____

23. The AV valves are attached by fibrous strands of tissue to small muscular projections from the inner surface of each ventricle. What is the name of these fibrous strands of tissue? What is the name of the muscular projections to which they attach? What function do these tissue strands serve?

_____
_____
_____
_____

24. What does it mean when we say a valve is "stenosed"?

_____
_____
_____
_____

25. What does the term *valvular regurgitation* mean?

_____
_____
_____

26. What blood vessels provide blood and oxygen to the myocardium? From what structure do these blood vessels arise?

_____
_____
_____

27. During which phase of the cardiac cycle (systole or diastole) do these vessels fill with blood?

_____
_____
_____

28. What blood vessel provides most of the blood flow to the anterior surface of the left ventricle?

_____

_____

_____

29. What blood vessel provides most of the blood flow to the lateral surface of the left ventricle?

_____

_____

_____

30. What blood vessel provides most of the blood flow to the right ventricle and to the inferior surface of the left ventricle?

_____

_____

_____

31. Coronary circulation may be referred to as being *left dominant*. This terminology is specific to the blood supply of the inferior wall of the left ventricle. Based on your knowledge of coronary artery anatomy and physiology, what do you believe this means?

_____

_____

_____

32. Coronary circulation may be referred to as being *right dominant*. This terminology is specific to the blood supply of the inferior wall of the left ventricle. Based on your knowledge of coronary artery anatomy and physiology, what do you believe this means?

_____

_____

_____

33. What blood vessel provides most of the blood flow to the AV node?

_____

_____

_____

34. What is the normal pathway of an impulse through the electrical conducting system of the heart?

_____

_____

_____

35. What is the intrinsic rate of firing of pacemaker sites in the following: the SA node; the AV node; the ventricular conduction system?

_____

_____

_____

36. What part of the cardiac conduction system normally acts as the heart's pacemaker? Why?

_____

_____

_____

37. What effect will stimulation of the vagus nerve have on the rate of firing of the SA node? What effect will it have on the rate of conduction through the AV node?

_____

_____

_____

38. What effect will stimulation of the sympathetic nervous system have on the following: the rate of firing of the SA node; the rate of impulse conduction through the AV node; the force of contraction of the ventricles?

_____

_____

_____

39. What is preload?

_____

_____

_____

40. Based on what you learned about preload and myocardial contractility in both this chapter and prior chapters, how can these factors interact to increase stroke volume? What is the name given to this phenomenon?

_____

_____

_____

41. Combining what you learned about muscle contraction in Chapter 7 and your new knowledge of Starling's law, synthesize answers for the following questions. Why does increasing the amont of 'stretch' in the heart result in a greater contraction? Is there a limit to this mechanism of increasing the force of contraction? If so, why?

_____

_____

_____

42. What is afterload?

_____

_____

_____

43. What is stroke volume?

_____

_____

_____

44. Based on what you learned in this chapter and in Chapter 7, predict the effect on stroke volume if preload increases.

_____

_____

_____

_____

45. Based on what you learned in this chapter and in Chapter 7, predict the effect on stroke volume if preload decreases.

_____

_____

_____

_____

46. Based on what you learned in this chapter and in Chapter 7, predict the effect on stroke volume if contractility increases.

_____

_____

_____

47. Based on what you learned in this chapter and in Chapter 7, predict the effect on stroke volume if contractility decreases.

_____

_____

_____

_____

48. Based on what you learned in this chapter and in Chapter 7, predict the effect on stroke volume if afterload increases.

_____

_____

_____

_____

49. Based on what you learned in this chapter and in Chapter 7, predict the effect on stroke volume if afterload decreases.

_____

_____

_____

_____

50. Based on what you learned in this chapter and in Chapter 7, what is the relationship between stroke volume, heart rate, and cardiac output?

_____

_____

_____

51. Based on what you learned in this chapter and in Chapter 7, if stroke volume increases, what will happen to cardiac output?

_____

_____

_____

52. Based on what you learned in this chapter and in Chapter 7, if stroke volume decreases, what will happen to cardiac output?

_____

_____

_____

53. Consider what you learned about cardiac output in both Chapter 7 and this chapter. When applying the principles of the formula for cardiac output, what effect would an increasing heart rate have on cardiac output?

_____

_____

_____

54. Clinically, an increase in heart rate will produce the effect above only to a point. Then the opposite effect occurs. Applying the principles represented by the formula for cardiac output, as well as what you learned in both Chapter 7 and this chapter, why does this occur?

_____

_____

_____

55. In Chapter 7 you learned about the factors that make up a blood pressure. Referring to that chapter as needed, what is the relationship between cardiac output, peripheral vascular resistance, and blood pressure?

_____

_____

_____

56. What effect will constricting the arterioles have on the peripheral vascular resistance?

_____

_____

_____

57. What effect will dilating the arterioles have on the peripheral vascular resistance?

_____

_____

_____

58. Integrating the formula you learned for blood pressure in Chapter 7 and the principles you learned in this chapter, what do you believe would happen to the blood pressure if peripheral vascular resistance increases?

_____

_____

_____

_____

59. Integrating the formula you learned for blood pressure in Chapter 7 and the principles you learned in this chapter, what do you believe would happen to the blood pressure if peripheral vascular resistance decreases?

_____

_____

_____

60. What effect will an increase in heart rate usually have on myocardial oxygen demand?

_____

_____

_____

_____

61. What effect will a decrease in heart rate usually have on myocardial oxygen demand?

_____

_____

_____

_____

62. Forceful, prolonged episodes of coughing can produce dizziness and light-headedness. Utilizing your knowledge of anatomy, physiology, and cardiology, what explanation can you provide for this phenomenon?

_____

_____

_____

_____

63. Applying what you learned about left ventricular failure and pulmonary edema, why do patients with this condition benefit from sitting up and dangling their lower extermities?

_____

_____

_____

_____

64. Utilizing your prior knowledge of pharmacology from Chapters 11-13, and applying that knowledge to patients experiencing a cardiac emergency, what kind of drug is epinephrine?

_____

_____

_____

_____

65. As you learned in pharmacology, epinephrine has many cardiac effects. What effect will administration of epinephrine have on the following: heart rate, myocardial contractility, peripheral vascular resistance, blood pressure, myocardial oxygen demand?

_____

_____

_____

_____

66. Applying your knowledge of anatomy, physiology, and pharmacology to the cardiac patient, consider the following. Isoproterenol (Isuprel) is a beta adrenergic agonist that affects both beta 1 and beta 2 receptors and has minimal to no alpha effects. Knowing this, what effect will administration of isoproterenol have on the following: heart rate, myocardial contractility, peripheral vascular resistance, myocardial oxygen demand?

_____

_____

_____

_____

67. With the information given about isoproterenol in the above question, what effect(s) can isoproterenol potentially produce on the blood pressure?

_____

_____

_____

_____

68. Integrating your prior knowledge of the mechanism of action of nitroglycerine, and your knowledge of cardia anatomy and physiology and acute coronary syndromes, please provide two mechanisms by which nitroglycerine may relieve the pain of angina pectoris.

_____

_____

_____

_____

69. What effect does nitroglycerin have on the peripheral vascular resistance? What effect does nitroglycerin have on the blood pressure?

_____

_____

_____

_____

70. Use your knowledge of the mechanism of acion of nitroglycerine, and your knowledge of cardiac anatomy and physiology to answer the following questions. What effect can administration of nitroglycerin have on the heart rate? Why should this effect be taken into consideration when giving nitroglycerin to patients with myocardial ischemia?

_____

_____

_____

_____

71. Utilizing your prior knowledge of pharmacology from Chapters 11-13, and applying that knowledge to patients experiencing a cardiac emergency, what kind of drug is norepinephrine?

_____

_____

_____

_____

72. As you learned in pharmacology, norepinephrine has many cardiac effects. What effect will norepinephrine have on the following: heart rate, myocardial contractility, peripheral vascular resistance, blood pressure, and myocardial oxygen demand?

_____

_____

_____

_____

73. In a patient with an acute MI, bradycardia may be left untreated if the patient shows no signs of decreased cardiac output. Why?

_____

_____

_____

_____

74. In a patient with left ventricular failure, what might happen if preload is increased by rapidly infusing IV fluids? Why?

_____

_____

_____

_____

75. Utilizing your prior knowledge of pharmacology from Chapters 11-13, and applying that knowledge to patients experiencing a cardiac emergency, what kind of drug is Inderal (propanolol)?

_____

_____

_____

76. Combining your knowledge of pharmacology, the autonomic nervous system, and cardiology, what effect will administration of Inderal have on the following: heart rate; myocardial contractility; cardiac output; blood pressure; myocardial oxygen demand?

_____

_____

_____

_____

77. The administration of Inderal is contraindicated in congestive heart failure. Based on your knowledge of the medication and the cardiovascular system, why is this the case?

_____

_____

_____

_____

78. Integrating what you have learned about the cardiovascular system and left ventricular failure, why are medications that cause vasodilation, such as nitroglycerine, useful in the management of left ventriculare failure?

_____

_____

_____

_____

79. Why is morphine sulfate useful in the management of acute MI?

_____

_____

_____

_____

80. If a patient having an acute MI presents with AV conduction defects, what coronary artery would you anticipate being the site of the blockage?

_____

_____

_____

_____

81. Based on what you have learned about cardiac anatomy and physiology, left ventricular failure, and coronary artery perfusion, what coronary artery would you suspect is blocked if a patient having an acute myocardial infarction presents with signs and symptoms of left ventricular failure, pulmonary congestion, and poor peripheral perfusion?

_____

_____

_____

82. Is it possible for a patient to infarct both the inferior and the posterior walls of the heart as a result of only one thrombus? What condition must exist in the coronary circulation for this to happen?

_____

_____

_____

_____

83. Considering the pathophysiology of a right ventricular infarction and its systemic effects, what might happen to the patient's cardiac output and blood pressure if you administer medications with vasodilatory effects, such as nitroglycerine or morphine? What accounts for this phenomenon?

_____

_____

_____

_____

84. Consider the role of the right ventricle, and the effects on the heart of a ventricular infarction. If you suspect that a patient is having a right ventricular infarct, what action should you consider before giving medications that cause vasodilation?

_____

_____

_____

_____

85. Consider the functions of the left side of the heart. Based on this knowledge what effect do you suspect mitral stenosis would have on left ventricular preload? What will happen to the cardiac output? What can happen to the pressure in the pulmonary capillary beds? What problem could result from this?

_____

_____

_____

_____

86. Much like in hypertrophic cardiomyopathy of the left ventricle, mitral valve stenosis can lead to increased pressures in the left atrium. In this situation what can happen to the left atrium over time?

_____

_____

_____

_____

87. Consider the function of the mitral valve. If a patient has mitral regurgitation, what can happen to the cardiac output? What will happen to the pressure in the pulmonary capillary beds? What problem will result from this?

_____

_____

_____

_____

88. Applying your knowledge of blood flow through the heart, what might happen to the cardiac output in the setting of an aortic stenosis? Over time, what could happen to the left ventricle?

_____

_____

_____

_____

89. As you learned in Chapter 21 if a patient has emphysema or chronic bronchitis they can develop pulmonary hypertension. Integrating your knowledge of cardiology what effect will this have on the afterload of the right ventricle?

_____

_____

_____

_____

90. A patient with severe congestive heart failure is receiving infusions of dobutamine (a beta 1 adrenergic medication, see Appendix B for more information) and nitroglycerin. Why would dobutamine be beneficial in the management of congestive heart failure? What kind of drug is nitroglycerin? What effect does nitroglycerin have that potentiates the effects of dobutamine in congestive heart failure?

_____

_____

_____

_____

91. You have been summoned to a small community hospital to transfer a patient who has been diagnosed as having a dissecting aortic aneurysm secondary to severe uncontrolled hypertension. When you receive report from the nursing staff, you are told that the patient has received a beta blocker. Why do you think the physician ordered a beta blocker to this patient?

_____

_____

_____

_____

92. After receiving nitroglycerin for an episode of angina pectoris, a 72-year-old female felt dizzy and weak. Her pulse rate increased. Her skin became pale, cool, and diaphoretic. And she began to complain of *worsening* chest pain. What probably accounts for the pallor, dizziness, and weakness? What probably accounts for the increase in the patient's heart rate? Why did the patient's chest pain worsen after you gave the nitroglycerin? (HINT: Think about what nitroglycerin does, what component of the blood pressure is likely to be impacted most by this effect, and when the coronaries fill with blood.) How should you manage this patient? Why?

_____

_____

_____

_____

171

93. A patient has labored breathing, distended neck veins, tachycardia, rales in the lung bases, pedal edema, and a third heart sound (S$_3$). What problem do you suspect?

_____

_____

_____

_____

MULTIPLE CHOICE

1. A 62-year-old female complains of substernal tightness radiating to her left shoulder and to her jaw bilaterally. She has a history of poorly controlled diabetes mellitus and hypertension. A 12-lead ECG shows ST segment elevation in leads V$_1$-V$_3$. Initial vital signs are: BP—136/104 mm Hg; P—118 beats/min strong, regular; R—22 breaths/min shallow, regular. You have placed the patient on oxygen by nonrebreather mask, established a keep-open IV, and given 325 mg of ASA and 0.4 mg of nitroglycerin. About 2 minutes later the patient begins to complain of dizziness and weakness. She is pale, cool, and diaphoretic. Her radial pulses now are thready. BP is 86/50 mm Hg. Based on your knowledge of the cardiovascular system, and the mechanism of action of nitroglycerine, what would be your best action?

A. Place the patient supine; elevate her lower extremities; infuse D$_5$W.

B. Place the patient supine; elevate her lower extremities; infuse normal saline or Ringer's lactate.

C. Place the patient supine; elevate her lower extremities; start dopamine at 5 mcg/kg/min.

D. Place the patient supine; give the patient another 0.4 mg of nitroglycerin since her myocardial ischemia is worsening.

2. You arrive on the scene of a cardiac arrest to find the fire department doing quality CPR on a 65-year-old male. When you perform a quick look, you see this rhythm:

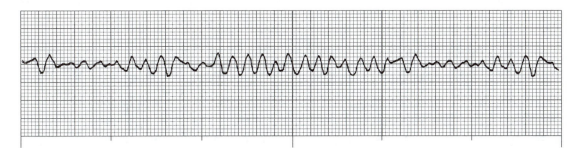

You are using a monophasic defibrillator. You should _____.
A. immediately charge the defibrillator to 200 J and defibrillate
B. immediately charge the defibrillator to 360 J and defibrillate
C. intubate; start an IV; give epinephrine 1.0 mg IV push; defibrillate at 200 J
D. intubate; start an IV; give amiodarone 300 mg IV push; defibrillate at 200 J

3. A 16-year-old female developed palpitations after an argument with her boyfriend. She is awake and alert. Her skin is warm and dry. Breath sounds are present and equal bilaterally with no adventitious sounds. Vital signs are: P—approximately 150 beats/min strong, regular; BP—128/84 mm Hg; R—18 breaths/min shallow, regular.

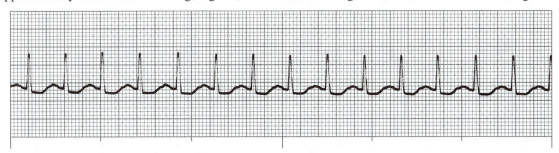

The initial treatment for this patient should be to _____.
A. cardiovert with 50 joules
B. give adenosine 6 mg IV push
C. have her do a vagal maneuver to decrease her vagal tone
D. have her do a vagal maneuver to increase her parasympathetic tone

4. The following is the ECG of a 45-year-old male complaining of an "empty" feeling in the center of his chest. He is awake and alert. His skin color and temperature are within normal limits. Breath sounds are present and equal bilaterally with no adventitious sounds. Vital signs are: P—150 beats/min; BP—130/70 mm Hg; R—16 breaths/min shallow, regular.

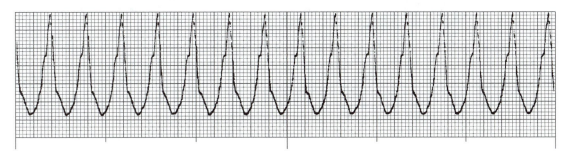

The initial treatment for this patient should be _____.
A. adenosine 6 mg IV push
B. amiodarone, 150 mg infused over 10 minutes, or lidocaine, 1 - 1.5 mg/kg IV push
C. cardioversion at 100 J
D. vagal maneuvers

5. The following is the ECG of a 57-year-old female who suddenly developed severe substernal chest pain, weakness, and dizziness about 10 minutes ago. She is extremely anxious and agitated. Her skin is pale, cool, and clammy. Breath sounds are present and equal bilaterally with no adventitious sounds. Vital signs are: P—180 beats/min weak, regular; BP—100/90 mm Hg; R—24 breaths/min shallow, regular.

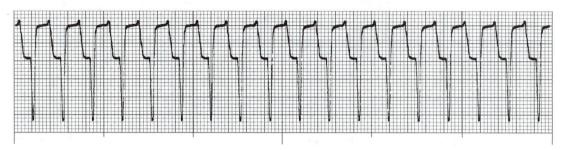

The initial management for this patient would be to give oxygen, start an IV, and _____.
A. give 5 mg of midazolam and perform synchronized cardioversion at 50–100 J
B. give adenosine 6 mg IV push
C. give amiodarone 50-100 mg IV push
D. have the patient do Valsalva's maneuver

6. The following is the ECG of a 73-year-old male complaining of crushing chest pain that began suddenly 15 minutes ago. He is lethargic and has diffiulty responding to questions. His skin is pale, cool, and dry. Breath sounds are present and equal bilaterally with no adventitious sounds. Vital signs are: P—approximately 210 beats/min, weak, and regular; BP—90/70 mm Hg; R—20 breaths/min shallow, regular.

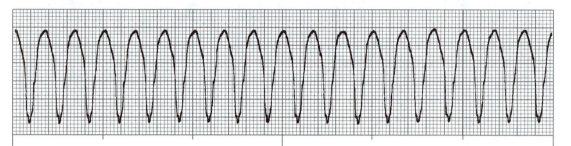

After giving oxygen and starting an IV, you should _____.
A. perform synchronized cardio version at 100 J
B. give adenosine 6 mg IV push
C. give lidocaine 1–1.5 mg/kg IV push, or 150 mg amiodarone over 10 minutes by IV infusion
D. have the patient do Valsalva's maneuver

7. Following resuscitation from ventricular fibrillation, a 48-year-old male has the ECG shown below. Vital signs are: P—consistent with monitor; BP—82 mm Hg/palpation; R—0 breaths/min, supported by bag-mask device.

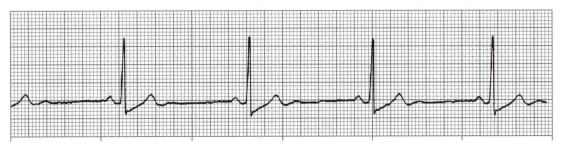

What sequence is the correct order of treatment?
A. Atropine 0.5 mg IV push; dopamine infusion at 5 mcg/kg/min; transcutaneous pacing; evaluate adequacy of oxygenation and ventilation
B. Dopamine infusion at 5 mcg/kg/min; atropine 0.5 mg IV push; transcutaneous pacing; evaluate adequacy of oxygenation and ventilation
C. Evaluate adequacy of oxygenation and ventilation; atropine 0.5 mg IV push; transcutaneous pacing; dopamine infusion at 5 mcg/kg/min
D. Evaluate adequacy of oxygenation and ventilation; transcutaneous pacing; dopamine infusion at 5 mcg/kg/min; atropine 0.5 mg IV push

8. The following is the ECG of a 67-year-old male with a history of COPD. He complains of shortness of breath, slight chest pain, and is sitting in a tripod position. His skin is flushed and warm. Wheezing is present in all lung fields. Vital signs are: P—75 beats/min weak, regular; BP—162/96 mm Hg; R—24 breaths/min shallow, regular. How would you manage this patient?

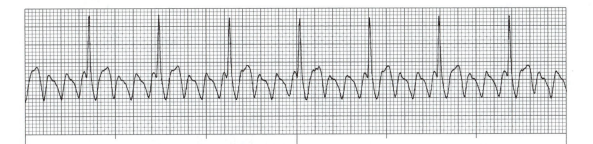

A. Oxygen, IV NS or LR, cardioversion at 50 J
B. Oxygen, IV NS or LR, nebulized albuterol via SVN
C. Oxygen, IV NS or LR, vagal maneuvers
D. Oxygen, IV NS or LR, verapamil 5 mg slow IV push

9. The following is the ECG of a 72-year-old female with severe dyspnea. She is awake and alert. Although she responds appropriately to questions, she is very frightened. Auscultation of the chest reveals rales and rhonchi in all lung fields. Pedal edema is present. She has a 3-month history of worsening dyspnea on exertion. The patient has had one previous MI approximately 3 months ago and chronic essential hypertension for approximately 20 years. Vital signs are: BP—110/76 mm Hg; R—28 breaths/min shallow, labored; P—consistent with rate of ECG.

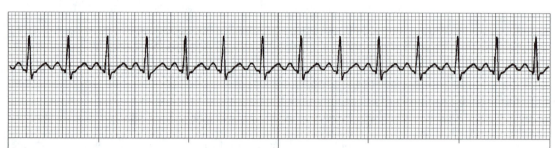

Your goals in managing this patient will be focused on _____.
A. decreasing preload; improving myocardial contractility; decreasing afterload
B. decreasing preload; improving myocardial contractility; increasing peripheral resistance
C. decreasing preload; increasing heart rate; improving myocardial contractility
D. increasing preload; decreasing myocardial oxygen demand; decreasing afterload

10. Initial management for the patient in the previous question should include _____.
A. oxygen, dopamine, furosemide after BP is >110 mm Hg systolic
B. oxygen, midazolam, cardioversion
C. oxygen, nitroglycerin, diltiazem, furosemide
D. oxygen, nitroglycerin, furosemide, morphine

11. The following is the ECG of a 72-year-old male who complains of nausea and of seeing yellow-green halos around lights. The patient has a history of congestive heart failure for which he takes furosemide and digitalis. Vital signs are: P—consistent with rate of ECG; BP—146/92 mm Hg; R—16 breaths/min shallow, regular.

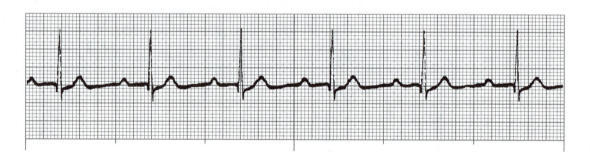

What is the dysrhythmia?
A. Normal sinus rhythm
B. Sinus dysrhythmia
C. Sinus bradycardia
D. Sinus rhythm with first-degree AV block

12. Integrating what you learned in chapter 12, which of the following drugs is most likely to be causing the dysrhythmia in the patient in the previous question?
A. Captopril
B. Digitalis
C. Diltiazem
D. Furosemide

13. The following is the ECG of a 59-year-old male who lost consciousness at work. The patient's co-workers report that he was complaining of squeezing substernal chest pain just before he passed out. Physical examination reveals pale, cool, diaphoretic skin; jugular vein distention; and equal breath sounds bilaterally with no adventitious sounds. Vital signs are: BP—50 mm Hg; P—consistent with rate of ECG; R—32 breaths/min shallow, regular.

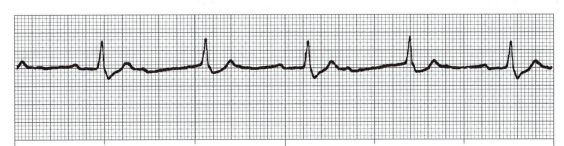

A lesion in which of this patient's coronary arteries probably has caused his problem?
A. Circumflex artery
B. Left anterior descending artery
C. Left main coronary artery
D. Right coronary artery

14. Which of the following changes would you anticipate seeing on the 12-lead ECG of the patient in the previous question?
A. ST segment depression in V_1, V_2, V_3, and V_4
B. ST segment elevation in I, aV_L, V_5, and V_6
C. ST segment elevation in II, III, aV_F, and V_4R
D. ST segment elevation in V_1, V_2, V_3, and V_4

15. A 16-year-old male was involved in a motor vehicle crash. He is pulseless, apneic, and presents in the rhythm shown below. The fire department is performing CPR. Breath sounds are present and equal bilaterally. The patient's neck veins are flat. His abdomen is distended with bruising over the right lower chest and right lower abdomen.

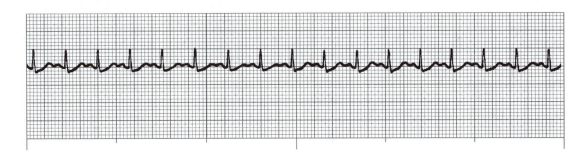

The most appropriate action would be to continue CPR and _____.
A. give adenosine 6 mg IV push
B. perform a needle decompression of the right chest
C. perform synchronized cardioversion at 50 J
D. transport immediately; establish two large-bore IVs with NS or LR

16. A 75-year-old female complains of a sudden onset of nausea, weakness, and severe chest pain. The ECG is shown below. Vital signs are: BP—76/42 mm Hg; R—18 breaths/min shallow, regular; P—consistent with ECG.

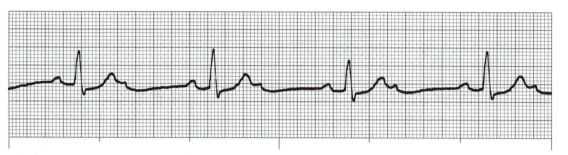

Your best course of action would be to provide supplemental oxygen to maintain an oxygen saturation of 94%, start an IV, and _____.
A. give atropine 0.5 to 1 mg IV push over 3 to 4 minutes
B. give lidocaine 1 mg/kg IV push over 1 to 2 minutes
C. give morphine 1 to 3 mg, slow IV push, titrated to pain relief
D. initiate transcutaneous pacing

17. You are called to a private residence for a "possible code." You find a 72-year-old female unresponsive on the floor. Initial assessment shows her to be apneic and pulseless. An EMT has inserted an oral airway and is ventilating the patient with a bag-mask device. Your partner has started chest compressions. The ECG shows the following rhythm:

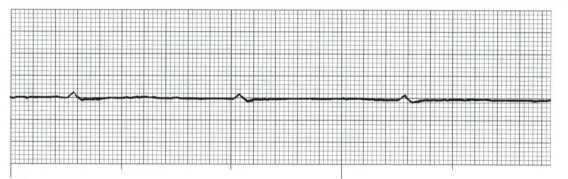

Your next action should be to _____.
A. confirm the rhythm in another lead
B. consider termination of resuscitation efforts
C. defibrillate immediately at 200 J
D. start an IV and administer 1 mg of epinephrine

18. A 52-year-old female complains of shortness of breath, palpitations, and severe chest pain that began about 15 minutes ago. She is pale, cool, and diaphoretic. Rales and wheezing are present over all lung fields. Vital signs are: P—172 beats/min weak, irregular; BP—74/50 mm Hg; R—24 breaths/min labored, regular.

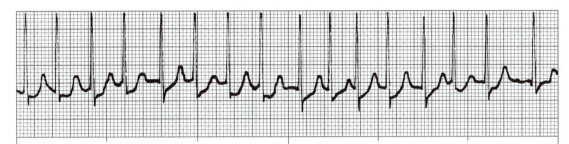

How should you manage this patient?
A. Oxygen, IV, dopamine infusion at 5 mcg/kg/min titrated to BP
B. Oxygen, IV, nitroglycerin, furosemide, morphine
C. Oxygen, IV, synchronized cardioversion at 120 to 200 J
D. Oxygen, IV, verapamil or diltiazem to control rate

19. A 76-year-old female complains of severe shortness of breath, weakness, and dizziness. Bilateral rales and expiratory wheezing are present in both lung bases. Pedal edema is present. Vital signs are: BP—76 mm Hg /palpation; P—90 beats/min weak, irregular; R—28 breaths/min labored, regular.

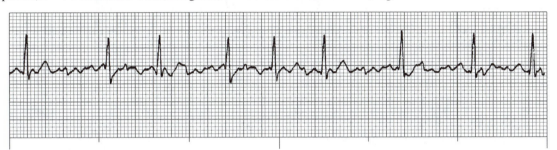

How should you manage this patient?
A. Oxygen IV, dopamine infusion at 5 mcg/kg/min titrated to BP
B. Oxygen, IV, synchronized cardioversion at 120 to 200 J
C. Oxygen, IV, nitroglycerin, furosemide, morphine
D. Oxygen, IV, verapamil or diltiazem to control rate

20. A 60-year-old male has the rhythm shown below after receiving a defibrillator shock. You have not been able to place an endotracheal tube or start an IV. Therefore administration of IV or endotracheal medications will be delayed.

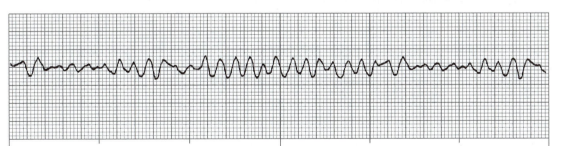

What is the most appropriate next step?
A. Deliver a precordial thump.
B. Continue CPR while attempting to obtain vascular access and defibrillate after 2 minutes of CPR.
C. Give intramuscular epinephrine using an autoinjector.
D. Obtain vascular access using the intraosseous route before giving the second defibrillator shock.

21. Which of the following patients who is having an acute MI would be most likely to show atypical, unusual, or vague signs and symptoms?
A. A 45-year-old female diagnosed with type 1 diabetes 22 years ago
B. A 48-year-old male who is 6-weeks status post coronary artery bypass surgery
C. A 56-year-old male with no prior history of heart disease
D. A 65-year-old female with a history of typical stable angina and moderate coronary artery disease according to a prior angiogram

22. For which of the following patients with pulseless electrical activity is sodium bicarbonate therapy most likely to be effective?
A. A patient who has been in cardiac arrest less than 5 minutes
B. A patient who is in respiratory acidosis following treatment of a tension pneumothorax
C. A patient with documented severe hypokalemia
D. A patient with documented tricyclic antidepressant toxicity

23. You decide to cardiovert a patient who has an unstable tachycardia. You place the cardioverter/defibrillator in synchronization mode and give the patient a sedative and an analgesic. Suddenly, the patient becomes unresponsive. A carotid pulse is absent, and you see this rhythm:

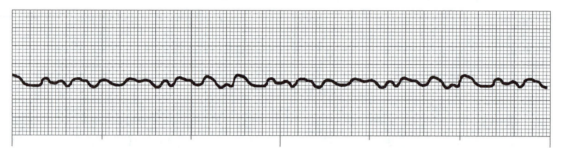

When you attempt to deliver a countershock, the defibrillator will not discharge. What is the explanation for the failure to deliver the shock?
A. The cardioverter/defibrillator's battery has failed.
B. The defibrillator will not deliver a shock because it is attempting to synchronize the shock with an R wave.
C. The monitor cannot synchronize the shock because a lead has come loose.
D. The SYNCH switch is not functioning properly.

24. The following is the ECG of a 48-year-old male with crushing substernal chest pain. He is anxious and confused. His skin is pale, cool, and moist. The patient's neck veins are flat when he is in a seated position. Breath sounds are present and equal bilaterally with crackles in the lung bases bilaterally. Vital signs are: BP—86/50 mm Hg; R—26 breaths/min shallow, regular; P—consistent with monitor, irregular. As you monitor the patient you notice that the ectopic beats appear to be varying in shape and size.

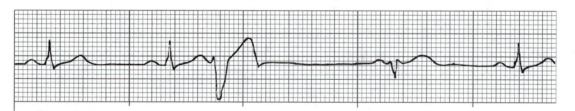

After giving oxygen and starting an IV, the next treatment should be _____.
A. atropine or transcutaneous pacing to increase cardiac output and blood pressure by raising the heart rate
B. dopamine to increase cardiac output and blood pressure by increasing myocardial contractility and peripheral vascular resistance
C. lidocaine to suppress the ectopic beats by decreasing myocardial irritability
D. nitroglycerin to reduce myocardial workload by decreasing preload

25. The following is the ECG of a 55-year-old male with a history of three episodes of syncope in the past hour. He says that he began to experience epigastric pain just before the fainting spells started. His pulse is irregular at 90 to 95 beats/min. His blood pressure is 90/50 mm Hg.

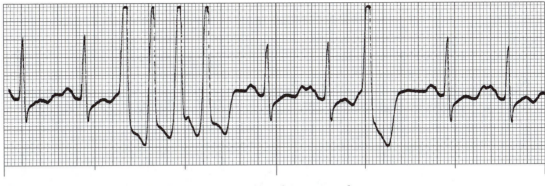

The rhythm being experienced by this patient may be a forerunner of _____.
A. paroxysmal atrial tachycardia
B. pulseless electrical activity
C. ventricular asystole
D. ventricular tachycardia or fibrillation

26. The following is the ECG of a 42-year-old male who is complaining of crushing substernal chest pain and nausea that began about 10 minutes ago. He is awake, alert, and afraid that he will die. The patient has a history of chronic essential hypertension for which he takes "blood pressure pills." His skin is warm and dry. Capillary refill time is less than 2 seconds. His chest is clear to auscultation. Neck veins are flat with the patient in a semi-sitting position. Vital signs are: BP—128/92 mm Hg; P—70 beats/min strong, regular; R—20 breaths/min shallow, regular.

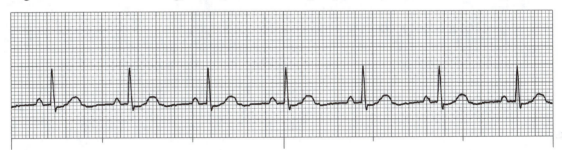

Management of the patient should include _____.
A. oxygen, aspirin, IV fluid bolus, atropine, nitroglycerin, and morphine only if rate increases
B. oxygen, aspirin, IV fluid bolus, nitroglycerine, and morphine if pain continues
C. oxygen, aspirin, IV, nitroglycerine, atropine, and morphine if pain continues
D. oxygen, aspirin, IV, nitroglycerine, and morphine if pain continues

27. An 82-year-old female has been experiencing "fainting spells" for approximately one hour. She is restless and confused. Her skin is pale, cool, and moist. Vital signs are: BP—100/60 mm Hg; R—26 breaths/min shallow, regular. Her pulse is weak and irregular. When you attach the ECG monitor, you see this rhythm.
    The rhythm is _____.
    A. atrial synchronous pacemaker with failure to capture
    B. atrial synchronous pacemaker with failure to sense
    C. ventricular pacemaker with failure to capture
    D. ventricular pacemaker with failure to sense

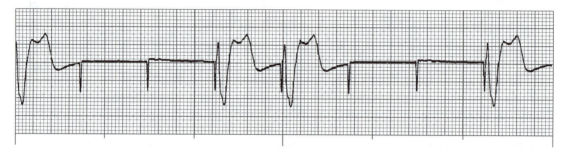

28. A 75-year-old male complains of light-headedness and palpitations that have been occurring for about 1 week. Vital signs are: BP—100/70 mm Hg; P—160 beats/min weak, irregular; R—16 breaths/min regular. Breath sounds are present and equal bilaterally. Skin is cool and dry. Capillary refill time is 2 seconds. There is no jugular vein distention or pedal edema. The ECG shows this rhythm:

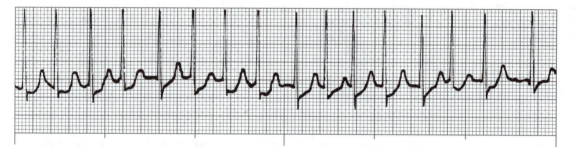

Referring to your knowledge of pharmacology and cardiology, the most appropriate treatment for this patient would be _____.
    A. IV amiodarone in an attempt to convert to sinus rhythm
    B. IV digoxin to slow ventricular response
    C. IV diltiazem to slow ventricular response
    D. synchronized cardioversion

29. A 65-year-old male complains of severe shortness of breath that awakened him 25 minutes ago. He is in acute distress. Peripheral cyanosis is present. His respirations are noisy and labored. He is coughing up pink, frothy sputum. Wheezing and rales are present in both lung fields. Vital signs are: P—75 beats/min; R—36 breaths/min gasping, labored; BP—146/100 mm Hg. The patient's wife tells you he has been awakening short of breath for several weeks. When the monitor is applied, you see the rhythm shown here:

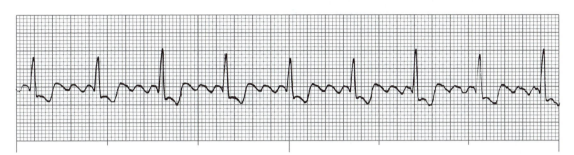

What is the dysrhythmia?
A. Atrial fibrillation
B. Atrial flutter
C. Atrial tachycardia with 2:1 AV block
D. Ventricular tachycardia

30. Management of the patient in the previous question should include _____.
A. adenosine and diltiazem
B. adenosine and furosemide
C. nitroglycerine and furosemide
D. midazolam and cardioversion

31. The patient is a 63-year-old female complaining of "tightness" in her chest accompanied by dull pain in her neck and jaw bilaterally beginning about 5 minutes ago. She is in moderate distress. Vital signs are: BP—146/96 mm Hg; R—22 breaths/min regular; P—110 beats/min weak, regular. She says the pain is unchanged by coughing, swallowing, deep breathing, or positional changes. She has taken 3 nitroglycerin tablets with substantial relief of the pain, but states her previous episodes of pain always have responded to 1 nitroglycerin. She also tells you that previous episodes occurred only when she climbed stairs, not when she walked on a level surface as she was today. She is awake and alert. Her skin is cool and moist. The remainder of the physical examination is unremarkable. A 12-lead ECG shows ST segment depression in leads V_1-V_4. You should suspect _____.
A. acute MI
B. CHF
C. stable angina pectoris
D. unstable angina pectoris

32. A 52-year-old female complains of pain and tenderness in her right calf. She also complains of fever, chills, and malaise. Examination of the affected extremity reveals that the calf is edematous, warm, and red. The pain in her calf increases upon dorsiflexion. What problem should be suspected?
A. Acute arterial occlusion
B. Deep vein thrombosis
C. Intermittent claudication
D. Peripheral arterial insufficiency

33. Combining what you learned in Chapter 21 and this chapter, which of the following conditions is this patient at greatest risk for?
A. Acute MI
B. Aortic aneurysm
C. Cerebrovascular accident
D. Pulmonary embolism

Chapter **22**

34. You are called to see a 73-year-old male with a history of hypertension and angina pectoris. The patient says he developed cramping pain in his lower extremities while climbing a flight of stairs. When he rested, the pain quickly subsided. Examination of his lower extremities shows that they are pale and cool to the touch. Pedal pulses are present but weak. Capillary refill is slowed in the toes, but is within normal limits in the fingertips. What problem should be suspected?
    A. Acute arterial occlusion
    B. Deep vein thrombophlebitis
    C. Peripheral arterial insufficiency with intermittent claudication
    D. Varicose veins

35. For several months, a 62-year-old male with a history of diabetes mellitus has been experiencing episodes of aching pain and weakness in his legs while walking. Two hours ago, he developed severe pain in his left leg accompanied by paresthesias. Motor and sensory functions in the leg were gradually lost. The affected extremity is pale and cool to the touch. Dorsal pedal and posterior tibial pulses are absent. You suspect the patient may have suffered _____.
    A. acute arterial occlusion
    B. deep vein thrombophlebitis
    C. dissecting aortic aneurysm
    D. intermittent claudication

36. A 54-year-old male with a history of COPD has been diagnosed as having cor pulmonale. Which of the following signs would you expect to find?
    A. Crackles and wheezing in the lung bases, distended neck veins, and decreased skin turgor
    B. Crackles in both lung bases, severe dyspnea, and pedal edema
    C. Distended neck veins and pedal edema
    D. Hypotension, tachycardia, and paroxysmal nocturnal dyspnea

37. A 52-year-old male with a history of diabetes mellitus complains of weakness, nausea, and shortness of breath that began about 10 minutes ago. He is awake and alert. His skin is pale, cool, and moist. Breath sounds are present and equal bilaterally without adventitious sounds. He has taken his insulin today and has eaten his normal diet. He has not experienced any abnormal levels of stress or activity. Vital signs are: BP—162/98 mm Hg; P—118 beats/min weak, irregular; R—22 breaths/min shallow, regular. This patient is most likely to be suffering from _____.
    A. acute MI
    B. diabetic ketoacidosis
    C. hypoglycemia
    D. pulmonary embolism

38. Combining your knowledge of cardiac anatomy and physiology from chapter 6, and your knowledge of cardiology from this chapter, which statement best describes the effect of increasing the heart rate on systole and diastole?
    A. Systole lengthens; diastole lengthens.
    B. Systole lengthens; diastole shortens.
    C. Systole shortens; diastole lengthens.
    D. Systole shortens; diastole shortens.

39. The major modifiable risk factors for developing atherosclerosis include _____.
    A. diabetes, male gender, and advanced age
    B. hypertension, smoking, elevated serum lipid levels
    C. smoking, positive family history, and hypertension
    D. smoking, male gender, and elevated serum lipid levels

40. Combinig your knowledge of cardiac anatomy and physiology from chapter 6, and your knowledge of cardiology from this chapter, what effect would increasing the preload have on a heart that is in congestive failure?
    A. The congestive failure will improve.
    B. The congestive failure will worsen.
    C. The congestive failure will worsen and then improve gradually.
    D. There will be no change in the patient's condition since a heart in CHF loses the ability to respond to changes in preload.

41. A 52-year-old male is not oriented to person, place, or time. His wife tells you he began complaining of chest pain 2 hours ago but refused to let her call the ambulance. He has a history of three previous acute MIs. His skin is pale, cool, and diaphoretic. His radial pulses are absent and he has a weak carotid pulse matching the rhythm shown below. He is also complaining of respiratory distress and presents with crackles (rales) to all lung fields. The blood pressure is 64/40 mm Hg. The patient's ECG is shown here:

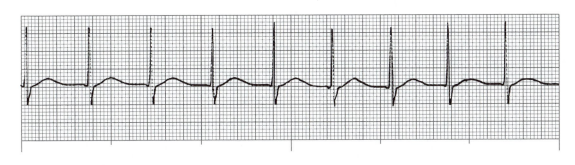

Management of this patient should include _____.
A. aspirin
B. morphine
C. nitroglycerin
D. norepinephrine

42. A 52-year-old male is in ventricular fibrillation that has persisted after two DC countershocks. An IV is started, epinephrine is administered, and the patient was shocked for a third time. After the third shock, a carotid pulse is palpated at 72 beats/min. The blood pressure is 76/54 mm Hg. The rhythm shown here is present on the monitor:

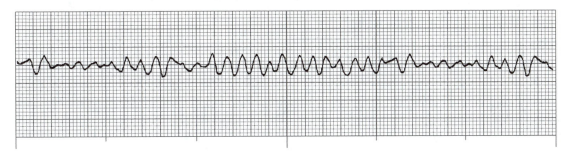

The most appropriate action at this point would be to _____.
A. administer 1 mg/kg lidocaine and hang a lidocaine drip at 2 mg/min
B. cardiovert at 100 J
C. check the placement of the ECG leads
D. start a dopamine infusion at 5 to 10 mcg/kg/min

Case one

A 65-year-old male complains of severe shortness of breath that awakened him about 25 minutes ago. He is in acute distress. Peripheral cyanosis is present. His respirations are noisy and labored, and he is coughing up pink, frothy sputum. Auscultation of the chest reveals wheezing and rales in both lung fields. His neck veins are distended when he is placed in a semi-sitting position. Vital signs are: BP—160/96 mm Hg; R—28 breaths/min shallow, gasping. When you attach the ECG monitor, you see the following rhythm. Pulse rate corresponds to the ECG. Integrating your knowledge of anatomy and physiology, cardiology, pulmonology, airway management, and pharmacology, please synthesize answers to the following questions.

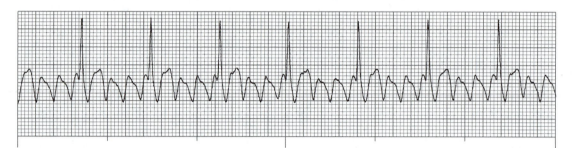

1. Identify the cardiac rhythm.

   _____

2. From what problem is the patient suffering?

   _____

3. Why are the patient's neck veins distended?

   _____

4. Involvement of which heart chamber is producing the patient's respiratory distress? Explain the pathophysiology.

   _____

5. Describe your management of this patient. Include the rationale for selecting each medication that you administer.

   _____
   _____
   _____
   _____
   _____
   _____
   _____
   _____
   _____

Case two

A 36-year-old male has a 6-hour history of weakness and nausea. The patient is awake and alert. He denies any history of heart disease. However, he does have a history of type 1 diabetes for approximately 22 years. The patient's vital signs are: BP—106/86 mm Hg; P—90 to 100 beats/min weak, regular; R—22 breaths/min shallow, regular. His skin is pale, cool, and moist. The jugular veins are distended with the patient in a semi-seated position. Breath sounds are present and equal bilaterally with no adventitious sounds. Blood glucose level is 130 mg/dL. The patient's 12-lead ECG appears below. Integrating your knowledge of anatomy and physiology, cardiology, pulmonology, airway management, and pharmacology, please synthesize answers to the following questions.

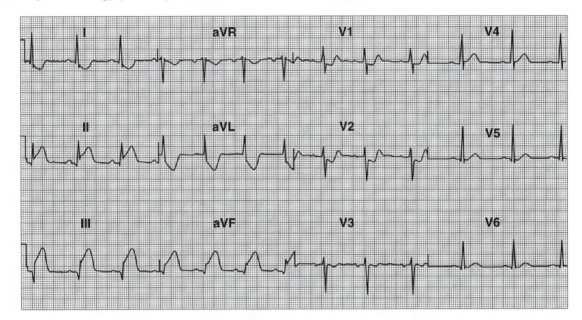

1. Is the patient's history of type 1 diabetes significant? Why or why not?

   _____
   _____
   _____
   _____

2. The patient's 12-lead ECG suggests what problem?

   _____

3. Where is the probable location of the vascular lesion that is producing this problem?

   _____

4. Are there any other ECG leads you should acquire? Why or why not?

   _____
   _____
   _____
   _____

5. Describe your management of this patient.

   _____
   _____
   _____
   _____
   _____
   _____
   _____

Case three

The patient is an 82-year-old female with a 3-day history of weakness and vomiting. Her visiting granddaughter called you when she became concerned with her grandmother's appearance. The patient keeps insisting she is fine and that she only has "the flu." Her skin is pale, cool, and moist. Crackles are present in both lung bases. Blood pressure is 160/90 mm Hg. The patient has a history of chronic essential hypertension and is compliant in taking her medications. The patient's 12-lead ECG appears below. Integrating your knowledge of anatomy and physiology, cardiology, pulmonology, airway management, and pulmonology, please synthesize answers to the following questions.

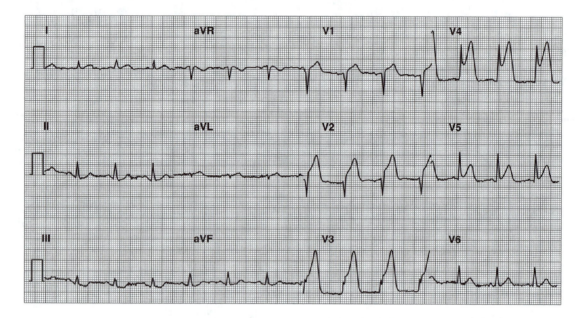

1. The patient's 12-lead ECG suggests what problem?

2. Why is the patient's age significant in evaluating her complaint and possible problem?

3. Where is the probable location of the vascular lesion that is producing this problem?

4. Describe your management of this patient.

Case four

You are summoned to a political rally where a 40-year-old candidate for city council became ill while delivering a speech. You find the patient in the backstage area of a large auditorium, sitting in a chair with his tie pulled loose and his shirt collar open. He says that while he was making his most crucial point about the dangers of inflation, he began to feel a "squeezing" pain in his chest and became sick to his stomach. He denies any significant medical history, has no allergies, and takes no medications regularly. On physical examination, he is pale, diaphoretic, and anxious. Vital signs are: BP—150/80 mm Hg; R—18 breaths/min full, regular; P—consistent with ECG strong, regular. The patient's 12-lead ECG appears here:

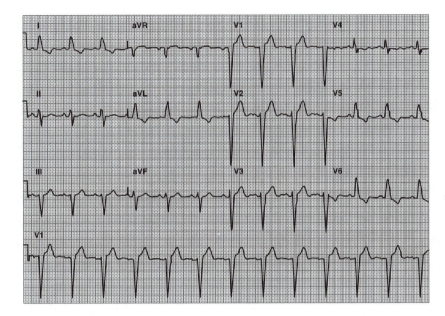

1. Interpret the patient's 12-lead ECG.

   _____

2. What is the significance of this interpretation to your attempts to diagnose this patient's problem?

   _____
   _____
   _____
   _____

Case five

The patient is a 72-year-old male who began to experience nausea and epigastric pain approximately 30 minutes ago. He has a history of poorly controlled chronic essential hypertension and two previous acute myocardial infarctions. Vital signs are: BP—98/50 mm Hg; R—23 breaths/min labored, regular; P—consistent with ECG. The patient's skin is pale, cool, and moist. He is confused and restless. Crackles are present in the lower lobes of both lungs. When you acquire a 12-lead ECG, you see the rhythm shown below. Integrating your knowledge of anatomy and physiology, cardiology, pulmonology, airway management, and pharmacology, please synthesize answers to the following questions.

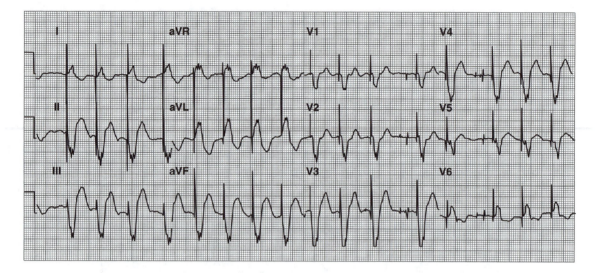

1. Interpret the 12-lead ECG.

2. What is the significance of this interpretation to your attempts to diagnose this patient's problem?

3. How would you manage this patient?

Case six

A 56-year-old male is complaining of substernal chest pain. His 12-lead ECG appears here:

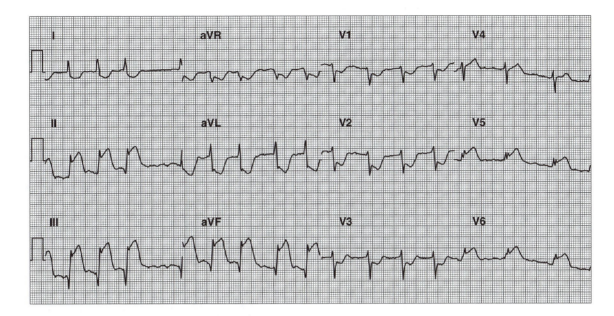

1. Assuming that there is only one vascular lesion responsible for this patient's problem, what will the cardiologist discover about the coronary circulation when he or she images the coronary arteries?

_____
_____
_____
_____

Case seven

A third-string high school quarterback kicked a 55-yard field goal in the last 5 seconds of a game that decided a district championship. His 45-year-old coach screamed, clutched his chest, and collapsed unconscious on the sidelines. When you arrive, an assistant coach is performing CPR. The patient is cyanotic. He has no pulse, no respirations, and no blood pressure. His ECG rhythm follows:

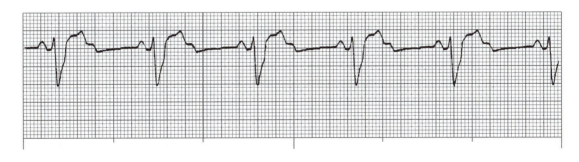

1. Identify the cardiac rhythm.

_____

2. Describe your prehospital management of the patient.

_____

_____

_____

_____

_____

_____

3. List the problems you should consider when you are trying to identify the cause of this rhythm.

_____

_____

_____

_____

23 Disorders of the Nervous System

READING ASSIGNMENT

Chapter 23, pages 891-944, in *Paramedic Practice Today: Above and Beyond*.

OBJECTIVES

After completing this chapter, you will be able to:

1. Discuss the anatomy and physiology of the organs and structures related to the nervous system.
2. Discuss indications for a neurologic assessment.
3. Discuss and practice the components of the neurologic assessment, including the following:
   - Posture and gait
   - Mental status
   - Examination of the cranial nerves
   - Sensory examination
   - Motor examination
   - Deep tendon reflexes
   - Meningeal examination
   - Glasgow Coma Scale
4. Describe the etiology, epidemiology, history, and physical findings for the following neurologic conditions or situations:
   - Altered mental status
   - Delirium
   - Dementia
   - Seizures
   - Status epilepticus
   - Syncope
   - Headache
   - Brain tumor
   - Brain abscess
   - Stroke
   - Transient ischemic attack
5. With the patient history and physical examination findings, develop a treatment plan for a patient having any of the following neurologic conditions or situations:
   - Altered mental status
   - Delirium
   - Dementia
   - Seizures
   - Status epilepticus
   - Syncope
   - Headache
   - Brain tumor
   - Brain abscess
   - Stroke
   - Transient ischemic attack
6. Identify risk factors that may affect the nervous system.
7. Describe the etiology, epidemiology, history, and physical findings for any of the following infectious neurologic diseases:
   - Meningitis
   - Encephalitis
   - Shingles
   - Poliomyelitis
8. With the patient history and physical examination findings, develop a treatment plan for a patient having any of the following infectious neurologic diseases:
   - Meningitis
   - Encephalitis
   - Shingles
   - Poliomyelitis
9. Describe the etiology, epidemiology, history, and physical findings for the following degenerative neurologic diseases:
   - Alzheimer's disease
   - Parkinson's disease
   - Amyotrophic lateral sclerosis
   - Multiple sclerosis
   - Guillain-Barré syndrome
   - Myasthenia gravis
   - Huntington's disease
10. With the patient history and physical examination findings, develop a treatment plan for a patient having any of the following degenerative neurologic diseases:
    - Alzheimer's disease
    - Parkinson's disease
    - Amyotrophic lateral sclerosis
    - Multiple sclerosis
    - Guillain-Barré syndrome
    - Myasthenia gravis
    - Huntington's disease
11. Describe the etiology, epidemiology, history, physical findings, and management of spinal cord disorders.
12. Describe the etiology, epidemiology, history, physical findings, and management of autonomic dysreflexia.
13. Describe the etiology, epidemiology, history, physical findings, and management of hydrocephalus.
14. Describe the etiology, epidemiology, history, physical findings, and management of spina bifida.

15. Define the following:
    a. Muscular dystrophy
    b. Dystonia
    c. Trigeminal neuralgia
    d. Bell's palsy

CHAPTER SUMMARY

- The most basic portion of the nervous system is the neuron, or nerve cell.
- Each neuron has three parts: the dendrites, cell body, and axon.
- Neurons send impulses to other cells by neurotransmitters, chemicals that cross the synapse.
- The central nervous system is composed of the brain and spinal cord.
- The central nervous system is covered by three layers of connective tissue called the *meninges*.
- The meninges contain cerebrospinal fluid (CSF), which circulates throughout the central nervous system.
- All nervous tissue not in the brain or spinal cord comprises the peripheral nervous system.
- The peripheral nervous system has two parts: the somatic, which controls voluntary muscle movements and sensation from the skin; and the visceral, which comprises the autonomic nervous system (ANS).
- The spinal nerves branch off of the spinal cord and are named for the vertebra level where they exit.
- The ANS has two divisions that work against each other: the sympathetic, or fight-or-flight response; and the parasympathetic, or rest-and-digest response.
- Twelve cranial nerves branch off of the brain and spinal cord.
- Perform a complete neurologic assessment if your patient has or has had altered mental status, a loss of consciousness, an alteration in strength or sensation, or a loss of function of an extremity.
- One of the primary goals of the neurologic assessment is to find focal deficits—absent or altered functions of sensations of a body part caused by damage to a portion of the nervous system.
- All patients with altered mental status should have their blood glucose levels monitored.
- Dementia is a slow, progressive decline in mental functions; delirium is an acute, temporary state of mental confusion and/or fluctuating level of consciousness.
- Disruption of blood flow to an area of brain tissue is known as a *cerebrovascular accident* or *stroke*.
- A seizure is massive, excessive neuronal firing in the brain that alters behavior.
- Seizures are divided into partial seizures, which only affect part of the brain, and generalized seizures, which affect the entire brain.
- After a generalized seizure, the patient goes through a postictal period in which he or she may be combative, confused, and fearful.
- Status epilepticus is a single seizure lasting longer than 30 minutes or repeated seizures without full recovery of responsiveness between seizures and lasting longer than 30 minutes. It is a life-threatening condition requiring aggressive care.
- Syncope is a transient loss of consciousness, often resulting in a ground-level fall.
- Headaches are either vascular (caused by dilation of blood vessels within the head) or nonvascular (caused by something else).
- A brain neoplasm is a tumor within the brain that may be benign or malignant.
- A brain abscess is a collection of pus within the brain.
- An ischemic stroke is caused by a blocked blood vessel in the brain.
- A hemorrhagic stroke is caused by a ruptured, bleeding blood vessel in the brain.
- Hypertension, bradycardia, and abnormal respirations are the hallmarks of Cushing's triad, signifying rising intracranial pressure (ICP).
- A transient ischemic attack (TIA) shows the same signs and symptoms as a stroke but resolves within 24 hours.
- Alzheimer's disease is a degenerative, progressive decline in memory, reasoning, and cognition. It is the most common cause of senile dementia in the elderly.
- Parkinson's disease is a degenerative nervous disorder affecting fine motor control and the extrapyramidal system.
- Any injury to the spinal cord will affect sensation and movement below the site of injury.

SHORT ANSWER

1. What is the basic unit of the nervous system?
   _____
   _____
   _____
   _____

2. What are dendrites? What is their function?
   _____
   _____
   _____
   _____

3. What are axons? What is their function?
   _____
   _____
   _____
   _____

4. Where is the myelin sheath located? What is its function?
   _____
   _____
   _____
   _____

5. What are the nodes of Ranvier? What is their function?
   _____
   _____
   _____
   _____

6. How do nerve impulses move on the neurons?

_____

_____

_____

_____

7. What are the gaps between the axons of one neuron and the dendrites of the next called?

_____

_____

_____

_____

8. How do nerve impulses cross these gaps?

_____

_____

_____

_____

9. What effect does the neurotransmitter gamma-aminobutyric acid (GABA) have when it is released into the synapse?

_____

_____

_____

_____

10. What structures compose the CNS?

_____

_____

_____

_____

11. What are the three membranes that surround the structures of the CNS?

_____

_____

_____

_____

12. What is the function of CSF? Where is CSF normally located?

_____

_____

_____

_____

13. What portion of the brain is responsible for controlling the vegetative functions such as breathing, heart rate, and vasomotor tone?

_____

_____

_____

_____

14. Where in the brain is body temperature controlled?

_____

_____

_____

_____

15. What is the reticular activating system (RAS)?

_____

_____

_____

_____

16. If the connection is lost between the cerebral cortex and the RAS how does the patient respond?

_____

_____

_____

_____

17. What part of the brain controls posture, balance, and equilibrium?

_____

_____

_____

_____

18. What part of the brain controls conscious perception and action and is the seat of conscious thought and personality?

_____

_____

_____

_____

19. What functions are localized in the frontal lobe?

_____

_____

_____

_____

20. What functions are localized in the parietal lobe?

_____

_____

_____

_____

21. What functions are localized in the temporal lobe?

_____

_____

_____

_____

22. What functions are localized in the occipital lobe?

_____

_____

_____

_____

23. What is the relationship between the location of a sensory or motor center in the brain and the area of the body it serves?

_____

_____

_____

_____

24. Where is the speech center usually located?

_____
_____
_____
_____

25. What is the role of thiamine in the functioning of neurons?

_____
_____
_____
_____

26. What is a cranial nerve?

_____
_____
_____
_____

27. List, in order and with their number, all of the cranial nerves and describe the function of each nerve.

Nerve	Name	Function
I		
II		
III		
IV		
V		
VI		
VII		
VIII		
IX		
X		
XI		
XII		

28. What is the function of the spinal cord?

_____
_____
_____
_____

29. What level of sensation on the body surface corresponds to each of the following levels of the spinal cord?
a. C3

_____
_____
_____

b. T4

_____
_____
_____

c. T10

_____
_____
_____

d. L1

_____
_____
_____

30. What division of the peripheral nervous system controls functions that take place below the level of consciousness?

_____
_____
_____

31. What portion of the peripheral nervous system controls responses to stress?

_____
_____
_____

32. What is the postganglionic neurotransmitter for the portion of the peripheral nervous system that controls responses to stress?

_____
_____
_____

33. What portion of the peripheral nervous system controls vegetative or routine housekeeping functions?

_____
_____
_____

34. What principal nerve acts to control the portion of the peripheral nervous system that regulates routine housekeeping functions?

_____

_____

_____

_____

35. What is the postganglionic neurotransmitter for the portion of the peripheral nervous system that controls routine housekeeping functions?

_____

_____

_____

36. What is the name for the type of receptor site to which this neurotransmitter binds?

_____

_____

_____

_____

37. What is the neurotransmitter released by the portion of the peripheral nervous system that controls voluntary movement of the skeletal muscles?

_____

_____

_____

_____

38. What is the name of the type of receptor site to which this neurotransmitter binds?

_____

_____

_____

_____

39. What do the letters in the mnemonic AEIOU TIPS signify?

_____

_____

_____

_____

40. What is the initial priority in the management of all patients who present with coma of unknown cause?

_____

_____

_____

_____

41. Why is thiamine indicated before administration of glucose to unconscious patients who may be intoxicated or alcoholic?

_____

_____

_____

_____

42. List three causes of cerebrovascular accident (CVA).

_____

_____

_____

_____

43. List four factors that increase a patient's risk of having a CVA.

_____

_____

_____

_____

44. What is a transient ischemic attack?

_____

_____

_____

_____

45. Why are transient ischemic attacks significant?

_____

_____

_____

_____

46. What is an aura?

_____

_____

_____

_____

47. Why is it important to obtain information about the aura in a first-time seizure?

_____

_____

_____

_____

48. List in order the phases of a tonic-clonic (grand mal) seizure.

_____

_____

_____

_____

_____

49. If a patient who is experiencing generalized seizure activity makes asymmetric or purposeful movements or can recall things done or said during the seizure, what do you know about the origin of the seizure?

_____

_____

_____

_____

50. What is the name for the form of seizure in which a patient is conscious and displays tonic-clonic movements of one part of the body such as an arm or leg?

_____

_____

_____

_____

51. What is the name for the form of seizure characterized by loss of consciousness and apparently purposeful movements such as lip-smacking or repetitive movements of a hand or arm?

_____

_____

_____

_____

52. What is status epilepticus?

_____

_____

_____

_____

53. What is the drug of choice in the prehospital management of status epilepticus?

_____

_____

_____

_____

54. What is the most common cause of death from seizures?

_____

_____

_____

_____

MULTIPLE CHOICE

1. Unequal pupils, as may be seen in a patient with increased ICP, indicate the possibility of _____.
   A. a periorbital fracture
   B. an ischemic stroke
   C. pressure on the third cranial nerve
   D. pressure on the vagus nerve

2. The phase of a generalized seizure characterized by fatigue, confusion, and a possible headache is called the _____.
   A. aura phase
   B. postictal phase
   C. prodrome phase
   D. tonic phase

3. A significant characteristic differentiating hemorrhagic stroke from ischemic stroke is _____.
   A. a history of recent trauma
   B. confusion or altered mental status
   C. the presence of hemiplegia
   D. the rapid onset of severe symptoms

4. Which of the following is Cushing's triad?
   A. Abnormal breathing pattern, bradycardia, hypertension
   B. Bradycardia, unequal pupils, abnormal respiratory pattern
   C. Hypertension, unequal pupils, abnormal respiratory pattern
   D. Unequal pupils, bradycardia, abnormal respiratory pattern

5. Petit mal seizures are most common in _____.
   A. children
   B. children of parents with seizure disorders
   C. newborn babies of diabetic mothers
   D. patients with recent stroke or head injury

6. You are called to a seizure patient. Witnesses say the man was clutching his head, collapsed to the floor, and immediately began to have a convulsion. He has no medic alert tags and no one nearby knows the man. He seems very healthy and there is no evidence of drug use; the 28-year-old man responds only to painful stimuli by moaning. Your examination reveals the following: no obvious injuries; eyes deviated to the left; BP—184/94 mm Hg; P—64 beats/min; skin—warm, dry; ventilations—24 breaths/min; lung sounds clear and equal. Which of the following diagnoses has the most supporting evidence?
   A. Seizure and now in a postictal state
   B. Seizure caused by alcohol withdrawal
   C. Seizure caused by CVA
   D. Seizure caused by drug overdose

7. A 58-year-old woman has fainted while on the toilet. She states she has been constipated lately and had difficulty with bowel movements. She was having a difficult time when she suddenly "passed out." Her husband heard the noise and found her awake but on the floor. She is now awake and alert. The most probable cause of her syncope is _____.
   A. excessive vagal tone
   B. hypovolemia
   C. micturition syncope
   D. tussive syncope

8. Your patient is experiencing tremors of his left arm and hand. He tells you he has a seizure disorder that causes this. You observe what appears to be tonic-clonic activity of the left arm only. This seizure is referred to as a _____.
   A. complex partial seizure
   B. hysterical seizure
   C. petit mal seizure
   D. simple partial seizure

9. Which of the following actions would be appropriate in caring for a patient who is actively seizing?
   A. Forcibly restraining the patient to keep him from injuring himself
   B. Gently supporting and guiding the patient's movements to keep him from injuring himself
   C. Placing the patient in a prone position so he will not aspirate if he vomits
   D. Placing something in the patient's mouth to keep him from swallowing his tongue

10. Focal motor seizures (simple partial seizures) are characterized by _____.
    A. altered personality states and repetitive movements that appear to be purposeful
    B. brief loss of consciousness without loss of postural tone
    C. generalized tonic-clonic activity followed by unconsciousness
    D. tonic-clonic movements of one part of the body

11. Status epilepticus is _____.
    A. a major motor (grand mal) seizure that will not respond to antiseizure medications
    B. a very violent seizure that can cause brain death
    C. seizures produced by an unknown cause
    D. two or more seizures without an intervening period of consciousness

12. A type of seizure characterized by brief loss of consciousness without loss of postural tone is _____.
    A. focal (simple partial)
    B. grand mal (major motor)
    C. petit mal (absence)
    D. psychomotor (complex partial)

13. During the postictal phase of a seizure, a patient most probably will _____.
    A. be restless and anxious
    B. complain of a headache and wish to sleep
    C. engage in rambling conversation
    D. have an aura

14. A CVA may be caused by _____.
    A. a ruptured artery in the brain or blockage of an artery by a thrombus
    B. blockage of an artery by a thrombus or an embolus.
    C. blockage of an artery by an embolus or rupture of an artery in the brain.
    D. rupture of an artery in the brain or blockage of a cerebral artery by a thrombus or embolus

Case one

A 17-year-old male responds to painful stimuli with nonspecific movement and incomprehensible sounds. His right pupil is dilated and unreactive. His left pupil is mid-position and responds sluggishly to light. He does not respond when painful stimuli are applied to his left arm or left leg. The patient's family tells you he has had the "flu" for 3 days and has been complaining of a severe headache, nausea, and vomiting. Vital signs are BP—210/130 mm Hg; P—40 beats/min, bounding, regular; R—24 breaths/min deep, regular. His ECG is shown here:

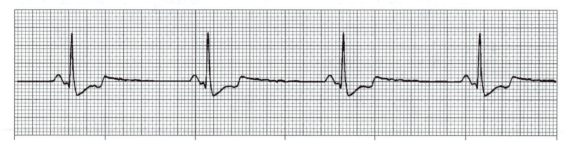

1. What problem do you suspect?

_____
_____
_____
_____

2. What are the three pathophysiologic mechanisms that produce this problem?

_____
_____
_____
_____

3. Which mechanism is probably producing this problem in this patient?

_____
_____
_____
_____

4. What do the patient's signs and symptoms suggest about the location of his problem?

_____
_____
_____
_____

5. What accounts for the changes in the patient's vital signs?

_____
_____
_____
_____

6. How would you manage this patient?

_____
_____
_____
_____

Case two

At 1000 hours, you are dispatched to a medical emergency at a middle school. On arrival, you and your partner are led to the school nurse's office. The patient is a 13-year-old male who appears to be unconscious. He is lying on his side on a cot. His respirations are slow and shallow, and his skin is very cool, moist, and very pale. Radial pulses are rapid and weak. The school nurse tells you that about 15 minutes ago she was called to the patient's classroom. She found the patient on the floor beside his desk having what she describes as a generalized seizure. She stayed with the patient and protected his airway until the seizure activity ceased. He was then taken on a stretcher to her office where he had two more seizures. The patient does not have a history of a seizure disorder, but recently he was diagnosed with type 1 diabetes, and he now takes insulin. Vital signs are BP—92/60 mm Hg; P—130 beats/min, weak, regular; R—10 breats/min, shallow, regular.

1. Is it likely that the patient's seizure activity is related to his diabetes? Explain your response.

   _____
   _____
   _____
   _____

Case three

A 76-year-old male fell when he tried to stand after taking an afternoon nap. He is awake, and oriented. Vital signs are P—78 beats/min, strong, regular; R—16 breaths/min, regular; BP—146/92 mm Hg. The patient has a history of hypertension for which he takes hydrochlorothiazide (HydroDIURIL). He also had a total right hip replacement 2 years ago. The patient is unable to move his left leg. His left arm moves weakly, and he is unable to grasp with his left hand. He says he does not know where his left arm and leg came from. He moves his right arm and leg at will. Breath sounds are present and equal bilaterally without adventitious sounds. Blood glucose level is 100 mg/dL.

1. From what problem is this patient suffering?

   _____
   _____
   _____
   _____

2. What are the three pathophysiologic mechanisms that can cause this problem?

   _____
   _____
   _____
   _____

3. Which mechanism probably is causing the problem in this patient?

   _____
   _____
   _____
   _____

4. What part of this patient's brain is affected?

   _____
   _____
   _____
   _____

5. Why is this patient's speech not affected?

   _____

   _____

   _____

   _____

6. How does hypertension predispose to this problem?

   _____

   _____

   _____

   _____

7. What is significant about the patient's statement that he does not know where his left arm and leg came from?

   _____

   _____

   _____

   _____

8. Why would it be important to find out how long ago the patient laid down for his nap?

   _____

   _____

   _____

   _____

9. How would you manage this patient?

   _____

   _____

   _____

   _____

24 Endocrine Emergencies and Nutritional Disorders

READING ASSIGNMENT

Chapter 24, pages 945-971, in *Paramedic Practice Today: Above and Beyond*.

OBJECTIVES

After completing this chapter, you will be able to:

1. Describe the incidence, morbidity, and mortality rates of endocrine emergencies, including the need for rapid assessment and intervention.
2. Discuss the anatomy and physiology of the organs and structures involved in endocrinologic diseases.
3. Describe normal glucose metabolism.
4. Describe the pathophysiology of type 1 and type 2 diabetes.
5. Discuss the pathophysiology of diabetic metabolism.
6. Describe the assessment findings of the hypoglycemic patient.
7. Develop a treatment plan based on the assessment findings of the hypoglycemic patient.
8. Describe the assessment findings of the hyperglycemic patient.
9. Develop a treatment plan based on the assessment findings of the hyperglycemic patient.
10. Describe the assessment findings of the patient with diabetic ketoacidosis.
11. Develop a treatment plan based on the assessment findings of the patient with diabetic ketoacidosis.
12. Describe the assessment findings of the patient with hyperosmolar hyperglycemic nonketotic coma.
13. Develop a treatment plan based on the assessment findings of the patient with hyperosmolar hyperglycemic nonketotic coma.
14. Discuss the pathophysiology of pituitary gland disorders.
15. Describe the assessment findings of patients with pituitary gland disorders.
16. Develop a treatment plan based on the assessment findings of the patient with a pituitary gland disorder.
17. Discuss the pathophysiology of thyroid gland disorders.
18. Describe the assessment findings of patients with thyroid gland disorders.
19. Develop a treatment plan based on the assessment findings of the patient with a thyroid gland disorder.
20. Discuss the pathophysiology of parathyroid gland disorders.
21. Describe the assessment findings of patients with parathyroid gland disorders.
22. Develop a treatment plan based on the assessment findings of the patient with a parathyroid gland disorder.
23. Discuss the pathophysiology of adrenal gland disorders.
24. Describe the assessment findings of patients with adrenal gland disorders.
25. Develop a treatment plan based on the assessment findings of the patient with an adrenal gland disorder.
26. Discuss the etiology of nutritional disorders.
27. Discuss the pathophysiology of nutritional disorders.
28. Describe the assessment findings of patients with nutritional disorders.
29. Develop a treatment plan based on the assessment findings of the patient with a nutritional disorder.

CHAPTER SUMMARY

- The endocrine system, along with the neurologic system, is responsible for helping the body maintain homeostasis. Although the neurologic system is able to respond more rapidly to changes and the endocrine system takes longer to respond, those changes may remain in effect longer. The endocrine system communicates with tissues throughout the body through the release of hormones by eight main endocrine glands: the hypothalamus, pituitary, thyroid, parathyroid, thymus, pancreas, adrenal, and gonads. Hormones interact with target tissues in all parts of the body to effect changes to balance body systems and maintain homeostasis.

- The most prominent endocrine disorders you will encounter will be related to diabetes mellitus. In the patient with type 1 diabetes, the beta cells, found in the islets of Langerhans located in the pancreas, have ceased producing insulin. Insulin is responsible for aiding the movement of glucose across the cell wall and into the cell for metabolizing. It also prompts the liver to convert circulating glucose into glycogen for later use. In type 2 diabetes, either insulin production has diminished to the point where it can no longer meet metabolic demands or cellular receptor sites have decreased sensitivity and no longer respond effectively to current insulin levels. Glucagon is released by the alpha cells in the pancreas. Glucagon acts on the liver to convert glycogen back to glucose, a process called glycogenolysis.

- Although rare, some endocrine disorders besides diabetes may prove rapidly fatal to the patient. Thyrotoxicosis, or thyroid storm, is caused by overactivity of the thyroid gland. Signs and symptoms of a thyroid storm include tachypnea, tachycardia, shock, hyperthermia, and delirium. Treatment includes dysrhythmia management, shock management, airway support, beta-blockers, and steroids. The other rare but lethal endocrine disorder you may encounter is myxedema. Myxedema is an underactivity of the thyroid gland. Signs and symptoms include unexplained hypothermia, unexplained hypoglycemia, hypotension, respiratory depression, and coma. Prehospital treatment includes supportive care, airway management, temperature regulation, and treatment for shock.

■ Other than diabetes, most metabolic and nutritional disorders are not life threatening. They build over a period and are diagnosed by the patient's family physician. You usually become aware of these conditions during the history component of the patient assessment. Be aware of the pathophysiology of these disorders, how they interact with other disease processes, and what modifications you may need to make to current protocols to accommodate these interactions.

SHORT ANSWER

1. What is an endocrine gland?

_____
_____
_____
_____

2. What is the name of the substances secreted by endocrine glands?

_____
_____
_____
_____

3. What term is used to describe the site at which the products of an endocrine gland produce their effects?

_____
_____

4. What is the role of the hypothalamus in the endocrine system?

_____
_____
_____
_____

5. Describe the pathophysiology of diabetes insipidus.

_____
_____
_____
_____

6. What endocrine gland is called the *master gland*? Why?

_____
_____
_____
_____

7. List the names and functions of the hormones produced by the anterior portion of the gland from question 6.

_____
_____
_____
_____

8. List the names and functions of the hormones released by the posterior portion of the gland from question 6.

_____
_____
_____
_____

9. What effect will an excess of thyroid hormone (thyroxine) have on a patient's metabolic rate?

_____
_____
_____
_____

10. List the signs and symptoms of hyperthyroidism.

_____
_____
_____
_____

11. What is the cause of myxedema coma?

_____
_____
_____
_____

12. List the signs and symptoms of myxedema.

_____
_____
_____
_____

13. What gland releases calcitonin?

_____
_____
_____

14. What is the function of calcitonin?

_____
_____
_____
_____

15. Where are the parathyroid glands located?

_____

16. What hormone is released by the parathyroid glands?

_____

17. What problem(s) will be caused by an excess of the hormone from question 16?

_____
_____
_____
_____

18. What problem(s) will be caused by a deficiency of the hormone from question 16?

_____
_____
_____
_____

19. What hormone is released by the adrenal medulla?

_____

20. Where is aldosterone produced?

_____

21. What is the effect of aldosterone?

_____

22. Where are the glucocorticosteroids produced?

_____

23. What effect is produced by the glucocorticosteroids?

_____

24. What is Addison's disease?

_____
_____
_____
_____

25. Describe the effects of an addisonian crisis on a patient.

_____
_____
_____
_____

26. How would you manage a patient in addisonian crisis?

_____
_____
_____
_____

27. What is the name of the structures in the pancreas that function as endocrine glands?

_____

28. What type of cell produces insulin?

_____

29. What is the principal effect of insulin?

_____

30. What type of cell produces glucagon?

_____

31. What is the principal effect of glucagon?

_____

32. What hormone is absent or deficient in diabetes mellitus?

_____

33. Compare and contrast type 1 and type 2 diabetes.

_____
_____
_____
_____

34. What change in the extracellular fluid pH would you expect to find in a patient with diabetic ketoacidosis? What acid-base imbalance would this change reflect?

_____
_____
_____
_____

35. What are the "polys" of diabetic ketoacidosis?

_____
_____
_____
_____

36. What is a silent myocardial infarction (MI)? Why are patients with diabetes prone to having silent MIs?

_____
_____
_____
_____

37. What is the principal pathophysiologic difference between diabetic ketoacidosis and hyperglycemic hyperosmolar nonketotic coma (HHNC)?

_____
_____
_____
_____

38. What group of patients with diabetes is particularly prone to HHNC?

_____

39. What is gestational diabetes? What physiologic effect is responsible for gestational diabetes?

_____
_____
_____
_____

MULTIPLE CHOICE

1. The body attempts to compensate for the acidosis associated with diabetic ketoacidosis by _____.
   A. decreasing the heart rate and ventilatory rate
   B. decreasing urine output
   C. increasing heart rate and contractility
   D. increasing the rate and depth of ventilations

2. The islets of Langerhans secrete _____.
   A. glucagon from alpha cells, which decreases the blood glucose level
   B. glucagon from beta cells, which increases the blood glucose level
   C. insulin from alpha cells, which increases the blood glucose level
   D. insulin from beta cells, which decreases the blood glucose level

3. Your patient is a 45-year-old man with a 3-year history of diabetes mellitus. He was found unresponsive and hyperglycemic. He has been ill recently with an infected toe. Based only on this information, which of the following is the most accurate statement about this patient?
   A. He has type 1 diabetes.
   B. He is experiencing diabetic ketoacidosis.
   C. He is experiencing HHNC.
   D. He will need to be placed on insulin injection therapy for the remainder of his life.

4. Which of the following statements regarding the pathophysiology of osmotic diuresis in the diabetes patient is correct?
   A. Because the kidneys can only concentrate urine to a certain osmotic pressure, they must excrete more water than usual.
   B. Hypoglycemia decreases the osmotic pressure of the blood.
   C. Hypoglycemia increases the osmotic pressure of the blood.
   D. The kidneys begin to excrete glucose, thus decreasing the osmotic pressure in the urine.

5. The functions of the endocrine system overlap with those of other body systems. The body system that has the most significant interaction with the functions of the endocrine system is the _____.
   A. autonomic nervous system
   B. central nervous system
   C. digestive system
   D. lymphatic system

6. The presence of a thyroid goiter, tachycardia, fever, and weight loss are typically associated with _____.
   A. adrenal insufficiency
   B. calcitonin storm
   C. Graves' disease
   D. hypothyroidism

7. You respond to a 50-year-old woman who is complaining of dizziness, N/V, and weakness. She denies pain. You learn she was recently diagnosed with a tumor on top of her kidney. Your examination reveals: BP—98/62 mm Hg supine, 90/54 mm Hg sitting; P—96 beats/min supine, 114 beats/min sitting; ventilatory rate—24 breaths/min; lung sounds clear and equal; no JVD; ECG—sinus rhythm varying to sinus tachycardia; skin—cool and clammy. Based upon this information, your differential diagnosis should include which of the following?
   A. Addisonian crisis
   B. Cushing's disease
   C. Graves' disease
   D. Myxedema

8. You are called to the residence of a 22-year-old female with type 1 diabetes who is reportedly unconscious. She apparently did not eat her lunch. She responds to pain by moaning only. Her vital signs are: BP—118/78 mm Hg; P—110 beats/min; R—20 breaths/min; skin—cool and clammy; blood glucose—30 mg/dL. After administering oxygen, your next steps are to _____.
   A. administer ½ tube of glucose paste into the cheek while attempting to establish IV access
   B. administer 1 mg of glucagon IM and then obtain IV access
   C. establish IV access and administer 1 mg of glucagon IV
   D. establish IV access and administer 25 g of 50% glucose IV

9. You are seeing a 40-year-old woman complaining of headache and dizziness. In your examination, you find a swelling (hump) between the shoulder blades, a moon-shaped face, and excessive facial hair growth. You suspect this woman has a condition known as _____.
   A. Addison's disease
   B. Cushing's syndrome
   C. hepatic encephalopathy
   D. myxedema

10. Of the following diabetes conditions, which is associated with an autoimmune origin?
    A. Diabetes insipidus
    B. Diabetic ketoacidosis
    C. Type 1 diabetes
    D. Type 2 diabetes

11. Calcitonin is responsible for _____.
    A. decreasing the amount of calcium in the blood by inhibiting breakdown of bone
    B. increasing the amount of calcium in the blood by breaking down calcium stored in the bone
    C. increasing thyroid-stimulating hormone levels in the blood
    D. stimulating the release of epinephrine from the adrenal medulla

12. Your patient is reported to have a history of myxedema coma episodes. Based on this information you expect his cardiovascular examination to result in findings of _____.
    A. bradycardia and hypertension
    B. bradycardia and hypotension
    C. tachycardia and hypertension
    D. tachycardia and hypotension

CASE STUDIES

Case one

The patient is a 14-year-old female who has been sick with pneumonia for approximately 1 week. The pneumonia responded to a course of antibiotics that was completed 3 days ago. The patient then began complaining of headache, abdominal pain, nausea, and vomiting, which worsened over the last 2 days. The patient responds to questions with a weak voice. Her skin is dry, pale, and cool. Her respirations are deep and rapid, and her breath smells like rotten apples. Vital signs are: BP—94/60 mm Hg; P—136 beats/min weak, regular; R—32 breaths/min deep, regular. The patient has not taken any other medications since completing her antibiotic therapy.

1. From what endocrine disease is this patient suffering?
   _____

2. This disease occurs in two types (type 1 and type 2). From which type is this patient probably suffering?
   _____

3. What is the difference between the two types of this disease?
   _____
   _____
   _____
   _____

4. What is the patient's acute problem?
   _____

5. Why are the patient's respirations deep and rapid?
   _____
   _____
   _____
   _____

6. What is this respiratory pattern called?
   _____

7. What is the cause of the patient's unusual breath odor?
   _____

8. Why are the materials producing this unusual breath odor present in her body?
   _____
   _____
   _____
   _____

9. Would you expect this patient's blood sugar level to be too high or too low? Why?

_____
_____
_____
_____

10. Would her blood pH be increased or decreased? Why?

_____
_____
_____
_____

11. From what acid-base imbalance is the patient suffering?

_____

12. From what type of shock is this patient suffering?

_____

13. Describe your prehospital management of this patient.

_____
_____
_____
_____

14. Based on the pathophysiology of the patient's underlying disease process, justify your selection of an IV fluid.

_____
_____
_____
_____

15. The patient's ECG shows tall, peaked T waves. What electrolyte imbalance does this suggest? Why is this electrolyte imbalance present?

_____
_____
_____
_____

16. What drug would you give to correct this problem?

_____

17. As this patient's acute problem resolves, what is likely to happen to the amounts of this electrolyte in the extracellular fluids? Why?

_____
_____
_____
_____

Case two

You are called to a nursing home to see a 68-year-old female who is 10-days status postsurgical amputation of the right leg below the knee because of diabetes. The patient has been complaining of weakness and fatigue. She now responds only to painful stimuli with nonpurposeful movement of her arms and legs. The patient's skin is pale, cool, and dry. Her tongue and mucous membranes are dry. She does not have any unusual breath odors, and her respirations are rapid and shallow. Her blood sugar level is 950 mg/dL. Vital signs are: BP—88/50 mm Hg; P—128 beats/min weak, irregular; R—22 breaths/min shallow, regular. Her ECG shows atrial fibrillation with a rapid ventricular response.

1. From which type of diabetes is this patient probably suffering?

   _____

2. What is the patient's acute problem?

   _____

3. Why is this patient not exhibiting the respiratory pattern seen in the patient in Case One?

   _____
   _____
   _____
   _____

4. Why does this patient not have the unusual breath odor seen in the patient in Case One?

   _____
   _____
   _____
   _____

5. Why do patients with this condition develop blood sugar levels that are much higher than those seen in patients such as the one in Case One?

   _____
   _____
   _____
   _____

6. From what type of shock is this patient suffering?

   _____

7. Why has this patient developed this form of shock?

   _____
   _____
   _____
   _____

8. Because of the patient's very high blood sugar levels, what problem can you anticipate concerning blood flow in the vascular system?

   _____
   _____
   _____
   _____

9. Over time, what change will you anticipate seeing in this patient's blood pH? Why?

   _____
   _____
   _____
   _____

10. From what acid-base imbalance is the patient suffering?

   _____

11. Describe your prehospital management of this patient.

   _____
   _____
   _____
   _____

Case three

Your patient is a 24-year-old male with a history of diabetes who is experiencing syncopal episodes, dizziness, and headache. He has a BP of 130/80 mm Hg and a full, regular pulse of 120 beats/min. His skin is pale, cool, and moist. He says he took his insulin this morning but has not eaten all day.

1. From what problem is the patient probably suffering?

2. How does the brain differ from other tissues in its demand for and its ability to process sugar?

3. Why does this patient have tachycardia, pallor, and diaphoresis?

4. How should this patient be managed?

Case four

A 23-year-old woman (gravida 1, para 0) has developed increasing urinary output. She also complains of headache, nausea, and weakness. A check of her blood sugar level shows that she is hyperglycemic with a blood glucose level of 300 mg/dL. She has no previous history of diabetes mellitus.

1. From what problem is this patient suffering?

2. What is the relationship between this problem and the patient's pregnancy? (Be specific about the hormone involved.)

3. Why are the effects of this hormone on blood glucose levels normally useful during pregnancy?

4. What other mechanism can produce this problem in women?

Case five

A 62-year-old male with a history of diabetes mellitus developed nausea and shortness of breath. He also complained of feeling dizzy and weak. The patient's blood glucose level was found to be 170 mg/dL. Vital signs are: P—56 beats/min weak, regular; BP—96/50 mm Hg; R—24 breaths/min shallow, regular. The monitoring lead showed a sinus bradycardia. A 12-lead ECG showed ST segment elevation in leads II, III, and aVF.

1. What problem do you suspect is present?

   _____

2. Why is this problem common in patients with diabetes?

   _____

   _____

3. In what other group does this problem commonly occur?

   _____

Case six

You are called to see a 24-year-old male who has been arrested for driving while intoxicated. The patient exhibits confusion, slurred speech, and an ataxic gait. You can smell the odor of beer on his breath. His pupils are dilated and react sluggishly to light. His skin is pale, cool, and moist. Vital signs are: P—124 beats/min strong, regular; BP—138/96 mm Hg; R—18 breaths/min shallow, regular. The patient complains of a headache and double vision, but swears that he only had "one beer." When you check the patient's blood glucose level, it registers at 40 mg/dL. When the patient is given oral glucose, his symptoms rapidly resolve. A blood alcohol level registers at 5 mg/dL (0.05), well below the legal limit. The patient has no history of diabetes and takes no medications.

1. What explains the decrease in this patient's blood sugar levels?

   _____

   _____

   _____

   _____

Case seven

You are called to see a 28-year-old female who has reportedly "gone crazy." The patient is not oriented to place and time and has rapid, confused speech. She is extremely restless and anxious with fine tremors of her hands. Her skin is flushed, warm, and moist. The patient has a recent history of delivering her first child 4 weeks ago. The symptoms began after delivery. She is scheduled to see her internist because her obstetrician is concerned about recent weight loss and a mass near the base of her neck. Her ECG shows atrial fibrillation with a rapid ventricular response. Vital signs are: BP—176/84 mm Hg; P—138 beats/min weak, irregularly irregular; R—28 breaths/min shallow, regular; temperature—102.4° F.

1. From what problem is this patient suffering?

   _____

2. What complications can result from this problem?

   _____

   _____

   _____

   _____

3. How can this problem be managed?

   _____

   _____

   _____

   _____

Case eight

A 68-year-old female underwent a thyroidectomy to treat Graves' disease about 5 weeks ago. Her neighbors had not seen her for 3 days, so they called the police, who forced entry into the patient's home. It is winter, and the temperature of the apartment was 66°F. The patient was found lying on the couch. She responds to painful stimuli by moaning. Vital signs are: P—58 beats/min weak, regular; R—8 breaths/min shallow, regular; BP—92/56 mm Hg. The patient's skin is pale, cool, and dry. Nonpitting edema of the face and extremities is present. An unfilled prescription for levothyroxine (Synthroid) was found on the kitchen table.

1. From what problem is this patient suffering?

2. How would you manage this patient?

Case nine

A 55-year-old female has been experiencing syncopal episodes. She tells you that she has been experiencing extreme weakness and fatigue during the past month, and that her sleep patterns have become altered. Physical examination reveals an unusually full face and truncal obesity with a large intrascapular deposit of fat. The patient's extremities are thin and fragile looking with numerous bruises.

1. The patient's signs and symptoms probably are a result of a problem with which endocrine gland?

2. If you measured the patient's blood glucose levels, what change probably would be present? Why?

3. If you took the patient's blood pressure, what would you probably discover?

4. What accounts for this change in the patient's blood pressure?

5. What change would you probably notice in the patient's serum potassium levels?

6. Over time, some female patients with this problem develop increased growth of facial hair. Why?

_____

_____

_____

_____

Case ten

A 15-year-old male with a history of asthma was receiving treatments with hydrocortisone in an attempt to reduce the severity of the attacks. After 2 months he discontinued the medication without telling his physician or his parents. About 36 hours later he complained of a headache, became nauseated, and began to experience vomiting and diarrhea. He is now restless and confused. His respirations are rapid and shallow. His skin is pale, cool, and dry. Vital signs are: P—130 beats/min weak, regular; BP—88/46 mm Hg; R—24 breaths/min shallow, regular.

1. From what problem is the patient suffering?

_____

2. Why is he developing signs of hypoperfusion?

_____

_____

_____

_____

3. If you asked about the patient's urine output over the last couple of days, what would you find?

_____

_____

_____

_____

4. What change would you anticipate in the patient's blood glucose levels?

_____

_____

_____

_____

5. What change would you anticipate in the patient's serum potassium levels?

_____

_____

_____

_____

6. How should this patient be managed?

_____

_____

_____

_____

25 Immune System Disorders

READING ASSIGNMENT

Chapter 25, pages 972-996, in *Paramedic Practice Today: Above and Beyond.*

OBJECTIVES

After completing this chapter, you will be able to:

1. Review the specific anatomy and physiology of the immune system and pathophysiology pertinent to immune system disorders.
2. Describe characteristics of the immune system, including the categories of white blood cells, the reticuloendothelial system, and the complement system.
3. Describe the processes of the immune system defenses, including humoral and cell-mediated immunity.
4. Define *natural* and *acquired immunity.*
5. Define *antigens* and *antibodies.*
6. Discuss the formation of antibodies in the body.
7. Define specific terminology identified with immune system disorders.
8. Discuss the following relative to the human immunodeficiency virus: causative agent, body systems affected and potential secondary complications, modes of transmission, the sero-conversion rate after direct significant exposure, susceptibility and resistance, signs and symptoms, specific patient management and personal protective measures, treatments, and research exploring possible immunization.
9. Discuss the following autoimmune disorders: systemic lupus erythematosus, type 1 diabetes mellitus, rheumatoid arthritis, celiac disease, chronic active hepatitis, and multiple sclerosis.
10. Define *allergic reaction.*
11. Define *anaphylaxis.*
12. Describe the incidence, morbidity, and mortality rates of anaphylaxis.
13. Identify the risk factors most predisposing to anaphylaxis.
14. Discuss the anatomy and physiology of the organs and structures related to anaphylaxis.
15. Describe the prevention of anaphylaxis and appropriate patient education.
16. Discuss the pathophysiology of allergy and anaphylaxis.
17. Describe the common methods of entry of substances into the body.
18. List common antigens most frequently associated with anaphylaxis.
19. Describe physical manifestations and pathophysiologic principles of anaphylaxis.
20. Differentiate manifestations of an allergic reaction from for anaphylaxis.
21. Recognize the signs and symptoms related to anaphylaxis.
22. Differentiate the various treatment and pharmacologic interventions used in the management of anaphylaxis.
23. Describe the clinical significance of abnormal findings in the patient with anaphylaxis.
24. Develop a treatment plan for the patient with allergic reaction and anaphylaxis.
25. Discuss the principles of and disorders related to transplantation surgery.
26. Discuss public health principles relevant to immune system disorders.

CHAPTER SUMMARY

- The immune system includes both internal and external defenses to protect against pathogens.
- Pathogens include prions, viruses, bacteria, parasites, and fungi.
- Internal defenses are divided into natural and acquired immunity. Natural immunity is nonspecific and defends against all potential pathogens in a similar way (e.g., inflammatory response). Acquired immunity is specific to a particular pathogen (e.g., vaccination).
- The immune system can fail, causing immunodeficiencies, which may be acquired or congenital. Congenital immunodeficiencies, such as severe combined immunodeficiency syndrome, are present at birth and often are genetic. Acquired immunodeficiencies, such as HIV, must be transmitted to a patient and usually are infectious.
- Autoimmune diseases are present when the immune system response attacks its own tissue (e.g., MS and lupus).
- Hypersensitivity disorders manifest themselves as excessive responses to an antigen that are uncomfortable or dangerous for the patient. They are divided into four types: type I (immediate), type II (cytotoxic), type III (immune complex–mediated), and type IV (delayed).
- Anaphylaxis is a good example of type I hypersensitivity. Drug reactions are an example of type II. Poststreptococcal glomerulonephritis is an example of type III, and tuberculosis skin testing is a good example of type IV hypersensitivity.
- Transplant recipients can have two different types of problems involving the immune system. Their immune

system can function too well and reject the transplanted organ. On the other hand, when the immune system is suppressed to avoid rejection, other opportunistic infections can develop because of the lack of normal immune response.

■ Meticulous attention to personal protective equipment and body substance isolation are important when treating all patients, especially those with communicable immune system disorders. This also includes complying with vaccination requirements for health providers and specific missions and encouraging the public to comply with universal vaccination recommendations.

SHORT ANSWER

1. Which type of immunoglobulin is responsible for most allergic reactions?

_____

2. Name the chemical released by mast cells that produces signs and symptoms of anaphylaxis.

_____

3. List the three effects produced by this substance that account for these signs and symptoms.

_____

_____

_____

4. What is the preferred IV solution for the management of anaphylaxis? Why?

_____

_____

_____

_____

5. What are the two first-line drugs other than oxygen used in the management of anaphylaxis?

_____

_____

6. In what general class of drugs is diphenhydramine (Benadryl) a member?

_____

7. By what two routes is diphenhydramine given in the prehospital setting?

_____

_____

8. Which route should be used for medication administration if a patient is suffering from anaphylaxis? Why?

_____

_____

_____

9. Why are the alpha effects of epinephrine beneficial in the management of anaphylactic shock?

_____

_____

_____

_____

10. Why are the beta effects of epinephrine beneficial in the management of anaphylaxis?

_____

_____

_____

_____

11. Should epinephrine or diphenhydramine be given first during the management of anaphylaxis? Why?

_____

_____

_____

_____

12. Why are corticosteroids sometimes given during follow-up care of patients who have had severe allergic reactions?

_____

_____

_____

_____

13. What group of cells produces antibodies?

_____

14. What organ is responsible for promoting the development of T-cells?

_____

15. What is the role of the helper T-cell in the functioning of the immune system?

_____

_____

_____

_____

16. What is the role of the macrophage in the functioning of the immune system?

_____

_____

_____

_____

17. What are the signs and symptoms of a mild allergic reaction?

_____

_____

_____

_____

18. What are the signs and symptoms of a moderate allergic reaction?

_____

_____

_____

_____

19. What are the signs and symptoms of a severe allergic reaction (anaphylaxis)?

_____

_____

_____

_____

20. What is systemic lupus erythematosis?

_____

_____

_____

_____

21. Describe the major problems likely to result in a patient with systemic lupus erythematosis seeking care from EMS.

_____

_____

_____

_____

MULTIPLE CHOICE

1. Administration of epinephrine can correct urticaria associated with anaphylaxis. This can best be explained by epinephrine's effects on _____.
   A. alpha-receptor sites
   B. beta$_1$-receptor sites
   C. beta$_2$-receptor sites
   D. dopaminergic receptor sites

2. The release of histamine causes _____.
   A. arteriolar constriction and hypovolemia
   B. bronchospasm and increased circulating blood volume
   C. constriction of vascular smooth muscle and hypoxemia
   D. increased vascular membrane permeability and bronchospasm

3. You are called for a 24-year-old woman with a rash. You find the patient sitting in a chair, alert and oriented to person, place, and time. She is covered with a rash and states she itches all over. She states that she has been ill with a cold and saw her physician yesterday. She was given an antibiotic prescription. She took the first dose yesterday morning and the second dose 30 minutes ago. Auscultation of the chest reveals clear lung sounds. The patient's BP is 128/74 mm Hg, pulse is 92 beats/min and regular, and respirations are 18 breaths/min. Management of this patient should include oxygen followed by _____.
   A. 0.3 mg of epinephrine 1:1000 Sub-Q
   B. 2.5 mg of albuterol by small volume nebulizer
   C. 50 mg of diphenhydramine IM
   D. 125 mg of methylprednisolone IM

4. Antibodies or immunoglobulins are a component of _____.
   A. cell-mediated immunity and produced by the B-lymphocytes
   B. cell-mediated immunity and produced by the T-lymphocytes
   C. humoral immunity and produced by the B-lymphocytes
   D. humoral immunity and produced by the T-lymphocytes

5. IgE-type antibodies are primarily bound to mast cells in the _____.
   A. blood
   B. bone marrow
   C. lymphatic system
   D. tissues

6. The T-lymphocytes that coordinate the activities of the immune system's other components are the _____.
   A. helper T-cells
   B. killer T-cells
   C. memory T-cells
   D. suppressor T-cells

7. A 20-year-old man is experiencing an anaphylactic reaction. After administration of oxygen, the first drug that should be administered to this patient is _____.
   A. diphenhydramine
   B. epinephrine
   C. hypotonic fluids
   D. Solu-Medrol

8. Your patient is a 38-year-old woman who originally experienced a syncopal episode witnessed by her family. The patient is now complaining of mild shortness of breath, facial swelling, and abdominal pain. In your examination, you find that the patient has a positive orthostatic test and her skin is very warm and red. You suspect this patient is experiencing _____.
   A. a mild allergic reaction
   B. a moderate allergic reaction
   C. an anaphylactic reaction
   D. hemorrhagic shock

9. The most dramatic hypersensitivity reactions are classified as type I reactions. In a type I hypersensitivity reaction, the IgE antibody is bound to _____.
   A. basophils or mast cells
   B. histamine or chemotactic substances
   C. immunoglobulins
   D. opsonins or leukocytes

10. Mast cells release _____.
    A. heparin, leukotrienes, and macrophages
    B. histamine, heparin, and leukotrienes
    C. leukotrienes, histamine, and macrophages
    D. macrophages, histamine, and heparin

11. Your patient is a 45-year-old man whose medical history includes a disorder of the GI system that also involves his immune system. Which of the following is the most likely GI disease included in this man's history?
    A. Crohn's disease
    B. Diverticulitis
    C. Myasthenia gravis
    D. Type 1 diabetes

12. Of the following diabetic conditions, which is associated with an autoimmune origin?
    A. Diabetes insipidus
    B. Diabetic ketoacidosis
    C. Type 1 diabetes
    D. Type 2 diabetes

13. Diphenhydramine should be avoided in which of the following patients?
    A. A 20-year-old patient with myasthenia gravis who is having an anaphylactic reaction
    B. A 30-year-old patient with asthma who is having a moderate allergic reaction
    C. A 40-year-old patient with a history of dystonic reactions
    D. A 50-year-old patient with congestive heart failure who is presently having a mild allergic reaction

14. Abdominal pain associated with an allergic reaction occurs because of _____.
    A. smooth muscle spasm
    B. sympathetic nervous system response
    C. the release of eosinophils
    D. vasodilation

15. Oxygen should be given to a patient who is having an allergic reaction _____.
    A. by nasal cannula at 4 L/min
    B. by nonrebreather mask at 15 L/min
    C. by nonrebreather mask at 6 L/min
    D. only if wheezing or stridor are present

16. When a nebulized bronchodilator is given to a patient, which of the following effects should be anticipated?
    A. Drowsiness; tremors
    B. Increased pulse rate; drowsiness
    C. Nervousness; decreased pulse rate
    D. Tremors; increased pulse rate

17. The classic signs and symptoms of anaphylaxis include
    _____.
    A. bradycardia and hypotension
    B. hypertension and bradycardia
    C. hypertension and tachycardia
    D. tachycardia and hypotension

CASE STUDY

You are dispatched to a report of "difficulty breathing." The patient is a 38-year-old male who was mowing his lawn when he was stung on his right arm by a bee. He has a history of severe allergic reactions to Hymenoptera sting. He is unresponsive. His respirations are rapid and shallow. Inspiratory stridor and expiratory wheezing are present. The patient's face and nailbeds are cyanotic. Radial pulses are absent. The carotid pulse is rapid and weak. Capillary refill is greater than 5 seconds. The bee's stinger is visible on the patient's right forearm.

1. What is your first priority in managing this patient?

   _____
   _____

2. Should you remove the bee's stinger? If your answer is yes, how should this be done?

   _____
   _____
   _____
   _____

3. Why is the patient hypoperfusing?

   _____
   _____
   _____
   _____

4. What type of IV solution should be used to manage this patient? Why?

_____

_____

_____

_____

5. What route should be used to administer medications to this patient? Why?

_____

_____

_____

_____

6. What is the first drug other than oxygen that should be given to this patient? Why?

_____

_____

_____

_____

7. After this drug is administered, what drug should be given next?

_____

8. What is the therapeutic effect of this drug?

_____

_____

_____

_____

9. Why would Solu-Medrol be given to this patient?

_____

_____

_____

_____

10. Why should Solu-Medrol be administered last during the management of this patient?

_____

_____

_____

_____

26 Gastrointestinal Disorders

READING ASSIGNMENT

Chapter 26, pages 997-1031, in *Paramedic Practice Today: Above and Beyond*.

OBJECTIVES

After completing this chapter, you will be able to:

1. Describe the incidence, morbidity, and mortality rates of gastrointestinal emergencies.
2. Identify the risk factors most predisposing to gastrointestinal emergencies.
3. Discuss the anatomy and physiology of the organs and structures related to gastrointestinal diseases.
4. Discuss the pathophysiology of inflammation and its relation to acute abdominal pain.
5. Define *somatic pain* as it relates to gastroenterology.
6. Define *visceral pain* as it relates to gastroenterology.
7. Define *referred pain* as it relates to gastroenterology.
8. Differentiate hemorrhagic from nonhemorrhagic abdominal pain.
9. Discuss the signs and symptoms of local inflammation relative to acute abdominal pain.
10. Discuss the signs and symptoms of peritoneal inflammation relative to acute abdominal pain.
11. List the signs and symptoms of general inflammation relative to acute abdominal pain.
12. Based on assessment findings, differentiate local, peritoneal, and general inflammation as they relate to acute abdominal pain.
13. Describe the questioning technique and specific questions the paramedic should ask when gathering a focused history in a patient with abdominal pain.
14. Describe the technique for performing a comprehensive physical examination on a patient with abdominal pain.
15. Define *abdominal wall hernia*.
16. Define *incarcerated hernia*.
17. Define the etiology of an incarcerated hernia.
18. Describe signs and symptoms of an incarcerated hernia.
19. Describe the treatment for an incarcerated hernia.
20. Define *esophagitis*.
21. List the common causes of esophagitis.
22. Describe the signs and symptoms of esophagitis.
23. Describe the treatment of esophagitis.
24. Define *candidiasis of the esophagus*.
25. Describe the etiology of candidiasis esophagitis.
26. Describe the signs and symptoms of candidiasis esophagitis.
27. Describe the treatment for candidiasis esophagitis.
28. Describe gastroesophageal reflux.
29. Define the cause of gastroesophageal reflux.
30. Describe the symptoms of reflux and explain how they differ from other forms of esophagitis.
31. Describe the treatment for gastroesophageal reflux.
32. Define *caustic substances*.
33. Provide examples of caustic substances.
34. Define the type of necrosis that occurs with acidic and alkali substances.
35. Describe the importance of obtaining a history in caustic ingestion.
36. Describe the pertinent parts of the physical examination in caustic ingestion.
37. Define treatment for caustic ingestion.
38. Define *Boerhaave syndrome*.
39. Describes the signs and symptoms of Boerhaave syndrome.
40. Describe the treatment of Boerhaave syndrome.
41. Define *esophageal foreign body*.
42. Describe the signs and symptoms of an esophageal foreign body.
43. Describe the appropriate treatment for esophageal foreign body.
44. Define *hiatal hernia*.
45. Describe the signs and symptoms of a hiatal hernia.
46. Define *Mallory-Weiss syndrome*.
47. Describe the signs and symptoms of Mallory-Weiss syndrome.
48. Describe the appropriate treatment for Mallory-Weiss syndrome.
49. Define *esophageal stricture* and *stenosis*.
50. Describe the signs and symptoms of esophageal stricture and stenosis.
51. Describe the appropriate treatment for esophageal stricture and stenosis.
52. Define *tracheoesophageal fistula*.
53. Describe the signs and symptoms of a tracheoesophageal fistula.
54. Describe the appropriate treatment for tracheoesophageal fistula.
55. Define *esophageal varices*.
56. Discuss the pathophysiology of esophageal varices.
57. Describe the signs and symptoms related to esophageal varices.
58. Describe the appropriate management for esophageal varices.
59. Integrate pathophysiologic principles and assessment findings to formulate a field impression and implement a treatment plan for the patient with esophageal varices.

60. Define *cirrhosis*.
61. Describe the pathophysiology of cirrhosis.
62. Describe the signs and symptoms of cirrhosis.
63. Describe the appropriate treatment of cirrhosis.
64. Define *hepatorenal failure*.
65. Describe the signs and symptoms of hepatorenal failure.
66. Describe the appropriate treatment of hepatorenal failure.
67. Define *acute hepatitis*.
68. Discuss the pathophysiology of acute hepatitis.
69. Recognize the signs and symptoms related to acute hepatitis.
70. Describe the management of acute hepatitis.
71. Integrate pathophysiologic principles and assessment findings to formulate a field impression and implement a treatment plan for the patient with acute hepatitis.
72. Define *hepatic tumors*.
73. Describe the signs and symptoms of hepatic tumors.
74. Describe the appropriate treatment of hepatic tumors.
75. Define *cholecystitis, cholelithiasis, cholangitis*, and *choledocholithiasis*.
76. Discuss the pathophysiology of cholecystitis.
77. Recognize the signs and symptoms related to cholecystitis.
78. Describe the management of cholecystitis.
79. Integrate pathophysiologic principles and assessment findings to formulate a field impression and implement a treatment plan for the patient with cholecystitis.
80. Define *pancreatitis*.
81. Discuss the pathophysiology of pancreatitis.
82. Recognize the signs and symptoms related to pancreatitis.
83. Describe the management of pancreatitis.
84. Integrate pathophysiologic principles and assessment findings to formulate a field impression and implement a treatment plan for the patient with pancreatitis.
85. Define *pancreatic tumors*.
86. Define *adenocarcinoma, cyst adenoma*, and *neuroendocrine tumors*.
87. Describe the signs and symptoms of pancreatic tumors.
88. Describe the appropriate treatment of pancreatic tumors.
89. Define *peritonitis*.
90. Describe the signs and symptoms of peritonitis.
91. Describe the appropriate treatment for peritonitis.
92. Define *gastritis*.
93. Describe signs and symptoms of gastritis.
94. Describe the appropriate treatment for gastritis.
95. Define *peptic ulcer disease*.
96. Discuss the pathophysiology of peptic ulcer disease.
97. Recognize the signs and symptoms related to peptic ulcer disease.
98. Describe the management of peptic ulcer disease.

99. Integrate pathophysiologic principles and assessment findings to formulate a field impression and implement a treatment plan for the patient with peptic ulcer disease.
100. Define *upper gastrointestinal bleeding*.
101. Discuss the pathophysiology of upper gastrointestinal bleeding.
102. Recognize the signs and symptoms related to upper gastrointestinal bleeding.
103. Describe the management of upper gastrointestinal bleeding.
104. Integrate pathophysiologic principles and assessment findings to formulate a field impression and implement a treatment plan for the patient with upper gastrointestinal bleeding.
105. Define *lower gastrointestinal bleeding*.
106. Discuss the pathophysiology of lower gastrointestinal bleeding.
107. Recognize the signs and symptoms related to lower gastrointestinal bleeding.
108. Describe the management of lower gastrointestinal bleeding.
109. Integrate pathophysiologic principles and assessment findings to formulate a field impression and implement a treatment plan for the patient with lower gastrointestinal bleeding.
110. Define *acute gastroenteritis*.
111. Discuss the pathophysiology of acute gastroenteritis.
112. Recognize the signs and symptoms related to acute gastroenteritis.
113. Describe the management of acute gastroenteritis.
114. Integrate pathophysiologic principles and assessment findings to formulate a field impression and implement a treatment plan for the patient with acute gastroenteritis.
115. Define *bowel obstruction*.
116. Discuss the pathophysiology of bowel obstruction.
117. Recognize the signs and symptoms related to bowel obstruction.
118. Describe the management of bowel obstruction.
119. Integrate pathophysiologic principles and assessment findings to formulate a field impression and implement a treatment plan for the patient with bowel obstruction.
120. Define *appendicitis*.
121. Discuss the pathophysiology of appendicitis.
122. Recognize the signs and symptoms related to appendicitis.
123. Describe the management of appendicitis.
124. Integrate pathophysiologic principles and assessment findings to formulate a field impression and implement a treatment plan for the patient with appendicitis.
125. Define *colitis*.
126. Discuss the pathophysiology of colitis.
127. Recognize the signs and symptoms related to colitis.
128. Describe the management of colitis.

129. Integrate pathophysiologic principles and assessment findings to formulate a field impression and implement a treatment plan for the patient with colitis.
130. Define *Crohn's disease*.
131. Discuss the pathophysiology of Crohn's disease.
132. Recognize the signs and symptoms related to Crohn's disease.
133. Describe the management of Crohn's disease.
134. Integrate pathophysiologic principles and assessment findings to formulate a field impression and implement a treatment plan for the patient with Crohn's disease.
135. Define *diverticulitis*.
136. Discuss the pathophysiology of diverticulitis.
137. Recognize the signs and symptoms related to diverticulitis.
138. Describe the management of diverticulitis.
139. Integrate pathophysiologic principles and assessment findings to formulate a field impression and implement a treatment plan for the patient with diverticulitis.
140. Define *hemorrhoids*.
141. Discuss the pathophysiology of hemorrhoids.
142. Recognize the signs and symptoms related to hemorrhoids.
143. Describe the management of hemorrhoids.
144. Integrate pathophysiologic principles and assessment findings to formulate a field impression and implement a treatment plan for the patient with hemorrhoids.
145. Integrate pathophysiologic principles of the patient with a gastrointestinal emergency.
146. Differentiate gastrointestinal emergencies on the basis of assessment findings.
147. Correlate abnormal findings in the assessment with the clinical significance in the patient with abdominal pain.
148. Develop a patient management plan based on field impression in the patient with abdominal pain.

CHAPTER SUMMARY

- Abdominal pain is one of the most common reasons that patients seek emergency care.
- Etiology of abdominal pain varies with the patient's age and risk factors.
- The gastrointestinal (GI) system includes all organs responsible for the ingestion and digestion of food.
- Pain that is well localized is called *somatic pain*.
- Pain that is poorly localized is called *visceral pain*.
- Pain that is felt at a distant location is called *referred pain*.
- Pain assessment should follow the OPQRST mnemonic.
- The assessment should contain open-ended questions.
- Management of GI symptoms should include a primary survey, a secondary survey, pain and nausea management, and fluid replacement.
- Local protocols should be followed for appropriate treatment and management.

- Hernias that become strangulated or incarcerated can pose a serious medical condition.
- Esophagitis is inflammation of the esophagus and has many causes.
- Gastroesophageal reflux disease (GERD) is a common disorder that leads to esophagitis.
- Caustic ingestions can cause trauma to the esophagus.
- Historical facts such as time of ingestion, chemical ingestion, and amount ingested are important.
- Airway control is very important in caustic ingestions.
- Esophageal obstruction can occur with caustic ingestions.
- Most foreign objects will pass through the GI tract if they enter the stomach.
- Vomiting may lead to longitudinal tears in the esophagus called Mallory-Weiss tears.
- Hematemesis (frank bloody emesis) may occur with a Mallory-Weiss tear.
- Esophageal stenosis can occur from esophagitis.
- Tracheoesophageal fistula and esophageal atresia are congenital conditions.
- Tracheoesophageal fistula can lead to aspiration of food and liquids into the lungs.
- Esophageal varices can be caused by portal hypertension.
- Hematemesis may occur with varices and may be serious.
- Cirrhosis can lead to liver failure.
- Cirrhosis is caused by damage to the liver cells.
- Cirrhosis can lead to ascites or fluid in the abdominal cavity.
- Ascites can become infected and lead to sepsis (small-bowel perforation [SBP]).
- Cirrhosis often can cause encephalopathy, or altered consciousness or coma.
- Renal failure may follow liver failure.
- Hepatitis is an inflammatory condition of the liver.
- Hepatitis may be self-limiting or progress to liver failure.
- Hepatitis A is transmitted by the fecal-oral route.
- Hepatitis B is transmitted by sexual contact, body fluid, tattoos, and blood transfusions.
- Hepatitis C is transmitted by infected blood or body fluids.
- Cholelithiasis is the presence of stones in the gallbladder.
- Cholelithiasis has an incidence of 10% to 20% of the population in developed countries.
- Pancreatitis is inflammation of the pancreas.
- Pancreatitis can present with severe abdominal pain, nausea, and vomiting.
- Peritonitis occurs when the lining of the abdominal cavity becomes inflamed.
- Rebound tenderness may be present with peritonitis.
- Gastritis is inflammation of the gastric mucosa.
- Gastritis can present with significant abdominal pain.
- Peptic ulcers can cause significant GI bleeding.
- GI bleeding has many causes.
- Treatment begins with a primary survey for GI bleeding.
- Appendicitis usually begins with periumbilical pain.
- Appendicitis can lead to sepsis if the luminal cavity ruptures.

- Ulcerative colitis typically affects the rectum. Ulcerative colitis is an inflammatory condition that involves the mucosal lining of the GI tract.
- Crohn's disease can affect the small and large intestines. It can cause erosion through all layers of the bowel, leading to fistula formation.
- Patients who have Crohn's disease may have arthritis, skin conditions, and inflammatory conditions of the eye in addition to bowel symptoms.
- Diverticular disease is caused by stretching of the bowel during straining and low-fiber diets. Diverticulosis is the disease of colonic diverticula (small outpouchings of the colon). Diverticulitis is inflammation of one or more of the outpouchings.
- Hemorrhoids are distended veins either internal or external to the anal opening.

SHORT ANSWER

1. Indicate the QUADRANT of the abdomen in which each of these organs is located. Also indicate whether the organ is HOLLOW or SOLID.

_____	_____	Appendix
_____	_____	Liver
_____	_____	Stomach
_____	_____	Spleen
_____	_____	Gallbladder
_____	_____	Pancreas
_____	_____	Sigmoid colon
_____	_____	Right kidney

2. What is the visceral peritoneum?

_____

_____

3. What is the parietal peritoneum?

_____

_____

4. What is visceral pain?

_____

_____

5. What is somatic pain?

_____

_____

6. What is referred pain?

_____

_____

7. Name three organs that can refer pain to the abdomen.

_____

_____

_____

8. What is a dark, tarry, foul-smelling stool called?

_____

9. What is the significance of a dark, tarry, foul-smelling stool?

_____

_____

_____

_____

10. What does the presence of bright red blood in the stool indicate about the location of hemorrhaging into the gastrointestinal tract?

_____

_____

_____

_____

11. Should you palpate a patient's abdomen before or after auscultating? Why?

_____

_____

_____

_____

12. What are esophageal varices?

_____

_____

13. Why are patients with a history of alcohol abuse at increased risk of developing esophageal varices?

_____

_____

_____

_____

14. What is Mallory-Weiss syndrome?

_____

_____

15. The patient complains of severe cramping abdominal pain associated with nausea and vomiting. The abdomen is markedly distended. Auscultation of the abdomen reveals high-pitched "tinkling" bowel sounds that peak at the moment of the patient's greatest pain. What problem do you suspect?

_____

16. Patients with acute abdominal pain generally should not be given anything by mouth. Why?

_____

_____

_____

_____

17. Patients 30 years of age or older who complain of acute abdominal pain, especially in the epigastric area, should be placed on an ECG monitor. Why?

_____

_____

_____

_____

18. What IV fluid should be used for a patient experiencing acute abdominal pain and diffuse tenderness? Why?

_____
_____
_____
_____

19. What is McBurney's point?

_____
_____

20. What is Murphy's sign?

_____
_____

MULTIPLE CHOICE

1. A 52-year-old businessman is complaining of mid-epigastric pain and nausea. He states the pain is constant and radiates to his mid-back. The patient admits to drinking an average of 4 to 5 alcoholic beverages every evening to unwind. This patient's pain is most characteristic of _____.
   A. cholecystitits
   B. esophagitis
   C. kidney stones
   D. pancreatitis

2. A 45-year-old man is complaining of a sudden onset of acute lower abdominal pain and dizziness. He appears pale and fatigued. When obtaining a history from this patient, it would be most important to ask about the chronic use of which of the following groups of medications?
   A. Antihypertensives, aspirin, diuretics
   B. Aspirin, anticoagulants, NSAIDs
   C. Cardiac antidysrhythmics, antidepressants, anticoagulants
   D. Sedatives, laxatives, antilipidemics

3. The pain of acute appendicitis most often begins as _____.
   A. diffuse abdominal pain
   B. nonspecific periumbilical pain
   C. pain after eating a fatty meal
   D. right lower quadrant pain

4. You are called to a residence for a 55-year-old man who has had a syncopal episode. He is awake and oriented to person, place, and time, but is complaining of right upper and lower quadrant pain that radiates down his right leg. He states that his right leg also feels numb. He has no other complaints. His history includes a past myocardial infarction only, with no previous surgeries. He takes no regular medications. Considering this information, the single most likely diagnosis for this patient is _____.
   A. abdominal aortic aneurysm
   B. acute appendicitis
   C. diverticulitis
   D. renal calculus

5. Uniform inflammation of the mucosal lining of the colon and rectum that results in bloody diarrhea and abdominal pain is most likely the result of _____.
   A. colitis
   B. Crohn's disease
   C. diverticulosis
   D. esophageal varices

6. A 45-year-old male complains of severe burning pain in his upper abdomen that began suddenly 15 minutes ago. About 5 minutes before the onset of the pain, he vomited a small amount of bright red blood. For the last 6 months, he has been experiencing burning pain in the upper abdomen during periods of increased stress. His bowel movements have become dark "like tar." He is pale and diaphoretic. His epigastric area is tender to palpation. Vital signs are: BP—90/50 mm Hg; P—120 beats/min weak, regular; R—22 breaths/min shallow, regular. What problem should you suspect?
   A. Abdominal aortic aneurysm
   B. Duodenal ulcer with bleeding into the GI tract
   C. Gallbladder disease
   D. Kidney stone

7. A 42-year-old male complains of severe, constant abdominal pain. He is lying very still and says it is painful to move. His skin is warm and moist. His abdomen appears to be slightly distended, rigid, and diffusely tender. Bowel sounds are absent. Vital signs are: BP—96/50 mm Hg; P—120 beats/min weak, regular; R—26 breaths/min shallow, regular. You suspect _____.
   A. appendicitis
   B. kidney stone
   C. peritonitis
   D. ruptured aortic aneurysm

8. A 39-year-old male has experienced persistent abdominal pain for the past 12 hours. He has a history of alcoholism but takes no medications. He says he has been vomiting and that it looks "funny." You notice the vomitus in a trashcan, and it resembles coffee grounds. Vital signs are: P—126 beats/min weak, regular; R—24 breaths/min shallow, regular; BP—110/88 mm Hg. You should _____.
   A. allow the patient to drink, but only if the liquid is at room temperature
   B. avoid giving the patient anything by mouth
   C. encourage the patient to drink as much as possible to replace lost fluids
   D. give the patient water, but less than 1 cup

9. Pain and tenderness that begin around the umbilicus and move to the right lower abdominal quadrant are characteristic of _____.
   A. appendicitis
   B. cholecystitis
   C. kidney stone
   D. peptic ulcer

225

10. What is the most common cause of cholecystitis?
    A. Alcohol abuse
    B. Diabetes
    C. Gallstones
    D. Low-fiber diets

11. Which of the following patients would be most likely to develop cholecystitis?
    A. A 46-year-old male who drinks a six-pack of beer every evening
    B. A 49-year-old air traffic controller
    C. A 58-year-old male who works at a job requiring physical activity
    D. An overweight 42-year-old female with five children

12. Which of the following statements about peptic ulcer disease is correct?
    A. Duodenal ulcers are more common in persons under stress.
    B. Duodenal ulcers tend to occur in males older than 50 years.
    C. Pain from duodenal ulcers usually does not occur at night.
    D. Pain from gastric ulcers tends to occur when the stomach is empty.

13. Which of the following are risk factors for developing diverticulitis?
    A. Advanced age and alcohol abuse
    B. Alcohol abuse and low-fiber diets
    C. Female gender and being overweight
    D. Low-fiber diets and advanced age

14. The most common causes of pancreatitis are _____.
    A. diabetes and low-fiber diets
    B. excessive consumption of fatty foods and low-fiber diets
    C. gallstones and alcohol abuse
    D. low-fiber diets and advanced age

15. What type of pain is caused by stimulation of nerve fibers in the parietal peritoneum?
    A. Radiating
    B. Referred
    C. Somatic
    D. Visceral

16. What type of pain is caused by distention of a hollow organ?
    A. Radiating
    B. Referred
    C. Somatic
    D. Visceral

17. A 43-year-old female complains of abdominal pain radiating from the right upper quadrant around her right side to the angle of the scapula. What is the most likely cause of the pain?
    A. Cholecystitis
    B. Duodenal ulcer
    C. Kidney stone
    D. Pancreatitis

18. What is hematochezia?
    A. Bright red blood in the stool
    B. Dark, tarry stool
    C. Vomiting bright red blood
    D. Vomiting of material that looks like coffee grounds

19. You are called to a nursing home to transfer an 83-year-old male who is complaining of weakness and dizziness. The nurse tells you that when the patient had a bowel movement 30 minutes ago melena was present. This means that _____.
    A. bright red blood was present in the stool
    B. the stool was clay colored
    C. the stool was dark and tarry
    D. the stool was green because excess bile was present

CASE STUDIES

Case one

A 13-year-old male complains of abdominal pain that began in the periumbilical area and moved to the right lower quadrant. He also is nauseated and has been vomiting. The RLQ is tender, and the patient wants to lie on one side with his right leg drawn up. The patient denies any bleeding, melena, or significant medical history. Vital signs are: P—104 beats/min strong, regular; R—20 breaths/min shallow, regular; BP—130/70 mm Hg.

1. From what problem is this patient suffering?

   _____

2. What is the pathophysiologic mechanism that produces this problem?

   _____

226

3. Why does the pain associated with this problem begin in the periumbilical area?

_____

_____

4. Why do patients with this problem usually prefer to lie on their right side with their leg drawn up?

_____

_____

_____

_____

When you complete your examination, the patient tells you that the pain has disappeared and that he does not need to go to the hospital.

5. What should you tell this patient?

_____

_____

_____

_____

6. How should you manage him at the scene and en route to the hospital?

_____

_____

_____

_____

_____

_____

Case two

A 42-year-old male was watching television when he felt nauseated. He went to the bathroom where he vomited bright red blood. He then became dizzy and slumped to the floor. His wife called EMS. The patient is lying on the floor. He is awake but does not know where he is or what day it is. His respirations are rapid, shallow, and regular. Breath sounds are present and equal bilaterally with no adventitious sounds. The patient's radial pulse is slow and weak. The patient has a history of high blood pressure for which he takes enalapril (Vasotec). He has been experiencing intermittent episodes of "burning" epigastric pain for about 6 months. The pain is triggered by stress and drinking coffee and is relieved by taking antacids and eating bland food. The patient denies melena. Vital signs are: P—88 beats/min weak, regular; R—22 breaths/min shallow, regular; BP—106/76 mm Hg. The epigastric region is tender to palpation.

1. From what problem is the patient probably suffering?

_____

2. Is the patient's pulse rate consistent with the suspected problem? If not, why?

_____

_____

_____

_____

3. Why does this patient not have melena?

_____

_____

_____

_____

When the patient was moved to a sitting position, he became diaphoretic and complained of dizziness. His systolic BP dropped to 82 mm Hg and his radial pulses disappeared.

4. What is the significance of the changes noted in the patient's vital signs?

_____

_____

_____

_____

5. How would you treat the patient?

_____

_____

_____

_____

_____

_____

Case three

A 72-year-old female complains of severe, cramping abdominal pain. She is awake, alert, and very anxious. Her respirations are rapid and shallow. The patient's radial pulses are rapid and weak. Her skin is pale, cool, and moist. She has a history of surgery 8 months ago for treatment of diverticulosis. She has been unable to move her bowels for 3 days. Vital signs are: P—122 beats/min weak, regular; R—22 breaths/min shallow, regular; BP—96/72 mm Hg. Her abdomen is severely distended. Auscultation of the abdomen reveals high-pitched bowel sounds that peak at the moment of the patient's greatest discomfort.

1. What problem do you suspect?

_____

2. Why is the history of surgery significant?

_____

_____

_____

_____

3. What problem is suggested by the patient's vital signs? What mechanism is producing this problem?

_____

_____

_____

_____

4. The patient denies any vomiting. Combined with the severe abdominal distention, what does the absence of vomiting suggest about the location of this patient's problem?

_____

_____

_____

_____

5. When the patient begins vomiting, what can you predict about the character of the vomitus?

_____

_____

_____

_____

6. How would you manage this patient?

_____

_____

_____

_____

_____

_____

27 Renal and Urogenital Disorders

READING ASSIGNMENT

Chapter 27, pages 1032-1058, in *Paramedic Practice Today: Above and Beyond*.

OBJECTIVES

After completing this chapter, you will be able to:

1. Discuss the anatomy and physiology of the urogenital organs and structures.
2. Describe the questioning technique and specific questions the paramedic should use when gathering a focused history in a patient with abdominal pain.
3. Describe the techniques used in performing a comprehensive physical examination of a patient reporting abdominal pain associated with the urologic system.
4. Describe the incidence, morbidity, and mortality rates and risk factors predisposing to urologic emergencies.
5. Describe the etiology, history, and physical findings of acute renal failure.
6. With the patient history and physical examination findings, develop a treatment plan for a patient in acute renal failure.
7. Describe the etiology, history, and physical findings of chronic renal failure.
8. With the patient history and physical examination findings, develop a treatment plan for a patient in chronic renal failure.
9. Define *renal dialysis*.
10. Discuss the common complications of renal dialysis.
11. Describe the etiology, history, and physical findings of renal calculi.
12. With the patient history and physical examination findings, develop a treatment plan for a patient with renal calculi.
13. Describe the etiology, history, and physical findings of urinary retention.
14. With the patient history and physical examination findings, develop a treatment plan for a patient with urinary retention.
15. Describe the etiology, history, and physical findings of a urinary tract infection.
16. With the patient history and physical examination findings, develop a treatment plan for a patient with a urinary tract infection.
17. Describe the internal and external male anatomy.
18. Describe the incidence and signs and symptoms associated with genital lesions, including genital herpes, syphilis, chancroid lesions, granuloma inguinale, lymphadenoma, genital warts, and molluscum contagiosum.
19. Discuss the signs and symptoms associated with blunt genital trauma in the male patient.
20. Describe the prehospital care for blunt genital trauma in the male patient.
21. Discuss male genitourinary infections, including epididymitis, orchitis, Fournier's gangrene, prostatitis, and urethritis.
22. Describe the signs and symptoms of male genitourinary infections, including epididymitis, orchitis, and Fournier's gangrene.
23. Describe the etiology, history, and physical findings of phimosis and paraphimosis.
24. With the patient history and physical examination findings, develop a treatment plan for a patient with paraphimosis.
25. Describe the etiology, history, and physical findings of priapism.
26. With the patient history and physical examination findings, develop a treatment plan for a patient with priapism.
27. Discuss the epidemiology of benign prostatic hypertrophy.
28. Discuss the effects of an enlarged prostate gland, including urinary retention, increased risk of urinary tract infections, and renal failure.
29. Discuss the etiology of testicular masses.
30. Describe the etiology, history, and physical examination findings of testicular torsion.
31. With the patient history and physical examination findings, develop a treatment plan for a patient with testicular torsion.

CHAPTER SUMMARY

- Patients complaining of abdominal pain or discomfort pose a challenge to paramedics. One source of the patient's chief complaint is the urinary system.
- Functions of the urinary system include water and electrolyte regulation, acid-base balance, excretion of waste products and foreign chemicals, hormone excretion, arterial blood pressure regulation, erythrocyte production, and gluconeogenesis.
- Conditions including renal failure (acute or chronic plus end-stage renal disease [ESRD]), renal calculi, urinary retention, urinary system infections, and male genitourinary problems (including structural problems) can contribute to acute abdominal discomfort.
- A thorough assessment coupled with an understanding of the urinary system can help identify the nature of

the patient's condition and lead to the best course of treatment.

SHORT ANSWER

1. What are the major functions of the kidney?

   _____
   _____
   _____
   _____

2. What is a nephron?

   _____
   _____
   _____
   _____

3. What structure secretes aldosterone?

   _____

4. What effect does aldosterone have on the kidney?

   _____
   _____
   _____
   _____

5. What structure secretes antidiuretic hormone?

   _____

6. What effect does antidiuretic hormone have on the kidney?

   _____

7. What structure secretes atrial natriuretic peptide?

   _____

8. What effect does atrial natriuretic peptide have on the kidney?

   _____
   _____
   _____
   _____

9. What is the mechanism by which each of the following diuretics increases urine output?
   Mannitol:_____
   Lasix: _____
   Hydrochlorothiazide: _____

10. Describe the mechanism by which a decrease in renal blood flow produces an increase in systemic blood pressure.

    _____
    _____
    _____
    _____

11. Why do patients with extensive loss of renal tissue become anemic?

    _____
    _____
    _____
    _____

12. What distinguishes acute from chronic renal failure?

    _____
    _____
    _____
    _____

13. What is end-stage renal disease?

    _____
    _____
    _____
    _____

14. What are the three types of acute renal failure?

    _____
    _____
    _____

15. What is the pathophysiology of prerenal acute renal failure?

    _____
    _____
    _____
    _____

16. What is the pathophysiology of intrarenal acute renal failure?

    _____
    _____
    _____
    _____

17. What is the pathophysiology of postrenal acute renal failure?

    _____
    _____
    _____
    _____

18. Explain why renal failure will produce each of the following signs or symptoms:
    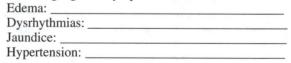
    Edema: _____
    Dysrhythmias: _____
    Jaundice: _____
    Hypertension: _____

19. Patients who develop renal failure will tend to develop what electrolyte imbalance? Why?

    _____
    _____
    _____
    _____

20. Patients who develop renal failure will tend to develop what acid-base imbalance? Why?

_____
_____
_____
_____

21. A patient has a dialysis fistula in his right arm. What precautions should you take regarding the management of the fistula?

_____
_____
_____
_____

22. A renal patient presents in cardiac arrest. What two drugs not normally used in the management of cardiac arrest should you consider administering? Why are these drugs indicated in the management of cardiac arrest in renal patients?

_____
_____
_____
_____

23. How can you quickly determine whether blood flow through a dialysis graft or fistula is obstructed?

_____
_____
_____
_____

24. What is disequilibrium syndrome?

_____
_____
_____
_____

25. Which gender is more prone to developing urinary tract infections? Why?

_____

26. What is priapism?

_____

27. List five causes of priapism.

_____
_____
_____
_____
_____

28. What is benign prostatic hypertrophy?

_____
_____
_____
_____

29. What complications can result from benign prostatic hypertrophy?

_____
_____
_____
_____

MULTIPLE CHOICE

1. Signs and symptoms of renal failure include _____.
   A. coffee ground emesis, left lower quadrant pain, and decreased urine output
   B. edema, low urine output, and signs of heart failure
   C. fever, flank pain and frequent urination
   D. hematuria, flank pain, and high cholesterol levels

2. A 24-year-old male is complaining of testicular pain. He states that he has noticed a urethral discharge and has pain on urination for the past couple of days. The scrotum is red and warm to the touch. You suspect this patient is suffering from _____.
   A. epididymitis
   B. testicular torsion
   C. urethritis
   D. urinary tract infection

3. You are dispatched to a dialysis center for a patient complaining of chest pain. As you arrive, the patient is being disconnected from the dialysis machine. He is complaining of jaw and chest pain. He is also short of breath. The patient has a history of diabetes, hypertension, emphysema, and renal failure. Based upon this information, you are concerned that this patient may be experiencing _____.
   A. cardiac ischemia
   B. disequilibrium syndrome
   C. hypertension
   D. pneumonia

4. Hyperkalemia is associated with _____.
   A. a short P-R interval
   B. atrial fibrillation
   C. premature atrial contraction
   D. peaked T waves

5. A 22-year-old female complains of right flank pain, nausea, and vomiting. She has been experiencing dysuria and urinary frequency for about a week. Her vital signs are: P—108 beats/min strong, regular; R—18 breaths/min shallow, regular; BP—136/92 mm Hg; T—102.4 ° F. What problem most likely is present?
   A. Appendicitis
   B. Cholecystitis
   C. Pyelonephritis
   D. Tubal ectopic pregnancy

6. The most common causes of chronic renal failure are _____.
   A. autoimmune reactions and shock
   B. hypertension and diabetes
   C. hypertension and acute myocardial infarction
   D. pyelonephritis and sepsis

7. Cardiac arrest in a patient with chronic renal failure usually is associated with what electrolyte imbalance?
   A. Hypercalcemia
   B. Hyperkalemia
   C. Hypocalcemia
   D. Hypokalemia

8. A patient with chronic renal failure would be most likely to develop which of the following problems?
   A. Congestive heart failure
   B. Hypoglycemia
   C. Hypotension
   D. Metabolic alkalosis

9. Your 34-year-old male patient is complaining of severe right-sided flank pain that radiates to his groin. He says the pain started this morning. He has been working hard building his house but does not believe he strained any muscles. He denies nausea, vomiting, and diarrhea. He states he has not been eating or drinking well because he is too busy. The patient is unable to sit or lie still. His vital signs are: BP—122/74 mm Hg; P—112 beats/min; ventilations—24 breaths/min; lung sounds clear and equal; skin—warm, dry, pink; blood glucose level—90 mg/dL. Which of the following should definitely remain in your differential diagnosis for this patient?
   A. Cholecystitis
   B. Esophagitis
   C. Pancreatitis
   D. Urinary calculus

10. Which of the following mechanisms would result in prerenal acute renal failure?
    A. Acute glomerulonephritis
    B. Ethylene glycol toxicity
    C. Hypovolemia
    D. Urethral obstruction

11. Which of the following mechanisms would result in intrarenal acute renal failure?
    A. Acute pyelonephritis
    B. Hypotension secondary to acute myocardial infarction
    C. Obstruction of the ureter by a kidney stone
    D. Stenosis of the renal artery

12. A 67-year-old male has developed acute renal failure after his urethra became obstructed secondary to prostate cancer. The mechanism that produced renal failure in this patient would be _____.
    A. intrarenal.
    B. postrenal
    C. primary
    D. secondary

13. A patient receiving dialysis has become restless and confused. He complains of a headache and nausea. He then loses consciousness and begins to seize. What problem should you suspect?
    A. Acute myocardial infarction
    B. Air embolism
    C. Disequilibrium syndrome
    D. Hypotension secondary to hemorrhage

CASE STUDIES

Case one

The patient is a 58-year-old male with a history of chronic renal failure who is in cardiac arrest. He reportedly missed his last two appointments for dialysis. CPR is in progress. When you attach the ECG leads, you see the following ECG.

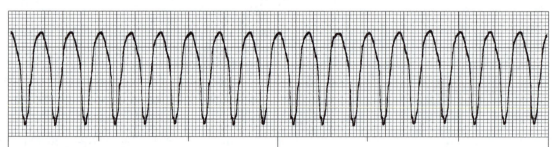

1. This ECG is characteristic of cardiac arrest secondary to what electrolyte imbalance?

   _____

2. What acid-base imbalance would you expect this patient to have? Why?

   _____
   _____
   _____
   _____

3. In addition to standard therapy for cardiac arrest, what two other drugs might you anticipate being ordered early in the management of this patient?

_____
_____
_____
_____

4. What problems would these drugs correct?

_____
_____
_____
_____

5. Would you expect this patient to be volume-depleted or in volume overload? Why?

_____
_____
_____
_____

You are having difficulty obtaining vascular access. You notice that the patient has a dialysis fistula that is readily visible.

6. What rule generally applies to starting an IV in a dialysis fistula? Why?

_____
_____
_____
_____

7. Does this rule hold true in this situation? Why?

_____
_____
_____
_____

Case two

A 50-year-old male has been experiencing "twinges" in his right lower back for about a week. At 0300 hours today, he awoke with excruciating pain in his back, unresponsive to a hot water bottle, liniment rub, and aspirin. He spent 3 hours pacing the house with intermittent bouts of emesis. Finally his wife persuaded him to call EMS. The patient reports no prior medical illnesses or surgical procedures. He takes no medications, does not use tobacco or alcohol, and is very active on his farm, working 12 to 14 hours a day. He reports that his father and grandfather occasionally "passed blood in their water." No cause for this problem was ever sought. The patient is pacing and wincing in acute discomfort. His skin is pale, cool, and moist. The patient continues to experience moderate to severe right flank pain. Vital signs are: P—140 beats/min strong, regular; R—28 breaths/min shallow, regular; BP—138/78 mm Hg.

1. From what problem is the patient probably suffering?

_____

2. What is the most potentially damaging side effect of this problem?

_____

3. Why is this patient's skin pale, cool, and moist?

_____
_____
_____
_____

4. This problem tends to occur commonly in the South and Southwest, particularly among persons who work outside for long hours. What explains this phenomenon?

_____
_____
_____
_____

5. This problem also is more common in persons who consume large amounts of dairy products; meats such as chicken, pork, and beef; salmon; and vegetables such as spinach, rhubarb, asparagus, parsley, garlic, and tomatoes. What explains this phenomenon?

_____
_____
_____
_____

6. How would you manage this patient?

_____
_____
_____
_____
_____
_____

7. What precautions could this patient take to prevent recurrence of this problem in the future?

_____
_____
_____
_____

Case three

A 15-year-old male complains of sudden onset of severe pain in the right testicle that is worsened by elevation of the scrotum. The pain radiates to the right flank and is accompanied by nausea, vomiting, and testicular edema. The patient denies hematuria and melena. He has no significant medical history. Vital signs are: P—88 beats/min strong, regular; R—22 breaths/min shallow, regular; BP—148/100 mm Hg.

1. What problem do you suspect?

_____

2. What is the pathoanatomy that makes a patient susceptible to this problem?

_____
_____
_____
_____

3. This problem is rare in people elder than 20 to 24 years. Why?

_____
_____
_____
_____

4. Are the patient's vital signs consistent with the problem you suspect and the rest of the patient's presentation? Why or why not?

_____
_____
_____
_____

5. If the vital signs are not consistent with the presentation, what might explain this? (HINT: What could you ask the patient?)

_____

_____

_____

_____

28 Musculoskeletal Disorders

READING ASSIGNMENT

Chapter 28, pages 1059-1073, in *Paramedic Practice Today: Above and Beyond*.

OBJECTIVES

After completing this chapter, you will be able to:
1. Discuss and describe the basic anatomy and function of the musculoskeletal system.
2. Discuss the general assessment, physical examination findings, and treatment of patients with musculoskeletal conditions.
3. Discuss the causes, identification, and prehospital management of acute and chronic low back pain.
4. Discuss the causes, identification, and prehospital management of acute and chronic neck pain.
5. Discuss the causes, identification, and prehospital management of overuse injuries.
6. Discuss the causes, identification, and prehospital management of generalized muscle disorders.
7. Discuss the causes, identification, and prehospital management of generalized joint disorders.
8. Discuss the causes, identification, and prehospital management of infectious diseases of the musculoskeletal system.
9. Discuss the causes, identification, and prehospital management of neoplastic disorders of the musculoskeletal system.
10. Discuss the causes, identification, and prehospital management of a child with a limp not associated with trauma.

CHAPTER SUMMARY

- In addition to fractures, the musculoskeletal system is subject to many other injuries and disease processes.
- In the prehospital setting, making the exact diagnosis for most musculoskeletal disorders is usually not possible, or necessary, because treatment principles generally are the same.
- A careful history and physical examination may provide clues to a more serious condition, such as an infectious or neoplastic disease.
- The majority of musculoskeletal diseases and injuries are not life-threatening, and prehospital treatment can be directed toward appropriate analgesia and comfort measures such as splinting, ice packs, elevation, and transportation in a position of comfort.
- When evaluating the patient with back pain, be sure to consider nonmusculoskeletal causes of pain, including cardiac, pulmonary, and abdominal conditions.

MATCHING

1. Match the bones with the correct classification.
   - ____ Carpals, metacarpals, tarsals, metatarsals, phalanges
   - ____ Humerus, radius, ulna, femur, tibia, fibula
   - ____ Sternum, ribs, bones of cranium
   - ____ Vertebrae, bones of face

   A. Flat bones
   B. Irregular bones
   C. Long bones
   D. Short bones

SHORT ANSWER

1. What are the principal functions of the musculoskeletal system?

2. The axial skeleton is made up of what structures?

3. The appendicular skeleton is made up of what structures?

4. What term is used to describe a bone that develops inside a tendon?

5. What is the name of the fibrous outer covering of the bone?

6. Name the anatomic structure that connects bone to bone.

7. Name the anatomic structure that connects muscles to bone.

8. What is the origin of a muscle?

9. What is the insertion of a muscle?

_____
_____
_____
_____

10. What is the difference between a strain and a sprain?

_____
_____
_____
_____

11. Morning stiffness and pain that improve with light movement suggest what problem?

_____

12. Fever associated with a tender, swollen joint suggests what problem?

_____

13. How is passive range of motion tested?

_____
_____
_____
_____

14. How is active range of motion tested?

_____
_____
_____
_____

15. What problems may be indicated by a difference between passive and active range of motion?

_____
_____
_____
_____

16. What is sciatica?

_____
_____
_____

17. What is cauda equina syndrome?

_____
_____
_____
_____

18. What characteristics distinguish cauda equina syndrome from sciatica?

_____
_____
_____
_____

19. List four conditions not associated with the musculoskeletal system that can produce pain in the mid-back.

_____
_____
_____
_____

20. List three conditions that can cause nontraumatic neck pain.

_____
_____

21. What is the pathophysiology of carpal tunnel syndrome?

_____
_____
_____
_____

22. What are the signs and symptoms of carpal tunnel syndrome?

_____
_____
_____
_____

23. What is rhabdomyolysis?

_____
_____
_____
_____

24. Why can rhabdomyolysis produce renal failure?

_____
_____
_____
_____

25. What is compartment syndrome?

_____
_____
_____

26. What are the signs and symptoms of compartment syndrome?

_____
_____
_____
_____

27. What are the three principal forms of arthritis?

_____
_____
_____

28. What is osteomyelitis?

_____
_____
_____
_____

29. What are the principal risk factors for developing osteomyelitis?

_____
_____
_____
_____

30. What is a pathologic fracture?

_____
_____
_____
_____

MULTIPLE CHOICE

1. Which of the following structures is part of the axial skeleton?
   A. Clavicle
   B. Femur
   C. Scapula
   D. Sternum

2. Which of the following structures is part of the appendicular skeleton?
   A. First rib
   B. Seventh cervical vertebra
   C. Scapula
   D. Sternum

3. Which of the following is a sesamoid bone?
   A. Calcaneus
   B. Mandible
   C. Patella
   D. Scapula

4. The pain associated with a herniated lumbar disk is most likely to be described as _____.
   A. aching, and localized in the lower back
   B. cramping and radiating around the flank to the groin
   C. shooting and radiating down the posterior aspect of one leg
   D. throbbing and radiating through to the anterior abdominal wall

5. Cauda equina syndrome is characterized by _____.
   A. numbness and tingling in both lower extremities without motor deficits
   B. sharp pain that radiates down the posterior aspect of both legs
   C. sharp pain that radiates down the posterior aspect of one leg
   D. weakness of the muscles of the buttocks and posterior thighs, sensory deficits, and loss of bladder and bowel continence

6. The principal risk factor for developing osteoarthritis is _____.
   A. age
   B. alcohol abuse
   C. female gender
   D. IV substance abuse

7. A 25-year-old female developed a syndrome characterized by morning stiffness, fatigue, low-grade fever, weight loss, and bilateral swelling and tenderness of her wrist, metacarpophalangeal, and proximal interphalangeal joints that has persisted for 6 weeks. Which of the following disease processes is most likely to be the cause of her signs and symptoms?
   A. Gouty arthritis
   B. Osteoarthritis
   C. Rheumatoid arthritis
   D. Septic arthritis

8. What joint is most commonly affected by gout?
   A. First metacarpophalangeal joint
   B. First metatarsophalangeal joint
   C. Distal interphalangeal joints
   D. Proximal interphalangeal joints

9. Fever associated with tenderness, swelling, and redness of a single joint indicates the presence of _____.
   A. gouty arthritis
   B. osteoarthritis
   C. rheumatoid arthritis
   D. septic arthritis

Case one

The neighbors of a 24-year-old male with a history of alcohol and drug abuse had not seen him for several days. The police were summoned. After forcing entry into the patient's apartment, they found the patient on his left side on the floor, unconscious and unresponsive. Several empty wine bottles and an empty bottle of a prescription benzodiazepine were present. The patient's respirations were slow and shallow. Peripheral pulses were slow and weak. Pupils were dilated and reacted sluggishly to light. EMS was called, and the patient was transported to the local hospital. After initial treatment in the emergency department, he was admitted to the ICU.

It now is 8 hours later. You have been called to the local hospital to transfer the patient to a tertiary care facility. The transfer was requested after the nurses in the ICU noticed that the patient's left arm and leg were edematous, pale, and cool. Closer assessment revealed that distal pulses and capillary refill were absent. Just before you arrived, the patient's indwelling catheter began to drain reddish brown urine.

1. What problem probably is present?

   _____

2. Describe the pathophysiology of this problem.

   _____
   _____
   _____
   _____

3. Describe the treatment that should be performed to manage the effects of this problem on the patient's kidneys.

   _____
   _____
   _____
   _____
   _____
   _____

Case two

A 55-year-old man complains of pain in his right lower back that radiates down his right leg. He also states that his right leg is numb and feels weak. He has no other complaints. His history includes a past myocardial infarction only with no previous surgeries. He takes no regular medications. The patient's skin is pale, cool, and moist. His right lower extremity is mottled and cool with absent dorsal pedal and posterior tibial pulses. The left lower extremity is pale and cool with weak distal pulses. The patient's vital signs are: BP—108/80 mm Hg; P—130 beats/min weak, regular; R—26 breaths/min shallow, regular.

1. What problem do you suspect?

   _____

2. What signs and symptoms suggest that this is not a musculoskeletal problem such as lumbar disk disease?

   _____
   _____
   _____
   _____

3. How would you manage this patient?

   _____
   _____
   _____
   _____

29 Cutaneous Disorders

READING ASSIGNMENT

Chapter 29, pages 1074-1097, in *Paramedic Practice Today: Above and Beyond.*

OBJECTIVES

After completing this chapter, you will be able to:
1. Describe the three layers of the skin, their composition, and their functions.
2. Describe the morphology of primary skin lesions.
3. Describe the morphology of secondary skin lesions.
4. Describe the recognition and treatment of skin cancer.
5. Describe malignant melanoma and explain how it is best recognized.
6. Recognize and treat decubitus ulcers.
7. Recognize and treat atopic dermatitis.
8. Recognize and treat contact dermatitis.
9. Recognize and treat psoriasis.
10. Recognize and treat impetigo.
11. Recognize and treat folliculitis.
12. Recognize and treat furuncles and carbuncles.
13. Recognize and treat cellulitis.
14. Recognize and treat fungal infections.
15. Recognize and treat *Candida* species infections.
16. Recognize and treat pediculosis.
17. Recognize and treat scabies.
18. Recognize and treat common warts.
19. Recognize and treat *Varicella* species infections.
20. Recognize and treat herpes simplex.
21. Recognize and treat herpes zoster.
22. Recognize and treat urticaria.
23. Recognize and treat erythema multiforme.

CHAPTER SUMMARY

- As with any type of exposure, personal protective equipment is extremely important and acts as a barrier between infectious materials and the skin, mouth, nose, and eyes (mucous membranes).
- A primary skin lesion is best described as a lesion that has not been altered by scratching, rubbing, scrubbing, or other types of trauma.
- A secondary skin lesion is best described as any lesion that has been altered by scratching, scrubbing, or other types of trauma.
- Describing skin lesions by using the names of primary and secondary lesions enables the clearest communication between paramedic and the medical director and makes documentation of skin lesions the most accurate.
- Learn the ABCDE rule to distinguish melanoma from less harmful lesions.
- Decubitus ulcers, also known as *pressure ulcers*, are localized areas of tissue damage that develop when soft tissue is compressed between a bony prominence and a firm external surface for a prolonged period.
- Atopic dermatitis is a chronic inflammatory skin disease that is considered familial with allergic features. Atopic dermatitis and eczema are often incorrectly used interchangeably.
- Contact dermatitis refers to any dermatitis arising from direct skin exposure to a substance; the cause may be allergic or irritant induced, the latter being more common.
- Psoriasis is a common chronic skin disorder characterized by erythematous papules and plaques with a silvery scale.
- Impetigo is a superficial vesicopustular skin infection that primarily occurs on exposed areas of the face and extremities from scratching infected lesions.
- Folliculitis is localized to hair follicles and is more common in immunocompromised patients.
- Furuncles (boils) are inflammatory nodules that involve the hair follicle (and many times follow an episode of folliculitis), whereas a carbuncle is a series of abscesses in the subcutaneous tissues that drain through hair follicles.
- Cellulitis may appear as a swollen, red area of skin that feels hot and tender and may spread rapidly. If untreated, the spreading bacterial infection can rapidly turn into a life-threatening condition.
- Most fungal infections are superficial and are identified by the word *tinea* and then followed with a term that denotes the location of the lesion. The most common result from a group of fungal infections is called *dermatophytes.*
- The most common symptom of candidiasis is itching and burning of the skin. *Candida* infections in the oral cavity are called *thrush.*
- Lice are ectoparasites that live on the body. Human infestation with lice is referred to as *pediculosis.*
- Scabies is a contagious skin disease of the epidermis marked by itching and small raised red spots caused by the itch mite.
- Warts are benign lesions caused by the papillomavirus.
- Varicella (chickenpox) is an acute contagious vesicular skin eruption caused by the varicella-zoster virus. It can be distinguished from smallpox by its clinical presentation.

241

- Herpes simplex is a skin eruption caused by the herpes simplex virus and is divided into two types: HSV-1 causes oral infections and HSV-2 causes genital infections.
- Herpes zoster, also known as *shingles,* is a skin eruption that follows a particular nerve distribution called a *dermatome.*
- Urticaria, also known as *hives*, is a condition of a wheal on the skin resulting from edema.
- Erythema multiforme is known for its "target" lesions with three zones of color, which makes the diagnosis. The epidermis may be normal or blistered and the dermis may be erythematous.

MATCHING

1. Match the primary skin lesion with its description.

_____ A flat, circumscribed, discolored lesion
_____ A firm, rounded elevation of the skin that is evanescent and pruritic
_____ A lesion that contains purulent material
_____ A localized, fluid-filled lesion greater than 0.5 cm in diameter
_____ An elevated lesion that contains clear fluid
_____ An elevated, solid lesion greater than 0.5 cm in diameter in the deep skin or subcutaneous tissues
_____ An elevated, solid lesion greater than 0.5 cm in diameter that lacks a deep component
_____ An elevated, solid lesion less than 0.5 in diameter

A. Bulla
B. Macule
C. Nodule
D. Papule
E. Plaque
F. Pustule
G. Vesicle
H. Wheal

2. Match the secondary skin lesion with its description.

_____ A collection of cellular debris or dried blood
_____ A collection of new collective tissue resulting from dermoepidermal damage
_____ A full-thickness crater that involves the dermis and epidermis with loss of the surface epithelium
_____ A linear erosion caused by scratching
_____ Partial focal loss of epidermis that usually heals without scarring

A. Crust
B. Erosion
C. Excoriation
D. Fissure
E. Scale
F. Scar
G. Ulcer

_____ Thick stratum corneum resulting from hyperproliferation or increased cohesion of keratinocytes
_____ A vertical loss of epidermis and dermis with sharply defined walls forming a crack in the skin

3. Match the dermatophyte infection with its location.

_____ Tinea capitis
_____ Tinea corporis
_____ Tinea cruris
_____ Tinea manuum
_____ Tinea pedis
_____ Tinea unguium
_____ Tinea versicolor

A. Body
B. Feet
C. Groin
D. Hands
E. Nails
F. Scalp
G. Trunk

SHORT ANSWER

1. What are the functions of the skin?

_____
_____
_____
_____

2. What are the three layers that make up the skin?

_____
_____
_____

3. Which layer of the skin contains the hair follicles, sebaceous glands, and sweat glands?

_____
_____
_____
_____

4. What are the two types of skin cancer?

_____
_____

5. Which of the two types of skin cancer is more dangerous?

_____
_____

6. What is a decubitus ulcer?

_____
_____
_____
_____

7. What are the major factors that contribute to the formation of decubitus ulcers?

_____
_____
_____
_____

8. What is atopic dermatitis (eczema)?

_____
_____
_____
_____

9. What are the clinical features that must be present to make the diagnosis of atopic dermatitis?

_____
_____
_____

10. What is contact dermatitis?

_____
_____
_____
_____

11. What are the two causes of contact dermatitis?

_____
_____

12. Describe the lesion that characterizes psoriasis.

_____
_____
_____
_____

13. What organism causes impetigo?

_____

14. Describe the lesion that characterizes impetigo.

_____
_____
_____
_____

15. What is a furuncle?

_____
_____
_____
_____

16. What is a carbuncle?

_____
_____
_____
_____

17. What organism is the most common cause of furuncles and carbuncles?

_____

18. What are lice?

_____
_____
_____
_____

19. What are the three types of lice that affect humans?

_____
_____
_____

20. What problem should be suspected if pubic lice are found on a child?

_____

21. What organism causes scabies?

_____

22. What areas of the body are most likely to be affected by scabies?

_____
_____
_____

23. What causes warts?

_____

24. Describe the rash that characterizes varicella (chickenpox).

_____
_____
_____

25. What causes herpes simplex?

_____

26. Describe the skin lesion associated with herpes simplex.

_____
_____
_____

27. What is shingles?

_____
_____
_____
_____

28. What is the typical distribution of the skin lesions associated with shingles?

_____
_____
_____

29. What is the common name for urticaria?

_____

30. What is erythema multiforme?

_____
_____
_____
_____

31. What is the most common cause of erythema multiforme?

_____
_____
_____
_____

32. An 18-month-old male has complained of a headache since yesterday. Over the last 2 to 3 hours, he has become increasingly drowsy. His mother was about to take him to the hospital when he experienced a generalized seizure that lasted about 3 minutes. Vital signs are: P—168 beats/min weak, regular; BP—82/66 mm Hg; R—34 breaths/min regular, unlabored. When you examine the patient, you find small, reddish-purple spots on the upper chest and shoulders that look like small collections of blood under the skin. What are these lesions called? What problem do you suspect is present?

_____
_____
_____
_____

33. While examining a 57-year-old male with a long history of alcohol abuse, you notice numerous small, red, threadlike lines on the bridge of the nose and cheeks. What are these lesions called? What is producing them?

_____
_____
_____
_____

34. During a physical examination on a patient who has a 20-year history of type 1 diabetes, you find a lesion on the right foot that is purplish and circular and appears to extend into the dermal tissues. What would this lesion be called?

_____

35. A child with chickenpox presents with lesions that consist of small, clear, elevated bumps that appear to be filled with a clear fluid and are surrounded by a reddened area. What would these lesions be called?

_____

36. A 4-year-old female developed a stuffy nose, headache, and malaise yesterday. She also complained that bright lights hurt her eyes. About 1 hour ago, she began to develop small, flat, reddish spots on her chest that rapidly spread to the abdomen and extremities. What would these lesions be called?

_____

37. A 26-year-old male complains of severe pain at the proximal end of his left thumbnail. On examination, the area is reddened, warm, and tender. The tissues overlying the proximal and lateral nailbeds have swollen to the point that the cuticle is no longer visible. What would this lesion be called?

_____

38. You are transporting the loser of a knife fight. The patient is stable and his wounds are superficial, so you are passing the time listening to his tales of previous exploits. At one point he shows you an old injury and tells you, "This is where Bubba Jones cut me back in'91." You notice that the scar from the previous injury appears unusually thick and extends well beyond the margins of the original wound. What would this lesion be called?

_____

MULTIPLE CHOICE

1. What distinguishes a primary skin lesion from a secondary skin lesion?
   A. A primary skin lesion does not contain fluid-filled spaces of any kind.
   B. A primary skin lesion has not been altered by scratching, scrubbing, or other trauma.
   C. A primary skin lesion involves only the epidermis while a secondary skin lesion extends into the dermis.
   D. A secondary skin lesion has not been altered by scratching, scrubbing, or other trauma.

2. Most cancerous skin lesions are caused by _____.
   A. exposure to ultraviolet light
   B. human papillomavirus
   C. occupational exposure to carcinogens
   D. recurrent staphylococcal skin infections

3. The most common form of skin cancer is _____.
   A. basal cell carcinoma
   B. malignant melanoma
   C. nonmelanoma skin cancer
   D. squamous cell carcinoma

4. Which statement about atopic dermatitis (eczema) is correct?
   A. Atopic dermatitis is most common in rural areas of underdeveloped countries.
   B. Atopic dermatitis typically appears in early adulthood.
   C. Atopic dermatitis does not have a genetic component.
   D. Atopic dermatitis often coincides with asthma and allergic rhinitis.

5. Which statement about contact dermatitis is correct?
   A. Contact dermatitis affects both sexes equally.
   B. Contact dermatitis is more common in males than females.
   C. Contact dermatitis most commonly is caused by exposure to irritants.
   D. Contact dermatitis most commonly results from allergic reactions.

6. The typical lesion produced by psoriasis is _____.
   A. erythematous papules and plaques with a silver scale
   B. large nodules in the subcutaneous tissues
   C. pustules on an erythematous base
   D. small vesicles on an erythematous base

7. Most of bacterial skin infections are caused by _____.
   A. *Escherichia coli*
   B. *Pseudomonas aeruginosa*
   C. *Staphylococcus aureus* and group A beta-hemolytic streptococci
   D. tinea versicolor

8. Which statement about impetigo is correct?
   A. A thick, golden crust tends to form as the primary lesions rupture.
   B. Impetigo is caused by group A beta-hemolytic streptococci.
   C. Impetigo tends to be more common in cool, dry environments.
   D. The lesions of impetigo occur most commonly on the hands and arms.

9. The organisms that most commonly cause folliculitis are _____.
   A. *E. coli* and *Pseudomonas aeruginosa*
   B. *P. aeruginosa* and *S. aureus*
   C. *S. aureus* and group A beta-hemolytic streptococci
   D. tinea versicolor and *S. aureus*

10. A painful inflammatory nodule that involves a hair follicle and drains pus is a _____.
    A. bulla
    B. carbuncle
    C. furuncle
    D. vesicle

11. A dermatophyte infection on the trunk that produces pink, tan, or white patches with fine desquamating scale is called _____.
    A. tinea corporis
    B. tinea cruris
    C. tinea manuum
    D. tinea versicolor

12. Which of the following statements about pediculosis is correct?
    A. Body lice live in clothing but move to the skin to lay their eggs.
    B. Head lice are most common among African Americans.
    C. Head lice occur commonly among schoolchildren.
    D. Pubic lice occur only in the genital region of the body.

13. Which statement about scabies is correct?
    A. Scabies is caused by an insect that burrows in the skin.
    B. The lesions of scabies are most commonly found on the head.
    C. The most common finding is small papules that do not itch.
    D. Transmission is usually from person to person by direct contact.

14. Cauliflower-like lesions that form on and around the rectum, perineum, inguinal folds, and external genitalia are _____.
    A. condylomata acuminata
    B. herpes simplex type 1
    C. herpes simplex type 2
    D. molluscum contagiosum

15. Chickenpox is characterized by a rash that _____.
    A. occurs primarily on the extremities and consists of a mixture of macules, papules, vesicles, and crusting lesions
    B. occurs primarily on the extremities and consists of only one type of lesion at any point during the infection
    C. occurs primarily on the trunk and consists of a mixture of macules, papules, vesicles, and crusting lesions
    D. occurs primarily on the trunk and consists of only one type of lesion at any point during the infection

16. What distinguishes herpes simplex virus type 1 (HSV-1) from herpes simplex virus type 2 (HSV-2)?
    A. HSV-1 causes genital infection; HSV-2 causes oral infection.
    B. HSV-1 causes oral infection; HSV-2 causes genital infection.
    C. HSV-1 causes recurrent infections; HSV-2 does not.
    D. HSV-1 does not cause recurrent infections; HSV-2 does.

17. Which of the following drugs is used to treat herpes simplex virus infections?
    A. Acyclovir
    B. Nystatin
    C. Penicillin
    D. Tetracycline

18. Which statement best describes the lesions of herpes zoster (shingles)?
    A. Vesicles that follow a particular nerve distribution on the extremities on one side of the body
    B. Vesicles that follow a particular nerve distribution on the extremities bilaterally
    C. Vesicles that follow a particular nerve distribution on the trunk or face on one side of the body
    D. Vesicles that follow a particular nerve distribution on the trunk or face bilaterally

19. The medical term used for *hives* is _____.
    A. allergic vesicles
    B. allergic wheals
    C. papules
    D. urticaria

20. The most common cause of erythema multiforme is _____.
    A. allergic reactions to drugs
    B. dermatophyte infection
    C. exposure to occupational irritants
    D. ultraviolet light

21. Large areas of reddish purple blotches on the skin associated with specific disease states are called _____.
    A. angiomas
    B. hemangiomas
    C. petechiae
    D. purpura

30 Toxicology

READING ASSIGNMENT

Chapter 30, pages 1098-1136, in *Paramedic Practice Today: Above and Beyond*.

OBJECTIVES

After completing this chapter, you will be able to:
1. Describe the extent of injury and death associated with toxicologic emergencies.
2. Define *poison, toxicology*, and *toxicologic emergency*.
3. Describe the role of the poison control center in the treatment of toxicologic emergencies.
4. List the four routes of entry of poisons into the body and how they affect managed care of the poisoned patient.
5. Understand the need for an accurate scene size-up to ensure responder safety at toxicologic emergencies.
6. List and use available reference materials for poisonings involving household and industrial chemicals.
7. Describe the general toxidromes that can be used to classify and treat the poisoned patient.
8. Understand the importance of decontaminating patients.
9. Identify the difference between internal and external decontamination.
10. Describe the appropriate uses of activated charcoal for internal decontamination.
11. Identify the available antidotes to poisons and how they are used to treat patients.
12. Identify medications commonly involved in toxicologic emergencies and be able to list common signs and symptoms and treatment procedures that will benefit the patient.
13. Identify chemicals commonly involved in toxicologic emergencies and be able to list common signs and symptoms and treatment procedures that will benefit the patient.
14. Identify wildlife commonly involved in toxicologic emergencies and be able to list common signs and symptoms and treatment procedures that will benefit the patient.
15. Identify plants and mushrooms commonly involved in toxicologic emergencies and be able to list common signs and symptoms and treatment procedures that will benefit the patient.
16. Identify illegal drugs commonly involved in toxicologic emergencies and be able to list common signs and symptoms and treatment procedures that will benefit the patient.
17. Understand the toxicologic effects of alcohol and alcohol abuse and how to treat the signs and symptoms of alcohol abuse.

CHAPTER SUMMARY

- Toxicologic emergencies can cover a wide range of signs and symptoms depending on the toxin.
- Toxins can affect any organ system in the body.
- In an unknown medical emergency, you must quickly assess the signs and symptoms and determine the nature of the emergency.
- If an underlying medical condition seems implausible, a good patient history or examination of the area may reveal the source of illness as poisoning.
- Poisons can be found almost anywhere—in the home, in the workplace, and in nature.
- Poisonings may be accidental or intentional.
- You must always be cautious when responding to a toxicologic emergency.

SHORT ANSWER

1. If a patient has ingested an unknown toxic substance, on what should your management efforts focus?

   _____
   _____
   _____
   _____

2. How should a patient be treated if a toxic or corrosive substance has been introduced into the patient's eyes?

   _____
   _____
   _____
   _____

3. Based on the principles you learned in this chapter, list at least five questions that you feel should be asked when obtaining a history about a poisoned or overdosed patient.

   _____
   _____
   _____
   _____
   _____

4. What acid-base imbalance can be induced by methanol or ethylene glycol poisoning? What drug might be considered to correct this imbalance?

_____
_____
_____
_____

5. What are the color and odor of carbon monoxide?

_____
_____
_____
_____

6. What is the toxic action of carbon monoxide?

_____
_____
_____
_____

7. A patient suddenly becomes ill after ingesting several peach seeds. He is responsive only to deep pain and has rapid, gasping respirations. His lips are cyanotic. He has muscle spasms and twitching of his extremities. When you attempt to start an IV, the blood return is bright red, but it flows steadily like venous blood. With what substance is the patient poisoned?

_____
_____
_____
_____

8. What substances are used as antidotes to the toxin present in the previous question?

_____
_____
_____
_____

9. What group of chemicals produces a toxic syndrome characterized by salivation, tearing, increased gastrointestinal motility, urinary and fecal incontinence, vomiting, bradycardia, and pinpoint pupils?

_____
_____
_____
_____

10. What drug is used to immediately reverse the effects from the previous question? What agent is the definitive antidote for this group of poisons?

_____
_____
_____
_____

11. Why should catecholamines be avoided in the management of hypotension associated with ingestion of hydrocarbons?

_____
_____
_____
_____

12. What is the drug of choice for management of a patient who is bradycardic, hypotensive, or in congestive heart failure secondary to calcium channel blocker toxicity?

_____
_____
_____
_____

13. What is the principal danger associated with inhalation of Freon (which is a hydrocarbon compound)?

_____
_____

MULTIPLE CHOICE

1. The antidote for acetaminophen overdose is _____.
   A. activated charcoal
   B. ethyl alcohol
   C. *N*-acetylcysteine
   D. naloxone

2. A 24-year-old man is found unresponsive in his apartment by a neighbor. He has been depressed lately because of a recent breakup with his girlfriend. He is breathing shallowly at 6 to 8 breaths/min. His blood pressure is 114/70 mm Hg with a pulse rate of 92 beats/min. Integrating everything you have learned in this and previous chapters, which of the following represents the *most appropriate actions* in the proper sequence of implementation assuming each therapy does not improve the patient's spontaneous respiratory rate?
   A. Bag-mask ventilation, IV access, intubate, ventilate, check glucose level
   B. Bag-mask ventilation, IV access, Narcan 2 mg × 2, check glucose level, intubate, ventilate
   C. Intubate, ventilate, IV access, dextrose, thiamine, Narcan 2 mg × 2, check glucose level
   D. Intubate, ventilate, IV access, Narcan 2 mg × 2, check glucose level

3. Which of the following would be considered an early sign of most tricyclic antidepressant overdoses?
   A. Respiratory arrest
   B. Blurred vision
   C. Ventricular tachycardia/fibrillation
   D. Widened QRS

4. A 3-year-old male ingested the contents of a bottle of verapamil, which is, as you remember from the pharmacology chapters, a calcium channel blocker. During your assessment, you would anticipate finding _____.
   A. hypertension, tachycardia
   B. hypotension, bradycardia
   C. tachycardia, hypertension
   D. tachycardia, hypotension

5. Which of the following drugs would you anticipate giving to the patient in the previous question?
   A. Calcium chloride
   B. Magnesium sulfate
   C. Narcan
   D. Sodium bicarbonate

6. Hypertension and tachycardia will be associated with ingestion of _____.
   A. amphetamines, cocaine, phencyclidine
   B. iron, theophylline, sedative-hypnotics
   C. mushrooms, digoxin, parasympathomimetics
   D. organophosphates, beta-blockers, calcium channel blockers

7. Consider what you learned about treating toxicological emergencies (for example what you learned about activated charcoal in this chapter and the pharmacology chapters) and apply that knowledge in answering the following question. Why is it important to ascertain the time of ingestion of a drug in a suspected overdose or poisoning?
   A. Patients with a psychiatric history are more likely to attempt an overdose in the morning.
   B. The decision to transport the patient for physician evaluation is often determined by the time elapsed since the ingestion.
   C. The possibility of ingestion of additional substances, such as alcohol, can be determined largely by the time of day of the ingestion.
   D. Treatment decisions will be affected by the time that has elapsed since ingestion.

8. Signs and symptoms of organophosphate poisoning include _____.
   A. muscle weakness, hypertension, tachycardia
   B. paralysis, urinary retention, muscle fasciculations
   C. urinary incontinence, salivation, dilated pupils
   D. urinary incontinence, wheezing, paralysis

9. The police find an unconscious middle-aged male in an abandoned building. He is unresponsive. His skin is cool and dry. Vital signs are: BP—198/122 mm Hg; P—56 beats/min strong, regular; R—8 breaths/min shallow, regular. A broken wine bottle is found nearby. Based on these findings, do you believe alcohol intoxication alone is responsible for his presentation?
   A. Yes, he is expriencing isolated ethanol intoxication.
   B. No, while he may be intoxicated his presentation is not consistent with isolated intoxication.

10. Integrating what you learned in this chapter and in the pharmacology chapters, what is the goal when administering naloxone (Narcan)?
    A. To administer a dose of naloxone that is equal to the amount of narcotic introduced to the body
    B. To improve blood pressure
    C. To improve respirations to an acceptable rate and tidal volume
    D. To return the patient to an alert and oriented mental status

11. A man was working in an enclosed garage with a running gasoline-powered engine. You respond to a call from his wife who found him seizing. Before the seizures began, he was complaining of a headache and nausea. He now is unresponsive with dilated pupils and a bounding pulse. The substance to which he has been exposed is toxic because it _____.
    A. binds to hemoglobin and interferes with oxygen transport
    B. blocks the use of oxygen in metabolic processes at the cellular level
    C. increases myocardial sensitivity to catecholamines
    D. interferes with acetylcholine breakdown at the neuromuscular junction

12. When you apply a pulse oximeter to the patient in the question 11, it reads 99% with the patient receiving oxygen by bag-mask. Integrating what you know about how the pulse oximeter works, and what you know about carbon monoxide, which of the following would be the most appropriate course of action?
    A. Continue ventilating, but decrease the oxygen flow since the oxygen saturation is too high.
    B. Discontinue oxygenating and ventilating since the oxygen saturation is adequate.
    C. Disregard the oximeter since carbon monoxide may cause inaccurate readings.
    D. Increase the ventilation rate until the pulse oximeter indicates 100% saturation.

13. The administration of sodium nitrite and amyl nitrite to a cyanide-poisoned patient results in hemoglobin converting to _____.
    A. carboxyhemoglobin
    B. cytohemoglobin
    C. methemoglobin
    D. nitrohemoglobin

14. A 24-year-old male was found slumped over in a chair at home. An empty prescription bottle for thirty 100-mg amitriptyline (Elavil) tablets with an issue date of 5 days ago was found nearby. The patient is unresponsive. Knowing this medication is a tricyclic antidepressant, which of the following signs and symptoms would you anticipate finding?
    A. Diaphoresis
    B. Dilated pupils
    C. Heavy salivation
    D. Urinary incontinence

15. Applying your knowledge of naloxone, please formulate an answer to the following statement: Naloxone works by competing for the _____.
    A. cholinergic receptors of the CNS
    B. dopamine receptors of the CNS
    C. opiate receptors of the CNS
    D. serotonin receptors of the CNS

16. A 55-year-old alcoholic complains of weakness, nausea, difficulty breathing, and blurry vision. He admits to drinking windshield washer fluid. Vital signs are: BP—130/70 mm Hg; R—28 breaths/min deep, regular; P—122 beats/min weak, regular. The antidote that would be given to this patient works because it _____.
    A. binds with the toxin to neutralize its effects
    B. competes with the toxin for receptors in the heart and CNS
    C. inhibits metabolism of the toxin
    D. speeds metabolism of the toxin

17. The acid-base imbalance most likely to develop in the patient in the previous question is _____.
    A. metabolic acidosis because the toxin is metabolized to an acid
    B. metabolic alkalosis because the toxin is metabolized to a base
    C. respiratory alkalosis because the respirations are rapid and deep
    D. respiratory alkalosis because the toxin will cause hypocalcemia

18. Tinnitus is a common symptom of _____.
    A. acetaminophen overdose
    B. cyanide overdose
    C. ethanol overdose/poisoning
    D. salicylate overdose

19. Benzodiazepines affect the CNS by binding to the _____.
    A. dopaminergic receptors
    B. GABA receptors
    C. muscarinic receptors
    D. nicotinic receptors

20. Combining your knowledge of the autonomic nervous system and toxicology, please answer the following question: A farmer was riding a tractor when a crop duster accidentally sprayed him. He responds only to pain. He is salivating heavily, his pupils are pinpoint, and he has heavy rhinorrhea. Auscultation of his chest reveals rales, rhonchi, and wheezing. These symptoms are a result of _____.
    A. decreased parasympathetic tone
    B. decreased sympathetic tone
    C. increased parasympathetic tone
    D. increased sympathetic tone

21. Your patient is a 24-year-old woman who reportedly took an overdose of her diazepam (Valium) pills. She has no significant medical history but does have a history of depression for which she is being treated with a prescription medication. You find the patient with slow, snoring respirations at 8 breaths/min. Vital signs are: BP—100/60 mm Hg; P—110 beats/min; skin—cool, dry; pupils—dilated, equal and slow to react. After beginning bag mask ventilations and establishing IV access, what medication might be considered?
    A. Naloxone
    B. Dextrose
    C. Flumazenil
    D. Thiamine

22. The most dramatic form of alcohol withdrawal is referred to as _____.
    A. acute withdrawal syndrome
    B. alcohol deprivation syndrome
    C. an alcoholic seizure
    D. delirium tremens

23. In a tricyclic antidepressant overdose, toxcity is primarily attributed to _____.
    A. alpha-adrenergic blockade
    B. cholinergic stimulation
    C. inhibition of sodium channels
    D. metabolic acidosis

24. A 25-year-old female was moving wood from a woodpile when she felt a sharp pain on her hand "like a pin stuck me." Her hand became numb, and she began to experience intense pain and muscle spasms in her arm, shoulder, and chest muscles. What creature bit or stung her?
    A. Black widow spider
    B. Brown recluse spider
    C. Coral snake
    D. Scorpion

25. The police found an unconscious 24-year-old female in the alley behind the Salvation Army building. She is unresponsive to verbal or painful stimuli. Her skin is pale and cool. Her pupils are pinpoint. Vital signs are: BP—96/40 mm Hg; R—4 breaths/min shallow, regular; P—60 beats/min weak, regular. What problem should you suspect?
    A. Alcohol intoxication
    B. Amphetamine overdose
    C. Barbiturate overdose
    D. Narcotic overdose

26. A 28-year-old female was working in the warehouse of an agricultural chemical firm when the contents of a pesticide container were accidentally spilled over her. The pesticide has completely saturated her clothing and exposed skin. She is conscious but is confused and experiencing respiratory difficulty. She is salivating heavily, and her nose is running. You should _____.
    A. give activated charcoal to absorb any poison she might have ingested
    B. move her to fresh air, give oxygen, and transport without removing her clothing
    C. remove her contaminated clothing and wash her with large amounts of water
    D. transport immediately "code 3"

250

27. Applying your knowledge of airway management to the overdose patient, how would you treat the follwing patient? A 16-year-old female has ingested 60 propoxyphene (Darvon) pills, 100 diazepam (Valium) pills, 15 methaqualone (Quaalude) pills, 81 birth control pills, and 10 aspirin. She is unconscious and unresponsive. Her pupils are dilated. Peripheral cyanosis is present. Vital signs are: P—50 beats/min weak, regular; BP—60/40 mm Hg; R—6 breaths/min shallow, regular. You should _____.
    A. open the airway, assist ventilation with a bag-mask device and oxygen, and transport
    B. open the airway, give oxygen by nonrebreather mask at 15 L/min, and transport
    C. open the airway, insert an oral airway, give oxygen by nonrebreather mask at 15 L/min, and transport
    D. open the airway, insert an oral airway, assist venti-lation with a bag-mask device and oxygen, and transport

28. When you are managing a patient who has ingested an unknown poison, particular attention should be paid to _____.
    A. the color of the patient's vomitus
    B. the patient's airway, breathing, and circulation
    C. the presence of burns around the mouth
    D. unusual breath odors

29. The most immediate indication that a patient has been bitten by a pit viper is _____.
    A. drooping eyelids
    B. hematuria
    C. pain and swelling at the site of the bite
    D. respiratory arrest

30. Delirium tremens results from _____.
    A. alcohol withdrawal
    B. head injury
    C. narcotic withdrawal
    D. stimulant withdrawal

31. What can be done to reduce the severity of a Portuguese man-of-war sting?
    A. Apply ice packs to the area.
    B. Wash the area of the sting with salt water.
    C. Pour warm water over the area.
    D. Rub the area with sand.

32. Oxycodone, codeine, fentanyl, morphine, methadone, and meperidine are _____.
    A. barbiturates
    B. hallucinogens
    C. narcotics
    D. stimulants

33. Contraindications to administration of activated charcoal include _____.
    A. altered mental status; ingestion of diazepam
    B. inability to swallow; ingestion of digitalis
    C. ingestion of acids or alkalis; inability to swallow
    D. ingestion of aspirin; altered mental status

34. Applying to your knowledge of pharmacology to the treatment of an overdose patient, what is the dose range for adult administration of activated charcoal?
    A. 12.5 to 25 g
    B. 25 to 50 g
    C. 50 to 100 g
    D. either 50 to 100 g or 12.5 to 50 g

35. Inhaled poisons such as carbon monoxide are best treated with _____.
    A. activated charcoal to reduce blood gas levels of the toxin
    B. removal to fresh air
    C. removal to fresh air and either supplemental oxygen or assisted ventilation
    D. supplemental oxygen and assisted ventilation

36. Which statement about the coral snake is correct?
    A. It has fixed (non-erectile) fangs.
    B. It is a pit viper slightly smaller than a copperhead.
    C. It is a triangular-headed snake with hinged (erec-tile) fangs.
    D. It is closely related to the rattlesnake.

Case one

At 1440 hours, you are dispatched to a report of an "unconscious 2 year old, possible overdose." When you arrive on the scene, a woman in her 60s runs out of the house, carrying a flaccid, unresponsive 2-year-old child. The child appears pale with a cyanotic/gray face. The patient is unresponsive to voice and pain. Respirations are very slow and irregular. The patient's skin is cool, dry, and pale. Peripheral pulses are not detectable. Grandma reports she put the child down for a nap at 2:00 PM. At 2:30 PM she checked on him and found him on the floor, unresponsive with a bottle of her "heart pills" beside him. She then called EMS. The prescription bottle is for verapamil (Isoptin) 120 mg. The bottle of 60 pills is empty. The child has no muscle tone. Pupils are equal, dilated, and slow to react. The child weighs approximately 25 lb. The patient's ECG shows a complete atrioventricular block with a ventricular rate of 50. Knowing this medication is a calcium channel blocker, and integrating your knowledge of anatomy, physiology, airway management, pharmacology, cardiology, cardiac electrophysiology, body systems, and toxicology, please work through the following case and questions.

1. What are your immediate priorities?

2. What size endotracheal tube should you use with this patient?

3. Should chest compressions be started on this patient? (Refer to Chapter 37 as needed.)

4. What effect does verapamil have on the rate of the SA node?

5. What effect does verapamil have on ventricular contractility?

6. What effect does verapamil have on the peripheral blood vessels?

7. Is this rhythm consistent with what you would expect in verapamil toxicity?

8. How would you manage this patient?

Case two

A 5-year-old female ate a cup of apple seeds. She is unresponsive to verbal and painful stimuli. Vital signs are: P—146 beats/min weak, regular; BP—104/76 mm Hg; R—28 breaths/min deep, gasping. When you start an IV on the patient, you notice that her venous blood is bright red.

1. What toxin has the patient ingested?

2. Why is this substance toxic?

_____
_____
_____
_____

3. Why is the patient's venous blood bright red?

_____
_____
_____
_____

4. What are the antidotes given for this toxin?

_____
_____
_____

5. How do they work?

_____
_____
_____
_____

Case three

You respond to a report of an "unconscious person—police on location." Behind some abandoned buildings, the police have found an emaciated male who appears to be in his early 20s. He is unresponsive. His skin is pale, cool, and moist. His pupils are pinpoint. There are needle tracks on his arms. Vital signs are: P—60 beats/min weak, regular; BP—92/50 mm Hg; R—4 breaths/min shallow, regular.

1. What is the most probable cause of this patient's problem?

_____
_____
_____
_____

2. Why are the patient's pupils pinpoint?

_____
_____
_____
_____

3. What antidote should be given to this patient?

_____

4. How does this antidote work?

_____
_____
_____
_____

5. What things do you have to consider when administering this medication?

_____
_____
_____
_____

After you give the antidote, the patient's respiratory rate increases to 16 breaths/min. En route to the hospital, his respirations slow to 6 breaths/min.

6. What has happened?

_____
_____
_____
_____

7. What should you do?

_____
_____
_____
_____

Case four

At 1230 hours you are dispatched to a report of an "unconscious child, medical problem, nature unknown." The patient is a 13-year-old female who is lying on her bedroom floor. Pain elicits nonpurposeful movements. Respirations are slow and shallow. Radial pulses are present, rapid, and weak. Her skin is cool and dry. An empty bottle of thirty 100-mg amitriptyline (Elavil) tablets with an issue date of 5 days ago is found nearby. The patient's pupils are dilated and react sluggishly to light. Her mucous membranes are dry. Vital signs are: P—120 beats/min weak, regular; R—8/min shallow, regular; BP—96/52 mm Hg.

1. What type of drug is amitriptyline?

_____

2. Why does the patient have dilated pupils, dry skin, and a rapid heart rate?

_____
_____
_____
_____

3. What effects does this drug have on the heart?

_____
_____
_____
_____

4. What drug can be given to reverse the cardiotoxic effects of this agent?

_____
_____
_____
_____

Case five

A 35-year-old male alcoholic complains of weakness, nausea, difficulty breathing, and blurry vision. He admits to "taking a little nip of antifreeze" because he did not have enough money to buy "the good stuff." Vital signs are: BP—132/74 mm Hg; R—28 breaths/min deep, regular; P—122 beats/min weak, regular.

1. What is the principal component of antifreeze?

_____

2. What are the toxins produced by the metabolism of this component?

_____
_____
_____
_____

3. What is the antidote given when managing ingestions of this substance?

_____

4. Why is this antidote effective?

_____
_____
_____
_____

5. Referring to your prior knowledge of acid base balance, what is the acid-base imbalance most likely to develop in this patient?

_____
_____
_____
_____

6. Why does this patient have rapid, deep respirations?

_____
_____
_____
_____

7. What drug can be given in the management of this acid-base imbalance?

_____
_____
_____
_____

31 Infectious and Communicable Diseases

READING ASSIGNMENT

Chapter 31, pages 1137-1166, in *Paramedic Practice Today: Above and Beyond*.

OBJECTIVES

After completing of this chapter, you will be able to:
1. Review the specific anatomy and physiology pertinent to infectious and communicable diseases.
2. Define specific terminology identified with infectious and communicable diseases.
3. Discuss public health principles relevant to infectious and communicable diseases.
4. Identify public health agencies involved in the prevention and management of disease outbreaks.
5. For specific diseases, identify and discuss the issues of personal isolation.
6. Describe and discuss the rationale for the various types of personal protective equipment.
7. Discuss what constitutes a significant exposure to an infectious agent.
8. List and describe the steps of an infectious process.
9. List and describe the stages of infectious diseases.
10. List and describe infectious agents, including bacteria, viruses, fungi, protozoans, helminths (worms), and prions.
11. Describe host defense mechanisms against infection.
12. Describe the processes of the immune system defenses, including humoral and cell-mediated immunity.
13. Describe characteristics of the immune system, including the categories of white blood cells, the mononuclear phagocyte system, and the complement system.
14. Describe the assessment of a patient suspected of, or identified as having, an infectious or communicable disease.
15. Discuss the proper disposal of contaminated supplies (sharps, gauze sponges, tourniquets).
16. Discuss the following relative to the human immunodeficiency virus: causative agent, body systems affected and potential secondary complications, modes of transmission, the seroconversion rate after direct significant exposure, susceptibility and resistance, signs and symptoms, specific patient management and personal protective measures.
17. Discuss hepatitis A (infectious hepatitis), including the causative agent, body systems affected and potential secondary complications, routes of transmission, susceptibility and resistance, signs and symptoms, patient management and protective measures, and immunization.
18. Discuss hepatitis B (serum hepatitis), including the causative agent, the organ affected and potential secondary complications, routes of transmission, signs and symptoms, patient management and protective measures, and immunization.
19. Discuss the susceptibility and resistance to hepatitis B.
20. Discuss hepatitis C, including the causative agent, the organ affected, routes of transmission, susceptibility and resistance, signs and symptoms, patient management and protective measures, and control measures.
21. Discuss hepatitis D (hepatitis delta virus), including the causative agent, the organ affected, routes of transmission, susceptibility and resistance, signs and symptoms, patient management and protective measures, and control measures.
22. Discuss hepatitis E, including the causative agent, the organ affected, routes of transmission, susceptibility and resistance, signs and symptoms, patient management and protective measures, and control measures.
23. Discuss tuberculosis, including the causative agent, body systems affected and secondary complications, routes of transmission, susceptibility and resistance, signs and symptoms, patient management and protective measures, and control measures.
24. Discuss meningococcal meningitis (spinal meningitis), including causative organisms, tissues affected, modes of transmission, susceptibility and resistance, signs and symptoms, patient management and protective measures, and immunization and control measures.
25. Discuss other infectious agents known to cause meningitis, including *Streptococcus pneumoniae, Haemophilus influenzae* type b, and other varieties of viruses.
26. Discuss pneumonia, including causative organisms, body systems affected, routes of transmission, susceptibility and resistance, signs and symptoms, patient management and protective measures, and immunization.

27. Discuss tetanus, including the causative organism, the body system affected, modes of transmission, susceptibility and resistance, signs and symptoms, patient management and protective measures, and immunization.
28. Discuss rabies and hantavirus as they apply to regional environmental exposures, including the causative organisms, the body systems affected, routes of transmission, susceptibility and resistance, signs and symptoms, patient management and protective measures, and control measures.
29. Identify pediatric viral diseases.
30. Discuss chickenpox, including the causative organism, the body system affected, mode of transmission, susceptibility and resistance, signs and symptoms, patient management and protective measures, and immunization and control measures.
31. Discuss mumps, including the causative organism, the body organs and systems affected, mode of transmission, susceptibility and resistance, signs and symptoms, patient management and protective measures, and immunization.
32. Discuss rubella (German measles), including the causative agent, the body tissues and systems affected, modes of transmission, susceptibility and resistance, signs and symptoms, patient management and protective measures, and immunization.
33. Discuss measles (rubeola, hard measles), including the causative organism; the body tissues, organs, and systems affected; mode of transmission; susceptibility and resistance; signs and symptoms; patient management and protective measures; and immunization.
34. Discuss the importance of immunization and diseases, especially in the pediatric population, that warrant widespread immunization.
35. Discuss pertussis (whooping cough), including the causative organism, the body organs affected, mode of transmission, susceptibility and resistance, signs and symptoms, patient management and protective measures, and immunization.
36. Discuss influenza, including causative organisms, the body system affected, mode of transmission, susceptibility and resistance, signs and symptoms, patient management and protective measures, and immunization.
37. Discuss mononucleosis, including the causative organisms; the body regions, organs, and systems affected; modes of transmission; susceptibility and resistance; signs and symptoms; patient management and protective measures.
38. Discuss the characteristics of and organisms associated with febrile and afebrile respiratory disease, including bronchiolitis, bronchitis, laryngitis, croup, epiglottitis, and the common cold.

39. Discuss syphilis, including the causative organism; the body regions, organs, and systems affected; modes of transmission; susceptibility and resistance; stages of signs and symptoms; patient management and protective measures.
40. Discuss gonorrhea, including the causative organism, the body organs and associated structures affected, mode of transmission, susceptibility and resistance, signs and symptoms, patient management and protective measures.
41. Discuss chlamydia, including the causative organism; the body regions, organs, and systems affected; modes of transmission; susceptibility and resistance; signs and symptoms; patient management and protective measures.
42. Discuss herpes simplex type 1, including the causative organism, the body regions and system affected, modes of transmission, susceptibility and resistance, signs and symptoms, patient management and protective measures.
43. Discuss herpes simplex 2 (genital herpes), including the causative organism; the body regions, tissues, and structures affected; mode of transmission; susceptibility and resistance; signs and symptoms; patient management and protective measures.
44. Discuss scabies, including the etiologic agent, the body organs affected, modes of transmission, susceptibility and resistance, signs and symptoms, patient management and protective measures.
45. Discuss lice, including the infesting agents, the body regions affected, modes of transmission and host factors, susceptibility and resistance, signs and symptoms, patient management and protective measures, and prevention.
46. Describe Lyme disease, including the causative organism, the body organs and systems affected, mode of transmission, susceptibility and resistance, phases of signs and symptoms, patient management and control measures.
47. Discuss gastroenteritis, including the causative organisms, the body system affected, modes of transmission, susceptibility and resistance, signs and symptoms, patient management and protective measures.
48. Discuss the local protocol for reporting and documenting an infectious or communicable disease exposure.

CHAPTER SUMMARY

■ When treating patients with communicable diseases and infections, first protect your partner and yourself; then treat the patient while protecting the public from a widespread outbreak.
■ Wearing personal protective equipment and staying up to date with inoculations against infections are important aspects of patient care.

- Transmission of an infectious disease depends on a number of factors, including virulence, correct mode of entry into the body, and the immune status of the host.
- The stages of an infectious disease are the incubation period, window period, communicable period, latent period, and disease period.
- A disease may be caused by a bacterium, virus, fungus, protozoan, helminth, or prion.
- The body has multiple defense mechanisms, including the skin, white blood cells, the reticuloendothelial system (RES), and the complement system.
- A detailed history and physical examination of the patient should alert you to clues that an infectious disease may be present.
- HIV has two strains, HIV-1 and HIV-2. Both are communicable through unprotected sexual intercourse and contact with infected secretions or blood.
- HIV is incurable and has no vaccination.
- Hepatitis affects the liver and is communicable sexually and by infected blood and secretions.
- Hepatitis has no cure, although vaccinations are available for some strains.
- TB primarily affects the lungs but can affect other organs. It is spread through respiratory secretions from an infected person and may be treated with antibiotics.
- Meningitis may be caused by many pathogens. Bacterial meningitis is caused by bacteria reaching the meninges through the blood.
- Treatment for bacterial meningitis is antibiotic therapy based on the type of bacterium responsible for the infection.
- Bacterial pneumonia is a lung infection caused by bacteria and is transmissible through respiratory droplets or prolonged direct contact with an infected person.
- Bacterial pneumonia is treated with antibiotics.
- Tetanus is caused by a spore that enters the body through a wound, burn, or other injury to the skin.
- Tetanus is treated by vaccination.
- Herpes is a viral infection that may affect many organ systems.
- Herpes has no cure and no vaccination and may be spread through direct contact with infected persons.
- Gonorrhea is primarily a sexually transmitted disease that can affect different body systems depending on the site of exposure.
- Gonorrhea is treated with antibiotics.
- Syphilis is a sexually transmitted disease that begins as a chancre at the site of infection.
- Syphilis is treated with antibiotics and is spread through direct contact.
- Chickenpox is a common childhood disease that is highly communicable through contact with infected persons and is airborne. Chickenpox usually is self-limiting and currently has a vaccination, though no cure.

- Mumps is an infection that affects the parotid and salivary glands. Mumps infection is self-limiting and has a vaccination.
- Rubella is a viral infection spread through contact with infected persons. Rubella is self-limiting and has a vaccination.
- Measles is a highly contagious viral infection that has no cure, is self-limiting, and has a vaccination.
- Pertussis, meaning *forceful cough*, is a disease caused by a gram-negative bacterial infection. Pertussis is spread through infected respiratory secretions and may be treated in its early stages with antibiotics. Pertussis does have a vaccine, but its effectiveness has been shown to wane over time.
- Influenza is one of the most common and contagious infectious diseases that commonly affects the respiratory system. It has no cure, and vaccines are released yearly based on predictions of which strain will affect the general population that year.
- Avian influenza (H5N1) is an emerging strain of influenza A that has primarily been shown to be contagious from bird to human being; only limited cases of human-to-human transmission have been documented. Avian influenza in human beings has an extremely high mortality rate, and scientists warn that mutation of the virus could cause a worldwide pandemic.
- Mononucleosis is caused by a virus spread through infected secretions. Mononucleosis has no cure or vaccination, and symptoms may persist for several months.
- HSV-1 is a viral infection that affects the oropharynx, mouth, lips, skin, fingers and toes, and possibly the central nervous system. No cure or vaccination is available, and infection is lifelong.
- Acute afebrile respiratory distress can cause multiple upper and lower airway infections. Antibiotics are used only for bacterial infections with resistant strains.
- Respiratory syncytial virus (RSV) is a major viral infection in children younger than 2 years. RSV is largely spread from April to November. It can be prevented in children with a medication called *RespiGam*.
- Scabies is an infectious parasitic disease caused by the infestation of a mite. Females of the species invade the upper layer of the skin, causing irritation. Scabies is spread by person-to-person contact and infected linens in a 24-hour window. Infestation occurs at any site of female burrowing where eggs have been laid. Lesions form at sites of infestation. It is treated with a topical solution taken as perscribed by the physician to avoid toxicity.
- Lice infect the head, body, and pubic reigon. Lice have been known to spread typhus, relapsing fever, and trench fever (during World War I). Lice can be spread through direct and indirect contact, with pubic lice spread through sexual contact. Lice leave a febrile host, so overcrowded populations favor transmission for spread of lice. Itching is the primary symptom.

Topical solutions and mechanical removal of eggs are the only treatments available.

- Gastroenteritis is any infection that causes swelling to the stomach or its lining. Gastroenteritis is responsible for morbidity and mortality worldwide, especially in developing countries. Gastroenteritis is caused by multiple pathogens and is transmissible through contaminated food and water and fecal-oral contamination. Gastroenteritis manifest with abdominal pain and cramps, nausea and vomiting, diarrhea, fever, and frank shock.
- Standard precautions and hand-washing should be practiced when in contact with infected persons and in disaster areas. In the latter situation, a source of potable water must be ensured.
- Chlamydia is the most commonly spread sexually transmitted disease in the world today. The bacteria can only survive in the host using the cell's adenosine triphosphate. Chlamydia affects the eyes, respiratory tract, and sexual organs. Chlamydia is spread through sexual contact, hand-to-hand contact, and contaminated towels and clothes. No acquired immunity to chlamydia is possible, and symptoms depend on the site and stage of the disease. Chlamydia is the leading cause of preventable blindness worldwide.
- EMS personnel who come in contact with infected persons should practice standard precautions and hand-washing.
- Lyme disease is a bacterial infection spread by ticks and is most common in the United States, Europe, and Russia. Lyme disease often appears in stages, with the first stage presenting as a rash around the site of inoculation. The second and third stages begin the systemic infection. No vaccination against Lyme disease is available, and no immunity is acquired after infection. Lyme disease may be treated with antibiotics.
- Any exposure to potentially infectious diseases or materials should be immediately reported to the designated officer.
- Further medical testing and treatment are provided at no cost to the employee as appropriate.

SHORT ANSWER

1. What does the term *standard precautions* mean?

2. What is the most common cause of accidental needle stick? How can most accidental needle sticks be prevented?

3. What is the most important procedure for limiting the spread of infectious disease?

4. What infectious disease is characterized by headache, nausea, vomiting, stiff neck, and a rash consisting of pinpoint hemorrhages under the skin?

5. How is the disease described in question 4 transmitted?

6. What precautions should you take if you care for a patient with this disease?

7. What infectious disease is characterized by nausea, malaise, loss of appetite, jaundice, dark urine, and clay-colored stools?

8. By what route is hepatitis A typically transmitted?

9. By what route is hepatitis B typically transmitted?

10. By what route is hepatitis C typically transmitted?

11. Why does immunization against hepatitis B also provide immunity against hepatitis D?

12. How is tuberculosis transmitted?

13. If EMS personnel are exposed to a patient with active tuberculosis, what should they do?

14. A patient who is in late-term pregnancy tells you that she is infected with herpes simplex and that she has active lesions. How will this affect the delivery of her baby?

_____
_____
_____
_____

15. What is acquired immunodeficiency syndrome (AIDS)?

_____
_____
_____
_____

16. What pathogen produces AIDS?

_____
_____
_____
_____

17. How is the pathogen that produces AIDS transmitted?

_____
_____
_____
_____

18. By definition, when has a patient who is HIV positive developed AIDS?

_____
_____
_____

19. What precautions should you take when caring for a patient who is HIV positive?

_____
_____
_____
_____

20. What is *Pneumocystis carinii*?

_____
_____
_____
_____

21. Why is *Pneumocystis* significant to patients who are HIV positive?

_____
_____
_____
_____

22. Why should EMS personnel ensure they are immune to rubella (German measles)?

_____
_____
_____
_____

23. How is gonorrhea transmitted?

_____
_____
_____
_____

24. What are the signs and symptoms of gonorrhea?

_____
_____
_____
_____

MULTIPLE CHOICE

1. Which of the following poses the greatest risk of hepatitis C infection?
   A. Direct contact with the feces of an infected person
   B. Drinking from a glass used by an infected person
   C. Living in the same residence as an infected person
   D. Performing hemodialysis on an infected person

2. Which of the following medications is commonly used to treat symptoms of HSV?
   A. Acyclovir
   B. Fluconazole
   C. Kwell
   D. Zithromax

3. The hepatitis B virus may survive outside a human host on an inanimate surface for as long as approximately _____.
   A. 1 day
   B. 1 hour
   C. 1 month
   D. 1 week

4. The drug of choice in the prophylactic treatment of tuberculosis is _____.
   A. acyclovir
   B. ethambutol
   C. isoniazid
   D. vancomycin

5. Your patient is a 20-year-old college student who is complaining of abdominal pain. He was evaluated at the university clinic earlier today and diagnosed with hepatitis. The physician stated the transmission route for this type of hepatitis is the fecal–oral route. From which of the following types of hepatitis is this patient suffering?
   A. Hepatitis A
   B. Hepatitis B
   C. Hepatitis C
   D. Hepatitis D

6. The most common sign of syphilis in the *primary stage* is _____.
   A. a chancre
   B. a fever
   C. a rash on the palms/soles
   D. mental deterioration

7. For an EMS provider, the best method of minimizing your risk of disease transmission is to _____.
   A. always wear gloves
   B. ask the patient if he or she has any infectious diseases
   C. assume all body fluids and secretions are infectious
   D. assume all body fluids and secretions of homeless people and IV drug users are infectious

8. The lesions associated with Lyme disease initially appear as _____.
   A. large and circular lesions called *erythema migrans*
   B. large scabs
   C. small pink dots
   D. small red lesions

9. Which of the following is considered a vehicle for transmission of a communicable disease?
   A. Airborne droplets from an infected person
   B. Blood from an infected person
   C. Insect carrying a communicable disease
   D. Stretcher side rails of an ambulance

10. A 23-year-old male complains of nausea, vomiting, and generally feeling weak. He also says he has no appetite. Physical examination reveals that the sclerae are yellow, the right upper quadrant of the abdomen is diffusely tender, and a low-grade fever is present. You should suspect the patient has _____.
    A. AIDS
    B. hepatitis
    C. meningitis
    D. tuberculosis

11. A 20-year-old female military recruit responds only to pain. Before losing consciousness, she complained of a severe headache and nausea. Physical examination reveals a stiff neck and a rash consisting of pinpoint areas of subcutaneous hemorrhage over the shoulders and upper chest. You should suspect the patient has _____.
    A. AIDS
    B. hepatitis
    C. meningitis
    D. tuberculosis

12. Hepatitis A can be transmitted by _____.
    A. fecal–oral contamination
    B. fecal–oral contamination and needle stick
    C. needle stick
    D. sexual intercourse

13. Hepatitis B can be transmitted by _____.
    A. fecal–oral contamination
    B. needle stick
    C. needle stick and sexual intercourse
    D. sexual intercourse

14. EMS personnel should observe standard precautions _____.
    A. when a patient is bleeding
    B. when caring for any patient
    C. when HIV infection is suspected
    D. when starting an IV

15. Which of the following is the most common mode of transmission for meningitis?
    A. Fecal–oral contamination
    B. Inhalation of infected airborne droplets
    C. Needle stick
    D. Sexual intercourse

16. HIV is transmitted through which of the following body fluids _____.
    A. blood, semen, vaginal secretions
    B. blood, vaginal secretions
    C. urine, blood, semen
    D. urine, semen

17. Lyme disease is transmitted by _____.
    A. flies
    B. mites
    C. mosquitoes
    D. ticks

Case one

You are dispatched to a boarding school dormitory for a 17-year-old girl who is not acting appropriately. The patient's roommate states the girl has not been feeling well the past 2 days. Earlier today, she complained of a severe headache and backache. The patient tried to take a nap but could not. The patient's roommate called 9-1-1 when the patient began to cry without stopping. According to the roommate, the patient has no significant medical history and takes no medications. She does not use recreational drugs. You find the girl on a bed with her knees flexed up to her chest. She is awake, crying, and easily agitated. She answers questions by repeating that her head hurts.

1. What problem do you suspect?

   _____

2. What precautions should you take?

   _____
   _____
   _____
   _____

Case two

You are dispatched to a homeless shelter for a 50-year-old Russian immigrant with difficulty breathing. Witnesses state the patient was attempting to sleep but was unable to sleep because of coughing and shortness of breath. He appeared to be shaking as though he was chilled. The fire department first responders are on the scene and relay the following report to you: "50 y/o male c/o SOB and coughing. Onset was 3 hours ago. He is a smoker. Unknown past medical history because patient does not speak English. The patient is awake and alert. He is coughing and has a respiratory rate of 28 breaths/min with 'junky' lung sounds. Vital signs are: BP—140/88 mm Hg; P—110 beats/min; skin—hot and dry." The first responders are concerned the patient may have a gastrointestinal bleed because he is coughing up blood. They ask if there is anything further you would like them to do before your arrival.

1. What problem do you suspect?

   _____

2. What precautions should you take?

   _____
   _____
   _____
   _____

32 Psychiatric Disorders and Substance Abuse

READING ASSIGNMENT

Chapter 32, pages 1167-1240, in *Paramedic Practice Today: Above and Beyond*.

OBJECTIVES

After completing this chapter, you will be able to:

1. Define *behavior* and distinguish between normal and abnormal behavior.
2. Define *behavioral emergency*.
3. Discuss factors that may alter the behavior or emotional status of an ill or injured individual.
4. Discuss the pathophysiology of psychiatric disorders.
5. Describe appropriate measures to ensure the safety of the patient, paramedic, and others.
6. Correlate the abnormal findings in assessment with the clinical significance in patients using the most commonly abused drugs.
7. Define the following terms:
   - Affect
   - Anxiety
   - Fear
   - Open-ended question
   - Posture
   - Phobia
   - Dysphoria
   - Euphoria
8. Describe the circumstances when relatives, bystanders, and others should be removed from the scene.
9. Describe the techniques that facilitate the systematic gathering of information from the disturbed patient.
10. Identify techniques for physical assessment in a patient with behavioral problems.
11. Be able to recognize various psychiatric disorders on the basis of assessment and history of present illness.
12. Integrate pathophysiologic principles with the assessment of the patient with psychiatric disorders.
13. Discuss the prevalence of behavior and psychiatric disorders.
14. Describe the history and physical findings associated with psychiatric disorders.
15. Describe management strategies for various psychiatric disorders.
16. List the clinical uses, street names, pharmacologic characteristics, assessment findings, and management for patients who have taken or been exposed to the following substances:
    - Cocaine
    - Marijuana
    - Methamphetamines
    - Barbiturates
    - Sedative-hypnotics
    - Narcotics or opiates
    - Common household substances
    - Drugs abused for sexual purposes or gratification
    - Alcohols
    - Hydrocarbons
    - Psychiatric medications
    - Newer antidepressants and serotonin syndromes
    - Lithium
    - Monoamine oxidase inhibitors
    - Club drugs
    - Hallucinogens
    - Dissociatives
17. List situations in which you may have to transport a patient forcibly and against his or her will.
18. List the risk factors for suicide.
19. List behaviors that indicate a patient may be at risk for suicide.
20. Describe the verbal techniques useful in managing the emotionally disturbed patient.
21. Describe methods of restraint that may be necessary in managing the emotionally disturbed patient.
22. Describe the medical and legal considerations for management of emotionally disturbed patients.
23. Describe the condition of restraint asphyxia and why you must never restrain a patient in a prone position.
24. Define the following terms:
    - Substance or drug abuse
    - Tolerance
    - Withdrawal
    - Addiction
25. List the most commonly abused drugs by chemical name and street name.
26. Discuss the incidence of drug abuse in the United States.
27. Describe the pathophysiology of commonly abused drugs.
28. Differentiate the various treatments and pharmacologic interventions in the management of the most commonly abused drugs.
29. Integrate pathophysiologic principles and the assessment findings to formulate a field impression and implement a treatment plan for patients using the most commonly abused drugs
30. Discuss the signs and dangers of clandestine drug manufacturing labs.

CHAPTER SUMMARY

- The most essential skill for dealing with behavioral emergencies is listening.
- "Normal" behavior usually is measured against the standards and expectations of society.
- A behavioral emergency results when a patient's ideas or actions are harmful or potentially harmful to self or others.
- The majority of human emotional experience originates in the limbic system of the brain.
- Organic behavioral emergencies have biologic causes (e.g., stroke, hypoglycemia).
- Alterations in the concentrations or actions of neurotransmitters in the brain are linked to many psychiatric and substance abuse disorders.
- Psychosocial factors are life changes and events that may worsen psychiatric problems.
- Events during childhood help cause mental illness and are called *developmental factors.*
- The biopsychosocial concept of mental illness proposes that mental illnesses result from a complex interaction among biologic makeup, behavior, and a person's environment.
- For the majority of behavioral emergencies, such as a violent or suicidal patient, you should stay away from the scene and wait for law enforcement before entering.
- Careful study of a patient's residence and surroundings can yield important clues about his or her state of mind and illness.
- When interviewing a patient with a behavioral emergency, maintain a quiet, nonthreatening environment with equal, open access to exits for you and the patient.
- Do not be afraid to request bystanders, family, or friends to leave the scene, or move the patient to your ambulance to create a private, quiet setting.
- Open-ended questions about how the patient has been feeling and acting yield the best results.
- Assess and treat all reports of pain or discomfort per local protocols; do not dismiss somatic complaints of patients with behavioral emergencies.
- Always suspect organic illness in patients with a sudden-onset behavioral emergency and no prior history.
- Perform a neurologic examination as well as a detailed interview in all patients with behavioral emergencies.
- Speech patterns and mannerisms can be assessed to learn more about a patient's form of thought, specifically rate of speech and looseness of associations.
- Psychosis is a state of highly distorted perceptions of reality with hallucinations and delusions.
- A hallucination is false sensory information that originates within the brain; a delusion is a false perception or interpretation of events and situations.
- Preoccupations are ideas that consistently and constantly return to a patient's mind.
- Affect is the outward expression of a patient's emotions as observed and described by the interviewer.

- Mood is the dominant, sustained emotional state of a patient and is the lens through which he or she sees the world.
- Affect can be thought of as emotional weather that fluctuates around mood, the emotional climate.
- Dysphoria is an extremely depressed, low mood; euphoria is an exaggerated feeling of joy and happiness.
- Schizophrenia is a neurologic illness marked by psychotic symptoms, disorders of thought, and a decrease of social interactions.
- *Anhedonia* is defined as the lack of enjoyment of activities and people patient used to find pleasurable.
- Long-term use of antipsychotic medications often leads to tardive dyskinesia, a neurologic disorder characterized by involuntary movements of the mouth and face.
- Mood runs a continuum from melancholy at the low end to mania at the high end.
- Dysthymia is a chronic, constant, low-grade depression.
- Patients who have melancholic episodes are said to have unipolar depression, whereas patients whose melancholic episodes alternate with hypomania, mania, or mixed episodes have bipolar disorder.
- Cyclothymia is a lesser form of bipolar disorder.
- Fear is the physical and emotional reaction to a real or perceived threat; anxiety is apprehension and worry about a future event.
- Panic attacks are sudden, severe, paralyzing anxiety reactions.
- Phobias are intense fears of specific objects or situations.
- Excessive, persistent worrying about everyday events is termed *generalized anxiety disorder.*
- Episodes of vivid, disturbing memories and dreams alternating with periods of emotional numbness after a traumatic event define posttraumatic stress disorder.
- Obsessive-compulsive disorder consists of unwanted, intrusive ideas (obsessions) and specific, repetitive rituals that the patient feels he or she must perform (compulsions).
- Somatoform disorders are characterized by abnormal preoccupations with bodies and physical symptoms.
- Patients with factitious disorder intentionally produce signs and symptoms of an illness to assume the sick role.
- Faking an illness for a tangible gain is called *malingering.*
- Patients with anorexia nervosa consistently see themselves as overweight, take drastic measures to become thin, and have strange behaviors and rituals associated with food and eating.
- Eating large amounts of food in one setting (binging) and then forcing oneself to vomit or use laxatives (purging) to avoid gaining weight is characteristic of bulimia.
- Personality disorders are abnormal and damaging ways of thinking about and interacting with the world that are always present.
- Three groupings of personality disorders exist: odd and eccentric disorders (cluster A), emotional and

dramatic disorders (cluster B), and anxious and fearful disorders (cluster C).

- Suicide is the act of ending one's own life. Thoughts of suicide are called *suicidal ideations*, and unsuccessful tries to end one's own life are known as *suicide attempts*.
- Cutting, burning, or hurting oneself is known as self-injury and is an unhealthy coping mechanism for overwhelming and troubling emotions.
- To care for behavioral patients, you must move out of a mindset characterized by invasive procedures and drugs and into one of observation, evaluation, and emotional support.
- Stop violent situations by preventing them.
- Physical and chemical restraints are last resorts used only to prevent the patient from harming himself or others.
- Patient restraint carries medical, legal, and ethical risks.
- Patients should never be restrained in the prone position and should never be transported while handcuffed.
- Chemical restraint should be used after physical restraint to prevent continued struggling and the development of excited delirium.
- Restraint asphyxia results from an inability to expand the chest cavity and create a negative pressure for inspiration.
- Using a substance for any reason other than its approved, accepted purpose is known as *abuse*.
- Addiction, or dependence, is an uncontrollable need to use a substance despite negative consequences.
- Long-term use of a drug makes its receptors in the brain less sensitive, forcing users to take more of the substance to achieve the same effects, known as *tolerance*.
- Withdrawal symptoms result when a patient abruptly stops using a drug after his or her body has adapted to its constant presence.
- Those who abuse drugs rarely only choose one; poly-substance abuse and overdose are common, making assessment and treatment difficult.
- The intoxicating agent in alcoholic beverages such as wine, beer, and liquor is called ETOH.
- Stimulant drugs such as cocaine, methamphetamine, and 3,4-methylenedioxymethamphetamine (MDMA) are highly addictive and carry high risks of side effects and withdrawal syndromes.
- Excited delirium can produce wildly abnormal behavior characterized by aggression, paranoia, hyperthermia, superhuman strength, and insensitivity to pain.
- Excited delirium is related to the use of stimulant drugs and often ends in sudden death.
- Drugs that relax, relieve anxiety, and/or induce sleep are called *sedative-hypnotics*.
- Opioids are powerful pain-killing drugs with a high potential for abuse and addiction.
- Sedative-hypnotics, gamma-hydroxybutyrate (GHB), ketamine, and ETOH are used separately or together to facilitate sexual assault.
- Marijuana is the dried and shredded leaves, stems, and seeds of the hemp plant, which is smoked or eaten to cause euphoria and relaxation.

- Abuse of inhalants causes a rush of euphoria of short duration and is most common among older children and teenagers.
- Hallucinogens, such as lysergic acid diethylamide (LSD), psilocybin mushrooms, peyote, and mescaline, cause hallucinations and distort perceptions of reality.
- Dissociatives, such as ketamine, phencyclidine hydrochloride (PCP), and dextromethorphan, create a feeling of detachment (dissociation) of the mind, body, and the user's surroundings.

MATCHING

1. Match the personality disorder with its description.

_____ Acute discomfort with close relationships, eccentric behavior, cognitive distortions

_____ Detachment from social relationships

_____ Disregard for the rights of others

_____ Distrust and suspiciousness

_____ Excessive emotions and attention seeking

_____ Instability in interpersonal relationships and self-image, impulsivity

_____ Preoccupation with orderliness, perfectionism, control

_____ Social inhibition, feelings of inadequacy, hypersensitivity to criticism

_____ Submissive or clinging behavior, excessive need to receive care

A. Antisocial
B. Avoidant
C. Borderline
D. Dependent
E. Histrionic
F. Obsessive-compulsive
G. Paranoid
H. Schizoid
I. Schizotypal
J. Narcissistic

SHORT ANSWER

1. What is a behavioral (psychiatric) emergency?

_____
_____
_____
_____

2. What is *affect*?

_____
_____

3. Compare and contrast delirium and dementia.

_____

_____

_____

_____

4. List and describe the four major types of schizophrenia.

_____

_____

_____

_____

5. What is bipolar disorder?

_____

_____

_____

_____

6. What medication commonly is used to treat bipolar disorder?

_____

7. Compare and contrast anorexia nervosa and bulimia nervosa.

_____

_____

_____

_____

8. Your patient is a 28-year-old female whose neighbors called you because she is "acting funny." When you enter her apartment, she begins to scream that you are Russian G-men who have come to get her. She runs to the kitchen and returns with a butcher knife. What should you do?

_____

_____

_____

_____

9. You are transporting a patient who has been placed in restraints because he smashed the windows of several cars with a baseball bat. The patient now appears to be calm and is asking you to loosen the restraints because they are hurting him. What should you do?

_____

_____

10. After talking to a depressed, suicidal patient for 30 minutes, you finally convince her to go to the hospital. She tells you that she needs to go to the bedroom to get some things before you transport her. What should you do?

_____

_____

11. Your ambulance is the first unit on a scene where a 22-year-old male is threatening to jump from a building. What should your first action be in this situation?

_____

_____

12. List five organic (nonpsychologic) causes of altered behavior.

_____

_____

_____

_____

_____

13. What question should you always ask every patient with clinical depression?

_____

_____

14. List at least four factors that increase the risk of a successful suicide attempt.

_____

_____

_____

_____

15. If you must interview a bystander or relative about a patient who is having paranoid delusions, what is the best way to conduct the interview?

_____

_____

_____

_____

MULTIPLE CHOICE

1. A car struck a utility pole and burst into flames. When you arrive on the scene, a police officer tells you the occupants of the car are dead and burned beyond recognition, but there is a bystander you "need to check out." The patient is a 23-year-old male who is sitting in his vehicle. When you make contact with him, he says, "I wanted to help them. I could hear them screaming. I wanted to help, but I can't see anything. I've gone blind." As the patient talks to you, he seems unusually calm for someone who has experienced acute loss of eyesight. This patient may be suffering from _____.
   A. conversion hysteria
   B. depression
   C. over-reaction
   D. paranoia

2. Characteristics of depression may include _____.
   A. helpless or hopeless feelings, increased risk of suicide, loss of interest in hobbies
   B. helpless or hopeless feelings, increased risk of suicide, loss of interest in hobbies, paranoia
   C. helpless or hopeless feelings, increased risk of suicide, paranoia
   D. helpless or hopeless feelings, paranoia

3. You respond to a call to "assist the police" on the scene of a "behavioral emergency." When you arrive at the scene, a 22-year-old male who has wrapped his body in aluminum foil and is wearing a colander on his head greets you. He tells you that CIA agents are following him and plotting to kill him because he is able to intercept messages from aliens who have signed a secret treaty with the Trilateral Commission to take over the Earth. The metal objects are to protect him against the ozone that the government agents are directing against him. The police officers with the patient tell you they "believe this is a job for EMS." You suspect the patient is suffering from _____.
   A. bipolar disorder
   B. clinical depression
   C. paranoia
   D. paranoid schizophrenia

4. As you interview the patient in the previous question, he asks you, "Where do you plan to take me?" The most appropriate response to this question would be _____.
   A. "Either to jail or to the hospital. It's up to you!"
   B. "I think it is important for you to go to the hospital."
   C. "To a safe house where the aliens and CIA can't get you."
   D. "Would you like to go to the hospital?"

5. A 17-year-old female is standing on top of a building and threatening to jump. What is the first action you should take?
   A. Leave until the police secure the situation and the scene is safe.
   B. Shock the patient back to reality by daring her to jump.
   C. Tell the patient if she really meant to kill herself she would have jumped already.
   D. Try to get the patient to talk to you.

6. After applying restraints to a combative patient, you should _____.
   A. loosen the straps if the patient appears to be rational.
   B. loosen the straps if the patient complains they are hurting.
   C. not loosen the restraints until the patient reaches a medical facility.
   D. not loosen the straps unless the patient loses consciousness.

7. What is the best option available if you cannot calm a hostile, aggressive patient?
   A. Ask the patient to sign a form refusing treatment.
   B. Obtain appropriate assistance from law enforcement personnel.
   C. Quickly subdue the patient using whatever force is necessary.
   D. Try to disarm the patient immediately if he has a weapon.

8. Which of the following conditions may produce behavioral changes?
   A. Cerebrovascular accident; depression or schizophrenia
   B. Hypoglycemia; cerebrovascular accident
   C. Schizophrenia or depression; hypoglycemia
   D. Schizophrenia or depression; hypoglycemia; cerebrovascular accident

9. Which action would be most appropriate in handling a noncombative emotionally disturbed patient?
   A. Allowing the patient adequate time to discuss his feelings
   B. Obtaining police assistance to subdue the patient as soon as possible
   C. Transporting the patient to the hospital as quickly as possible
   D. Using restraints immediately because your safety may be at risk

10. You are managing a 23-year-old female patient who is actively threatening suicide. You should _____.
    A. allow her to remain at home with family members if she claims the suicidal feelings have decreased
    B. dare the patient to do it to shock her into reality
    C. encourage the patient to think about alternatives and the effects her suicide might have on others
    D. tell the patient she does not really want to commit suicide

11. Which of the following factors indicates the greatest risk for successful suicide?
    A. Chronic substance abuse
    B. Female gender
    C. Strong ties with family and friends
    D. Vague suicide plans

12. The word that best describes a patient with paranoia is _____.
    A. bizarre
    B. sad
    C. suspicious
    D. trusting

13. Which technique would be most effective in managing a patient with paranoia?
    A. Agreeing with delusional statements to calm the patient
    B. Attempting to convey as much warmth and concern for the patient as possible
    C. Avoiding discussions with bystanders and family members in the patient's presence
    D. Being truthful with the patient

14. A patient who exhibits dizziness, tremors, tachycardia, dyspnea, and sweating _____.
    A. probably has a psychologic problem only
    B. probably has a physiologic problem only
    C. may have either a psychologic problem or a physiologic problem, but should be assessed and treated for the psychologic problem first
    D. may have either a physiologic problem or a psychologic problem, but should be assessed and treated for the physiologic problem first

15. A call comes in for a "man who has gone crazy." When you arrive, you discover the call has originated from a pay phone at a convenience store. The caller is a very excited young woman with three small children huddled around her. She gestures to the house across the street and states that her husband is inside with a gun, threatening to kill anyone who comes near him. She tells you he came home from work today "completely crazy." She never has seen him this way before. What should you do?
    A. Enter the house and try to reason with the patient.
    B. Inform the caller this is a not a medical problem and that there is nothing you can do to help.
    C. Keep the woman and her children in a safe place and request a response by the police.
    D. Remain with the woman and her children while your partner enters the house with the patient's wife and tries to reason with him.

16. A patient with a history of clinical depression recently purchased a gun. When assessing this behavior in terms of suicide risk, you should remember that _____.
    A. no assumptions should be made based on an isolated behavior such as this one
    B. suicide usually happens without warning
    C. this action indicates a high degree of intent to commit suicide that probably cannot be deterred
    D. this action may indicate suicidal intentions and should signal a need for therapeutic intervention

17. Which of the following is an example of an open-ended question?
    A. Do you take any medications?
    B. Have you done anything else to hurt yourself?
    C. Have you had feelings like this before?
    D. When did you begin feeling like you want to die?

Questions 18 to 25 relate to the following scenario:

You are called to a disturbance involving an "emotionally disturbed person." The patient is a 32-year-old male who became violent when told he was being laid off his job. On arrival, you find the patient and his supervisor in the patient's office. The patient is pointing a sharp letter opener at the supervisor, and you hear the following:

Patient: "I'm going to get you all. You aren't going to do this to me!"

Supervisor: "Settle down, Fred. No one is out to get you."

Patient: "Yes they are! They're talking about me . . . spreading rumors about me. I'm going to show them . . . and I'll start with you!"

Supervisor: "Don't you threaten me, you lunatic!"

At this point, the patient lunges at his supervisor, misses, and steps back to his original position. The police have been called, but have not yet arrived.

18. Given the preceding scenario, your most appropriate initial action would be to _____.
    A. attempt to restrain the patient
    B. identify yourself and step between the patient and the supervisor
    C. ignore the conversation between the patient and supervisor, and start taking a history
    D. remove the supervisor from the room

19. Which of the following would be the best response to the patient's actions?
    A. "Give me that letter opener!"
    B. "I can see you're very angry. What are you so angry about?"
    C. "I see you don't like your boss."
    D. "You better put down that letter opener. The police will be here in a minute."

20. The patient asks, "Who are you and what are you doing here?" What would be the best response?
    A. "I'm a paramedic with EMS. I am here to help you."
    B. "I'm a paramedic, and I'm here because your friends called me to come help you."
    C. "I'm a paramedic, and I'm here to take you to the hospital."
    D. "Who are you, and what are you doing?"

21. Choose the response that would most likely calm the patient.
    A. "Fred, I would like you to put down the letter opener so you and I can talk."
    B. "Fred, trust me. I'm not going to let them get you."
    C. "Fred, you're going to the hospital. You can decide whether it will be the easy way or the hard way."
    D. "You better calm down before you get into trouble."

22. What would be the most appropriate response if the patient asks you if you think he is right?
    A. Be completely honest; let the patient know when you think he is delusional.
    B. Tell him you agree with him.
    C. Tell him you do not take sides.
    D. Tell him you understand he feels he is right and you respect his point of view, even though you may not always agree with him.

23. What would be the best way to ask the patient to go to the hospital?
    A. "Do you want to go with us or with the police?"
    B. "Fred, I think a doctor could help you if you will go with us to the hospital."
    C. "Fred, would you like to go with us to the hospital?"
    D. "Fred, you've got to go to the hospital for medication to treat your mental illness."

24. Fred responds by saying, "You're just a nobody, a stupid ambulance driver! Why should I listen to you?" How should you respond?
    A. Acknowledge that Fred may feel angry and wonder why he should trust you; then repeat your offer to help.
    B. Ask Fred how he would feel if you called him stupid.
    C. Explain you are a highly trained healthcare professional who knows what is best for him.
    D. Ignore his remarks and repeat your offer to help.

25. Fred replies, "No! I will not go with you. You're out to get me too!" What should you do?
    A. Ask him to sign a form refusing treatment.
    B. Offer to take him home.
    C. Remain calm and continue to talk to him while waiting for police assistance.
    D. Try to get him to agree to take some medicine to "calm his nerves," and then give him haloperidol.

CASE STUDIES

Case one

Your patient is a 52-year-old female who is experiencing crushing substernal chest pain that radiates to her left shoulder and down the medial aspect of her left arm. She is pale and diaphoretic and complains of nausea. When you tell her she needs to go to the hospital, she becomes increasingly anxious and tells you that she has not gone outside in 15 years. When you become increasingly insistent about her need to go to the hospital, she tells you, "I can't go outside! I'll die if I go outside!"

1. From what psychiatric problem is the patient suffering?

   _____

2. How should you manage a patient suffering from this problem who requires transport to the hospital?

   _____
   _____
   _____
   _____

Case two

You respond to a report of a car crashing into a utility pole. When you arrive, you discover that the vehicle burst into flames following the impact, and the two female occupants burned to death. A police officer tells you that he thinks you need to "check out" one of the people who witnessed the crash. You find this patient sitting in the back of a police patrol car. When you ask him what is wrong, he replies, "I could hear them screaming. I wanted to help them. I wanted to do something. But I couldn't. I've gone blind." On physical examination, you discover that the patient does not appear to be aware of any visual stimuli. However, until just after he witnessed the accident, he had no problems with his vision. You also notice that the patient seems to be unusually calm for someone who has suddenly lost his eyesight.

1. From what psychiatric problem is this patient suffering?

   _____

2. What are the psychodynamics that produce this problem?

   _____
   _____
   _____
   _____

3. Why is the patient so unusually calm when he is suffering from a problem (loss of sight) that would be expected to produce significant anxiety?

_____

_____

_____

_____

4. How would you manage this patient?

_____

_____

_____

_____

Case three

A 72-year-old female is being transported from a nursing home to the hospital for evaluation. En route, she keeps calling you "conductor" and asking how long it will be until the train reaches St. Louis.

1. From what problem is this patient suffering?

_____

_____

_____

_____

2. Why is this problem particularly common in the geriatric population?

_____

_____

_____

_____

3. Whenever a patient develops this problem acutely, what other possibilities should you consider?

_____

_____

_____

_____

4. If this problem develops acutely, how should you manage it?

_____

_____

_____

_____

5. If this problem has been present chronically, does this change the way you manage it?

_____

_____

33 Hematologic Disorders

READING ASSIGNMENT

Chapter 33, pages 1241-1254, in *Paramedic Practice Today: Above and Beyond*.

OBJECTIVES

After completing this chapter, you will be able to:
1. Identify the anatomy of the hematopoietic system.
2. Describe the components of blood and volume and volume control in relation to the hematopoietic system.
3. Identify and describe the blood-forming organs and how and where blood is formed.
4. Describe normal red blood cell production, function, lifespan, and destruction.
5. Explain the significance of the hematocrit regarding red blood cell size and number.
6. Explain the correlations of the red blood cell count, hematocrit, and hemoglobin values.
7. Describe normal white blood cell production, function, and destruction.
8. Identify the characteristics of the inflammatory process.
9. Identify alterations in immunologic response.
10. Describe the number, normal function, types, and lifespan of leukocytes.
11. Identify the difference between cellular and humoral immunity.
12. Describe platelets in regard to normal function, lifespan, and numbers.
13. Describe the components of the hemostatic mechanism.
14. Describe the function of coagulation factors, platelets, and blood vessels necessary for normal coagulation.
15. Describe the intrinsic and extrinsic clotting systems in regard to identification of factor deficiencies in each stage.
16. Define *fibrinolysis*.
17. Describe disseminated intravascular coagulation and its precipitating factors.
18. Identify blood groups.
19. Define *anemia*.
20. Describe the pathology and clinical manifestations and prognosis associated with:
    - Aplastic anemia
    - Hemoglobinopathy (including sickle cell disease)
    - Hemolytic anemia
    - Iron-deficiency anemia
    - Methemoglobinemia
21. Describe the pathology and clinical manifestations associated with disorders of hemostasis: platelet dysfunction, thrombocytopenia, decreased production, platelet destruction, sequestration, and hemophilia.
22. Describe the pathology and clinical manifestations associated with leukocyte disorders: leukemia, lymphoma, and multiple myeloma.
23. Identify the components of physical assessment as they relate to the hematologic system and integrate pathophysiologic principles into the assessment of a patient with a hematologic disease.

CHAPTER SUMMARY

- Blood is a connective tissue that consists of cells and cell fragments. It comprises approximately 8% of the total body weight (5 to 6 L).
- Blood is composed of 55% plasma and 45% formed cellular fragments.
- Red blood cells (RBCs) are developed through a carefully regulated process known as *erythropoiesis*.
- White blood cells (WBCs) are the body's normal host defense. They include neutrophils, eosinophils, basophils, monocytes, and macrophages.
- Platelet function requires cohesion among the platelet, the vessel wall, von Willebrand factor, and fibrinogen.
- Agglutinogens are specific blood type antigens on the surface of the RBC membrane; antibodies are made to the agglutinogens (i.e., antigens). The A, B, O, and Rh agglutinogens must be matched before transfusion.
- Diagnosis of the specific cause of the patient's hematologic symptoms in the field is impossible. However, most patients with a hematologic disorder show symptoms of hypoxia, infection, and anemia.
- Each clinical disorder can present with acute life-threatening manifestations. As a result of limited information in the field, you must manage the ABCs and be prepared for aggressive resuscitation.

SHORT ANSWER

1. What are the three types of "formed elements" found in blood?

   _____

   _____

   _____

2. Which of the formed elements is responsible for transporting oxygen to the tissues?

_____
_____
_____
_____

3. What antigens will be found on the erythrocytes of a patient with each of the following blood types?
Type A:_____
Type B:_____
Type AB:_____
Type O:_____

4. What antibodies will be found in the plasma of a patient with each of the following blood types?
Type A:_____
Type B:_____
Type AB:_____
Type O:_____

5. Which blood type is the universal donor? Why?

_____
_____

6. Which blood type is the universal recipient? Why?

_____
_____

7. What is the function of the thrombocytes?

_____
_____
_____
_____

8. Contrast the mechanisms that trigger the intrinsic and extrinsic pathways of clot formation.

_____
_____
_____
_____

9. What is the function of plasmin in the process of hemostasis?

_____
_____
_____
_____

10. Why is sickle cell anemia most common in areas of the world where malaria is endemic?

_____
_____
_____
_____

11. How is a patient who is suffering from a sickle cell thrombo-occlusive (pain) crisis treated?

_____
_____
_____
_____

12. Why are patients with sickle cell anemia prone to having cerebrovascular accidents?

_____
_____
_____

13. What is the most common cause of death in patients who have hemophilia?

_____
_____
_____

14. What is the most common site of hemorrhages in patients who have hemophilia?

_____
_____
_____

15. Describe how bleeding from a wound in a patient with hemophilia should be managed.

_____
_____
_____
_____

16. What is leukopenia?

_____
_____
_____

17. Patients with leukopenia are at risk for what problem?

_____
_____
_____
_____

18. What is leukemia?

_____
_____
_____

19. Why are patients with leukemia prone to developing infections?

_____
_____
_____
_____

20. Why do patients with leukemia develop problems with bleeding?

_____
_____
_____
_____

21. Describe the pathophysiology of disseminated intravascular coagulation (DIC).

_____
_____
_____
_____

22. Describe two mechanisms that may trigger DIC in a pregnant patient.

_____
_____

23. Describe the pathophysiology of the process that makes administration of Rh-positive blood to an Rh-negative female a problem.

_____
_____
_____
_____

MULTIPLE CHOICE

1. Which of the following blood types is the "universal donor"?
   A. A
   B. AB
   C. B
   D. O

2. Which of the following blood types is the "universal recipient"?
   A. A
   B. AB
   C. B
   D. O

3. Which of the following are functions of eosinophils?
   A. Release of chemicals that fight parasitic infections; release of histamine
   B. Release of chemicals that inactivate the chemical mediators of allergic reactions; release of chemicals that fight parasitic infections
   C. Release of histamine; release of chemicals that fight parasitic infections
   D. Release of histamine; release of chemicals that inactivate the chemical mediators of allergic reactions

4. The principal function of neutrophils is to _____.
   A. ingest and destroy invading microorganisms
   B. produce antibodies
   C. release chemicals that modulate allergic reactions
   D. release histamine

5. Humoral immunity is mediated by _____.
   A. B-lymphocytes and involves direct attacks on cells carrying specific antigens
   B. B-lymphocytes and involves production of antibodies
   C. T-lymphocytes and involves direct attacks on cells carrying specific antigens
   D. T-lymphocytes and involves production of antibodies

6. T-lymphocytes are responsible for _____.
   A. cellular immunity through direct attacks on cells carrying specific antigens
   B. cellular immunity through production of antibodies
   C. humoral immunity through direct attacks on cells carrying specific antigens
   D. humoral immunity through production of antibodies

7. Giving Rh-positive blood to a female with Rh-negative blood creates what problem?
   A. Antibodies in the patient's blood will attack the transfused RBCs, causing hemolysis.
   B. Antibodies in the patient's blood will attack the transfused RBCs, causing agglutination.
   C. The patient may produce antibodies that could attack the RBCs of an Rh-positive fetus during a future pregnancy.
   D. The patient may produce antibodies that could attack the RBCs of an Rh-negative fetus during a future pregnancy.

8. Antibodies or immunoglobulins are a component of _____.
   A. cell-mediated immunity and produced by the B-lymphocytes
   B. cell-mediated immunity and produced by the T-lymphocytes
   C. humoral immunity and produced by the B-lymphocytes
   D. humoral immunity and produced by the T-lymphocytes

9. The type of leukocyte responsible for recognizing foreign antigens, producing antibodies, and developing memory is the _____.
   A. basophil
   B. eosinophil
   C. lymphocyte
   D. macrophage

10. One of the functions of the inflammatory response is _____.
    A. "walling off" the infected area
    B. attacking foreign substances
    C. causing allergic reactions to specific antigens
    D. developing memory for antigens

11. Which statement about patients with type AB blood is correct?
    A. The erythrocyte's cell membrane contains both A and B antibodies.
    B. The erythrocyte's cell membrane contains both A and B antigens.
    C. The plasma contains both A and B antibodies.
    D. The plasma contains both A and B antigens.

12. The extrinsic pathway of hemostasis is activated by _____.
    A. a decrease in the blood's oxygen-carrying capacity caused by a drop in blood pressure
    B. damage to platelets from turbulent blood flow
    C. exposure of the blood to external contaminants entering the vessel
    D. trauma to the vessel walls.

13. The most common cause of death in a patient with hemophilia is _____.
    A. bleeding from the heart that causes cardiac tamponade
    B. gastrointestinal tract bleeding that leads to exsanguinations
    C. intracranial bleeding that produces increased intracranial pressure
    D. laryngeal bleeding that results in loss of the airway

14. Which of the following situations is most likely to result in DIC in pregnancy?
    A. Activation of the clotting mechanism by dead fetal tissue or hemorrhage associated with the pregnancy
    B. Hemolysis of RBCs resulting from fetal enzyme release
    C. Reduced relative concentrations of thrombocytes associated with increased maternal blood volume
    D. Thromboembolism because pregnancy produces a hypercoagulable state

15. Hemophilia is inherited as _____.
    A. an autosomal dominant disorder
    B. an autosomal recessive disorder
    C. an X-linked dominant disorder
    D. an X-linked recessive disorder

16. Problems that can develop in patients with multiple myeloma include _____.
    A. anemia, increased risk of infection
    B. anemia, increased risk of infection, pathologic fractures
    C. pathologic fractures, increased risk of infection, polycythemia
    D. polycythemia, increased risk of infection

17. Patients with thrombocytopenia are at increased risk of _____.
    A. bleeding
    B. infection
    C. myocardial infarction and cerebrovascular accident
    D. pathologic fracture

18. The most common presenting sign of non-Hodgkin's lymphoma is _____.
    A. bleeding of the gums
    B. life-threatening opportunistic infections
    C. spontaneous bruising
    D. swelling of lymph nodes

19. Which statement about von Willebrand disease is correct?
    A. It involves both a clotting factor dysfunction and abnormal platelet function.
    B. It is inherited as an X-linked recessive trait.
    C. The associated bleeding is more severe than the bleeding caused by hemophilia A.
    D. The disease affects females more frequently than males.

CASE STUDY

A 36-year-old woman (gravida 4, para 3) G4P3 is in the seventh month of her pregnancy. She complains of a sudden onset of dizziness and weakness associated with severe, constant abdominal pain. She is pale and diaphoretic. Radial pulses are weak and rapid. The uterus is tender to palpation and is "rock-hard." A small amount of vaginal bleeding is present. Vital signs are: BP—84/68 mm Hg; P—126 beats/min weak, regular; R—22 breaths/min shallow, regular. The patient has a history of chronic essential hypertension controlled with diet and diuretics. You believe your patient is experiencing a placental abruption. Patients with this problem are susceptible to developing DIC.

1. What is DIC?

    _____
    _____
    _____
    _____

2. What is the pathophysiology of DIC?

_____
_____
_____
_____

3. Why are patients with this patient's underlying problem prone to developing DIC?

_____
_____
_____
_____

4. What is the clinical presentation of DIC?

_____
_____
_____
_____

5. How is DIC managed?

_____
_____
_____
_____

34 Shock and Resuscitation

READING ASSIGNMENT

Chapter 34, pages 1256-1282, in *Paramedic Practice Today: Above and Beyond*.

OBJECTIVES

After completing this chapter, you will be able to:
1. Discuss the anatomy and physiology of the cardiovascular system.
2. Discuss the stages and types of shock, including aerobic and anaerobic metabolism, and the ischemic, stagnant, and washout phases of shock.
3. Describe the etiology, history, and physical findings of hypovolemic shock.
4. Using the patient history and physical examination findings, develop a treatment plan for a patient in hypovolemic shock.
5. Describe the etiology, epidemiology, history, and physical findings of cardiogenic shock.
6. Using the patient history and physical examination findings, develop a treatment plan for a patient in cardiogenic shock.
7. Describe the etiology, epidemiology, history, and physical findings of distributive shock.
8. Using the patient history and physical examination findings, develop a treatment plan for a patient in distributive shock.
9. Describe the etiology, epidemiology, history, and physical findings of obstructive shock.
10. Using the patient history and physical examination findings, develop a treatment plan for a patient in obstructive shock.
11. Discuss dissociative shock.

CHAPTER SUMMARY

- The five primary types of shock are hypovolemic, cardiogenic, distributive, obstructive, and dissociative.
- Shock is a sign, not a diagnosis. If shock is not reversed, it will result in death.
- The three primary stages of shock are early (compensatory), late (progressive or decompensated), and irreversible.

- Treatment goals for a patient in shock include reperfusing tissue with oxygenated blood and repairing or stopping the cause.
- Definitive care for a patient in hypovolemic shock is not provided in the prehospital setting. These patients should be transported to the closest appropriate medical facility, such as a trauma center.
- IV fluids can increase perfusion pressures in a patient who is in shock but also can increase anemia, stop clotting, and lower body temperature.
- Age, drugs, existing medical conditions, and overall health status can affect the body's ability to compensate for shock.

MATCHING

1. What type of shock is present in each of the following patients?

____ 23 y.o. h/o vomiting and diarrhea × 4 days; BP—98/76 mm Hg; P—120 beats/min; R—22 breaths/min

____ 27 y.o. c/o abdominal pain following an incomplete abortion 3 days ago; skin— warm, flushed; BP—96/56 mm Hg; P—136 beats/min; R—26 breaths/min shallow; T—103° F

____ 30 y.o. c/o loss of lower extremity motor function following a motor vehicle collision; BP—96/40 mm Hg; P—72 beats/min; R—24 breaths/min shallow

____ 77 y.o. c/o substernal chest pain and SOB; BP—70/56 mm Hg; P—130 beats/min irregular; R—36 breaths/min

A. Cardiogenic
B. Hypovolemic
C. Neurogenic
D. Septic

SHORT ANSWER

1. What are the three elements of circulation that must be present for adequate tissue perfusion to occur?

_____

_____

_____

2. Define *shock*.

_____

_____

_____

_____

3. Is a falling blood pressure an early or a late sign of shock? Why?

_____

_____

4. What happens to cellular metabolism as a result of hypoperfusion? What substances are produced by the cells as a result of this change in metabolism?

_____

_____

_____

_____

5. What is the most important treatment that can be administered in the prehospital setting to a patient in shock?

_____

_____

_____

_____

6. Describe the physiologic mechanism that produces neurogenic shock. Why do these patient have dry skin and slow heart rates?

_____

_____

_____

_____

7. What type of fluid (hypotonic, isotonic, hypertonic) should be used if a patient is in hypovolemic shock? Applying the principle of osmosis, explain why this fluid is used.

_____

_____

_____

_____

8. What complication will result if fluid is rapidly infused into a patient with inadequate cardiac function?

_____

_____

_____

_____

9. Explain why an elderly patient may by hypoperfused at a blood pressure of 120/80 mm Hg.

_____

_____

_____

_____

10. How does the pediatric response to hypoperfusion differ from that of adults? Why does this happen?

_____

_____

_____

_____

11. What are the three therapeutic effects of pneumatic antishock garment (PASG)?

_____

_____

_____

12. What is the one absolute contraindication to applying and inflating PASG? Why?

_____

_____

_____

_____

13. What change will early shock produce in a patient's level of consciousness?

_____

14. What change will early shock produce in a patient's respirations? Why does this occur?

_____

_____

_____

15. You arrive at the hospital with a trauma patient who has had a PASG applied and inflated. The physician on-duty (a moonlighting proctology resident) tells you to "Get that inflatable underwear off so I can see the wound!" What should you tell the doctor regarding the proper removal of the PASG?

_____

_____

_____

16. You are called to see a patient who has an obvious head injury. The abdomen is also bruised and distended. Signs and symptoms of hypovolemic shock are also present. The patient has absent radial pulses. What do you know about the cause of the patient's shock? Why?

_____

_____

_____

_____

17. Could you apply the pneumatic anti-shock garment to the patient in the previous question and inflate it? Why or why not?

_____

_____

_____

_____

18. What substance released by the body primarily is responsible for causing anaphylactic shock? What are the effects of this substance on the peripheral vascular resistance, on capillary permeability, and on extravascular smooth muscle (bronchioles, gastrointestinal tract)? What three drugs can be given to counteract the effects of this substance?

_____

_____

_____

_____

19. Compare and contrast the skin signs in hypovolemic, cardiogenic, and distributive shock. Physiologically, why is the skin pale in some shock patients but not in others?

_____

_____

_____

_____

20. Why are patients in shock frequently restless and anxious?

_____

_____

_____

_____

21. What change occurs in the diastolic blood pressure in early hypovolemic shock? Why? What effect does this have on the pulse pressure (the difference between the systolic and diastolic blood pressure readings)?

_____

_____

_____

_____

22. Patients who are in shock frequently complain of feeling cold. Based on the effects of hypoperfusion on metabolism, explain why this symptom develops.

_____

_____

_____

_____

23. Describe why the use of a PASG may be contra-indicated in patients with chest injury.

_____

_____

_____

_____

24. Why should vasopressors not be used to raise blood pressure until hypovolemia is corrected?

_____

_____

_____

_____

25. Your initial assessment reveals an anxious, restless patient who has pale, cool skin; a weak, rapid pulse; flat neck veins in the supine position; and dilated, sluggish pupils. What problem do you suspect?

_____

_____

_____

_____

26. Why is blood pressure not a reliable indicator of hypoperfusion?

_____

_____

_____

_____

MULTIPLE CHOICE

1. You are called to see a patient with a closed head injury. The patient is pale, cool, and sweaty. Radial pulses are absent. The carotid pulse is weak and rapid. You should recall that _____.
   A. a patient cannot lose enough blood inside his skull to cause shock; the patient is bleeding elsewhere
   B. head injuries often produce shock from blood loss within the skull
   C. shock associated with closed head injury seldom causes complications
   D. the signs and symptoms of hypovolemic and neurogenic shock are similar and easily confused

2. A wasp stung a 45-year-old male. There was local swelling and redness at the sting site, but he continued working. About 15 minutes later, he developed tightness in his chest and severe breathing difficulty. He now is unresponsive, his skin is cyanotic, and his carotid pulse is rapid and weak. Blood pressure is 68/palpation. The patient is suffering from _____.
   A. anaphylactic shock
   B. cardiogenic shock
   C. neurogenic shock
   D. septic shock

3. An 18-year-old male was involved in a motor vehicle crash. He complains of weakness and tingling in his lower extremities and of severe pain in the mid lumbar region. His skin is cool and dry. Vital signs are: BP— 76/40 mm Hg; P—60 beats/min weak, regular; R—20 breaths/min shallow, regular. The patient probably is suffering from _____.
   A. cardiogenic shock
   B. hypovolemic shock
   C. neurogenic shock
   D. septic shock

4. A 72-year-old male was struck by an automobile. He has a possible fracture of his right femur. He is awake and alert. En route to the hospital, he becomes increasingly restless and anxious. He complains of being cold, thirsty, and dizzy. His radial pulses become increasingly rapid and weak, and his respirations become rapid and shallow. The patient probably is _____.
   A. dehydrated
   B. hyperventilating from anxiety caused by pain
   C. hypothermic
   D. hypovolemic

5. A 40-year-old female was struck by a automobile. Initially, her blood pressure is 156/92 mm Hg and her pulse is 116 beats/min, strong and regular. After 5 minutes, her blood pressure is 122/82 mm Hg and her pulse is 132 beats/min, weak, regular. After 10 minutes, her blood pressure is 116/72 mm Hg and her pulse is 148 beats/min and thready. You should suspect that _____.
   A. the patient could be going into shock from a closed head injury
   B. the patient could be going into shock from internal blood loss
   C. the patient initially was anxious and now her blood pressure is returning to normal
   D. the sphygmomanometer is malfunctioning because the blood pressure should be rising if the pulse is falling

6. Which set of vital signs leads you to suspect neurogenic shock?
   A. P—140 beats/min; BP—60/40 mm Hg; R—24 breaths/min shallow, irregular
   B. P—60 beats/min; BP—180/110 mm Hg; R—42 breaths/min deep, regular
   C. P—62 beats/min; BP—70/50 mm Hg; R—26 breaths/min shallow, regular
   D. P—72 beats/min; BP—120/80 mm Hg; R—16 breaths/min normal, regular

7. If you suspect that a patient is in hypovolemic shock, you should _____.
   A. place the patient in the supine position
   B. give oxygen at 4 to 6 L/min by nasal cannula
   C. give the patient fluids by mouth to help replace lost volume
   D. wrap the patient in blankets to raise the body temperature

8. The pneumatic antishock garment can be useful in prehospital care because it _____.
   A. applies pressure to bleeding from massive soft tissue injuries of the lower extremities
   B. immobilizes bone and joint injuries of the lower extremities
   C. will immobilize pelvic and lower extremity fractures, reduce internal blood loss, and compress lower extremity bleeding
   D. will immobilize pelvic injuries and help reduce internal blood loss

9. Shock can be caused by _____.
   A. dilation of the blood vessels or pump failure
   B. inadequate blood volume or dilation of the blood vessels
   C. inadequate blood volume, dilation of the blood vessels, or pump failure
   D. pump failure or inadequate blood volume

10. Shock may be produced by spinal cord injury because _____.
    A. spinal cord injury always involves internal bleeding, which rapidly produces hypovolemic shock
    B. the blood vessels below the injury become dilated and there is no longer enough blood to fill them
    C. the heart no longer receives electrical impulses to pump blood, resulting in a slow heart rate and low blood pressure
    D. the patient's skeletal muscles become paralyzed, which slows the return of blood to the heart

11. Shock may be produced by a systemic infection (sepsis) because toxins released by bacteria _____.
    A. constrict blood vessels, decreasing the size of the vascular space and causing "relative" hypovolemia
    B. constrict blood vessels, enlarging the vascular space and causing "relative" hypovolemia
    C. dilate blood vessels, decreasing the size of the vascular space and causing "relative" hypovolemia
    D. dilate blood vessels, enlarging the vascular space and causing "relative" hypovolemia

12. If signs of shock are present, use of the PASG would be indicated for _____.
    A. a pelvic injury with signs of intra abdominal bleeding
    B. an open wound to the chest with severe external bleeding
    C. blunt trauma to the chest with signs of internal bleeding
    D. an isolated, open head injury accompanied by severe external bleeding

282

13. Damage to the sympathetic nervous system caused by a spinal fracture can produce _____.
    A. hypothermia because of increased heat loss through dilated peripheral vessels
    B. peripheral vasodilation, leading to pooling of blood in the vascular system and a fall in blood pressure
    C. severe tachycardia
    D. both hypothermia because of increased heat loss through dilated peripheral vessels as well as peripheral vasodilation, leading to pooling of blood in the vascular system and a fall in blood pressure

14. The shock that follows spinal cord injury is due to _____.
    A. associated head injury
    B. hypovolemia
    C. loss of peripheral resistance
    D. pump failure

CASE STUDIES

Case one

A 25-year-old male is complaining of dizziness when he stands. He states he has been suffering from vomiting and diarrhea for about 3 days. A physical examination reveals poor skin turgor, a furrowed tongue, and sunken eyes. The patient's pulse is weak and rapid. The patient has a positive tilt test.

1. What problem do you suspect?
    _____

2. What IV fluid would you use to treat this patient? Why?
    _____
    _____
    _____
    _____

Case two

A 62-year-old male is complaining of substernal chest pain and shortness of breath that awakened him 20 minutes ago. Auscultation of his chest reveals rales in both lung bases. Bilateral pedal edema is present.

1. Is this patient overhydrated or dehydrated?
    _____

2. What would happen if you rapidly infused an isotonic crystalloid solution into this patient? Why?
    _____
    _____
    _____
    _____

3. What IV fluid would you use to treat this patient? Why?
    _____
    _____
    _____
    _____

4. What infusion rate would you use? Why?
    _____
    _____
    _____
    _____

Case three

A 35-year-old male has a gunshot wound to the right upper quadrant of the abdomen. His skin is pale, cool, and moist. He responds only to pain. Radial pulses are absent. Carotid pulses are rapid and thready. Breath sounds are present and equal bilaterally.

1. From what type of shock is he probably suffering?

   _____

2. What IV fluid would you use to treat him? Why?

   _____
   _____
   _____
   _____

3. What type of IV fluid administration set and what gauge of IV catheter would you use? Why?

   _____
   _____
   _____
   _____

4. What other modality of therapy would you consider using? Why?

   _____
   _____
   _____
   _____

Case four

A 19-year-old male fell from a ladder. He landed on his feet and then fell backwards onto his buttocks. When he attempted to stand, he developed severe mid lumbar pain that radiated to both lower extremities. He is now experiencing weakness and paresthesias in his lower extremities bilaterally. He is anxious and agitated. His skin is warm and dry. Vital signs are: BP—86/50 mm Hg; P—60 beats/min weak, regular; R—26 breaths/min shallow, regular.

1. From what type of shock is he suffering?

   _____

2. What IV fluid should be used to treat him? Why?

   _____
   _____
   _____
   _____

3. Why is he not diaphoretic and tachycardic even though he is in shock?

   _____
   _____
   _____
   _____

4. If IV fluid administration is not successful in raising his BP, what two other treatments may be used?

   _____
   _____

Appendix A: Answer Keys

CHAPTER 1: EMS SAFETY AND WELL-BEING OF THE PARAMEDIC

Short Answer

1. The three components of wellness are physical, mental, and emotional well-being. (Objective 1)
2. Cardiovascular endurance, also known as aerobic capacity, provides the ability to maintain a sustained level of activity without fatigue. Muscle strength provides the ability to exert the forces necessary for lifting and moving. Flexibility helps prevent injuries by allowing the muscles and joints to be used efficiently through an adequate range of motion. (Objective 3)
3. Circadian rhythms are the natural cycle of daytime activity and nighttime sleep during a 24-hour period. Shift work disrupts the circadian rhythm by requiring activity at unusual times of the 24-hour cycle. This can lead to sleep deprivation while on-duty and interfere with normal sleep while off-duty. (Objective 4)
4. Four steps you can take to reduce the effect of shift work on circadian rhythms include: avoid drinking caffeine for a few hours before attempting to sleep; take a break at the end of a shift to unwind before attempting to sleep; eat carbohydrates that may help induce sleep; as much as possible, maintain the same sleep schedule on- and off-duty. (Objective 4)
5. A risk assessment consists of assessing an individual's health status and behaviors for factors that increase the probability of specific diseases as well as performing screening examinations such as breast self-examinations, mammograms, prostate exams, and colonoscopies. Risk assessment and screening can lead to lifestyle modifications to prevent disease or result in identification of a disease process in an earlier, more treatable stage. (Objective 5)
6. Six steps that can reduce the risk of cardiovascular disease include: controlling high blood pressure, maintaining normal weight, keeping cholesterol and triglyceride levels within acceptable limits, controlling diabetes, getting regular physical examinations including risk assessments, and using estrogen with caution, if at all. (Objective 5)
7. Seven warning signs of cancer include: a change in bowel or bladder habits, a sore throat that will not heal, unusual bleeding or discharge, a thickening or lump in the breast or elsewhere, indigestion or difficulty swallowing, an obvious change in a wart or mole, and a nagging cough or hoarseness. (Objective 5)
8. Proper body mechanics for lifting and moving include: move a load only if you can safely handle it; ask for help when you need it for any reason; position the load close to your body and center of gravity; keep your palms up whenever possible; take the time to establish good footing and balance; keep a wide base of support with one foot ahead of the other; avoid twisting and turning; flatten your lower back and tighten your abdominal muscles; bend your knees and let the large leg muscles do the work of lifting, not your back; do not hold your breath, exhale during the lift; when possible, push, do not pull; whenever possible, move forward rather than backward; when a team is lifting a load, only one person should give commands. (Objective 6)
9. The stress response is nonspecific response of the body to any demand placed upon it. Stress results from environmental stimuli combining with an individual's physical, mental, and emotional state to trigger the need for an adaptive response. Stress can result from either positive or negative stimuli. Each person perceives different stimuli as stressors and may react differently to a stressor at different times. Fatigue, sleep deprivation, loss or fear of loss, poor health, poor nutrition, frustration, and injury or fear of injury can trigger stress responses. (Objectives 10, 11)
10. Cardiac rhythm disturbances: rapid, irregular; chest tightness or pain; palpitations; dyspnea; increased respiratory rate; nausea and/or vomiting; gastrointestinal problems: diarrhea, constipation; sleep disturbance: insomnia, nightmares, sleep all the time; sweating; headaches; increased blood pressure; aching muscles and joints. (Objectives 12, 13)
11. Difficulty making decisions; critical thinking slow or impaired; decreased level of awareness (others, self, scene); difficulty concentrating or focusing; memory problems; strange dreams or nightmares; confusion or disorientation. (Objectives 12, 13)

12. Examples of positive coping mechanisms include the following:
   - Exercising to reduce stress, clear the mind, and do something healthy.
   - Talking with friends or peers who understand what is causing the stress, which provides support and a safe place to vent.
   - Using time management techniques is a solid way to decrease stress, prevent overload, and practice learning to say "no" to extra shifts, new assignments, and so forth.
   - Getting plenty of rest because fatigue and sleep deprivation can significantly decrease the ability to manage stress well.
   - Following good nutrition, a foundation block for staying healthy and giving your body what it needs to recover and rebuild.
   - Scheduling time for fun activities, events, or hobbies that bring pleasure (e.g., music, concerts, sports, reading).
   - Reframing an event, situation, or attitude to lay out the facts and examine them from different perspectives.
   - Taking deep, slow, controlled breaths to decrease feelings of stress and increase the feeling of calmness or serenity.
   - Following guided imagery to take short "mental vacations" or breaks from the current stress.
   - Performing relaxation exercises to relax the body progressively.

   Examples of negative coping mechanisms include the following:
   - Smoking
   - Drinking
   - Use of other substances (Objective 11)
13. The stages of the grieving process (Kübler-Ross) include:
   - Denial: Feelings of disbelief and the sensation that the news cannot be true.
   - Anger: Feelings of anger directed at others over the question of "why me?"
   - Bargaining: An attempt to "cut a deal" with a higher power to be able to accomplish some unfinished task. Indicates the individual has admitted the condition or event.
   - Depression: Sadness, regret, or despair from revisiting past events.
   - Acceptance: Recognition of the inevitable with a reasonable level of comfort with the anticipated outcome. (Objective 14)
14. Methods of communicating death to survivors include:
   - Introducing yourself by name and function.
   - Stating that their loved one has died. Do not use euphemisms such as "passed on."
   - Stating that nothing more could have been done. (Objective 15)

15. An exposure is an occurrence in which blood or body fluids come into contact with nonintact skin or mucous membranes or enter the body through parenteral contact (needle stick). (Objective 7)
16. High-efficiency particulate air (HEPA) masks or N-95 respirators should be worn when caring for patients with confirmed or suspected diseases that can be transmitted through respiratory secretions. Caution should be taken when giving nebulized medications, suctioning, or inserting airway management devices. A face mask and protective eyewear should be worn during these procedures. Disposable resuscitation equipment should be used as the primary means of artificial ventilation. (Objectives 7, 8)
17. Disposable gloves should be applied before every patient encounter and changed between patients. Hands should be washed or cleaned following glove removal. Protective eyewear and a facemask should be worn to protect from blood and fluid splatters. Gowns should be worn to protect clothing from splashes. Contaminated uniforms should be removed as soon as possible and personnel should shower. Contaminated clothing should not be taken home for laundering. (Objectives 7, 8, 9)
18. Immediately wash the affected area with soap and water; notify your agency's infection-control officer; document the incident, including keeping a copy for your records; obtain a medical examination with appropriate baseline tests and screenings; receive any recommended immunizations or prophylactic medications; continue follow-up and evaluation as needed. (Objective 7)

Multiple Choice

1. D. A patient's blood splashing into your eye would be considered a significant communicable disease exposure. Contact between blood and intact skin would pose a lower risk of disease transmission. A clean needle stick would pose a still lower risk. Tuberculosis is not a blood-borne disease. (Objective 7)
2. B. Physical fitness reduces, but will not eliminate, the risk of injury. (Objectives 1, 2)
3. D. Reaching over your head for a heavy box at the station supply room would be most likely to result in a back injury. (Objective 6)
4. B. An N-95 or HEPA facemask is the most appropriate respirator for the paramedic to be provided in order to provide protection from tuberculosis. (Objective 7)
5. D. The most important infection-control practice for healthcare workers is frequent hand-washing. (Objectives 7, 8)
6. C. For an EMS provider, the best method of minimizing his or her risk of disease transmission is to assume all body fluids and secretions are infectious. A significant number of patients with

communicable diseases do not know they are infected or will not admit infection to healthcare providers. Gloves help prevent transmission of communicable disease but do not provide complete protection. (Objective 8)

7. A. You believe this behavior may also be due to the stage of grief referred to as depression. (Objective 14)

8. B. The most appropriate statement would be, "Your son has died. Can we call someone to come be with you?" Euphemisms such as "passed away" can prevent family members from receiving the message that a loved one has died. The statement that a patient "felt no pain" cannot be verified if a family member asks, "How do you know that?" Saying that it was someone's "time to go" is another statement that also cannot be verified and that may upset family members. (Objective 15)

9. A. Steps you can take to help yourself sleep more easily after ending a shift include attempting to maintain the same sleep schedule on- and off-duty. (Objective 2)

10. A. A person's age affects how they respond to death and dying. All persons do not pass through the stages of dealing with death in the same order and at the same rate. In some cases a person may move back to an earlier stage in the process. Responses to death are highly individual and are affected by ethnicity and culture. (Objective 14)

CHAPTER 2: PARAMEDIC ROLES AND RESPONSIBILITIES

Short Answer

1. An emergency medical services system is a comprehensive network of personnel, equipment, and resources established to provide emergency medical care to the community. An EMS system includes both out-of-hospital and in-hospital components. (Objectives 1, 4)

2. ■ Licensure represents permission granted to an individual by the state to perform certain restricted activities. Scope of practice represents the legal limits of the licensed individual's performance. States have a variety of mechanisms to define the margins of what an individual is legally permitted to perform.

   ■ Certification is an external verification of the competencies that an individual has achieved and typically involves an examination process. While certification exams can be set to any level of proficiency, in health care they are typically designed to verify that an individual has achieved minimum competency to assure safe and effective patient care.

   ■ Registration is the process of entering an individual's name and essential information into a record. NREMT offers examinations for each

level of EMS professional. If an individual passes the NREMT examination, his or her name is placed on a registry of EMTs. Currently, many states grant an EMS professional the ability to practice in his or her state through certification or licensure, if the individual is nationally registered. (Objectives 1, 5)

3. A profession is a group of similar jobs or fields of interest that require mastery of a specialized body of knowledge and skills. (Objective 1)

4. Professionalism is following the standards of conduct and performance for a particular field of occupation. (Objective 1)

5. Paramedics should follow accepted standards of conduct and performance both on- and off-duty because the public views them as representatives of the EMS profession. Unprofessional conduct by one paramedic can damage the reputation of the entire profession. (Objective 9)

6. Medical direction is the process used by the medical community to ensure quality and accountability in the delivery of prehospital care. (Objective 1)

7. Prospective medical control consists of development of guidelines and standards for personnel selection, training, equipment, supplies, and patient care. Prospective medical direction ensures that the structure and processes of an EMS system are consistent with safe, effective medical practice. (Objectives 16, 17)

8. On-line medical direction consists of advice or orders given by a physician to a paramedic either directly or by telecommunications while the paramedic is caring for a patient. (Objectives 16, 17)

9. Retrospective medical direction consists of a review of patient management and appropriate steps based on the results of that review to improve care of future patients. (Objective 18)

10. A protocol is a set of guidelines outlining appropriate assessment and management for a specific injury or illness. A standing order is the portion of a protocol that a paramedic may carry out without being in direct communication with a physician. (Objective 17)

11. The National Registry of EMTs is an organization that administers a standardized testing and certification process to ensure that graduates of EMS training programs have met standards for minimum competency necessary to protect the public. (Objective 3)

12. Emergency medical responder, emergency medical technician, advanced emergency medical technician, paramedic. (Objective 5)

13. This report is commonly referred to as the *White Paper.* (Objective 2)

14. The National Highway Safety Act of 1966 required states to develop effective EMS systems or risk losing federal highway construction funds. (Objective 2)

15. Manpower, training, communications, transportation, emergency facilities, critical care units, pubic safety agencies, consumer participation, access to care, patient transfer, standardized record keeping, public information and education, system review and evaluation, disaster management plans, mutual aid. (Objective 4)
16. The first EMT-Basic (EMT-A) curriculum was published in 1971. (Objective 2)
17. The first paramedic curriculum was published in 1977. (Objective 2)
18. 1. Regulation and policy
    2. Resource management
    3. Human resources and training
    4. Transportation
    5. Facilities
    6. Communications
    7. Public information and education
    8. Medical direction
    9. Trauma systems
    10. Evaluation
19. Integration of health services, EMS research, legislation and regulation, system finance, human resources, medical direction, education systems, public education, prevention, public access, communications systems, clinical care, information systems, evaluation. (Objectives 2, 4)
20. Preparation and safety, response, scene assessment, patient assessment, emergency care, determination of appropriate patient destination, transfer of care, documentation, returning to service. (Objective 12)
21. Patients, family members, and bystanders form an initial opinion of the paramedic's competence based on his/her appearance. This initial opinion can affect interactions essential to providing effective care. (Objectives 10, 11)
22. Continuing education helps ensure that a paramedic develops and maintains the knowledge and skills necessary for safe, effective, efficient practice. (Objectives 7, 8)
23. Critical care transport, primary care, industrial medicine, sports medicine, tactical medicine. (Objective 12)
24. Integrating paramedics into the healthcare system can help improve the health of the community, prevent injuries and illnesses, enhance patient compliance with treatment regimens, and ensure a more appropriate use of resources through public education. (Objective 14)
25. Your involvement with teaching in the community can have many benefits. These include enhancing the visibility and positive image of EMS professionals. Participating in illness and injury prevention courses also helps improve the overall health of the community. Teaching cardiopulmonary resuscitation and first-aid courses establishes your role as a resource in your community. Cooperative public education efforts improve the integration of EMS with other healthcare and public safety agencies. (Objective 13)
26. Citizen involvement creates informed, independent supports of the EMS system. It also provides an outside, objective view into quality improvement and problem resolution. (Objective 15)
27. Research validates existing treatments and protocols, verifies whether changes in protocol and procedure are helpful or harmful, and identifies ways to improve devices used by paramedics. In an environment of limited resources, research is essential to demonstrating that the resources entrusted by the community to the EMS system are being used as efficiently and effectively as possible. (Objectives 19, 20)

Multiple Choice

1. D. The creation of "Modern EMS" systems is often associated with the passage of the National Highway Safety Act in 1966. (Objective 2)
2. A. Standing orders, training programs, and case reviews are examples of off-line medical control and direction. (Objective 16)
3. C. Of the following, the *most significant advantage* to the paramedic who reads professional journals is the ability to learn from clinical research. (Objectives 19, 20)
4. B. The National Highway Safety Act of 1966 required states to develop effective EMS systems or risk losing federal highway construction funds. (Objective 2)
5. D. The paramedic is the on-scene authority in prehospital care. (Objective 12)
6. C. A protocol provides uniform guidelines for management of patients; standing orders are portions of protocols that may be used without direct radio contact with a physician. (Objectives 1, 16, 17)
7. C. Two elements that were not included in the components of an EMS system under the Emergency Medical Services Systems Act of 1973 were system financing and medical direction. (Objectives 2, 4)
8. C. Reciprocity is the process by which an EMS professional who is approved to practice in one state obtains approval to practice in another state. (Objective 6)
9. C. Doing the right thing, even when no one is looking, is integrity. (Objective 11)
10. D. Taking on and following through on tasks without constant supervision is an example of self-motivation. (Objective 11)
11. C. Referring to patients as "frequent flyers" or "turkeys" demonstrates lack of the professional attribute of respect. (Objective 11)
12. A. Always placing the needs of your patients above your own self-interest is an example of advocacy. (Objectives 10, 11)

13. C. Sympathy is sharing the feelings of another empathy is showing compassion to another with an appreation of their situation without feeling the same emotions. (Objective 11)

14. B. A paramedic's first priority when arriving at the scene of a call always is to identify and deal with any threats to his/her safety. (Objective 12)

15. C. The National Highway Traffic Safety Administration is the agency of the federal government that establishes national guidelines for education and training of emergency medical services personnel. (Objective 5)

16. C. Under the National EMS Scope of Practice Model, the minimum level of training that can provide transport of a patient to an acute care facility is emergency medical technician. (Objective 5)

17. A. A paramedic's primary responsibilities include documentation. (Objective 12)

18. C. The role of the National Registry of EMTs is to provide a uniform testing process to ensure that graduates of EMS training programs have met minimum standards for competent practice. (Objective 3)

CHAPTER 3: ILLNESS AND INJURY PREVENTION

Short Answer

1. Injury is intentional or unintentional damage to a person resulting from acute exposure to thermal, mechanical, electrical, or chemical energy or from the absence of such essentials as heat or oxygen. (Objective 1)

2. Primary injury prevention is keeping an injury from ever occurring. Secondary injury prevention is preventing further injury from an event that already has occurred. (Objective 1)

3. EMS personnel are high-profile role models. EMS personnel are considered champions of the healthcare consumer and are welcome in schools and other environments. Because they see the results of injury every day, EMS personnel are considered authorities on injury and prevention. (Objective 3)

4. The time after an injury has occurred when the patient and observers remain acutely aware of what has happened and may be more receptive to teaching about how the event or illness could have been prevented. (Objective 4)

5. Education: teaching the target population. Engineering: altering products or devices in ways that offer automatic protection without thought on the part of the user. Enforcement: using legislation, regulations, or litigation to modify behavior and ensure compliance. Environment: changing the physical environment or culture to enhance effectiveness of a program, product, or device. EMS: engaging EMS personnel in the program. (Objectives 3, 4, 5)

6. Problem: identification of a public health issue through data analysis. Program: strategies for implementing a variety of interventions, including a feedback component that provides continuous feedback on effectiveness. Partnership: collaboration among public and private organizations and agencies. Preparation: investment of time and resources in data collection, analysis of similar interventions cited in the literature, identification of resources, training of participants, and follow-up with community partners. Policy: advocacy for changes in the law or in public or private policy that addresses an issue. (Objectives 3, 7)

7. Epidemiology is the study of the causes, patterns, prevalence, and control of disease in groups of people. (Objective 1)

8. By properly documenting calls, EMS personnel can provide the data epidemiologists need to study the causes, distribution, and control of disease in populations. (Objective 5)

9. Narratives completed by EMS personnel provide first-hand information about the physical and emotional characteristics of a scene, the chronology of events during an incident, the conditions of the scene, and the actions and reactions of persons involved in an injury event. This information frequently is omitted from hospital or police reports that rely on third- or fourth-hand information and are completed hours to days later. (Objective 7)

Multiple Choice

1. D. The leading cause of death in persons from ages 1 to 44 is unintentional injuries. (Objective 1)

2. D. For all ages combined, injuries are the fourth leading cause of death. (Objectives 1, 2)

3. C. The leading cause of death among all age groups is heart disease. (Objective 1)

4. B. Applying a cervical collar, spine board, and head blocks to a patient involved in a motor vehicle collision is an example of secondary prevention because it is care provided after an injury to prevent the occurrence of further problems. (Objective 5)

5. D. Presenting a program to preschoolers on identifying poisons in their homes is an example of education as an injury prevention strategy. Concrete

barriers placed in highway medians are an engineering strategy. Increased traffic fines in highway work areas are an enforcement strategy. Sanding highway overpasses before ice storms is an environmental strategy. (Objectives 3, 4, 5, 7)

6. A. Presenting a program to students in the public school that is designed to encourage seat belt use is an example of primary injury prevention because seat belt use prevents the occurrence of injuries. The strategy being used for this primary injury prevention activity would be educational. (Objectives 3, 4, 5)

7. A. This is an example of EMS system involvement in primary prevention because it is designed to prevent the occurrence of injuries. (Objectives 4, 5, 6)

8. B. Discussing seat belt use with a parent who was just involved in a minor traffic collision with a child in his or her vehicle is the best example of taking advantage of a "teachable" moment to provide effective public health education because the information being supplied directly relates to an event that recently occurred. People are most receptive to information about preventing specific injuries when they have recently experienced an event that produced or could have produced the type of injury being discussed. (Objective 4)

9. C. Ongoing systematic collection, analysis, and interpretation of injury data for planning, implementing, and evaluating injury prevention efforts is an injury surveillance program. (Objectives 5, 7)

10. D. A situation that puts people in danger of sustaining injury is an injury risk. (Objective 1)

CHAPTER 4: LEGAL AND REGULATORY ISSUES

Short Answer

1. Statutory law (statutes and ordinances enacted by Congress, state legislatures, and city councils). Administrative law (rules adopted by executive agencies under authority granted by statutory law). Case law (interpretations of constitutional, statutory, or administrative law made by the courts). (Objectives 3, 4)

2. A tort is a civil wrong, other than a breach of contract, for which the law provides a remedy. (Objective 3, 5)

3. Battery is touching another person without consent or other just cause. Physical contact is necessary for battery to have occurred. Assault is placing another person in fear for his or her safety without consent or other just cause. Physical contact is not necessary for assault to have occurred, only the fear that bodily harm might occur. (Objectives 5, 15)

4. Slander is making untrue verbal statements about another person that damage the person's reputation. Libel is making untrue statements about another person in writing or by some other graphic representation (such as drawing a picture) that damage the person's reputation. (Objectives 5, 15)

5. An adult (a legally and mentally competent person, typically 18 years of age or older) or a legally emancipated minor.

6. A minor is a person under 18 years of age who is not married or who has not had his or her status as a minor removed by court order. In most states when a person under the age of 18 marries, he or she legally becomes an adult. A person who is less than 18 years old who has his or her status of minority removed by the court is considered a legal adult. (Objective 16)

7. Consent is permission granted for medical care by an adult or by a minor under circumstances where the minor may consent to his/her medical care. (Objective 16)

8. Involuntary consent is the rendering of care to a person under specific legal authority, even if the patient does not consent to the care. (Objective 16)

9. Involuntary consent may be used when patients pose a threat to themselves or others, as well as when patients are in the custody of law enforcement or incarcerated in a correctional facility. (Objective 16)

10. Implied consent is the legal principle in which you may presume that a patient who is ill or injured, and is for any reason is unable to give consent, (e.g., unconscious, incapacitated, patient is a minor) would consent to receiving the necessary emergency care for his or her condition. (Objective 16)

11. Unconsciousness or inability to communicate and the presence of what reasonably seems to be a life-threatening injury or illness. (Objective 16)

12. The person accused of negligence had a duty to follow a standard of care (duty). The standard of care was not followed (breach of duty). Damage occurred to the plaintiff (damages). The damages were a result of the failure to follow the standard of care (causation). (Objectives 11, 12)

13. What a reasonable, prudent paramedic would do under the same or similar circumstances. (Objective 6)

14. Good Samaritan Acts usually do not provide a defense for gross negligence. (Objective 14)

15. Yes, oxygen administration would be appropriate. A do not resuscitate order is a directive to withhold resuscitative measures if clinical death occurs. As long as the patient is breathing and has a pulse, steps can be taken to make the patient comfortable and support vital functions. (Objectives 21, 26)

16. Yes, you can treat and transport this patient based on involuntary consent provided by the police officer. A police officer is responsible for the health and safety of persons in his or her custody. An officer can be held civilly and criminally liable for failure to ensure a prisoner's health and safety. Because of this responsibility, law enforcement officers have limited authority to order emergency medical treatment for persons in their custody. (Objectives 15, 17)

17. Yes, you can treat and transport this patient. The patient is unable to communicate and appears to be suffering from a life-threatening illness, a stroke. You have his implied consent. (Objectives 16, 17, 20, 24)

18. You should remain with the patient until a nurse or physician can assume responsibility for his care. Leaving the patient without ensuring continued care by a person of equal or higher training is abandonment. (Objective 20)

19. As an adult, this patient has the right to refuse care. You should inform him of the nature of his injuries, the benefits and risks associated with receiving and refusing treatment and transport, and appropriate alternatives. The patient should be able to indicate to you that he understands the nature of his injuries and the potential consequences of refusing treatment and transportation by repeating the information you have provided back to you. You should thoroughly document the patient's condition, the information you have provided, and his understanding of this information. You should have the patient sign a refusal of care form that includes a release of liability. (Objectives 16, 17, 18, 19)

20. You are at risk of being sued for libel because you have written an untrue statement about the patient that could damage his reputation. (Objectives 5, 29, 30, 31)

Multiple Choice

1. C. The recognition of minimal competency and the completion of prescribed education or training in a profession or occupation is called licensure. Certification is the recognition of minimal competency in certain skills or tasks. (Objective 8)

2. B. Treatment of this patient is initiated using implied consent. (Objective 16)

3. D. If this statement is false, your partner may be guilty of slandering the physician. (Objective 5)

4. D. The conduct that would be expected of a reasonable, prudent individual with similar training and experience under similar circumstances is called the standard of care. (Objective 6)

5. A. Your best course of action will be to assume consent for treatment is implied and proceed with all appropriate emergency medical treatment. Because children can compensate for injuries for extended periods and then decompensate suddenly, considering almost any nontrivial injury to a child to be life-threatening is reasonable. (Objectives 16, 17)

6. A. Your partner is not liable because the patient is not competent to give consent due to his intoxication. (Objectives 15, 16, 17)

7. C. The family most probably will sue you for negligence. You have breached a standard of care established by your organization's policies and procedures that may have contributed to failure to resuscitate the patient. (Objectives 3, 5, 11, 12)

8. A. Your action is an example of breach of confidentiality. To commit slander or libel you must make a statement verbally or in writing that is untrue. Giving information about a patient to a person not legally entitled to receive it is breach of confidentiality. (Objectives 1, 3, 4, 5, 22)

9. D. By providing basic life support measures only, you and your partner are not following the standard of care for paramedics. The standard of care for resuscitation by paramedics includes use of advanced airway management, electrical therapy, vascular access, and administration of appropriate medications. (Objectives 5, 21)

10. C. You should stop all resuscitative efforts and honor the DNR order. (Objectives 5, 21, 26)

11. D. You should offer assistance, document the names of the parties involved, write a refusal document, and have the woman sign the refusal. A durable power of attorney for healthcare gives an individual the authority to act for an individual in making healthcare decisions. A refusal of care by a person holding a durable power of attorney should be handled using the same procedures as a refusal of care by the patient. (Objectives 18, 19)

12. B. This decision by the court is an example of case law. (Objective 2)

13. D. Simply stating that the patient was ill would not violate medical confidentiality. (Objective 22)

14. C. Giving information to other EMS personnel who did not participate in the care of the patient would be a breach of confidentiality. (Objective 22)

15. A. Caring for an adult who has suffered a humerus fracture and who is awake, alert, and refusing treatment could result in a lawsuit against a paramedic for battery. (Objective 15)

16. A. A paramedic's "standard of care" is judged by comparing his/her actions to the actions expected of a paramedic in the same situation. (Objective 6)

17. A. Your best protection from liability when a patient refuses treatment or transportation is a detailed written report that documents all attempts made to obtain consent. (Objectives 17, 18, 29, 30)

18. B. Release of information about a patient to law enforcement officers who are attempting to determine whether a patient was using drugs would be a breach of confidentiality. The police have no special status granting them access to a patient's medical information. (Objective 22)

19. C. For the purpose of consenting to medical treatment, a child becomes an adult at 18 years of age whether the patient is male or female. (Objective 4)

20. C. You should obtain consent from the guardian because he is authorized to consent for the patient. (Objective 16)

21. A. You probably will be sued for abandonment because you terminated your relationship with the patient without ensuring continued care for the patient at a level adequate for his medical needs. (Objectives 9, 20)

22. D. You should start CPR, and then contact on-line medical control for advice on how to proceed. On-line medical control can direct you to stop the resuscitation attempt. Because a DNR order is not present, you must have authorization from a

physician to terminate resuscitation. While you are seeking this order, CPR must be performed. (Objective 26)

23. B. Your comment to the neighbor could result in your being sued for slander because you have made an untrue statement that damages the patient's reputation. (Objectives 3, 4, 5, 22)

Case Studies

Case one (objectives 1, 2, 3, 4, 5, 16, 17)

1. Yes.
2. The patient is an adult and can consent to her own medical care. Her mother's wishes are not relevant legally.
3. Expressed consent.

Case two (objectives 1, 2, 3, 4, 5, 16)

1. Yes.
2. The patient is experiencing a seizure, which can be a life-threatening condition. It is expected that the child's parents would want treatment for this condition.
3. Implied consent, as it is assumed the parents of a minor would want their child treated for life-threatening conditions. The wishes of the sister and grandmother are not legally relevant in this case.

Case three (objectives 1, 2, 3, 4, 5, 16, 17)

1. No, you cannot treat and transport the patient because she has refused consent.
2. You should request a response by the police. You should continue to explain the risks associated with refusing care to the patient while waiting for the police to arrive. You might also wish to contact on-line medical control by telephone and have a physician talk to the patient. If the patient continues to refuse treatment and transportation, the police should be asked to take her into protective custody.
3. Until some form of consent is obtained the patient cannot be treated. If you can convince her to allow treatment you would be treating under expressed consent. If the patient becomes unresponsive you can treat with implied consent. If neither of these conditions occur you will have to involve the judicial system to provide care under involuntary consent. In most states, police officers are authorized to take individuals into protective custody if they appear to be a danger to themselves or others. The police officer who takes an individual into custody must have them transported to a facility where they can be evaluated by a physician. Some EMS systems have developed procedures for obtaining emergency court orders for treatment of persons refusing care.

Case four (objectives 1, 2, 3, 4, 5, 16)

1. No.
2. The patient's parent is present and refusing consent for care.

3. Request a response by the police and request that an officer take the child into protective custody. In most states, law enforcement officers are provided with broad powers to protect the safety of sick, injured, or abused children.
4. You cannot treat until involuntary consent is provided by the police officer.
5. A judge, a law enforcement officer, a child protection officer (an authorized agent of the state agency responsible for child protective services), and in some states a juvenile probation officer responsible for the patient.

Case five (objectives 1, 2, 3, 4, 5, 16)

1. Yes.
2. The patient is unconscious.
3. Implied consent. Implied consent is present when a patient is unconscious or unable to communicate and is suffering from what appears to be a life-threatening injury or illness. Unconsciousness can be considered to be life-threatening, regardless of its cause, because unconscious persons are unable to protect their airways.

Case six (objectives 1, 2, 3, 4, 5, 16, 17)

1. Yes
2. He is suffering from a potentially life-threatening problem, potential loss of his airway, and a parent has not refused consent.
3. Implied consent.
4. Presence of what reasonably appears to be a life-threatening injury or illness in a minor with no refusal of consent by a parent or legal guardian.

Case seven (objectives 1, 2, 3, 4, 5, 9)

1. Ask the individual to show appropriate documentation of licensure as a physician. Ask him whether he is willing to assume responsibility for the patient and accompany the patient to the hospital. If he is willing to do so, place him in contact with your on-line medical control. If there is any disagreement between the physician intervener and your on-line medical control, follow the orders of on-line medical control. Until directed otherwise by on-line medical control, continue to follow the protocols approved by your medical director.
2. You have a preexisting contractual relationship with your medical director that obligates you to follow the protocols he or she has established for patient management unless he or she directs otherwise.

Case eight (objectives 1, 2, 3, 4, 5, 16)

1. No.
2. She is not the patient's legal guardian.
3. No.
4. Although the cousin is an adult, this individual is not the patient's legal guardian.
5. Yes.

6. The patient has life-threatening injuries and there is no parental refusal. Therefore you have the implied consent of the parents.

CHAPTER 5: ETHICS

Short Answer

1. Ethics are societal principles of conduct that people or groups of people adopt as guidelines for personal behavior. (Objective 1)
2. Laws tend to have a narrower focus than ethics because they focus on defining and discouraging behaviors that a society considers wrong. Because ethics encourage ideal behavior, they tend to be more oriented to what is good or right. (Objective 5)
3. What is in the patient's best interest? (Objective 3)
4. Doing good for others. A healthcare professional has an obligation to act in the patient's best interests. (Objective 1)
5. Autonomy is the right of a competent adult to determine what happens to his or her body. In the context of healthcare this means that a competent adult has the right to consent to or refuse treatment. (Objective 3)
6. Justice is the obligation to treat all persons fairly. In the context of healthcare this means the same care should be provided to all persons without regard to gender, race, religion, cultural background, sexual orientation, or economic and social status. (Objective 3)
7. *Primum non nocere* means "first do no harm." (Objective 3)
8. To exercise autonomy, a patient must have information about the benefits and risks associated with consenting to or refusing the options available for care. The patient also must have the mental capacity to evaluate these risks and benefits and must be free from constraints that might interfere with his or her ability to determine what he or she thinks is the best option. (Objective 6)
9. For healthcare personnel to provide safe, effective care, patients must be willing to share private information with them. If the public came to believe that healthcare professionals would not hold private information in confidence, they might become unwilling to provide critical information essential to their care. (Objective 6)

Multiple Choice

1. D. The term "ethics" is best described as standards of conduct and behavior defined by society. (Objective 1)
2. A. By complying with the wishes of a mentally competent adult to refuse care, the paramedic recognizes the patient's right to autonomy. (Objective 6)
3. B. You should introduce the student, explain you are supervising him or her and will take over if there are any problems, and ask the patient's permission for the student to start the IV. The principle of autonomy

dictates that patients have the right to know the qualifications of those caring for them so they can make informed judgments about whether to accept or refuse care. Therefore patients always should be told when the person caring for them is a student, regardless of how skilled that student is. Patients have the right to refuse care by a student although the argument could be made that all persons have an ethical obligation to society to ensure that students receive adequate opportunities to learn. (Objective 6)
4. A. Treat the patient according to his signs and symptoms, following appropriate treatment for chest pain, including the administration of morphine if indicated. (Objectives 6, 9)
5. C. Differentiating care based on economic or social status is a violation of the ethical principle of justice. (Objectives 4, 9)
6. D. By advocating an action that would cause harm to a patient your partner is violating the principle of primum non nocere. Intentionally causing injury or pain or withholding care to "punish" a patient for behavior that the paramedic considers inappropriate is unethical. (Objectives 6, 9)
7. A. By following the wishes of the patient as expressed in his advance directives, you are respecting the fundamental principle of medical ethics known as autonomy. (Objective 8)
8. D. If a physician asks you to perform an act that is illegal or unethical, you should refuse to perform the act and report the physician to the appropriate authorities. The principles of beneficence (doing good) and doing no harm impose not only an obligation to refuse involvement in unethical or illegal acts but also a requirement to expose those who engage in unethical or illegal activities. (Objectives 6, 9)

CHAPTER 6: MEDICAL TERMINOLOGY REVIEW

Matching

1.

Q	a-, an-	D	hemi-
H	aden-	C	hyper-
O	bi-	P	hypo-
G	contra-	E	macro-
K	derma-	L	micro-
N	dia-	I	my-
B	dys-	F	poly-
M	edem-	A	retro
J	erythro-		

2.

M	arthr-	E	cyt-
A	brachi-	C	encephal-
F	bucc-	K	enter-
J	cardi-	G	faci-
R	carp-	H	fibr-
I	cephal-	O	gastr-
D	chondr-	Q	gloss-
N	cost-	L	gnath-
B	cyst-	P	hist-

3.
M	-algia	E	-osis
D	- cyte	W	-paresis
T	-dipsia	H	-phagia
G	-ectomy	N	-plegia
A	-emia	B	-pnea
R	-esthesia	S	-phasia
C	-genic	I	-phobia
O	-gram	P	-rhythmia
K	-itis	J	-rrhea
Q	-logy	L	-taxia
F	-ostomy	U	-uria
V	-oma		

Short Answer

1. Medical terminology is used to record and describe every aspect of patient care. Incorrect use of these words could result in ineffective or even harmful treatment at the hospital, which could even result in a lawsuit. (Objectives 1, 7)
2. Root words, prefixes, and suffixes. (Objective 2)
3. This can help you determine the meaning of an unfamiliar word. (Objective 3)

True/False

1. A. True. This is an example of unusual pronunciation. (Objective 4)
2. B. False. *G* is usually soft if it is before *e* or *i*. (Objective 4)

Multiple Choice

1. A. Antonyms. These words mean the opposite of each other. For example, *ad,* toward; *ab*, away. (Objective 6)
2. D. Synonyms. These words both mean "half." (Objective 6)
3. B. Myopathies. For nouns ending in a *y* preceded by a consonant, change the *y* to *i* and add *es*. (Objective 5)
4. C. Homonyms are words that sound alike, but are spelled differently and have different meanings. (Objective 6)
5. B. Eponyms are words that are named after specific people, places, or things. (Objective 6)
6. C. *Pinkeye* is an eponym. It is named after the actual appearance of the condition to which it applies. (Objective 6)
7. B. The prefix *my-* refers to muscle. (Objective 6)
8. D. Synonyms. These words both mean "lung." (Objective 6)
9. A. *Every day* is abbreviated *qd*.
10. B. *After* is abbreviated *p̄*.

CHAPTER 7: BODY SYSTEMS: ANATOMY AND PHYSIOLOGY

Labeling

1. A. Sagittal plane
   B. Anterior
   C. Transverse, horizontal, or axial plane
   D. Superior
   E. Coronal plane
   F. Posterior
   G. Medial
   H. Lateral
   I. Inferior

2. A. Hair shaft
   B. Epidermis
   C. Dermis
   D. Subcutaneous layer
   E. Sweat gland
   F. Cutaneous nerve
   G. Hair follicle
   H. Sweat gland opening
   I. Sebaceous (oil) gland
   J. Papilla of hair
   K. Arrector pili muscle

3. A. Cranium
   B. Mandible
   C. Clavicle
   D. Scapula
   E. Sternum
   F. Humerus
   G. Costal cartilage
   H. Ulna
   I. Radius
   J. Carpals
   K. Metacarpals
   L. Phalanges
   M. Femur
   N. Patella
   O. Tibia
   P. Fibula
   Q. Tarsals
   R. Metatarsals
   S. Phalanges
   T. Facial bones
   U. Ribs
   V. Vertebral column
   W. Hip bone
   X. Sacrum

4. A. Frontal bone
   B. Parietal bone
   C. Sphenoid bone
   D. Temporal bone
   E. Maxilla
   F. Mandible
   G. Lacrimal bone
   H. Nasal bone
   I. Nasal conchae
   J. Vomer
   K. Mastoid process

5. A. Cervical vertebrae
   B. Thoracic vertebrae
   C. Lumbar vertebrae
   D. Sacral vertebrae
   E. Coccyx (tailbone)
   F. C1; atlas
   G. C2; axis
   H. Cervical curve
   I. Thoracic curve
   J. Lumbar curve
   K. Sacral curve

6. A. True ribs
   B. False ribs
   C. Floating ribs
   D. Clavicle
   E. Manubrium
   F. Body
   G. Xiphoid process
   H. Sternum
   I. Costal cartilage
   J. L1 vertebra

7. A. Innominate bone
   B. Coccyx
   C. Symphysis pubis
   D. Sacrum
   E. Obturator foramen

8. A. Temporalis
   B. Orbicularis oculi
   C. Zygomaticus
   D. Buccinator
   E. Serratus anterior
   F. Rectus abdominis
   G. Transversus abdominis
   H. Internal oblique
   I. External oblique
   J. Rectus femoris
   K. Vastus lateralis
   L. Vastus medialis
   M. Frontalis
   N. Masseter
   O. Orbicularis oris
   P. Sternocleidomastoid
   Q. Deltoid
   R. Pectoralis major
   S. Brachialis
   T. Biceps brachii
   U. Linea alba
   V. Brachioradialis
   W. Iliopsoas
   X. Adductor longus
   Y. Adductor magnus
   Z. Sartorius
   AA. Tibialis anterior
   BB. Peroneus longus

9. A. Deltoid
   B. Triceps brachii
   C. Gluteus medius
   D. Gluteus maximus
   E. Adductor magnus
   F. Gracilis
   G. Trapezius
   H. Latissimus dorsi
   I. Biceps femoris
   J. Semitendinosus
   K. Semimembranosus
   L. Hamstring group
   M. Gastrocnemius
   N. Soleus
   O. Calcaneal (Achilles) tendon

10. A. Cerebrum
    B. Pituitary gland
    C. Brainstem
    D. Midbrain
    E. Pons
    F. Medulla
    G. Thalamus
    H. Hypothalamus
    I. Diencephalon
    J. Cerebellum
    K. Spinal cord

11. A. Parathyroids
    B. Adrenals
    C. Ovaries (female)
    D. Testes (male)
    E. Pituitary
    F. Thyroid
    G. Pancreas

12. A. Semilunar valves
    B. Pulmonic valve
    C. Right atrium
    D. Right ventricle
    E. Atrioventricular valves
    F. Left atrium
    G. Aortic valve
    H. Left ventricle
    I. Tricuspid valve
    J. Chordae tendineae
    K. Bicuspid (mitral) valve

13. A. Sinoatrial (SA) node or pacemaker
    B. Atrioventricular (AV) node
    C. Purkinje fibers
    D. Atrial conduction fibers
    E. Bundle of His
    F. Right and left bundle branches

14. A. Tonsils
    B. Thymus gland
    C. Spleen
    D. Pharyngeal tonsil
    E. Palatine tonsil
    F. Lingual tonsil
    G. Cervical nodes
    H. Subclavian vein
    I. Axillary nodes
    J. Lingual nodes

15. A. Primary bronchi
    B. Secondary bronchi
    C. Tertiary bronchi
    D. Bronchiole
    E. Superior lobe
    F. Middle lobe
    G. Inferior lobe
    H. Trachea
    I. Cartilaginous rings
    J. Apex
    K. Superior lobe
    L. Hilus
    M. Inferior lobe
    N. Base
    O. Terminal bronchiole
    P. Alveolar ducts
    Q. Alveolar sacs
    R. Capillaries
    S. Alveoli

16. A. Tongue
    B. Esophagus
    C. Liver
    D. Pancreas
    E. Colon
    F. Ileum
    G. Cecum
    H. Rectum
    I. Anal canal
    J. Stomach
    K. Spleen
    L. Duodenum
    M. Gallbladder
    N. Cystic duct
    O. Hepatic bile duct
    P. Pancreas

17. A. Rectum
    B. Vagina
    C. Kidney
    D. Ureter
    E. Bladder
    F. Pubic symphysis
    G. Urethra
    H. Urinary meatus
    I. Rectum
    J. Penis

Short Answer

1.

	Alpha	Beta
1	Vasoconstriction, mild bronchoconstriction	Increased heart rate, myocardial conductivity, myocardial contractility
2	Smooth muscle contraction, inhibition of insulin release, induction of glucagon release, neurotransmitter inhibition	Vasodilation, bronchodilation

(Objective 46)

2. The working unit of muscle cells, consists of overlapping filaments of proteins called actin and myosin. During muscle contraction, myosin forms cross-links to actin, which pull the actin filaments across the myosin filaments, causing the muscle to shorten. Increasing ventricular preload creates tension on the ventricular walls, stretching them. Stretching a muscle displaces the actin filaments toward the ends of the myosin filaments, increasing the distance over which they can be pulled when the muscle contracts. This increases the force the muscle can exert during contraction, a phenomenon known at the Frank-Starling effect. However, if the muscle is stretched too far it will begin to pull the actin filaments past the ends of the myosin filaments, so cross-linking can no longer take place. At this point, stretching the muscle no longer will increase its force of contraction. (Objective 46)

3.

Nerve	Name	Function
I	Olfactory	Sensory: smell
II	Optic	Sensory: sight
III	Oculomotor	Motor: pupil constriction; superior rectus, inferior oblique muscles of eye; raising eyelid
IV	Trochlear	Motor: superior oblique muscle of eye
V	Trigeminal	Sensory: orbital structures, nasal cavity, skin of forehead, upper eyelid, cornea, eyebrows, nose, lips, gums, teeth, cheek, palate Motor: chewing muscles (temporalis, masseter, pterygoids)
VI	Abducens	Motor: lateral rectus muscle of eye
VII	Facial	Sensory: taste from anterior two thirds of tongue Motor: muscles of facial expression, lacrimal gland, submandibular and sublingual salivary glands
VIII	Acoustic	Sensory: hearing, balance
IX	Glossopharyngeal	Sensory: taste from posterior third of tongue; portions of pharynx and palate Motor: pharyngeal muscles and parotid salivary gland
X	Vagus	Sensory: pharynx; external ear, diaphragm; thoracic and abdominal viscera Motor: palatal and pharyngeal muscles; thoracic and abdominal viscera
XI	Spinal accessory	Motor: voluntary muscles of palate, pharynx, larynx; sternocleidomastoid and trapezius muscles
XII	Hypoglossal	Motor: tongue muscles

(Objective 39)

4. The lungs expand and contract as a result of the changes in the intra-thoracic pressure during the respiratory cycle. During inspiration, the diaphragm, scalene muscles, and parasternal muscles contract. This action increases the volume in the thoracic cage, causing the intrathoracic pressure to decrease compared with the air pressure outside the body. This allows outside air to rush in. During exhalation, the diaphragm and the accessory muscles of respiration relax, enabling the intra-thoracic pressure to increase above the air pressure outside the body. This causes the air to exit the mouth and nose. (Objective 60)

5. At the level of the alveolar-capillary membrane, the air within the alveolus contains a higher partial pressure of oxygen and a lower partial pressure of carbon dioxide than the blood within the capillaries. The gases diffuse along the pressure gradients, with oxygen moving into the blood and carbon dioxide diffusing into the alveoli. At the level of the tissue capillary beds, the blood within the capillaries contains a higher partial pressure of oxygen and a lower partial pressure of carbon dioxide than the interstitial fluid surrounding the capillaries. The gases diffuse along the pressure gradients, with oxygen moving into the interstitial fluid and cells and carbon dioxide diffusing into the capillaries. (Objectives 13, 59)

6. Phase 4: The cell is in its polarized resting state, with more positively charged sodium outside the cell and more potassium and large negatively charged protein molecules on the inside. The inside of the cell is negative relative to the outside. Phase 0: stimulation of the cell causes sodium channels in the cell membrane to open. Positively charged sodium flows into the cell, causing the inside of the cell to become positive relative to the outside. The cell now is depolarized. Phase 1: potassium channels open in the cell membrane, causing positively charged potassium to flow out of the cell. The inside of the cell moves toward once again being more negative than the outside. Phase 2: movement of positively charged calcium into the cell through calcium channels offsets the effects of the outward flow of potassium, creating a "plateau" phase where the distribution of charges does not change. Calcium interacts with the actin and myosin filaments of the sarcomeres to cause contraction. Phase 3: the calcium channels close, and the outward flow of positively charged potassium out of the cell restores a state in which the inside of the cell is negative relative to the outside. Phase 4: the action of the sodium-potassium pump restores a normal distribution of sodium and potassium across the cell membrane. (Objective 52)

7. Inferior and superior vena cava, right atrium, tricuspid valve, right ventricle, pulmonic valve, pulmonary artery, pulmonary vascular bed, pulmonary veins, left atrium, mitral valve, left ventricle, aortic valve, aorta. (Objectives 49, 50)

8.   __High__   aortic arch
     __High__   pulmonary vein
     __Low__   inferior vena cava
     __Low__   right ventricle
     __High__   renal artery
     __High__   left atrium
     __Low__   pulmonary artery
     __High__   carotid artery
(Objective 50)

9. Sinoatrial (SA) node, internodal pathways, atrioventricular (AV) node, bundle of His, bundle branches, Purkinje fibers. (Objective 55)

10.   __Open__   aortic
     __Closed__   mitral
     __Closed__   tricuspid
     __Open__   pulmonic
(Objectives 49, 50)

11. Stroke Volume × Heart Rate = Cardiac Output. (Objective 47)

12. Cardiac Output × Peripheral Vascular Resistance = Blood Pressure. (Objective 47)

13. SA node: 60 to 100
AV node: 40 to 60
Purkinje system: 20 to 40
(Objective 55)

14. A decreased heart rate will decrease cardiac output and blood pressure if stroke volume and peripheral resistance do not change. (Objective 47)

15. Increasing the heart rate shortens the length of systole and diastole; however, the greater effect is on diastole. (Objective 47)

16. Increasing peripheral vascular resistance will increase blood pressure if cardiac output remains constant. (Objective 47)

17. Increases in heart rate are accomplished by shortening diastole, the period between beats. Because the heart fills during diastole, a severe tachycardia can result in a decrease in cardiac preload, which leads to a fall in cardiac output. (Objective 47)

18. Stimulation of the sympathetic nervous system increases the heart rate. (Objectives 40, 53)

19. Stimulation of the parasympathetic nervous system slows the heart rate. (Objective 40)

20. In the absence of oxygen the Krebs cycle, or aerobic metabolism, cannot occur. Because of this cellular respiration stops after glycolysis, or anaerobic respiration. This is a very inefficient form of cellular respiration, leading to the net production of 2 molecules of ATP and large amounts of lactic acid. If oxygen is not restored to the cells the body not only will become acidotic but also will not be able to keep up with its energy demands. (Objective 12)

21. Diffusion is a passive process in which particles move freely from an area of higher concentration to an area of lower concentration. In the human body particles that can freely cross the cell membrane (such as gases) move by diffusion. Osmosis involves the movement of water across a semipermeable membrane. In this situation the solutes (the particles) remain in place and the water (the solvent) moves across the membrane, resulting in an equal concentration on each side of the membrane. Although the concentration (or percent solution) is equal on both sides of the membrane, the actual number of particles and the amount of water on each side of the membrane are not equal. Active transport is the movement of a substance against its concentration gradient. This involves the expenditure of energy. An example of this is the sodium-potassium pump. (Objective 13)

22. Functions of the integumentary system include protection, sensation, excretion, fluid regulation, and temperature regulation. (Objective 19)

23. Movement (muscle cells), conductivity (nerve cells), metabolic absorption (kidney and intestinal cells), secretion (mucous gland cells), excretion (all cells), respiration (all cells), reproduction (most cells). (Objective 8)

24. Ribosomes are organelles in which new protein is synthesized. They are made of complex strands of macromolecules of protein and ribonucleic acid. Ribosome chains form the framework for the genetic blueprint and the synthesis of proteins. Ribosomes may be found free-floating within the cytoplasm, or attached to the endoplasmic reticulum. The endoplasmic reticulum (ER) is a chain of canals and sacs that wind through the cytoplasm, connecting the nuclear membrane to the cytoplasmic membrane. This system of canals and sacs works as a circulatory system within the cell that moves substances and proteins through the cell. The ER also plays a part in the detoxification process. ER is either smooth or rough based on the presence or absence of ribosomes on its surface. Smooth ER lacks ribosomes and is found in cells that handle or produce fatty substances and certain hormones such as the sex hormones. Rough ER has ribosomes on its surface and is found in cells that produce protein to be excreted for use outside the cell. After creation of proteins the ribosomes transfer the protein into the rough ER for transport to the Golgi apparatus where it will be further processed. The Golgi apparatus is a series of flattened sacs that resemble a stack of pancakes. They are often found attached to the ER and their function is to concentrate and package material for secretion out of the cell. When the material is ready to be secreted a small vesicle breaks off of the Golgi apparatus and travels to the cytoplasmic membrane, where its contents are released outside the cell. An example of a Golgi apparatus product is mucus. Vesicles are the shipping containers of the cell. They are very simple in structure, consisting of a single membrane filled with liquid. They transport a wide variety of substances both on the inside the cell, referred to as endocytotic vesicles, and to the exterior of the cell, referred to as *exocytotic vesicles*. Lysosomes, which contain

297

enzymes, are membrane-walled organelles that are created by breaking off from the Golgi apparatus. The enzymes contained within these structures aid in the digestion of nucleic acids, fats, proteins, polysaccharides, and lipids. Certain white blood cells (leukocytes) have large amounts of lysosomes that contain enzymes designed to digest bacteria. Lysosomes also digest nonfunctional organelles. Peroxisomes contain chemicals that combine hydrogen and oxygen to form hydrogen peroxide. This then detoxifies substances that would be harmful to the cell. As the main organ of detoxification, the liver contains a large amount of peroxisomes. Mitochondria are the power plants of the cell (and the body). They are the site of aerobic respiration, which results in the synthesis of ATP. The ATP that is formed serves as a source of energy throughout the body. The mitochondria are comprised of two membranes. The outer membrane gives the organelle its shape while the inner membrane creates several folds called cristae. These two membranes are important in the discussion of cellular respiration later in this chapter as they are the location of the two steps of aerobic respiration. Tissues of the body that have high energy needs, such as muscle and nerve tissue, typically have large numbers of mitochondria. Centrioles are paired, rodlike structures that lie at right angles to each other. These structures exist in a specialized area of the cytoplasm known as the centrosome. The centrioles play an important role in the process of cell division. Cilia are organelles that are hairlike projections from the cytoplasmic membrane of some epithelial cells. Their function is to create a wave of motion, or a current that moves fluid over the surface of the cell. For example, the cells that line the respiratory tract have a large number of cilia to move particles that have been inhaled and trapped in the mucus into the oropharynx to be swallowed or expelled. Flagella are singular organelles that project from the cell and are used for propulsion. The male sperm cell is the only cell in the human body that has a flagellum. Microvilli are projections from the cytoplasmic membrane that serve to increase surface area for absorption. The lining of the small intestine has a large amount of microvilli to increase the rate of absorption of digested food. (Objective 10)

25. Solutions that have an equal concentration are called isotonic. A solution with a higher concentration as compared with another solution is hypertonic, and a solution with a lower concentration as compared with another solution is hypotonic. (Objective 12)

26. Hormones work by stimulating or altering the actions of cells. This may include increasing or decreasing cellular production, increasing or decreasing the absorption of materials by the cells, or any number of other alterations in cellular metabolism. They exert this effect through negative feedback mechanisms. In this type of system an effort is made to negate a certain action or effect in the body. (Objective 46)

27. Adenosine triphosphate stores energy used by the cell to drive metabolic reactions. (Objective 8)

28. DNA and RNA are nucleic acids. (Objective 8)

29. RNA and DNA are considered the blueprint of the cell. Because of this the function, products, appearance, reproduction, and all other aspects of the cell are controlled by the nucleic acids. (Objective 8)

30. A phospholipid bilayer is a double layer of lipid molecules that forms the membranes of the cell and its organelles. (Objective 8)

31. Cytoplasm fills the interior of the cell. (Objective 8)

32. Catabolism. (Objective 5)

33. Anabolism. (Objective 12)

34. Negative feedback. (Objective 46)

35. Positive feedback. (Objective 46)

36. The sympathetic nervous system. (Objective 44)

37. Potassium. (Objective 55)

38. Sodium. (Objective 55)

39. Sympathetic. (Objective 44)

40. Cardiac output is the amount of blood pumped by the heart in 1 minute. (Objective 50)

41. Cardiac Output = Heart Rate × Stroke Volume. (Objective 50)

42. Cardiac output and peripheral (systemic) vascular resistance. (Objective 50)

43. Increasing preload stretches the walls of the ventricles and causes them to contract with greater force, a phenomenon called the *Frank-Starling effect*. (Objective 50)

True/False

1. B. False. Hemoglobin is found in erythrocytes. (Objective 49)

2. B. False. An isotonic solution has an osmotic pressure equal to that of normal body fluids. (Objective 73)

3. B. False. Surfactant serves to prevent alveolar collapse. (Objective 63)

Multiple Choice

1. D. At the end of a normal expiration, air pressure inside the lungs is equal to atmospheric pressure. Air moves in the respiratory tract because of differences in pressure. Air no longer moves at the end of either inspiration or expiration because intrapulmonary pressure and atmospheric pressure are equal. (Objective 63)

2. B. Small hairlike processes on the outer surface of some cells that produce motion or current in a fluid are called *cilia*. (Objective 8)

3. C. Sympathetic nervous system stimulation increases the heart's rate and force of contraction, increasing cardiac output. (Objective 44)

4. C. Parasympathetic stimulation of the heart causes a decrease in the rate of discharge of the SA node. (Objective 44)

5. A. The process that occurs when the cell membrane actively pumps sodium out of the cell and potassium into the cell is called *repolarization*. (Objective 55)

6. D. H⁺ concentration changes by a factor of 10 for each unit change in pH. pH is used to express hydrogen ion concentration. Normal pH for human blood is 7.35 to 7.45. A solution with a pH below 7 is acidic. (Objective 73)

7. C. During ventricular diastole the mitral and tricuspid valves are open as blood flows through them from the atria to the ventricles, and the ventricles fill. (Objective 52)

8. D. Bile is produced by the liver and stored in the gallbladder. (Objective 64)

9. A. The right and left nasal cavities are separated by the nasal septum. (Objective 60)

10. C. A pH of 7.70 and a PCO_2 of 20 indicate respiratory alkalosis. The pH is above 7.45, indicating an alkalosis. The decreased PCO_2 indicates the alkalosis is the result of hyperventilation, excessive carbon dioxide elimination. (Objective 73)

11. A. Movement of particles from an area of higher concentration to an area of lower concentration resulting in an even distribution is diffusion. Osmosis is a special case of diffusion that involves movement of solvent molecules across a semipermeable membrane from a less concentrated solution to a more concentrated solution. Active transport moves particles from an area of lower concentration to an area of higher concentration. (Objective 12)

12. D. Nose, nasal cavities, nasopharynx, oropharynx, laryngopharynx, larynx, trachea. (Objective 60)

13. B. The most numerous formed elements of blood are the erythrocytes. (Objective 49)

14. D. Water and carbon dioxide or bicarbonate and hydrogen ions (Objective 73)

15. D. A pH of 7.58 and a PCO_2 of 36 indicate metabolic alkalosis. The pH is above 7.45, indicating an alkalosis. The normal PCO_2 indicates that the alkalosis is of metabolic, rather than respiratory, origin. (Objective 73)

16. A. Carbon dioxide is transported in the body primarily as bicarbonate. (Objective 73)

17. A. The thyroid gland secretes calcitonin. Oxytocin and antidiuretic hormone are released from the posterior pituitary. Epinephrine is released from the adrenal glands. Norepinephrine is released from the neurons of the sympathetic nervous system. (Objective 46)

18. A. The islets of Langerhans secrete insulin from the beta cells, which decreases the blood glucose level. Glucagon, secreted from the alpha cells, raises the blood glucose level. (Objective 46)

19. C. The major electrolytes that influence cardiac function are potassium, sodium, and calcium. (Objective 55)

20. D. The abdominal cavity extends from the diaphragm to the pelvic bones. (Objective 7)

21. B. The semilunar valves of the heart are the aortic and pulmonic valves. (Objective 52)

22. C. A person in the anatomic position would be standing erect, facing forward, palms and feet facing forward. (Objective 4)

23. A. The part of a neuron that carries impulses away from the cell body is the axon. Dendrites carry impulses toward cell bodies. The myelin sheath insulates the axon and helps increase the speed of impulse conduction. (Objective 18)

24. C. This patient's PCO_2 should be higher than normal, and her pH should be lower than normal, resulting in an acid-base disorder called *respiratory acidosis*. (Objective 73)

25. B. Capillaries are thin-walled vessels that permit flow of glucose, oxygen, carbon dioxide, and other substance through their walls. The resistance vessels of the cardiovascular system are the arterioles. (Objective 56)

26. B. Acid-base balance is the regulation of hydrogen ion concentration in body fluids. (Objective 73)

27. C. Tidal volume is the amount of gas inhaled or exhaled during a normal breath. (Objective 63)

28. A. The meningeal layer that lies closest to the brain's surface is the pia mater. (Objective 35)

29. D. Blood pressure is influenced by cardiac output and peripheral vascular resistance. Stroke volume and heart rate influence cardiac output. (Objective 56)

30. B. The principal intracellular cation is potassium. (Objective 73)

31. A. The principal extracellular cation is sodium. (Objective 73)

32. D. The coronary arteries fill during ventricular diastole. (Objective 54)

33. C. The point at which the trachea divides into the right and left mainstem bronchi is the carina. (Objective 62)

34. D. The thickest part of the myocardium is located in the left ventricle. (Objective 52)

35. D. Substances whose molecules dissociate into electrically charged components when placed in water are called *electrolytes*. (Objective 73)

36. D. The outer boundary of the human cell is formed by the plasma membrane. The nucleus, cytoplasm, and organelles are located within the plasma membrane. (Objective 10)

37. A. Nervous tissue can conduct electrical signals called action potentials. (Objective 44)

38. A. The lungs are covered by a smooth, moist epithelial layer called the visceral pleura. The parietal pleura lies against the chest wall. The peritoneum lines the abdominal cavity. (Objectives 59, 63)

39. D. The three main components of a nerve cell are the axon, dendrite, and cell body. (Objective 34)

40. C. Epinephrine is used in some patients with respiratory distress primarily to relax bronchial smooth muscle. (Objective 44)

41. C. Effects of alpha$_1$-adrenergic receptor stimulation include peripheral vasoconstriction. (Objective 44)

42. B. The atrioventricular valves of the heart are the mitral and tricuspid. (Objective 52)

43. A. The heart is enclosed in a fibrous sac called the *pericardium*. (Objective 50)

44. D. Insulin lowers blood glucose levels by increasing glucose transport into the cells. (Objective 46)

45. A. Minute volume is the amount of gas moved in and out of the respiratory system per minute. (Objective 63)

46. D. The larynx is anterior to the esophagus. (Objectives 62, 64, 65)

47. C. Cardiac output is equal to heart rate × stroke volume. (Objective 50)

48. D. A pH of 7.55 and a PCO$_2$ of 40 indicate a metabolic alkalosis. Because the pH is above 7.45, the patient is alkalotic. The normal pH indicates the alkalosis is of metabolic rather than respiratory origin. (Objective 73)

49. B. The vessels that empty into the right atrium are the superior vena cava, the inferior vena cava, and the coronary sinus. (Objective 53)

50. C. The thin strands of fibrous tissue connecting the AV valves to the papillary muscles are the chordae tendineae. (Objective 52)

51. B. When the heart rate increases, ventricular filling time decreases, resulting in decreased stroke volume. (Objective 50)

52. B. A pH of 7.30 and a PCO$_2$ of 50 indicate respiratory acidosis. The pH below 7.35 indicates an acidosis. The pH above 45 indicates the acidosis is of respiratory origin. (Objective 73)

53. B. The junction between two neurons is called a *synapse*. (Objective 16)

54. C. Afterload is the resistance against which the left ventricle must eject blood volume. (Objective 50)

55. C. The sinoatrial (SA) node normally depolarizes at a rate of 60 to 100 per minute. (Objective 55)

56. C. The part of the brain responsible for balance and coordination is the cerebellum. (Objective 40)

57. B. The pharynx serves as a passageway for both the respiratory and digestive systems. (Objectives 59, 65)

58. D. If the respiratory rate is 12 breaths per minute and the tidal volume is 800 mL per breath, the minute volume is 9600 mL (800 × 12). (Objective 63)

59. B. The lymphatic system consists of lymph nodes, lymph vessels, and the thymus, spleen, and tonsils. (Objective 58)

60. B. The ability of cardiac cells to spontaneously depolarize is automaticity. (Objective 55)

61. A. The cerebrum is the largest part of the brain. Respiration, heart rate, and blood pressure are controlled by the brainstem, which includes the midbrain, pons, and medulla. The cerebellum controls posture and balance. (Objective 39)

62. D. During expiration the diaphragm and intercostal muscles relax, reducing the thoracic cavity's volume. (Objective 60)

63. C. The only complete cartilaginous ring in the larynx is the cricoid cartilage. (Objective 61)

64. C. The process that occurs when an electrical stimulus causes sodium to rush into a resting cell is called *depolarization*. (Objectives 33, 55)

65. B. A pH of 7.26 and a PCO$_2$ of 40 reflect metabolic acidosis. The pH below 7.35 indicates acidosis. The normal PCO$_2$ indicates the acidosis is of metabolic, rather than respiratory, origin. (Objective 7)

66. A. The primary neurotransmitter of the parasympathetic nervous system is acetylcholine. (Objective 34)

67. A. A type of extracellular fluid located outside the vascular bed and between the cells of the body is called interstitial fluid. (Objective 8)

68. D. The digestive organs are surrounded by a connective tissue membrane called the *peritoneum*. The pericardium surrounds the heart. The pleura surrounds the lungs. The perineum is the area between the anus and the external genitalia. (Objective 64)

69. A. The brainstem connects the spinal cord to the remainder of the brain. Personality, judgment, thought logic, visual reception, and visual association are located in the cerebrum. (Objective 39)

70. D. The medulla oblongata's functions include regulation of heart rate and blood vessel diameter. (Objective 37)

71. B. When the right ventricle contracts, blood is pumped into the pulmonary arteries. (Objective 53)

72. A. Effects of beta$_2$-adrenergic receptor stimulation include bronchial smooth muscle relaxation. (Objective 44)

73. B. Total body water composes approximately 60% of body weight in adults. It is divided into two fluid-containing compartments: intracellular fluid and extracellular fluid. (Objective 73)

74. D. The primary neurotransmitter of the sympathetic nervous system is norepinephrine. (Objective 44)

75. C. Cardiac output is the amount of blood expelled by the ventricles per minute. (Objective 50)

76. B. Alveoli contain thin epithelial linings and dense capillary networks, and are responsible for oxygen and carbon dioxide exchange. (Objective 62)

77. C. Neutrophils surround and digest infectious organisms. (Objective 49)

78. A. Components of the integumentary system include the skin, nails, hair, sweat, and oil glands. (Objective 18)

79. B. Blood contains three formed elements. These are the platelets, leukocytes, and erythrocytes. (Objective 49)

80. D. Cortisol is secreted by the adrenal cortex. (Objective 46)

81. A. Norepinephrine is an alpha-adrenergic receptor stimulator. (Objective 46)

82. D. The portion of the action potential in which a stronger than normal electrical stimulus is needed to cause the cardiac cells to respond is called the relative refractory period. (Objective 55)

83. B. The movement of water through a semipermeable membrane from a solution that has a lower solute concentration to one that has a higher solute concentration is osmosis. (Objective 73)

84. A. Inspiratory reserve volume is the amount of additional air that can be inhaled at the end of a normal inhalation. (Objective 63)

85. A. The thoracic and abdominal cavities are separated by the diaphragm. (Objective 7)

86. B. Thrombocytes (platelets) participate in blood clotting and help to seal leaks in injured blood vessels. (Objective 49)

87. B. Conditions that reduce alveolar ventilation can cause respiratory acidosis. (Objective 73)

88. B. The ability of cardiac cells to propagate an impulse from cell to cell is called conductivity. (Objectives 15, 55)

89. D. The sinoatrial (SA) node is located at the junction of the superior vena cava and the right atrium. (Objective 55)

90. A. An ion with a negative charge is an anion. (Objective 73)

91. A. Plasma is made up of water and dissolved molecules such as electrolytes and proteins (i.e. albumin, globulins, and fibrinogen). (Objective 49)

92. D. The trachea has a ciliated inner lining. (Objective 62)

93. C. Osmotic pressure is the force that causes water to move from an area of low particle concentration to an area of higher concentration. (Objective 73)

94. A. The right atrium and right ventricle make up a low-pressure pump whose purpose is to pump blood to the pulmonary circulation. (Objective 52)

95. C. The spinal cord passes through the vertebral foramen. (Objective 41)

96. D. Surfactant prevents the collapse of the alveoli when there is little or no air in them. (Objective 62)

97. C. The most inferior cartilage of the larynx is the cricoid cartilage. (Objective 60)

98. B. The middle layer of an artery is the tunica media. (Objective 57)

99. B. The inner membranous surface of the heart wall that lines the heart valves and chambers is called the endocardium. (Objective 52)

100. D. Increased heart rate is an effect of beta$_1$-adrenergic receptor stimulation. (Objective 44)

101. A. A solution with the same solute concentration as normal extracellular fluid is isotonic. (Objective 73)

102. D. The vagus nerve (cranial nerve X) is responsible for slowing the heart rate and accelerating peristalsis. (Objective 43)

103. D. The trachea, bronchi, bronchioles, and alveoli are found in the lower airway. (Objective 59)

104. D. During inspiration the diaphragm contracts and the intercostal muscles contract. (Objective 62)

105. A. The sinoatrial (SA) node normally is the dominant pacemaker of the heart. (Objective 55)

106. B. The corpus callosum connects the right and left cerebral hemispheres. (Objective 39)

107. C. Ca^{++} influx causes the "plateau" phase of the cardiac cycle. (Objective 58)

108. C. A hypertonic solution will cause water to move from the cells and interstitial space into the vascular space. (Objective 73)

109. A. The right mainstem bronchus is shorter and straighter than the left. (Objective 62)

110. B. The buffer system responds most rapidly to changes in pH. (Objective 73)

111. B. The normal arterial CO$_2$ pressure (PaCO$_2$) is 35 to 45 mm Hg. (Objective 73)

112. A. The Frank-Starling law states that when cardiac muscle is stretched, it contracts with greater force. (Objective 50)

113. C. A membrane that allows certain substances to pass from one side to another but does not allow others to pass is semipermeable. (Objective 8)

114. C. The lymphatic system includes the spleen. (Objective 58)

115. C. Building up and breaking down of biochemical substances collectively is called metabolism. Anabolism is the constructive phase of metabolism. Catabolism is metabolism's destructive phase. (Objective 8)

116. A. A process that works to reverse, or to compensate for, a physiologic change is called a negative feedback loop. A positive feedback loop amplifies the effect of a change. Homeostasis is the ability of an organism to maintain a stable internal environment. Hemostasis is the process of controlling bleeding. (Objective 46)

117. A. The constructive phase of metabolism is anabolism. (Objective 8)

118. A. Approximately 75% of all body water is intracellular. (Objective 12)

CHAPTER 8: PATHOPHYSIOLOGY

Matching

1. __A__ Negatively charged ions
   __B__ Positively charged ions
   __C__ Substances forming ions in water
   __F__ Water inside blood vessels
   __E__ Water contained inside cells
   __D__ Water outside the cells (Objective 5)

2. __B__ Hypertonic solution

   __A__ Hypotonic solution

   __C__ Isotonic solution (Objective 5)

3. __B__ 23 y.o. h/o vomiting & diarrhea × 4 days; BP—98/76 mm Hg, P—120 beats/min, R—22 breaths/min

   __D__ 27 y.o. c/o abdominal pain following an incomplete abortion 3 days ago; skin—warm, flushed, BP—96/56 mm Hg, P—136 beats/min, R—26 breaths/min shallow

   __C__ 30 y.o. c/o loss of lower extremity motor function following an MVC; BP—96/40 mm Hg, P—72 beats/min, R—24 breaths/min shallow

   __A__ 77 y.o. c/o substernal chest pain and short of breath; BP—70/56 mm Hg, P—130 beats/min irregular, R—36 breaths/min (Objective 12)

4. __C__ Caseous necrosis

   __A__ Coagulative necrosis

   __B__ Fatty necrosis

   __D__ Liquefactive necrosis (Objective 4)

Short Answer

1. Hypertrophy occurs when a tissue increases the size of its cells. Hyperplasia occurs when a tissue increases the number of cells in it. (Objective 1)

2. Hypoxia. (Objective 2)

3. Caseous. (Objective 4)

4. The affected cells become liquefied. This is also commonly referred to as "wet gangrene". (Objective 4)

5. Albumin changes from a gelatinous form to a firm, opaque substance. This is commonly referred to as "dry gangrene". (Objective 4)

6. Osmosis is movement of water across a semipermeable membrane from a less concentrated solution to a more concentrated solution. (Objective 5)

7. Potassium. (Objective 5)

8. Sodium. (Objective 5)

9. (1) Carbonic acid – bicarbonate buffering; (2) Protein buffering; (3) Renal buffering. (Objective 5)

10. An increase in hydrogen ion concentration will cause acidosis, represented by a decrease in the pH. (Objective 5)

11. A decrease in hydrogen ion concentration will cause alkalosis, represented by an increase in the pH. (Objective 5).

12. 7.35 to 7.45 (Objective 5)

13. They will develop tissue edema. (Objective 5)

14. The pH of a patient who is hyperventilating will rise, and the patient will develop a respiratory alkalosis. (Objective 5)

15. A diabetic patient who has not taken insulin for several days will have a decrease in pH. (Objective 5)

16. Metabolic acidosis. (Objective 5)

17. The pH of a patient who is hypoventilating will decrease. (Objective 5)

18. Respiratory acidosis. (Objective 5)

19. Excess bicarbonate administration will cause an increase in pH and will develop a metabolic alkalosis. (Objective 5)

20. Isotonic solution should be used if a patient is in hypovolemic shock. An isotonic solution will remain in the vascular space, increasing circulating blood volume. (Objectives 5, 11, 12)

21. An isotonic solution should be used if a patient is in neurogenic shock. In neurogenic shock, the vascular space has dilated. Because the blood volume cannot fill the enlarged vascular space, hypoperfusion results. Because an isotonic fluid will remain in the vascular space, it can be used to fill the dilated blood vessels and restore adequate perfusion. (Objectives 5, 11, 12)

22. Shock is a state of inadequate perfusion resulting in tissue hypoxia and anaerobic metabolism. (Objective 11)

23. (1) Adequate amount of hemoglobin. (2) Sufficient cardiac output. (3) Ability of the pulmonary system to load hemoglobin with oxygen and the ability of the tissues to offload oxygen. (Objective 11)

24. Hypoperfusion results in the cessation of aerobic metabolism, and the dependence on glycolysis. This not only results in a decrease in the amount of ATP produced, but also leads to metabolic acidosis. (Objective 11)

25. Lactic acid is the primary product of anaerobic glycolysis. As described in chapter 7 ATP is also produced yielding a net gain of 2 ATP molecules. (Objective 11)

26. When the kidney is hypoperfused it releases renin. Renin acts on angiotensinogen I, a protein produced by the liver, to convert it to angiotensin I. Angiotensin I is acted on by the angiotensin-converting enzyme (ACE), which is produced in the lungs, and converted to angiotensin II. Angiotensin II is a potent vasoconstrictor, which increases peripheral resistance and blood pressure. Angiotensin II also stimulates aldosterone release by the adrenal cortex. Increased aldosterone levels cause the kidney to recover an increased amount of sodium and water, which also raises blood pressure. (Objective 11)

27. An ACE inhibitor blocks formation of angiotensin II. Lower levels of angiotensin II will cause a drop in systemic resistance, which will lower blood pressure. Decreased angiotensin II levels also will cause a decrease in aldosterone release from the adrenal cortex, leading to increased urine output, a drop in intravascular volume, and a fall in blood pressure. (Objective 11)

28. Because angiotensin II is a vasoconstrictor, blocking its effects will cause a decrease in systemic vascular resistance and a fall in blood pressure. (Objective 11)

29. Because shock is failure of the circulatory system to deliver enough oxygen to the tissues to prevent anaerobic metabolism, the most important drug in the management of shock is oxygen. (Objective 11)

30. In neurogenic shock, injury to the spinal cord interrupts the output of the sympathetic nervous system, which arises from the thoracic and lumber segments of the spinal cord. Loss of sympathetic tone causes vasodilation and a decrease in systemic vascular resistance. Decreased systemic resistance leads to a drop in blood pressure and to hypoperfusion. (Objective 12)

31. Activation of the sympathetic nervous system causes sweating and an increased heart rate. In neurogenic shock, sympathetic tone is decreased by an injury to the spinal cord. Therefore patients in neurogenic shock do not exhibit diaphoresis or tachycardia. (Objective 12)

32. Anaphylactic shock is caused by release of histamine. Histamine produces peripheral vasodilation and increases capillary permeability, resulting in loss of fluid into the interstitial space. An isotonic fluid will remain in the vascular space, helping to fill the dilated vessels and replace the fluid lost into the interstitial spaces. (Objectives 5, 12)

33. Rapid infusion of fluid into a patient with inadequate cardiac function can result in a buildup of fluid in the pulmonary circulation, pulmonary edema, and respiratory failure. (Objectives 5, 12)

34. Hypoperfusion can damage the filtering tubules of the kidney, causing acute tubular necrosis and renal failure. (Objective 11)

35. Hypoperfusion can damage the hepatocytes, the liver's working cells, causing hepatic failure. (Objective 11)

36. Disseminated intravascular coagulation is a state of impaired blood clotting that results from widespread clot formation. Formation of large numbers of blood clots can deplete the body's stores of clotting factors. In addition, as clots break down, they release split fibrin products into the bloodstream, interfering with further clotting. Prolonged hypoperfusion can lead to DIC by producing diffuse tissue damage that triggers widespread formation of clots. (Objective 11)

37. Histamine. (Objective 12)

38. Histamine causes vasodilation, increased capillary permeability, and spasms of the bronchioles and GI tract. (Objective 12)

39. Epinephrine, diphenhydramine, Solu-Medrol. (Objective 12)

40. Inflammation is a general response to tissue injury. Immunity involves a response to a specific pathogen. (Objectives 14, 18)

41. Pathogens include bacteria, viruses, fungi, protozoa, parasites, prions. (Objective 3)

42. Redness, swelling, pain, and warmth of the affected area. (Objective 22)

43. The helper T-cell coordinates the activities of the immune system's other components. (Objective 14)

44. Macrophages ingest pathogens and then present the surface antigens from the pathogens to the helper T-cell to assist the immune system in recognizing and responding to the pathogen. (Objective 14)

45. Systemic lupus erythematosis is an autoimmune disease in which the body generates an antibody specific to its own nucleic acid. This antibody then causes widespread damage to the patient's tissues. (Objective 26)

46. The B-lymphocyte manufactures antibodies against specific pathogens. (Objective 14)

47. Killer T-cells directly attack and destroy cells that bear foreign antigens. (Objective 14)

48. Specialization of B-cell precursors takes place through the processes of clonal diversity and clonal selection. As the precursors of B-cells develop in the bone marrow, various strains (clones) of these precursors develop receptors for specific antigens. Eventually a clone exists with receptors for every possible type of antigen. When this antigen is encountered, the clone with receptors specific for it is activated and matures into lymphocytes capable of producing antibodies specific to that antigen. (Objective 14)

49. T-cells develop in the thymus. (Objective 14)

50. Type 1 diabetes develops when an antibody generated by the patient's immune system attacks and destroys the islets of Langerhans, leaving the patient unable to produce insulin. (Objective 26)

51. Most allergic reactions are produced by IgE. (Objective 25)

52. Acquired immunity develops either from generation of antibodies following exposure to an antigen or from transfer of antibodies from an outside source. (Objective 15)

53. In active immunity antibodies are produced as a result of exposure of the immune system to an antigen. In passive immunity, antibodies from some other source are transferred to the patient. (Objective 15)

54. A cytokine is a protein released in response to an immune stimulus that alters the function of cells.

55. IgM is the first antibody produced during the immune response. (Objective 15)

Multiple Choice

1. A. A decrease in cell size resulting from a decreased workload is called atrophy. (Objective 1)

2. C. An increase in the number of cells resulting from an increased workload is known as hyperplasia. (Objective 1)

3. D. Tissues such as skeletal muscle or the myocardium that cannot increase in number in response to an increased workload will undergo hypertrophy, or an increase in size.

4. C. The most common cause of cellular injury is hypoxia. (Objective 2)

5. C. *Necrosis* means cell death. Apoptosis is the process by which an injured cell destroys itself. (Objective 2).

6. D. The most prevalent extracellular cation is sodium. (Objective 5)

7. A. The principal buffer of the body is bicarbonate. (Objective 5)

8. D. The difference in concentration between solutions on opposite sides of a semipermeable membrane is called the osmotic gradient. (Objective 5)

9. B. When a solution on one side of a semipermeable membrane is hypotonic, it has a lesser concentration of solute molecules. (Objective 5)

10. D. The pressure exerted by the concentration of solutes on one side of a membrane that, if hypertonic, tends to "pull" water from the other side of the membrane is called osmotic pressure. (Objective 5)

11. A. The total amount of water lost from blood plasma across the capillary membrane into the interstitial space is called net filtration. (Objective 5)

12. B. Edema is caused by imbalance between hydrostatic and oncotic pressures. (Objective 5)

13. C. Ringer's lactate is an isotonic solution. (Objective 5)

14. A. A high concentration of hydrogen ions is known as acidosis. (Objective 5)

15. D. The fastest mechanism the body has for removing hydrogen ions is the bicarbonate buffer system. (Objective 5)

16. C. Impaired ventilation is the cause of respiratory acidosis. Impaired ventilation leads to a buildup of carbon dioxide in the bloodstream, causing a rise in carbonic acid levels and a fall in the pH. (Objective 5)

17. A. Vomiting, diarrhea, or diabetes can cause metabolic acidosis. Volume loss from vomiting and diarrhea can lead to hypovolemia, which can produce hypoperfusion and lactic acidosis. Untreated diabetes can result in a state of ketoacidosis and the body uses fat as an alternative metabolic fuel. (Objective 5)

18. B. As $[H^+]$ increases, pH decreases. (Objective 5)

19. C. pH is the negative logarithm of $[H^+]$. (Objective 5)

20. C. Normal pH is 7.40. (Objective 5)

21. B. Normal pCO_2 is 35 to 45 mm Hg. (Objective 5)

22. C. A pH of 7.00, a PCO_2 of 60, and a HCO_3^- of 24 indicates an acute respiratory acidosis. The pH is less than 7.35 indicating an acidotic state, the increased PCO_2 and normal HCO_3^- indicates this is an acute situation resulting from carbon dioxide retention." (Objective 5)

23. D. A pH of 7.50, a PCO_2 of 20, and a HCO_3^- of 26 indicates respiratory alkalosis. The pH is above 7.45 indicating an alkalosis, the PCO_2 is less than 35 and the HCO_3^- is normal indicating the alkalosis was caused by acute excessive elimination of carbon dioxide through the respiratory system. (Objective 5)

24. A. Given a pH of 7.20 and a PCO_2 of 40, you would suspect metabolic acidosis. The pH is below 7.35, indicating an acidosis. The normal carbon dioxide levels indicate that the acidosis does not have a respiratory cause. (Objective 5)

25. B. Given a pH of 7.50 and a PCO_2 of 60, you would suspect metabolic alkalosis. The pH is above 7.45, indicating an alkalosis. Because the carbon dioxide levels are elevated, excess elimination of carbon dioxide through the respiratory system is not causing the alkalosis. Therefore it must be metabolic in origin. (Objective 5)

26. D. Hemophilia is a clotting factor deficiency caused by an X-linked recessive gene. (Objective 6)

27. D. When blood $[H^+]$ is above normal, the respiratory center responds by increasing rate and increasing tidal volume. This increases the amount of carbon dioxide removed from the body per minute, helping to decrease the amount of hydrogen ion present. (Objective 5)

28. D. When baroreceptors detect a drop in blood pressure, the sympathetic nervous system releases norepinephrine. (Objective 11)

29. D. Inadequate tissue perfusion causes cells to produce lactic acid and pyruvic acid. (Objective 12)

30. D. Hemoglobin levels, cardiac output, and the ability of the pulmonary system to load the hemoglobin with oxygen and the ability of the tissue to offload oxygen all effect tissue perfusion. (Objective 11)

31. A. Anaerobic metabolism is 18 times less efficient than aerobic metabolism. (Objective 11)

32. B. Aldosterone acts on the kidneys to conserve sodium and water. (Objective 5)

33. C. Angiotensin II produces vasoconstriction and decreased rate of urine production. (Objective 5)

34. C. Disseminated intravascular coagulation initially begins with uncontrolled, widespread clot formation. (Objective 11)

35. B. The primary cause of anaphylaxis is the release of histamine. (Objective 12)

36. C. Pallor, diaphoresis, and tachycardia are absent in neurogenic shock as norepinephrine is not released because of decreased sympathetic tone. (Objectives 11, 14)

37. A. Protection from infection or disease that is developed by the body after exposure to an antigen is called acquired immunity. (Objective 14)

38. C. The type of leukocyte responsible for recognizing foreign antigens, producing antibodies, and developing memory is the lymphocyte. (Objective 14)

39. B. The type of leukocyte that does not produce antibodies but directly attacks antigens is the T_C cell, also called cytotoxic T-cells or "killer" T-cells. (Objective 14)

40. D. A universal donor has type O blood. Because type O erythrocytes do not carry either A or B antigens, they are not attacked by the antibodies present in the plasma of patient with blood types A or B. Persons with type AB blood do not have antibodies to either A or B antigens in their plasma. Therefore they are universal recipients. (Objective 15)

41. D. The development by B-cell precursors in the bone marrow of receptors that allow for the development of millions of single antigen responses from only several hundred to a few thousand genes is called clonal selection. (Objective 14)

42. D. The first antibody produced during the primary immune response is IgM. (Objective 15)

43. C. The cells that transfer delayed hypersensitivity and secrete proteins that activate other cells are called T_H cells, or "helper" T-cells. (Objective 14)

44. B. Proteins produced by white blood cells, known as the "messengers" of the immune response, are cytokines. (Objective 15)

45. B. The organ responsible for T-cell development is the thymus. (Objective 14)

46. D. One of the functions of the inflammatory response is walling off an infected area. Responses to specific antigens is a function of the immune response. (Objective 22)

CHAPTER 9: LIFE SPAN DEVELOPMENT

Matching

1 __B__ Become assertive, take initiative, and assert their independence

   __A__ Develop a unique personality and a strong set of likes and dislikes

   __C__ Master environment through information; develop self-discipline; self-esteem issues may develop; begin to develop morals

   __D__ Seeking self-determination; fragile self-esteem; very acute body image; establishes identity and autonomy (Objectives 1, 2)

2. __A__ Fanning of the toes outward when the sole of the foot is stroked

   __B__ Flinging of the arms up and out in response to being startled

   __C__ Grasping when an object is placed in the hand

   __E__ Lifting one foot after another when the feet are held flat on a surface

   __D__ Turning of the head toward anything that brushes the face (Objectives 1, 2)

Short Answer

1. At the end of the first year of life, children typically triple their birth weight of 3 to 3.5 kilograms. Therefore a normal 1-year-old child weighs approximately 10 kilograms (22 pounds). (Objective 1)

2. If an infant or small child is placed in a supine position, their neck will tend to flex, causing obstruction of the airway. This happens because the anterior-posterior diameter of an infant or small child's head is greater than the anterior-posterior diameter of the torso. This problem can be prevented by padding under the torso to bring it into alignment with the head and neck. (Objective 1)

3. The fontanels are soft spots in the skull that allow for compression during delivery and for rapid growth of the brain during early life. The anterior fontanel closes at 9 to 18 months after birth. Dehydration will cause the anterior *fontanel* to appear sunken. Increased intracranial pressure from cerebral edema, intracranial bleeding, or meningitis will cause the anterior fontanel to bulge. (Objective 1)

4. Infants are much more dependent on movement of the diaphragm for adequate ventilation than are older children or adults. Pressure by a distended stomach under an infant's diaphragm can seriously impair the ability to exchange air. (Objective 1)

5. Older infants and toddlers have more contact with other people, particularly other infants and small children, than younger infants. Therefore they have more exposures to potentially infectious pathogens. However, infants in the first 3 to 6 months of life have an immature immunologic system and are more susceptible than an older infant or child to severe infections and infections by unusual organisms. The infant's immune system is essentially limited to passive immunity, based on maternal antibodies, through the first 6 months of life.

6. An infant older than approximately 9 months is likely to become very anxious if taken from his or her caregivers. (Objective 1)

7. Older infants should be examined in their parent's arms or on their parent's laps. If time allows, the paramedic should play with the infant for a few minutes to build rapport. The examination should be performed from toe to head to avoid frightening the child. More invasive portions of the examination should be performed last. (Objectives 1, 2)

8. You should attempt to gain as much information as possible by observing the child from a distance and taking a history before making contact with the child. Consider examining infants and toddlers in their parent's arms or with them seated in the parent's lap. You should spend a few minutes playing with the child after making contact, allowing them to become used to your presence. With children younger than school age, the physical examination should be performed in a toe to head direction so you are touching the head and face last. The most invasive portions of the examination should be saved until last. Some procedures such as listening to the heart and lungs can be performed on a parent first to demonstrate that they are not painful. Equipment such as a stethoscope can be introduced initially by touching it to the child's hand, foot, elbow, or knee and then moving it to the torso. Based on the history, determine the portions of the physical examination that must be performed to help establish the field diagnosis, and limit the examination to these procedures. (Objectives 1, 2)

9. The pulse and respiratory rates of pediatric patients normally are faster than those of adults. (Objective 1)

10. A typical toddler will respond to an attempt to examine them by crying, becoming uncooperative, and fighting. (Objective 2)

11. Try to obtain as much information as possible by observation before beginning the examination. Have a parent hold the child in his/her lap during the examination. Use the history to focus the examination on essential steps that must be performed to establish a field diagnosis. Set clear

305

expectations for the child's behavior—it is OK to cry but not to kick or bite. Perform the examination from toe to head, focusing on the steps essential to establishing a field diagnosis. Do not attempt to reason with a frightened toddler; just determine what needs to be done and complete it. (Objective 2)

12. The minimum acceptable blood pressure is (age of child × 2) + 70. So the minimum acceptable blood pressure for a 5-year-old child would be (5 × 2) + 70 = 80. (Objective 1)

13. Adolescents tend to be modest and are uncomfortable about being undressed in the presence of adults. (Objective 2)

14. Exposure of an adolescent during a physical examination should be kept to an absolute minimum. The patient's modesty and privacy should be protected at all times. Ideally, during the physical examination of an adolescent, a third party who is the same gender as the patient should be present. (Objective 2)

15. The weight of the kidneys decreases with age. Most of the reduction in weight is because of a loss of the renal cortex (which contains the glomeruli, Bowman's capsule, and 85% of the nephrons) rather than a loss of the renal medulla (where the tubules and collecting ducts are located). Atherosclerosis contributes to renal artery narrowing and decreased renal blood flow, which results in a decrease in the filtering ability of the kidneys (glomerular filtration rate). The renal tubules decrease in length and volume with age, reducing the ability to concentrate or dilute urine.

16. The terminal drop hypothesis of aging states that mental and physical functioning decline dramatically only during the few years immediately preceding death. (Objective 4)

Multiple Choice

1. C. The flat neck veins and clear lung fields decrease the probability that this patient's pedal edema is caused by heart failure or kidney failure. It is more probable that the edema is due to prolonged immobility and the dependent position of her feet. (Objective 4)

2. D. Treating pediatric patients is different from treating adults because children may have difficulty communicating their complaints and symptoms. Generally children are less trusting of strangers than adults. They also are more fearful of unusual situations such as being transported in an ambulance. (Objective 3)

3. C. When a pediatric patient is suffering from a problem that is *not* life-threatening, you should take more time to perform the examination and, if necessary, spend time letting the child get used to your presence. Children are not small adults. Their anatomy and physiology is different. A thorough examination frequently is necessary to identify subtle signs of injury or illness. However, the examination must be modified to accommodate differences in a child's perceptions and behavior. (Objective 2)

4. D. When treating a sick or injured child, you should use the parents to assist you when appropriate. Involving the parents in the child's care wins their trust and cooperation and helps gain the trust and cooperation of the child. (Objective 2)

5. A. The pulse rate of a pediatric patient is normally faster than that of an adult. (Objective 1)

6. B. The fontanel of an infant may be sunken if an infant is dehydrated. An increase in intracranial pressure will cause the fontanel to bulge. (Objective 1)

7. A. In children younger than school age, the detailed physical examination should be performed toe to head to avoid frightening the patient. (Objective 2)

8. D. When examining older infants and toddlers, you should leave the child on the parent's lap. Separating an infant or toddler from his/her parents will cause extreme distress. If the patient's condition allows, take your time with the examination and give the child time to adjust to your presence. (Objective 2)

9. A. The child's tongue is larger in relation to the other structures in the airway. Other differences in pediatric airway anatomy include a relatively larger head with a small mandible attached to a tongue that is larger and more posterior than an adult's tongue. The glottic opening of a child is higher than that of an adult. (Objective 1)

10. A. Generally, children 2 to 3 years old would be expected to be uncooperative. (Objective 1)

11. C. The ideal initial approach for assessment of the conscious, non–acutely ill child is to gain as much information as possible through history and observation before touching the child. (Objective 2)

12. D. When you are assessing or managing an older patient, you should use physical contact when necessary to compensate for loss of sight or hearing. Older adults who do not have hearing loss frequently are offended when younger persons speak louder than normal when addressing them. Elders also may be offended when younger persons do not address them with proper respect. Separating an older person from friends and family can produce anxiety and disorientation. (Objective 4)

13. B. Preschoolers usually are cooperative and like to help the paramedic. Toddlers typically are uncooperative and do not like to be touched. School-age children usually are more comfortable when they are told what is being done to them. Adolescents frequently have fragile self-esteem and are concerned about whether lasting effects of injury or illness will make them different from their peers. (Objective 2)

Case Study

1. The history should be taken from the patient in a private location away from the patient's mother if at all possible. A strategy for accomplishing this is to have your partner collect information from the mother such as the family's address, telephone number, preferred hospital, and insurance carrier while you are interviewing the patient. You should assure the patient that all information she gives you is confidential and will not be shared with her parents by you or any of the other healthcare providers who care for her. Because of the patient's complaint, you should ask her about the date of her last menstrual period, use of contraception, and the possibility of pregnancy. (Objectives 1, 2)

2. Adolescents are usually uncomfortable about being disrobed in the presence of adults. The physical examination should be limited to procedures necessary to confirm your field diagnosis based on the history. The patient's modesty should be protected at all times. Another female besides the patient should be present as a witness during the physical examination, even if the paramedic performing the examination is female. (Objectives 1, 2)

CHAPTER 10: PUBLIC HEALTH AND EMS

Matching

1. __B__ A state of complete physical, mental, and social well-being, not merely the absence of disease or infirmity (Objective 1)

   __D__ Comparison of number and nature of medical cases to expected number at a given time and place to identify disease outbreaks (Objective 4)

   __C__ Evaluating a population for presence or absence of disease (Objective 2)

   __A__ Study of prevalence and spread of disease in a community (Objective 4)

   __E__ The science and practice of protecting and improving a community's health (Objective 1)

Short Answer

1. Most healthcare professionals focus on the needs of individual patients or clients. Public health professionals focus on the overall health of populations and on interventions that affect the health and improve the quality of life of the public rather than individual patients. (Objective 1)

2. EMS stations are located in areas of ready community access; the use of vehicles by EMS allows access to widely dispersed populations; EMS has a positive public image that may encourage access by groups reluctant to use services provided by other private or governmental entities. (Objective 2)

3. Training needs, vaccine procurement, liability issues. (Objective 2)

4. Direct reimbursement by patients on a fee-for-service basis, reimbursement by third-party payers, including Medicare and Medicaid. (Objective 2)

5. No, because the concept of health used in public health addresses a physical, mental, and social well-being rather than merely absence of disease; "screening" should address risk factors and other determinants impacting health. (Objective 2)

6. Because EMS personnel treat patients in the community, they can observe the environments and social conditions that may be placing individuals or populations at risk. (Objective 2)

7. Cardiovascular disease, diabetes mellitus, domestic violence, alcohol abuse, depression. (Objective 2)

8. The teachable moment is a time period immediately following an acute event when patients and their families are most receptive to receiving and acting on information provided through health education. (Objective 2)

9. EMS personnel frequently deal with patients and family members in high-acuity events that produce a sense of distress and danger. During and after these events, EMS personnel are perceived as caregivers and protectors whose advice should be followed. (Objective 2)

10. Advocacy is education of policy makers and their staffs about relevant issues. (Objective 2)

11. Seat belt and child vehicle restraint laws, alcohol use, tobacco use, domestic violence, firearm safety. (Objective 2)

12. To be effective public health educators and advocates, EMS personnel must serve as models for the behaviors they seek to promote. Actions tend to speak much more loudly than words in the minds of the public. (Objective 2)

13. EMS traditionally has viewed emergency response as involving incidents that are intense, short-lived, and time-limited. Public health professionals tend to focus on much more prolonged events and have a longer-term view of preparednes. These different perspectives, as well as an independence from each other during day-to-day operations, can lead to conflicts between EMS and public health professionals during major incidents that can be overcome only through advance planning. (Objective 4)

14. Because the healthcare system operates with finite resources, failure to contain costs in one sector of the healthcare industry can reduce the resources available to other sectors. This, in turn, can adversely affect the ability of the entire healthcare system to deliver adequate services. Because the health of the community as a whole is the concern of public health, any problem that adversely impacts delivery of healthcare services becomes a public health issue. (Objective 5)

Multiple Choice

1. A. Activities impacting public health take place in a variety of agencies, including the U.S. Department of Agriculture and the Environmental Protection Agency. Although the U.S. Department of Health and Human Services is the lead federal agency for health-related issues and houses the Office of the Surgeon General, other agencies also have functions that impact public health. These include the Environmental Protection Agency, which is an independent agency of the executive branch of the federal government. (Objective 1)

2. A. Every state has a designated state health official. In some states the state health official is the executive head of the state health department. In other states the state health official is part of a larger agency that deals with a wide range of public health and human service issues. At the local level, public health functions are performed by county and municipal governments and, in some areas, by multijurisdictional public health districts. State and local laws, rules, and agreements determine the relationship between state and local public health agencies. (Objective 1)

3. C. EMS agencies doing public health screening are not legally obligated to develop systems for ensuring follow-up action. However, for screening by EMS personnel to work, patients must be given information on community resources and resource agencies must be notified of potential referrals. Although EMS personnel typically have the time to perform screening, studies have shown that they frequently lack the training to do so. (Objective 2)

4. A. An "all hazards" approach means that emergencies resulting from all hazards present in the community are managed from a single plan that provides common terminology and structure rather than several plans written to address specific problems such as floods or tornadoes. (Objective 4)

5. B. Isolation is seclusion of persons with an illness to prevent transmission; quarantine is seclusion of asymptomatic individuals exposed to a disease for monitoring. (Objective 4)

6. A. Studies have shown that mandating aggressive cost containment and revenue generation strategies can adversely affect the actions and attitudes of EMS personnel. Requiring that patients be billed for EMS services has been shown to decrease patient willingness to seek care, leading to negative outcomes. Triaging of callers by EMS dispatchers has not conclusively been demonstrated to be a safe or effective cost containment strategy. Actions to control costs by EMS organizations can have a significant effect on other parts of the healthcare system. (Objective 5)

7. B. In an emergency management model that groups agencies by emergency services functions (ESFs), EMS is most likely to function as part of the health and medical care ESF headed by the local health officer. (Objective 4)

8. B. Discussing child restraint devices with a 26-year-old female who was involved in a minor motor vehicle collision with her 2-year-old daughter in the vehicle. The mother's concern for her daughter's safety after having just been involved in a traffic collision will make her receptive to a message regarding child restraint devices. (Objective 3)

Case Studies

Case one

1. EMS personnel can institute isolation procedures to reduce transmission of syndrome X during field care and transport. EMS personnel can begin to screen the elderly and persons with obstructive pulmonary disease for vaccination against pneumococcal pneumonia and either provide vaccination services or make referrals to appropriate immunization clinics. EMS dispatch can initiate a symptomatic surveillance system to identify an increase in calls involving patients with symptoms resembling those of syndrome X. EMS personnel and the EMS communications center can notify public health authorities of probable contacts with patients suffering from syndrome X, so public health authorities can initiate appropriate epidemiologic investigations and direct isolation of contacts when necessary. EMS personnel, the EMS communications center, the public health department, and the local hospital council can identify procedures to ensure that syndrome X is not spread through interfacility transfer of patients. (Objective 4)

Case two

1. Transporting special healthcare patients from homes to shelters and back. Transporting patients from hospitals and nursing homes in the evacuation area to reception points. Moving supplies between shelters and within the community. Supplying medical gases to oxygen-dependent patients. Performing medical screening exams on evacuees. Providing personnel to serve in primary care roles as shelter medical staff. Using ambulances to conduct on-scene surveys of storm damage. (Objective 4)

CHAPTER 11: BASIC PRINCIPLES OF PHARMACOLOGY

Matching

1. __H__   A medication consisting of an extract in an alcohol solution

   __B__   A drug dissolved in water with sugar, flavorings, and alcohol added

   __E__   Drug mixed in a firm base that melts at body temperature

   __F__   Medication suspended in a liquid, such as an oral antibiotic

   __A__   Gelatin containers enclosing a dose of a drug

__C__ One liquid suspended in another; usually oil in water

__G__ Powdered drugs molded or compressed into disks

__D__ Volatile substance dissolved in alcohol (Objective 13)

2. __C__ A condition or situation in which a drug is not given

__F__ A condition that is a reason to give a drug

__H__ A predictable effect of a drug other than its therapeutic action

__K__ Decreased intensity of drug effect after several doses

__A__ Enhancement of one drug's effects by those of a related drug with similar effects

__G__ A prolongation or increase in the effect of a drug by another drug

__D__ Increased intensity of drug effect after several doses

__I__ Joint action of two drugs when combined exceeds the sum of their individual effects

__B__ Opposing action between drugs

__E__ Response to a drug that is peculiar to an individual

__J__ The beneficial effect of a drug (Objective 15)

3. __A__ Description of drug's exact molecular composition

__D__ Name given to drug by a specific manufacturer

__B__ Name given to drug by first manufacturer before approval by government

__C__ Name listed in the *United States Pharmacopoeia* (Objective 2)

4. __C__ Establishes drug effectiveness, safety; approves new drugs for use

__A__ Enforces controlled substances laws and monitors the need for changing schedules of abused drugs

__B__ Suppresses misleading drug advertising (Objective 6)

5. __C__ Authorized government to determine drug safety/effectiveness

__A__ Authorized "scheduling" of drugs based on use and abuse potential

__D__ Controlled import, manufacture, sale of opium, cocaine, derivatives; required physicians, pharmacists, and manufacturers to register with government

__E__ Required accurate labeling of products; established *United States Pharmacopoeia* as official information source

__B__ Required prescriptions for dangerous drugs; created over-the-counter medications (Objectives 5, 6, 8)

6. __G__ albuterol

__H__ diazepam

__B__ diphenhydramine

__A__ epinephrine

__D__ furosemide

__I__ lidocaine

__E__ naloxone

__F__ procainamide

__C__ propranolol (Objective 2)

Short Answer

1. A drug with an accepted medical use and high abuse potential would be a Schedule II drug. (Objective 7)

2. A drug with no accepted use and a high abuse potential would be a Schedule I drug. (Objective 7)

3. Insulin was originally obtained from animal sources, specifically porcine and bovine insulin was used in humans. Today insulin is produced synthetically.

4. Digitalis and morphine are obtained from plant sources. (Objective 3)

5. Calcium, sodium bicarbonate, and magnesium are obtained from mineral sources. (Objective 3)

6. Drugs that are chemically developed in a laboratory are called *synthetic drugs*. Synthetic drugs are free of the impurities found in natural substances. Insulin is an example of a synthetic drug. (Objective 3)

7. Because the liver is responsible for deactivating drugs by metabolizing them, a patient with liver disease probably would have a prolonged duration of drug effects. (Objectives 10, 11, 17, 18)

8. Because the kidneys excrete drugs from the body, a patient with renal disease probably would have a prolonged duration of drug effects. (Objectives 10, 11, 17, 18)

9. An antagonist is a drug that interferes with or blocks the effects of another drug. (Objective 12)

10. Tolerance is present when a patient requires increasing doses of a drug to produce the same effect. (Objectives 15, 17)

11. Predictable effects of a drug other than its therapeutic effect are called *side effects*. (Objectives 12, 17)

12. Absorption, distribution, metabolism, and excretion. (Objectives 16, 17)

13. During facilitated transport, molecules move across a cell membrane from an area of higher concentration to an area of lower concentration with the assistance of a carrier protein that provides a pathway through the membrane. Facilitated transport does not require energy to be expended because molecules are being moved down a concentration gradient. (Objectives 16, 17)

14. During active transport, molecules move across a cell membrane from an area of lower concentration to an area of higher concentration through the action of a transporter protein. Active transport requires energy to be expended because molecules are being moved up a concentration gradient. (Objectives 16, 17)

15. *Diffusion* is a general term that describes the tendency of particles to move from an area of higher concentration to an area of lower concentration. Osmosis is a special case of diffusion in which water molecules move across a membrane permeable to

309

water (semipermeable membrane) from a less concentrated solution (less solute, more water) to a more concentrated solution (more solute, less water). (Objectives 16, 17)

Multiple Choice

1. D. A trade name is one of the four drug names. Another name for trade name is *proprietary name*. (Objective 2)
2. D. The four main sources for drugs include plants, minerals, and animals. (Objective 3)
3. C. For many years, the primary source of insulin was the extract of the porcine (pig) pancreas. (Objective 3)
4. C. The *Physicians' Desk Reference* is a commercially published compilation of information for more than 4000 medications including indications, interactions, mechanism of action, side effects, adverse effects, and other information. (Objective 5)
5. B. Name, classification, mechanism of action, and indications are examples of information found in a drug's profile. (Objective 21)
6. D. According to the Controlled Substances Act of 1970, a Schedule I drug has no accepted medical indications. Schedule I drugs also have high abuse potential. (Objective 7)
7. D. Drug legislation passed in the United States in 1906 to protect the public from adulterated or mislabeled drugs was the Pure Food and Drug Act. (Objective 9)
8. A. An assay determines the amount and purity of a given chemical in a pharmaceutical preparation. (Objective 8)
9. B. The process by which a drug is absorbed, distributed, metabolized, and eliminated is called pharmacokinetics. This may also be referred to as the path by which a medication gets to its target organs.
10. D. A medication that may deform or kill a fetus is called a *teratogenic drug*. A category A drug is an agent for which adequate studies in pregnant women have not demonstrated a risk to the fetus in the first or later trimesters. (Objectives 10, 12, 17, 18)
11. B. A drug's mechanism of action is described by its pharmacodynamics. (Objectives 16, 17)
12. B. The liver's partial or complete breakdown of a drug before it reaches the systemic circulation is called the *first-pass effect*. (Objectives 16, 17)
13. B. An example of a barrier that hampers the distribution of some medications is the blood-brain barrier. (Objectives 16, 17)
14. D. A liquid form of a drug prepared using an alcohol extraction process is called a *tincture*. (Objective 13)
15. A. The force of attraction between a drug and a receptor is affinity for the receptor. (Objectives 11, 12, 16, 17)
16. B. An agonist is a drug that binds to a receptor and causes a physiologic response. (Objectives 11, 12, 15, 16, 17)
17. B. Tolerance for other opioid agents acquired as a result of developing tolerance for morphine is cross-tolerance. (Objectives 11, 12)
18. D. An antagonist agent binds to a receptor but does not elicit a response. By blocking the receptor, the antagonist also prevents an agonist from binding to the site and producing a response. (Objectives 11, 12, 15, 16, 17)
19. B. The "lock and key" and "induced fit" analogies of drug action describe drugs that are specific to a certain receptor morphology. (Objective 11)

CHAPTER 12: DRUG AND CHEMICAL CLASSES

Matching

1. __D__ Alpha with some beta effects
   __F__ Beta-blocker
   __B__ Beta with some alpha effects
   __A__ Parasympathetic blocker
   __E__ Pure alpha
   __C__ Pure beta (Objective 17)

Short Answer

1. Class I: Sodium channel blockers
   Class Ia—procainamide
   Class Ib—lidocaine
   Class Ic—flecainide
   Class II: Beta-blockers—propranolol
   Class III: Potassium channel blockers—amiodarone
   Class IV: Calcium channel blockers—verapamil
   Miscellaneous: Adenosine, digoxin
   (Objective 18)
2. ACE inhibitors inhibit the conversion of angiotensin I to angiotensin II by the angiotensin-converting enzyme (ACE). Angiotensin is a potent vasoconstrictor that also promotes release of aldosterone from the adrenal cortex. Aldosterone promotes retention of sodium and water, increasing intravascular volume. The decrease in angiotensin II levels caused by an ACE inhibitor results in a decrease in peripheral resistance and an increase in loss of sodium and water through the kidneys, lowering blood pressure. (Objective 18)
3. Antihyperlipidemic agents are used to treat high blood cholesterol. (Objective 20)
4. Thrombolytic (fibrinolytic) agents are drugs that act directly on blood clots (thrombi) to break them down. (Objective 19)
5. Fast potentials occur in the cardiac muscle tissue and in the ventricular conducting system. (Objective 18)
6. Slow potentials occur in the pacemaker cells of the heart's SA and AV nodes. (Objective 18)
7. Administering a calcium channel blocker will decrease cardiac automaticity. (Objective 18)
8. Phase 0: sodium channels open, sodium enters cell. Phase 1: sodium channels close, potassium channels open, potassium leaves cells. Phase 2: calcium channels open, potassium channels remain open, calcium enters cell, potassium continues to leave cell. Phase 3: calcium channels close, potassium channels remain open, potassium leaves cell. Phase 4: sodium-potassium

pump restores normal distributions of sodium and potassium across cell membrane. (Objective 18)

9. **M**ad as a hatter, **R**ed as a beet, **D**ry as a bone, **H**ot as a hare (or **H**otter than hell), **B**lind as a bat. (Objective 16)

10. The brain and the spinal cord compose the central nervous system. (Objective 14)

11. Opioid agonist-antagonists relieve pain while having a minimal effect on respirations. (Objective 4)

12. Benzodiazepines and barbiturates are sedative-hypnotics. (Objective 11)

13. Methylphenidate is used to treat attention deficit–hyperactivity disorder. (Objective 14)

14. Diphenhydramine may be given to treat these effects. (Objective 11)

15. Fluoxetine (Prozac), paroxetine (Paxil), sertrailne (Zoloft). (Objective 11)

16. Depression. (Objective 11)

17. Phenelzine (Nardil), tranylcypromine sulfate (Parnate), isocarboxazid (Marplan). (Objective 11)

18. Depression. (Objective 11)

19. MAOIs inhibit the action of monoamine oxidase, the enzyme that breaks down serotonin and norepinephrine. This effect increases the availability of serotonin and norepinephrine for release into the synapses of the central nervous system, relieving the symptoms of depression. (Objective 11)

20. Heart rate: Heart rate will decrease. GI tract gland secretions: GI tract gland secretions will increase. Pupils: Pupils will constrict. Lower airway muscle tone: Muscle tone in the lower airway will increase, resulting in slight bronchospasm. (Objective 16)

21. Nicotinic and muscarinic. (Objective 16)

22. Muscarinic receptor sites are found on structures innervated by the parasympathetic nervous system. Nicotinic receptors are found on skeletal muscle. These are the nicotinic-M receptors. Another type of nicotinic receptor, the nicotinic-N receptor, is found in all of the ganglia of the autonomic nervous system. (Objective 16)

23. Muscarinic receptors. (Objective 16)

24. Salivation, lacrimation, urination, defecation, gastrointestinal distress, and emesis. (Objective 32)

25. SLUDGE suggests toxicity with an acetylcholinesterase inhibitor. (Objective 32)

26. Blood flow to the abdominal organs: Blood flow to the abdominal organs will decrease. GI tract peristalsis: Peristalsis in the GI tract will decrease. Urinary bladder wall muscle tone: Muscle tone in the urinary bladder wall will decrease. Liver glycogen stores: Glycogen stores in the liver will decrease as they are mobilized to increase blood glucose levels. (Objective 17)

27. Stimulation of dopaminergic receptors causes the blood vessels of the kidneys and intestinal tract to dilate. (Objective 17)

28.

	Alpha Effect	**Beta Effect**
Heart	No effect	Increased rate, contractility, automaticity
Lungs (bronchioles)	Dilation	Mild constriction
Blood vessels	Constriction	Dilation

(Objectives 16, 17)

29. Sympathetic. (Objective 17)

30. Parasympathetic. (Objective 16)

31. Sympathetic. (Objective 17)

32. Parasympathetic. (Objective 16)

33. Parasympathetic. (Objective 16)

34. Sympathetic. (Objective 17)

35. The heart, producing increased heart rate, contractility, automaticity, and impulse conduction velocity. (Objective 17)

36. Smooth muscle in the blood vessels and bronchioles, causing relaxation. This effect produces vasodilation and bronchodilation. (Objective 17)

37. Parasympathetic. (Objective 16)

38. Sympathetic. (Objective 17)

39. You would want to administer an agent with beta$_1$ effects. (Objective 17)

40. You would want to administer an agent with alpha$_1$ effects. (Objective 17)

41. Heart rate would decrease, blood vessels would not dilate and might constrict, bronchi would constrict, cardiac automaticity would decrease. (Objective 17)

42. Dopamine will not cross the blood-brain barrier. Levodopa, a precursor of dopamine, will cross the blood-brain barrier into the neurons of the basal ganglia, where it can be converted into dopamine. (Objective 15)

43. When H$_2$ receptors are stimulated by histamine, they increase the activity of H$^+$,K$^+$-ATPase, an enzyme that exchanges potassium, leading to increased gastric acid secretion. Blocking the binding of histamine to the H$_2$ receptors with an H$_2$-receptor antagonist slows H$^+$,K$^+$-ATPase activity and decreases gastric acid secretion. (Objective 23)

44. Stimulation of ACh receptors increases gastric acid secretion. Blocking ACh receptors decreases gastric acid secretion. (Objective 23)

45. The vomiting center, which stimulates vomiting directly, and the chemoreceptor trigger zone (CTZ), which stimulates vomiting indirectly. (Objective 23)

46. The vomiting center is stimulated by H$_1$ and ACh receptors in the pathway between itself and the

inner ear, by sensory input from the eyes and nose, and by anxiety or fear. The CTZ stimulates the vomiting center in response to stimulation from serotonin receptors in the stomach or from blood-borne substances such as ipecac or opioids. (Objective 23)

47. Serotonin antagonists (Zofran), dopamine antagonists (Compazine, Phenergen, Haldol, Reglan), anticholinergics, cannabinoids (Marinol, Cesamet). (Objective 23)
48. Insulin lowers the blood glucose levels. (Objective 25)
49. Glucagon raises the blood glucose levels. (Objective 25)
50. Glucocorticoids have an antiinflammatory effect that decreases the bronchial edema that contributes to narrowing of the lower airway during an asthma attack. (Objective 25)
51. The onset of glucocorticoid effects is very slow; therefore these drugs have little value in managing an acute asthma attack. However, they can prevent the reoccurrence of an episode of asthma that has been treated successfully with beta$_2$ agonists. (Objective 25)
52. By blocking histamine receptor sites, H$_1$ blockers can prevent histamine from triggering the vasodilation, increased capillary permeability, and nonvascular smooth muscle spasms that characterize allergic reactions. (Objective 21)
53. An antitussive is a drug that suppresses the stimulus to cough in the central nervous system. Codeine and dextromethorphan are common antitussives. (Objective 21)
54. An expectorant increases the productivity of a cough. Guaifenesin is an expectorant. (Objective 21)
55. A mucolytic makes mucus more watery and easier to cough up. *N*-Acetylcysteine (Mucomyst) is a mucolytic agent. (Objective 21)

Multiple Choice

1. C. The drug that best demonstrates the common properties of opioid agonists and illustrates their particular characteristics is morphine. (Objective 4)
2. B. Naloxone is an opioid antagonist. (Objective 4)
3. D. Opioid agonist-antagonist drugs decrease pain response and have few respiratory effects. (Objective 4)
4. D. Benzodiazepines and barbiturates are the two main pharmacologic classes in the functional class of sedative-hypnotics. (Objective 12)
5. D. Xanthines include theophylline. (Objective 21)
6. B. Methylphenidate is the most commonly prescribed drug for attention deficit–hyperactivity disorder. (Objective 14)
7. A. Chlorpromazine is a phenothiazine. (Objective 11)
8. C. Therapeutic effects of phenothiazines and butyrophenones result from their selectively blocking dopamine$_2$ receptors in the CNS. (Objective 11)
9. B. Acute dystonic reactions are treated with diphenhydramine. (Objective 11)
10. B. SSRIs are used primarily to treat depression. (Objective 11)
11. A. Nardil is an MAOI. (Objective 11)

12. D. Stimulation of the parasympathetic nervous system results in secretion by digestive glands. Parasympathetic stimulation also produces pupillary constriction, decreased heart rate, and bronchoconstriction. (Objective 16)
13. D. The two main types of cholinergic receptors are nicotinic and muscarinic. (Objective 16)
14. D. SLUDGE is an acronym used to remember the effects of overdose of cholinergics. (Objective 16)
15. C. Stimulation of the nerves in the sympathetic collateral ganglia of the abdominal cavity causes relaxation of the smooth muscle in the wall of the urinary bladder. Sympathetic stimulation also causes decreased blood flow to the abdominal organs, decreased digestive activity, and mobilization of sugar from the liver's glucose stores. (Objective 17)
16. D. Dopaminergic receptors are believed to cause dilation of the renal and mesenteric arteries. (Objective 17)
17. D. Terbutaline specifically targets beta$_2$ receptors. (Objective 21)
18. D. Lidocaine and phenytoin belong to the class of sodium channel blockers. (Objective 18)
19. A. ACE inhibitors decrease blood pressure by blocking the effects of a complex "cascade" system responsible for regulating fluid balance. (Objective 18)
20. B. Drugs used to treat high blood cholesterol are called antihyperlipidemics. (Objective 20)
21. A. Fibrinolytics are used to break down thrombi. (Objective 19)
22. C. Proventil (albuterol) is a beta$_2$-specific agonist. (Objective 18)
23. B. Drugs that suppress the stimulus to cough activated by the central nervous system are antitussives. (Objective 19)
24. C. The hormone oxytocin is released by the posterior pituitary. (Objective 27)
25. A. The pancreatic hormone that increases blood glucose level when released is glucagon. Insulin lowers the blood glucose level. (Objective 25)
26. D. A solution containing a modified pathogen that does not actually cause disease but still stimulates the development of antibodies specific to it is a vaccine. (Objective 7)
27. A. The antidote for organophosphate poisoning is atropine. (Objective 16)

Case Studies

Case one

1. Captopril is an angiotensin-converting enzyme inhibitor. By blocking conversion of angiotensin I to angiotensin II, ACE inhibitors decrease peripheral vascular resistance. They also cause a decrease in aldosterone release from the adrenal cortex, leading to increased urinary loss of water and sodium. (Objective 18)
2. ACE inhibitors cause a decrease in aldosterone release from the adrenal cortex, leading to increased urinary loss of water and sodium. (Objective 18)

312

Case two

1. He appears to have ingested an anticholinergic agent. (Objective 16)
2. Anticholinergic agents block the action of acetylcholine at its receptor sites. This effect decreases parasympathetic tone and produces signs and symptoms characteristic of overactivity in the sympathetic nervous system, such as tachycardia, dilated pupils, and decreased salivation. Although sweating normally is associated with increased sympathetic tone, patients suffering from anticholinergic toxicity do not sweat because the sympathetic nervous system uses acetylcholine to activate the sweat glands. (Objective 16)

Case three

1. MAO inhibitors are used to treat depression. (Objective 11)
2. MAO inhibitors prevent monoamine oxidase from breaking down serotonin and norepinephrine, making larger amounts of these neurotransmitters available for release into the synapses. Higher levels of norepinephrine and serotonin in the synapses elevate mood and reverse the symptoms of depression. (Objective 11)
3. Cheese, liver, and wine contain high levels of tyramine, a precursor of norepinephrine. (Objective 11)
4. Coffee, tea, and chocolate contain caffeine, a chemical that tends to promote the release of norepinephrine. (Objective 11)
5. Consuming tyramine- or caffeine-containing foods while taking an MAOI can cause a patient to have a hypertensive crisis secondary to a massive release of norepinephrine. (Objective 11)

Case four

1. This patient probably is a narcotic addict. (Objectives 3, 4)
2. Talwin, Stadol, and Nubain are narcotic agonist-antagonists that relieve pain without producing the euphoria and respiratory depression associated with narcotic agonists. Because these drugs have narcotic antagonist properties, they can produce symptoms of narcotic withdrawal in narcotic addicts. Therefore addicts frequently will claim they are "allergic" to these drugs. (Objectives 3, 4)

Case five

1. Lidocaine is a Class Ib agent. (Objective 18)
2. Sodium channel blockers. (Objective 18)
3. Because impulses move on neurons as action potentials created by the opening of sodium channels, lidocaine can slow nerve conduction velocity. This effect can result in numbness of the lips, decreased hearing acuity, and depression. (Objective 18)
4. Slowing nerve impulse conduction velocity in the peripheral nervous system can decrease pain sensation. (Objective 18)

Case six

1. Viagra is a phosphodiesterase inhibitor that prevents the breakdown of cyclic-GMP in vascular smooth muscle. Cyclic-GMP (c-GMP) is a smooth muscle relaxant, which causes vasodilation. An increase in c-GMP levels increases blood flow to the corpus cavernosum and corpus spongiosum of the body of the penis, improving an erection. (Objective 27)
2. Severe hypotension. (Objective 27)
3. Nitroglycerin is a vasodilator that produces its effects by forming nitric oxide. Nitric oxide binds to receptor sites on vascular smooth muscle and triggers increased intracellular levels of c-GMP. Because Viagra prevents breakdown of c-GMP, its combined effect with nitroglycerin is to cause massive vasodilation and profound hypotension. (Objective 27)
4. The patient should be kept in a supine position. High-concentration oxygen should be administered. At least two large-bore IVs should be started. Large volumes of isotonic crystalloid should be infused to fill the dilated vascular space and support blood pressure and perfusion. (Objective 27)

Case seven

1. Terbutaline is a beta$_2$ agonist. (Objective 21)
2. Beta$_2$ agonists relax smooth muscle. Because the uterus consists of smooth muscle, administration of a beta$_2$ agonist can interrupt preterm labor. (Objective 27)

Case eight

1. Elavil is a tricyclic antidepressant (TCA). (Objective 11)
2. TCAs have anticholinergic properties; therefore they produce some toxic effects that resemble those caused by atropine. (Objective 11)
3. TCAs have an alpha$_1$-blocking effect in the peripheral circulation; therefore they cause peripheral vasodilation, decreased systemic vascular resistance, and hypotension. (Objective 11)
4. TCAs act in the heart as Vaughn-Williams Class Ia agents. Because they have sodium channel blocking properties, TCAs slow impulse conduction and prolong ECG intervals. (Objective 11)
5. Sodium bicarbonate is used to antagonize the cardiotoxic effects of TCAs. (Objective 11)
6. Sodium bicarbonate is effective against the cardiotoxic effects of TCAs for two reasons. First, it raises the serum sodium level, allowing sodium to out-compete the TCA molecules for the sodium channels. Second, it alkalinizes the plasma. This effect changes the charge distribution on certain plasma proteins, causing them to bind TCA molecules, keeping the TCA molecules from reaching the membranes of the cardiac muscle cells. (Objective 11)

Case nine

1. Glucagon is produced by the alpha cells of the islets of Langerhans in the pancreas. (Objective 25)
2. Glucagon raises blood glucose levels by mobilizing sugar stored in the liver as glycogen. (Objective 25)
3. For glucagon to work, a patient must have adequate liver glycogen stores. Alcohol abusers frequently are malnourished; therefore this patient may have no sugar stores in the liver for glucagon to mobilize. (Objective 25)

Case ten

1. These symptoms are being produced by an excess of acetylcholine from the parasympathetic nervous system. (Objective 16)
2. Atropine should be given to block the muscarinic acetylcholine receptors and reverse these symptoms. (Objective 16)

CHAPTER 13: MEDICATION ADMINISTRATION

Short Answer

1. To replace lost extracellular fluid. To administer medications. (Objective 21)
2. Pulling a catheter backwards over a needle can cause the tip of the catheter to be sheared off, creating an embolus. (Objective 21)
3. Bright red blood moving up an IV line in pulsations indicates cannulation of an artery. The IV should be discontinued immediately and pressure should be applied to the site until bleeding stops. (Objective 21)
4. The patient is experiencing a pyrogenic reaction to contaminated IV fluid. You should discontinue the IV and reestablish the line with uncontaminated fluid. This complication of IV therapy can be prevented by carefully checking IV fluids to ensure they are in-date and show no evidence of contamination. (Objective 21)
5. The patient may be experiencing an air embolism. The patient's oxygenation and ventilation should be supported. The patient should be placed on his or her left side and tilted 30 degrees head down. This position causes air that has entered the heart to rise away from the pulmonary outflow tract and slows entry of air into the pulmonary circulation. (Objective 21)
6. A microdrip administration set delivers 1 mL of fluid per 60 drops infused. (Objectives 4, 5)
7. The constricting band should limit venous return from the extremity without restricting arterial flow. Allowing blood to enter normally while slowing the rate at which it leaves will distend the extremity's veins and facilitate starting the IV. (Objective 21)
8. Increasing the diameter of an IV catheter will increase the fluid flow through the catheter. (Objective 21)
9. Decreasing the length of an IV catheter will increase the fluid flow through the catheter. (Objective 21)

10. __4__ Subcutaneous
    __5__ Oral
    __3__ Intramuscular
    __1__ Intravenous
    __2__ Endotracheal (Objectives 12, 16, 19, 20, 21)
11. The intravenous route is the fastest and most dangerous because drugs are being placed directly into the bloodstream. (Objective 21)
12. Because vials are airtight, air must be injected into them to replace the volume of drug solution being withdrawn. (Objective 18)
13. The top of an ampule is tapped before it is broken off to ensure any drug solution trapped in the top of the ampule is knocked down into the lower portion where it can be withdrawn. (Objective 17)
14. By definition patients who are in shock have poor peripheral perfusion. Since blood flow through the muscles and subcutaneous tissues during shock is minimal, drugs injected into those areas will not be absorbed into the circulation at an adequate rate. (Objectives 19, 20)
15. If a physician gives you a drug order that is inappropriate, you should ask the physician to repeat the order. (Objectives 6, 7)
16. The purpose of aspirating before administering a drug by the IM or Sub-Q route is to ensure the needle has not entered a vein. (Objectives 19, 20)
17. Because IV tubing has a larger diameter than the IV catheter it is connected to, it provides less resistance to fluid flow. If the IV tubing is not pinched off during bolus administration of a drug, the drug will back up into the IV line rather than entering the patient's circulation. This will slow the onset of the drug's effects. (Objective 21)
18. Angle at which the needle is inserted: IM—90 degrees to skin surface, Sub-Q—45 degrees to skin surface. Whether the skin is pulled into a fold or held taut: IM—skin surface held taut, Sub-Q—skin surface pulled into a fold to avoid entering underlying muscle. (Objectives 19, 20)
19. Do you have any allergies? (Objectives 7, 12, 13, 14, 15, 16, 19, 20, 21)
20. Lidocaine, atropine, epinephrine, and Narcan. (Objective 16)
21. Attempting to recap needles. (Objective 11)
22. Drug administration by a route other than the gastrointestinal tract. (Objectives 15, 16, 19, 20, 21)
23. Drug administration by way of the gastrointestinal tract. (Objectives 12, 13, 14)
24. You probably are injecting a nerve. You should immediately stop the injection and withdraw the needle. (Objective 20)
25. Diazepam, acetaminophen, aspirin. (Objective 13)
26. Sublingual. (Objective 12)
27. Resistance decreases as the needle passes through the cortex of the bone. The needle stands by itself. Marrow can be aspirated through the needle. Fluid infuses easily without swelling of the surrounding soft tissues. (Objective 22)

314

28. Any medication or fluid that can be given safely by the intravenous route can be administered through an intraosseous line. (Objective 22)
29. Right medication, right dose, right time, right route, right patient, right documentation. (Objective 7)

Drug Dose Calculations

1. 0.5 g × 1000 mg/g × mL/50 mg = 10 mL (Objective 5)
2. 400 mg × 10 mL/500 mg = 8 mL (Objective 5)
3. 30 mg × 0.5 mL/10 mg = 1.5 mL (Objective 5)
4. 10 mL/1 g × 1 g/1000 mg × 250 mg = 2.5 mL (Objective 5)
5. 1 g/250 mL × 1000 mg/g = 4 mg/mL (Objective 5)
6. 200 mg/250 mL × 1000 mcg/mg = 800 mcg/mL (Objective 5)
7. 500 mL/2 g × 1 g/1000 mg × 2 mg/min = 0.5 mL/min (Objective 5)
8. 220 pounds × kg/2.2 pounds × 0.01 mg/kg × 10 mL/mg = 10 mL (Objective 5)
9. 1 mg/min × 1 g/1000 mg × 250 mL/1 g × 60 drops/mL = 15 drops/min (Objective 5)
   2 mg/min × 1 g/1000 mg × 250 mL/1 g × 60 drops/mL = 30 drops/min (Objective 5)
   3 mg/min × 1 g/1000 mg × 250 mL/1 g × 60 drops/mL = 45 drops/min (Objective 5)
   4 mg/min × 1 g/1000 mg × 250 mL/1 g × 60 drops/mL = 60 drops/min (Objective 5)
10. 0.04 g × 1000 mg/g × 1 tablet/5 mg = 8 tablets (Objective 5)
11. 2 tablets × 7.5 g/tablet × 1000 mg/g = 15,000 mg (Objective 5)
12. 1 cc = 1 mL (Objective 5)
13. 220 pounds × kg/2.2 pounds × 2 mcg/kg/min × mg/1000 mcg × 250 mL/200 mg = 0.25 mL/min (Objective 5)
14. 0.25 mL/min × 60 drops/mL = 15 drops/min (Objective 5)
15. 120 miles × 1 hr/60 miles × 60 min/hr × 10 gtt/min × 1 mL/10 gtt = 120 mL during the first 120 miles of the trip
    15 miles × 1 hr/30 miles × 60 min/hr × 10 gtt/min × 1 mL/10 gtt = 30 mL during the last 15 miles of the trip
    120 mL + 30 mL = 150 mL total for the trip
    Therefore only one 1000-mL bag of Ringer's lactate will be needed to complete the trip. (Objective 5)
16. 30 gtt/min × 1 mL/60 gtt × 400 mg/500 mL × 1000 mcg/mg × 1/220 pounds × 2.2 pounds/kg = 4 mcg/kg/min (Objective 5)
17. 12.5 mg × 1 mL/25 mg = 0.5 mL (Objective 5)
18. 320 mg × tablet/80 mg = 4 tablets (Objective 5)
19. 4 mg × 1 mL/10 mg = 0.4 mL (Objective 5)
20. 2 mg × 5 mL/5 mg = 2 mL (Objective 5)
21. 7.5 mL × 5 mg/5 mL = 7.5 mg (Objective 5)
22. 220 pounds × kg/2.2 pounds × 0.01 mg/kg × 10 mL/mg = 10 mL (Objective 5)
23. 220 pounds × kg/2.2 pounds × 1.5 mg/kg × 5 mL/100 mg = 7.5 mL (Objective 5)
24. 250 mL/g × 1 g/1000 mg × 2 mg/min × 60 gtt/mL = 30 gtt/min (Objective 5)
25. 0.3 mg × 1 mL/1 mg = 0.3 mL (Objective 5)
26. 25 mg × 1 mL/50 mg = 0.5 mL (Objective 5)

CHAPTER 14: AIRWAY MANAGEMENT

Matching

1.
   - __D__ Air sacs in which gas exchange occurs
   - __I__ Double membrane covering lungs
   - __A__ Flap covering windpipe's opening
   - __E__ Point where mainstem bronchi branch
   - __G__ Smaller airways without cartilage in their walls
   - __F__ Space between base of tongue and epiglottis
   - __H__ Throat
   - __B__ Voice box
   - __C__ Windpipe (Objective 3)
2.
   - __A__ Fine bubbling sounds caused by fluid in small airways
   - __D__ High-pitched crowing sounds on inspiration resulting from tight upper airway
   - __B__ Rattling sounds from mucus obstruction of large airways
   - __C__ Sounds produced by partial obstruction of upper airway by tongue
   - __E__ Whistling sounds on exhalation caused by narrow or tight lower airways (Objective 20)
3.
   - __B__ Curved
   - __B__ Placed into vallecula
   - __A__ Placed under epiglottis
   - __A__ Straight (Objective 60)
4.
   - __A__ Volume inhaled or exhaled in 1 minute
   - __D__ Volume inhaled or exhaled in one respiratory cycle
   - __E__ Volume left in lungs after maximum expiration
   - __C__ Volume remaining in lungs at end of normal expiration
   - __G__ Volume that can be maximally exhaled after a normal expiration
   - __B__ Volume that can be maximally expired after a maximum inspiration
   - __H__ Volume that can be maximally inhaled after a normal inspiration (Objective 19)

Short Answer

1. The respiratory center is located in the medulla oblongata of the brainstem. (Objectives 16, 17)
2. The phrenic nerve, which stimulates the diaphragm, originates at the levels of cervical vertebrae 3, 4, and 5. (Objectives 16, 17)
3. The intercostal nerves, which control the intercostal muscles, arise from the thoracic spinal cord. (Objectives 16, 17)

4. Respirations normally are stimulated by an increase in arterial carbon dioxide level. (Objective 16)

5. The backup system for controlling respirations is the hypoxic drive, which is triggered by a fall in arterial oxygen levels. (Objective 21)

6. In long-standing chronic obstructive pulmonary disease the arterial carbon dioxide concentration becomes elevated. (Objective 21)

7. Administration of high concentrations of oxygen to some COPD patients may depress their respirations. Because COPD patients retain carbon dioxide and develop high arterial carbon dioxide levels, over time the respiratory center in the brain becomes desensitized to changes in arterial carbon dioxide concentrations. At this point, the hypoxic drive takes over control of respirations. Giving high concentrations of oxygen to a patient who is breathing in response to decreases in arterial oxygen levels may satisfy the hypoxic drive and cause respiratory depression or arrest. However, because oxygen is essential to life, any patient who is hypoxic must receive supplemental oxygen. If a COPD patient receiving supplemental oxygen develops respiratory depression, his or her breathing should be assisted with a bag-mask device while oxygen continues to be administered. (Objective 25)

8. Inspiration is the active phase of the respiratory cycle, requiring contraction of the intercostal muscles and diaphragm. (Objective 16)

9. Expiration is the passive phase of the respiratory cycle, and does not require contraction of the intercostal muscles and diaphragm. (Objective 16)

10. Contraction of the diaphragm increases the volume of air in the lungs. (Objective 16)

11. The right mainstem bronchus is shorter and straighter than the left mainstem bronchus. If an endotracheal tube is inserted too far, it is more likely to enter the right mainstem bronchus than the left mainstem bronchus. (Objective 3)

12. The tidal volume is the amount of air inhaled or exhaled during a single breath. The tidal volume of a 70-kg patient is approximately 500 mL. (Objective 19)

13. Tidal volume × respiratory rate = minute volume; 500 mL/breath × 20 breaths/min = 10,000 mL/min. (Objective 19)

14. Anatomic dead space is the portion of the respiratory tract in which gas exchange with the blood does not take place. (Objective 12)

15. Physiologic dead space consists of areas of the respiratory tract where gas exchange should be occurring but is not because of inadequate alveolar ventilation or inadequate blood flow through the capillary beds. (Objective 12)

16. Atelectasis is a localized collapse of the alveoli, resulting in a small area of the lung where gas exchange does not occur. (Objective 6)

17. The normal $PaCO_2$ is 35 to 45 mm Hg. (Objective 11)

18. The normal PaO_2 is 80 to 100 mm Hg. (Objective 10)

19. If respiratory rate and tidal volume decrease, $PaCO_2$ will increase. This condition is called hypoventilation. (Objectives 13, 19)

20. If respiratory rate increases and tidal volume decreases, $PaCO_2$ will decrease. This condition is called hyperventilation. (Objectives 12, 19)

21. Cyanosis is a late sign of hypoxia. For cyanosis to be present, a patient must have 5 mg/dL of his/her hemoglobin not bound to oxygen. Because the normal hemoglobin concentration is approximately 15 mg/dL, a patient must have desaturated approximately one third of his/her hemoglobin before cyanosis appears. (Objective 18)

22. The earliest sign of hypoxia usually is restlessness and anxiety. (Objective 18)

23. The tongue is the most common cause of an obstructed airway in a unconscious person. If a patient's chest does not rise when ventilation is attempted, the head should be repositioned to ensure the tongue is not obstructing the airway. (Objective 29)

24. The airway should be removed. (Objective 41)

25. A nasopharyngeal airway should be inserted in a patient who will not tolerate an oral airway but who requires assistance to maintain his/her airway. (Objective 40)

26. A patient who has a partial airway obstruction with good air exchange will be able to cough, speak, and exchange sufficient air to remain awake and oriented. A partial airway obstruction with poor air exchange will result in inability to cough, speak, or exchange air adequately, even though some air movement still may be present. A patient with a partial airway obstruction who is exchanging air adequately should be encouraged to cough, given supplemental oxygen, and transported to the hospital. If the patient cannot cough or speak, or shows signs of altered mental status, abdominal thrusts should be performed to relieve the obstruction. (Objective 27)

27. A nonrebreather mask should be used with a young adult who is having an asthma attack. Asthma is a reversible obstructive pulmonary disease that results in episodes of inadequate alveolar ventilation. This can result in hypoxia. Giving high-concentration oxygen can help correct the hypoxia produced by an asthma attack. (Objective 25)

28. The Venturi mask, also called an *air-entrainment mask*, provides precise control over a patient's FiO_2 level. Because some patients with long-standing COPD may be breathing in response to decreases in their arterial oxygen concentrations, giving high concentrations of oxygen may depress their respirations. The Venturi mask allows controlled increases in the FiO_2 level to find the concentration that corrects hypoxia without depressing respirations. (Objective 25)

29. If a COPD patient who is receiving oxygen develops depressed respirations, you should assist his/her breathing with a bag-mask device. (Objective 25)

30. Dual-lumen airway devices should not be used if a patient has ingested a caustic agent. Because the esophagus has been burned, insertion of a dual-lumen device could cause esophageal perforation. (Objective 56)

31. Cirrhosis of the liver secondary to chronic alcohol abuse or hepatic disease can lead to formation of esophageal varices. Passing a tube into the esophagus of a patient with varices can produce massive upper gastrointestinal tract bleeding. (Objective 56)

32. The maximum time period that should elapse without ventilating during an intubation attempt is 30 seconds. (Objective 57)

33. The person attempting the intubation should hold his or her breath. When the person performing the intubation feels the need to breathe, the patient needs to be ventilated. If the patient is perfusing adequately, a pulse oximeter also can be used to monitor for a drop in oxygen saturation, which also indicates the need to stop the intubation attempt and begin ventilating. (Objective 57)

34. (Patient's age/4) + 4 = endotracheal tube size. (Objective 64)

35. The tube probably is in the right mainstem bronchus. After ensuring the endotracheal tube's cuff is deflated, the tube should be withdrawn slowly until breath sounds are equal bilaterally. (Objective 62)

36. The cuff of an endotracheal tube should be inflated with 6 to 10 mL of air. Periodically assess the pilot balloon to ensure the distal cuff is adequately inflated. The cuff is adequately inflated when air does not leak around it. (Objective 57)

37. You see the tube pass through the vocal cords. You see the chest rise when the patient is ventilated through the tube. You hear breath sounds in the lung fields bilaterally when the patient is ventilated through the tube. You do not hear breath sounds over the epigastrium when the patient is ventilated through the tube. You detect carbon dioxide returning through the tube. (Objective 62)

38. The most common complication of endotracheal suctioning is hypoxia. Hypoxia during endotracheal suctioning is prevented by adequately preoxygenating the patient and by limiting the time of suctioning. (Objective 38)

39. The trachea should not be suctioned for longer than 15 seconds without oxygenating. (Objective 34)

40. During an intubation attempt, the head should be in the sniffing position. The head should be slightly extended and the neck should be flexed forward by placing padding under the occiput. Hyperextending the neck during an intubation attempt can result in inability to visualize the glottic opening. (Objective 60)

41. A gastric tube holds the gastroesophageal sphincter open, increasing the risk of regurgitation of gastric contents and aspiration. Since an unconscious person cannot protect his or her own airway, an endotracheal tube must always be placed before a gastric tube is inserted. (Objective 51)

42. Mid-face trauma or basilar skull fracture may be associated with injury to the cribriform plate at the top of the nasal cavity. If the cribriform plate is fractured, an instrument passed into the nose might pass through the fracture into the cranial cavity and enter the brain. (Objectives 41, 51, 65)

43. A bag-mask and reservoir with oxygen flowing at 15 L/min will deliver 90% to 100% oxygen. (Objective 43)

44. Chest rise is the only reliable indicator that rescue breathing is inflating the lungs. (Objective 43)

45. Orthopnea is dyspnea that is more severe when a patient is lying down. (Objective 20)

46. Nasal flaring; movement of the larynx and trachea up and down as the patient breathes; use of the muscles of the neck and upper chest (respiratory accessory muscles) to assist breathing; retractions between the ribs, at the top of the sternum, or over the epigastrium as the patient inhales. (Objective 20)

47. Soft suction catheters clog too easily when suctioning blood or vomitus. (Objective 35)

48. Subcutaneous emphysema is a crackling sensation under the skin of the chest wall or neck caused by leakage of air into the soft tissues. (Objectives 16, 17, 18)

49. The most common cause of an elevated $PaCO_2$ is inadequate respiratory rate or tidal volume. This problem is corrected by assisting the patient's ventilations with a bag-mask device. (Objectives 11, 13)

50. The $PaCO_2$ of 50 indicates the patient is not being ventilated adequately, because the CO_2 level is above normal. The PaO_2 of 120 indicates that the patient is oxygenating adequately on supplemental oxygen. (Objectives 11, 13)

51. This patient has not been oxygenating or ventilating for an extended time. He should be oxygenated and ventilated first using a bag-mask, before endotracheal intubation is attempted. The need to ventilate is not the same as the need to intubate. (Objectives 43, 60)

52. Depolarizing neuromuscular blockers cause muscles to depolarize and then hold them in a depolarized state, preventing further contraction. Nondepolarizing neuromuscular blockers block the acetylcholine receptors on skeletal muscles, preventing them from depolarizing and contracting. (Objective 68)

53. Neuromuscular blockers do not affect level of consciousness. (Objective 67)

54. Patients who will be receiving neuromuscular blockers to facilitate endotracheal intubation should be sedated first with a benzodiazepine. If this is not done, the patient will be completely paralyzed and unable to breathe while remaining fully conscious. (Objective 69)

Multiple Choice

1. C. An endotracheal tube should be inserted to a depth of 19 to 23 cm. (Objective 57)

2. C. A jaw thrust or chin lift with the head and neck in neutral position should be used because this patient may have a cervical fracture. (Objective 31)

3. A. The lungs of a 5-year-old child who is not breathing but has a pulse should be ventilated once every 3 seconds. (Objective 44)

4. C. Snoring respirations indicate partial obstruction of the upper airway by the tongue. (Objective 29)

5. C. The most probable values for the blood gases of a patient who is breathing 6 times per minute would be low oxygen, high carbon dioxide. (Objectives 10, 11)

6. D. The patient's minute volume (minute ventilation) is 6000 mL (15 breaths/min × 400 mL/breath). (Objective 19)

7. B. Transmission of meningitis by droplet inhalation poses the greatest risk to the paramedic when performing endotracheal intubation. HIV and hepatitis B are not airborne. Tuberculosis is not transmitted by skin contact. (Objective 58)

8. C. The normal tidal volume for a 70-kilogram adult is 500 mL. (Objective 19)

9. B. Rhonchi suggest mucus partially obstructing the larger airways. (Objective 20)

10. A. Ventilations are normally stimulated by the carbon dioxide content of arterial blood. (Objective 16)

11. D. The respiratory center is located in the medulla oblongata. (Objective 16)

12. A. The purpose or objective of endotracheal intubation is to achieve complete control of the airway. (Objective 57)

13. C. When a stylet is used during endotracheal intubation, the tip of the stylet should be recessed about ½ inch from the distal end or Murphy's eye of the endotracheal tube. (Objective 57)

14. C. The partial pressure of oxygen in arterial blood (systemic) is normally 80 to 100 torr. (Objective 10)

15. D. The right bronchus is shorter and straighter than the left. (Objective 3)

16. B. If a patient has a normal tidal volume and a decreased arterial carbon dioxide level, the patient's ventilatory rate probably is fast. (Objective 11)

17. B. Localized, unilateral wheezing in the lung fields would most likely be caused by aspiration of a foreign body into the lower airway. Asthma, pulmonary edema, and allergic bronchospasm would more likely produce generalized wheezing in both lungs. (Objective 20)

18. D. The best course of action following two unsuccessful intubation attempts in a 12-year-old child with complete airway obstruction from epiglottitis would be to perform a surgical cricothyrotomy. Because the obstruction is produced by edema instead of a foreign body, abdominal thrusts are unlikely to be successful. Because the airway obstruction is complete, the patient will not be able to exhale through the trachea; therefore the larger lumen of an ET tube is needed for exhalation rather than the small lumen of a needle cricothyrotomy. (Objectives 7, 71)

19. C. The best choice of endotracheal tube size for a 4-year-old child is a 5.0-mm tube. (Objective 64)

20. C. The most appropriate depth of insertion for the endotracheal tube would be 14 to 15 cm at the teeth. (Objective 64)

21. B. The most reliable indication that rescue breathing is adequately inflating the lungs is rise of the chest wall during ventilation. (Objective 43)

22. B. Extensive atelectasis would be expected to cause PaO_2 to be decreased and $PaCO_2$ to be increased. (Objectives 6, 12, 13)

23. D. Before an endotracheal intubation attempt, assuming spinal injury is not suspected, the head and neck should be placed in the sniffing position. (Objective 57)

24. B. Administration of oxygen to some COPD patients may depress spontaneous ventilations. (Objectives 13, 16, 17, 25)

25. C. Oxygen cylinders are potentially dangerous because oxygen vigorously supports combustion and the oxygen in cylinders is under pressure. Oxygen is not a flammable gas. It supports combustion of materials that are flammable. (Objective 24)

26. A. Either the tube is in the right mainstem bronchus or there is a pneumothorax in the left bronchus. (Objective 62)

27. B. The nasal cavity warms, filters, and humidifies inhaled air. (Objective 4)

28. A. Assessment of peak expiratory flow is most useful in asthma. (Objective 14)

29. B. The preferred airway for use in the patient with severe facial injuries is orotracheal intubation. The laryngeal mask airway and Combitube do not adequately protect the lower airway from blood and fluids draining into the airway from facial injuries. Tubes should not be inserted into the nose of a patient with significant facial injuries because a cribriform plate fracture may be present. (Objective 53)

30. B. The most correct insertion depth for a 7.5-mm endotracheal tube would be 21 cm at the teeth. (Objective 57)

31. A. A 2.5-mm tube is the most appropriate size endotracheal tube for a preterm infant. (Objective 64)

32. C. Because this patient's history and physical findings include chronic obstructive pulmonary disease, you should consider the possibility that his ventilations are being stimulated by the oxygen content of his arterial blood. (Objective 16)

33. D. Your next step should be to reposition the head and try again to ventilate. The most common cause of airway obstruction in an unconscious person is the tongue. (Objectives 2, 28, 29, 39, 31)

34. C. The best device for initially maintaining the airway of a patient who will not tolerate an oral airway is a nasopharyngeal airway. (Objectives 5, 40)

35. C. The best course of airway management before transport would be to open the airway, assist ventilations with a bag-mask device and oxygen, endotracheally intubate, and then insert an 18-French orogastric tube during transport. Giving oxygen by mask is ineffective if a patient does not have an adequate respiratory rate or tidal volume. Intubation by the oral route is preferred to nasotracheal intubation because passage of the endotracheal tube through the vocal cords can be visualized. (Objective 57)

36. C. The maximum amount of time in which the procedure of endotracheal intubation should be accomplished is 30 seconds. (Objective 57)

37. A. One of the most serious errors committed during endotracheal intubation is attempting to intubate without first adequately oxygenating and ventilating. Failure to oxygenate and ventilate the patient first worsens hypoxia and hypercarbia. (Objective 57)

38. D. The dual-lumen airway should be used only for unconscious adults. The dual-lumen airway is contraindicated in patients who are very short because the tube may not be placed to the proper depth in the esophagus. Placement of a dual-lumen airway in a patient who has ingested a caustic substance may cause esophageal perforation. Alcohol abuse or liver disease can cause esophageal varices. Placement of a dual-lumen airway in these patients may cause severe bleeding. (Objective 56)

39. D. The most appropriate initial method to remove a complete foreign body airway obstruction when BLS techniques have failed is to perform direct laryngoscopy and use Magill forceps to remove the object if it is visualized. (Objectives 28, 30, 59)

40. B. Of these patients, the 12-year-old child probably would be easiest to ventilate. The 3-year-old child will have a large, posteriorly placed tongue that is difficult to move and will have to have her neck maintained in neutral alignment. The football player and the obese female are likely to have thick necks that make proper positioning of the head and neck more difficult. (Objective 57)

CHAPTER 15: THERAPEUTIC COMMUNICATION

Matching

1.
   __A__ Asking the speaker to help you understand
   __H__ Briefly reviewing the interview and your conclusions
   __G__ Echoing the patient's message using your own words
   __E__ Encouraging the patient to provide more information
   __B__ Focusing on a particular point made during the interview
   __D__ Sharing objective information related to the message
   __F__ Stating the conclusions you have drawn from the information
   __C__ Using body language to show you understand and care (Objective 7)

Short Answer

1. Communication is the use of words, writing, or other commonly understood symbols by a sender to send a message to a receiver who then provides feedback that indicates the receiver's interpretation of the message. (Objective 1)

2. Presence of multiple patients. Lack of privacy. Noisy environments. Dangerous or chaotic environments. Reactions by family members and bystanders. Influences from other responders. Ambient lighting, weather. (Objective 3)

3. Personal beliefs about a patient or group of patients. Personal experiences with a patient or group of patients. Educational and professional beliefs about a patient or group of patients. Personal relationship or financial troubles. Personal illness. Anger or hostility toward a co-worker, supervisor, or agency that is misperceived by a patient. (Objective 3)

4. Use the patient's name. Address the patient by the appropriate title. Modulate your voice, speaking quietly, slowly, and in low tones. Use a professional, but compassionate voice tone. Explain what you are doing and why you are doing it. Keep a kind, calm facial expression. Begin with a calm, reassuring demeanor, but if necessary become firm and authoritative. (Objective 2)

5. Social distance is the acceptable distance between strangers used for impersonal business transactions. In the United States, social distance is 4 to 12 feet. (Objectives 3, 5, 11)

6. Personal space is the area around an individual perceived as an extension of self. In the United States, personal distance is 1.5 to 4 feet. (Objectives 3, 5, 11)

7. Intimate space is the area within 1.5 feet of a person. (Objectives 3, 5, 11)

8. Although some portions of the history may be taken from social distance, most of the patient assessment is performed within the patient's personal space. Some activities may require entering the intimate space. (Objectives 3, 5, 11)

9. Because entry of an individual's personal or intimate space by a stranger is likely to trigger anxiety, you should introduce yourself to the patient and ask their name. You should ask permission to examine them and use their body language and facial expression as indicators of their level of comfort. Although most persons will grant permission to enter their personal space to healthcare providers more readily than to other strangers, you should always be monitoring the patient for signs of anxiety or discomfort during the physical examination. (Objectives 3, 5, 11)

10. Placing yourself at the same eye level as the patient indicates that you regard them as an equal. (Objectives 3, 5, 11)

11. Standing over or above a patient indicates you are in authority. This position can be very intimidating to some patients. Standing above or over a patient is appropriate when you need to demonstrate you are in control of the situation (e.g., when a patient is not appropriately controlling his or her behavior). (Objectives 3, 5, 11)

12. Dropping below a patient's eye level indicates you are willing to let them have some control over the situation. (Objectives 3, 5, 11)

13. Children and the elderly. (Objectives 3, 5, 11)

14. An open-ended question cannot be answered by simply saying "yes" or "no," or by providing short answers. It requires a patient to provide a detailed response. (Objective 6)

15. Open-ended questions are useful when you want to obtain detailed information about the patient's complaint in his/her own words. (Objective 6)

16. Some patients will tend to wander off the subject when asked open-ended questions. Patients who are inarticulate or who have a limited vocabulary may have difficulty responding to open-ended questions. Open-ended questions also are not useful with patients who are confused. (Objective 6)

17. A direct (closed-ended) question can be answered simply by saying "yes" or "no," or by providing a short answer consisting of only a few words. (Objectives 5, 6)

18. Direct (closed-ended) questions are useful when you are trying to obtain a history quickly in a situation where time is critical. Close-ended questions also are helpful in dealing with patients who have difficulty responding to open-ended questions. (Objectives 5, 6)

19. Direct (closed-ended) questions elicit only the information requested, rather than giving a patient the opportunity to provide an answer that expands on the question asked. Closed-ended questions also may inadvertently lead patients toward certain answers. (Objective 8)

20. Identify other sources of information such as family, bystanders, medication bottles, medical identification bracelets. Ensure privacy for the patient during the interview. Assure the patient you are there to help. Determine whether the patient has a medical problem that may be interfering with their ability to talk. Use closed-ended questions. (Objectives 4, 5, 11)

21. Ensure your personal safety. Request a response by law enforcement. The presence of law enforcement officers on a scene may discourage a hostile patient from escalating a situation. Identify and remove potential sources of stress from the scene. Maintain a safe distance from the patient at all times. Avoid making the patient feel cornered. Acknowledge that you understand the patient is upset. Speak in a clear, low, calm voice. Maintain eye contact with the patient, but avoid staring because this can be interpreted as a threat. Clearly explain the benefits and advantages of cooperation. Never leave the patient alone without adequate assistance. Keep a clear path to an exit. Position yourself so you can see others entering and leaving the area. (Objectives 5, 11)

22. Questions beginning with "why" can sound as if the paramedic is asking the patient to explain his or her actions and, therefore, can be confrontational. (Objective 11)

23. Children can interpret language very concretely. Saying you are going to "take" their pulse can imply you are going to somehow remove it and possibly not return it. Saying you are going to "count" or "measure" their pulse is less threatening. (Objective 8)

24. Your partner has used medical jargon. The danger of using jargon commonly understood by healthcare providers is that patients may place an entirely different interpretation on the words used. For example, this patient may interpret the phrase "bag her" as meaning she is about to be put in a body bag. As a result of this misinterpretation of medical jargon, she may become upset, anxious, or uncooperative. (Objectives 2, 8, 10, 11)

Multiple Choice

1. C. In the United States, social distance (the acceptable distance between strangers) is 4 to 12 feet. (Objectives 3, 5, 11)

2. B. In the United States, personal space (the distance from themselves that most people perceive as an extension of themselves) is 1.5 to 4 feet. Entering another person's personal space without their permission can make them anxious and uncooperative. (Objectives 3, 5, 11)

3. B. Most of patient assessment takes place at personal distance. EMS personnel should introduce themselves and use the patient's facial expressions and body language as indicators of permission before entering a patient's personal space. (Objectives 3, 5, 10, 11)

4. C. Extended arms, open hands, relaxed large muscles, and a nodding head characterize an open stance, which communicates warmth, attentiveness, and positive signals to the patient. (Objectives 3, 5, 10, 11)

5. B. Flexed arms and clenched fists characterize a closed stance, which sends negative signals to the patient and can communicate disinterest, discomfort, or fear. (Objectives 3, 5, 10, 11)

6. A. Positioning yourself below a patient's eye level indicates willingness to let the patient have some control over the situation. (Objectives 3, 5, 11, 12)

7. D. When you are communicating with an elderly patient, you should use physical contact when necessary to compensate for decreased vision. Elderly persons can be offended if you assume they are hearing-impaired and talk louder than normal. Elders can find use of terms such as "dear" or

"honey" disrespectful and offensive. Separating an older person from friends and family can increase anxiety and cause confusion. (Objectives 3, 5, 11, 12)

8. D. You should use the patient's first name only after obtaining permission to do so. Generally speaking, all patients should be addressed by last name and appropriate title unless they offer you permission to use their first name. Excessive use of medical terminology can confuse and upset patients. Use of "pet" names by strangers can offend children. Patients should be allowed to answer fully without interruption before you ask for clarification of points you do not understand. (Objective 8)

9. D. Rephrasing a patient's responses into your own words is reflection. Reflection allows the patient to check your understanding of what he or she just said to you and provide corrections or additional information if necessary. (Objective 7)

10. C. A question that guides the direction of a patient's answer is a leading question. Leading questions usually should be avoided during patient interviews because they can reinforce tunnel vision on your part and keep you from recognizing serious problems. (Objective 8)

11. B. A question such as "Did you take your insulin today?" is referred to as a direct (closed-ended) question because it can be answered "yes" or "no." (Objective 8)

12. D. "What would someone have to do to you to produce pain similar to what you are feeling?" is an open-ended question because it requires the patient to provide a detailed, unguided response. The other questions are direct (closed-ended) because they can be answered "yes" or "no." "Do you have a squeezing sensation in your chest?" also is a leading question because it provides an answer for the patient. (Objective 6)

13. C. Facilitation consists of feedback techniques to indicate you are listening and to encourage the patient to continue talking. (Objective 7)

Case Studies

Case one

1. Recognize that his understanding of the human female reproductive anatomy and physiology is likely to be very limited. Recognize that if he is a refugee from an area where there has been warfare or conflicts with officials of an authoritarian regime, your uniform may frighten him. Use simple language appropriate to the vocabulary of a 7-year-old. Phrase your questions carefully and be sure he understands them. Ask one question at a time. Address the patient and not the interpreter. Recognize that much of the information you receive may not be reliable. Account for possible cultural differences in perception. Recognize that anxiety and other emotional responses by the interpreter may affect communication. Be very patient. (Objectives 10, 11 12)

Case two

1. An individual who has grown up in the dominant cultural tradition of the United States tends to interpret unwillingness to answer questions or to make eye contact as a sign of untruthfulness. However, in many of the cultures of eastern Asia, silence and reluctance to make eye contact are signs of respect for authority. Be cautious about assuming that persons from other cultures who will not speak to you or will not look you in the eye "have something to hide." They may simply be acknowledging the power and authority they perceive you to hold. (Objectives 10, 11, 12)

CHAPTER 16: HISTORY TAKING

Short Answer

1. In most situations the history will provide the basis for the field diagnosis on which treatment will be based. The history also helps to guide the physical examination by suggesting specific observations that should be made. The manner in which the history is taken also helps establish rapport and trust between the paramedic and the patient. (Objective 1)

2. Identifying data, source of referral, source of history, reliability, chief complaint, history of present illness, past medical history, current health status, family history, psychosocial history, review of systems.

3. The chief complaint is the reason EMS was called, if possible stated in the patient's own words. (Objective 2)

4. The chief complaint should suggest a differential diagnosis—a list of possible causes for the chief complaint. Once possible causes of the patient's complaint are identified, questions can be asked or physical findings can be sought to eliminate problems from the list. The problem that cannot be eliminated through the history and physical examination is the working or field diagnosis. (Objective 2)

5. An open-ended question cannot be answered by simply saying "yes" or "no," or by providing short answers. It requires a patient to provide a detailed response. (Objective 3)

6. Open-ended questions are useful when you want to obtain detailed information about the patient's complaint in his/her own words. (Objective 3)

7. Some patients will tend to wander off the subject when asked open-ended questions. Patients who are inarticulate or who have a limited vocabulary may have difficulty responding to open-ended questions. Open-ended questions also are not useful with patients who are confused. (Objective 3)

8. A closed-ended question can be answered simply by saying "yes" or "no," or by providing a short answer consisting of only a few words. (Objective 3)

9. Closed-ended questions are useful when you are trying to obtain a history quickly in a situation where time is critical. Close-ended questions also are helpful in dealing with patients who have difficulty responding to open-ended questions. (Objective 3)

10. Closed-ended questions elicit only the information requested, rather than giving a patient the opportunity to provide an answer that expands on the question asked. Closed-ended questions also may inadvertently lead patients toward certain answers. (Objective 3)

11. The chief complaint is the reason EMS was called. The primary problem is the underlying cause of the complaint. For example, a patient with a chief complaint of "difficulty breathing" might have a primary problem of chronic obstructed pulmonary disease exacerbated by pneumonia. (Objective 2)

12. If a patient has difficulty describing pain, ask them what would have to be done to them to create a similar sensation—for example, stab them, squeeze them, burn them. (Objective 3)

13. Because a 10 is typically defined as the worst pain the patient ever has experienced, find out what the worst pain they ever experienced is. A patient who previously has passed several kidney stones might rate the pain of an acute myocardial infarction lower on a scale of 0 to 10 than a patient who has never experienced a significantly painful event. (Objective 3)

14. A differential diagnosis is a list of problems that could produce the patient's chief complaint. (Objective 1)

15. The differential diagnosis helps guide the history and physical examination. The goal of the history and physical examination is to narrow the differential diagnosis by eliminating possible causes of the patient's complaint until only one possibility, the field diagnosis, remains. (Objective 1)

16. O = onset; P = provocation/palliation; Q = quality; R= region, radiation; S = severity; T = timing. (Objective 3)

17. How long ago did the pain begin? Does anything make it worse or better? What does the pain feel like? Where do you hurt? Have you had pain like this before? Does the pain travel anywhere else in your body? On a scale of 0 to 10, how bad is the pain? Are there any other symptoms? If so, what is the sequence in which they occurred? (Objective 3)

18. The review of systems is performed to screen for problems that may not have been mentioned in the history of present illness. (Objective 2)

19. Did the patient's mother receive routine prenatal care? Were there any complications during pregnancy? Were there any complications during delivery? What was the method of delivery—vaginal or cesarean? If the mother had a cesarean section, why did she need one? Did the infant require resuscitation or any other special treatment in the delivery room or nursery? How long was the infant in the hospital before discharged home? Did any health problems surface during the neonatal period? Has the child received standard immunizations against infectious disease? (Objective 4)

Multiple Choice

1. B. A question such as "Are you having numbness in your left arm?" is referred to as a *closed-ended question* because it can be answered with "yes" or "no." (Objective 3)

2. C. If possible, question the patient before talking to relatives and bystanders. This shows respect for the patient. Generally, it is better to begin an interview with open-ended questions to avoid leading the patient. Suggesting answers to speed the history-taking process can lead to the acquisition of incomplete or inaccurate information. Generally, it is better to ask about an area before examining it to avoid creating the impression you have found a problem during the physical exam. (Objective 3)

3. D. The duration of the pain would be part of the history of the present illness of a patient complaining of abdominal pain. Medications, allergies, and general health are not part of the history of present illness. (Objective 2)

4. A. The first information you should obtain from a conscious patient is the chief complaint. The chief complaint guides the rest of the history and the physical examination. (Objectives 2, 3)

5. C. In developing a history of the present illness, you will need to know the duration of the headache. Although information about the patient's medications is important, it is not part of the history of the present illness. (Objectives 2, 3)

CHAPTER 17: PATIENT ASSESSMENT

Matching

1. __A__ Fine, popping sounds that indicate the presence of fluid in alveoli and small airways
   __C__ Harsh, high-pitched crowing sound that indicates a narrow upper airway
   __B__ Rattling sound produced by collections of mucus and other fluids in larger airways
   __D__ High-pitched whistling sounds produced by air flowing through narrow lower airways (Objective 68)

Short Answer

1. Don gloves for body substance isolation and size-up the scene for any hazards. (Objective 13)

2. The purpose of the initial assessment (primary survey) is to identify any immediately life-threatening problems. (Objective 23)

3. General impression, airway, breathing, circulation, disability (CNS function), expose and examine. (Objective 23)

4. Attempts should be made to correct the problem. If the problem cannot be corrected, the patient should be transported immediately while continuing support of oxygenation, ventilation, and circulation. (Objective 23)

5. To identify less obvious signs and symptoms that may not have been detected during the initial assessment. (Objectives 43, 44)

6. The patient's mental status. (Objective 32)

7. Normal capillary refill time is less than 2 seconds. (Objective 32)

8. *A*lert, responsive to *v*erbal stimuli, responsive to *p*ainful stimuli, *u*nresponsive. (Objective 11)

9. The cervical spine should be controlled manually at the same time the airway is opened. (Objective 25)

10. The pulse rate is counted during the focused or detailed physical examination (secondary survey). (Objectives 43, 44)

11. The respiratory rate is counted during the focused or detailed physical examination (secondary survey). (Objectives 43, 44)

12. The blood pressure measurement is taken by cuff during the focused or detailed physical examination (secondary survey). (Objectives 43, 44)

13. Right-sided heart failure; pulmonary embolism; tension pneumothorax; cardiac tamponade. (Objective 65)

14. Battle's sign. (Objective 54)

15. Nasal flaring; tugging of the trachea; use of respiratory accessory muscles; suprasternal, substernal, and intercostal retractions. (Objectives 63, 64, 66)

16. Rate, strength, and rhythm (Objective 7)

17. Scene size-up (body substance isolation, scene safety, patient location and number, mechanism of injury/nature of illness, need for additional resources), primary survey (general impression, airway, breathing, circulation, disability, expose and examine, determination of priority for transport), secondary survey (focused or detailed history and physical examination), ongoing assessment. (Objectives 14, 15, 20, 22, 24, 36, 43, 44, 90)

18. Inspection: to look. Palpation: to feel. Auscultation: to listen. Percussion: to tap. (Objective 3)

19. To listen to higher pitched sounds. (Objective 4)

20. To listen to lower pitched sounds. (Objective 4)

21. The fingertips should be used for palpation to detect size, consistency, masses, fluid, and crepitus. (Objective 4)

22. The palm should be used to palpate for vibrations or impulses because it provides a larger surface area than the fingertips. (Objective 4)

23. The back of the hand should be used to check for skin moisture and temperature because the skin there is thinner and more sensitive. (Objective 4)

24. Olfactory: Test ability to identify familiar odors, with one nostril at a time and the eyes closed.
    Optic: Test visual acuity with Snellen chart. Test visual fields by confrontation and extinction of vision.
    Oculomotor: Test eyelids for drooping. Test extraocular eye movements.
    Trochlear: Test extraocular eye movements.
    Trigeminal: Palpate jaw muscles for tone and strength when patient clenches teeth. Test pain and touch sensation over face. Test corneal reflex.
    Abducens: Test extraocular movements.

    Facial: Inspect symmetry of facial features with various expressions. Test ability to identify sweet and salty tastes on each side of tongue.
    Acoustic: Test sense of hearing.
    Glossopharyngeal: Test ability to identify sour and bitter tastes. Test gag reflex and ability to swallow.
    Vagus: Inspect palate and uvula for symmetry with speech sounds and gag reflex. Observe for swallowing difficulty. Evaluate for presence of nasal or hoarse voice quality.
    Spinal accessory: Have patient shrug shoulders and turn head to each side against resistance.
    Hypoglossal: Check tongue for symmetry when protruded. Check tongue movement toward nose and chin. Evaluate quality of lingual speech sounds *(l, t, d, n)*.
    (Objective 86)

25. Obtain patient pulse rate and blood pressure measurement while supine.
    Sit patient up with feet dangling. Wait 60 seconds.
    Obtain pulse rate and blood pressure measurement with patient seated.
    Have patient stand. Wait 60 seconds.
    Obtain pulse rate and blood pressure measurement with patient standing.
    If pulse rate increases by 10 to 20 beats per minute AND systolic blood pressure decreases by 10 to 20 mm Hg moving from supine to sitting OR from sitting to standing, the patient has orthostatic hypotension (a positive tilt test).
    If the patient experiences syncope or presyncopal symptoms (dizziness, weakness, dim vision) at any point during the procedure, orthostatic hypotension is present and vital signs do not need to be taken. (Objective 69)

26. The patient has a pneumothorax. (Objective 63)

27. The patient has a hemothorax. (Objective 63)

28. These terms do not have sufficiently precise meanings to allow tracking of changes in mental status over time. A more appropriate approach to describing mental status is to describe the patient's response to various verbal and tactile stimuli. (Objective 12)

29. The fingertips become clubbed. Clubbing is a result of an increase in the number of capillaries in the soft tissues as a compensatory response to chronic hypoxia in the peripheral circulation. (Objectives 47, 48)

30. These depressions are called *Beau's lines*. They are associated with a severe illness that temporarily interrupts nail formation. (Objective 50)

31. Place the patient 20 feet from the wall chart or 14 inches from the visual acuity card. Ask him or her to cover one eye and begin reading the lines. Record the visual acuity grade next to the smallest line in which he or she can read at least one half of the letters. (Objective 52)

32. Have the patient count your raised fingers or read from a distance something you have printed. (Objective 52)

Multiple Choice

1. B. Considering this information, the most appropriate examination for the paramedic to perform on this patient would be a focused examination on the injured extremity. The patient has suffered trauma from a mechanism of injury that involved a minimal amount of energy, is conscious, and is able to provide you with a history to focus the examination. (Objectives 43, 44)

2. D. Your *initial efforts* should be directed toward supporting his respirations and beginning therapy for shock. This patient has immediate life-threatening problems that must be corrected before a secondary survey is performed or orthopedic and soft tissue injuries are addressed. (Objectives 24, 35)

3. C. Based upon this information, the most descriptive and accurate assessment statement is that the patient responds to a painful stimulus with decerebrate posturing. Extension of the upper extremities in response to painful stimulation is decerebrate posturing. (Objective 87)

4. A. The purpose of the primary survey (initial assessment) is to identify any immediate life-threatening problems. (Objective 24)

5. D. The most accurate and complete way to document these findings is pupils are equal, round, reactive to light with accommodation intact (PERRLA). (Objective 56)

6. D. The spurting hemorrhage should be treated first because it indicates arterial hemorrhage, a life-threatening problem. (Objective 28)

7. D. The first step you should take when you arrive on the scene of a motor vehicle collision is to survey for any special problems or hazards. (Objective 13)

8. C. Partial airway obstruction with poor air exchange should be managed first. Securing an adequate airway takes priority over all other problems. (Objective 26)

9. C. The first step during the primary survey (initial assessment always is to check for an open airway. (Objective 26)

10. C. Vital signs should be reassessed several times during transport. The principal value of vital signs is in detecting trends over time. To detect trends several sets of vital signs must be taken. (Objective 6)

11. C. The purpose of the secondary survey (focused or detailed physical examination) is to detect less obvious signs. (Objectives 43, 44)

12. B. The first information a paramedic should obtain from a conscious patient is the chief complaint.

13. A. The best description of a patient's mental status is "the patient responded to a painful stimulus by opening his eyes, moaning, and trying to push my hand away." This description documents the patient's responses to specific stimuli precisely. Therefore it allows the examination to be duplicated precisely at a later time to detect changes. (Objective 12)

14. B. The carotid pulse would be the last to vanish in a patient with decompensated shock. (Objective 32)

15. C. When you are assessing a patient with a chief complaint of abdominal pain, auscultation of the abdomen should be performed primarily to detect presence or absence of bowel sounds. An accurate assessment of bowel sounds involves listening with the diaphragm of the stethoscope over each quadrant for 1 minute. Auscultation should take place before palpation because palpation can cause falsely hyperactive sounds. (Objective 74)

16. B. The most probable cause of these signs and symptoms is occlusion of the extremity's arterial supply. (Objectives 70, 85)

17. B. If a patient is unstable, an ongoing assessment should be performed every 5 minutes. (Objectives 89, 90)

18. A. If a patient is stable, an ongoing assessment should be performed every 15 minutes. (Objectives 89, 90)

19. A. Light popping, nonmusical lung sounds heard during inspiration are crackles. (Objective 68)

20. C. Clubbing of the nailbeds is associated with diseases causing chronic hypoxia. (Objective 50)

21. A. The cranial nerve associated with the sense of smell is cranial nerve I. (Objective 86)

22. C. The most descriptive and accurate assessment statement is that the patient is responsive to a painful stimulus with decorticate posturing.

23. A. When using the otoscope to view the tympanic membrane, a normal appearance would be for the membrane to be concave with a visible cone of light. (Objective 59)

24. A. Hemothorax of the left chest would most likely be responsible for these findings. A tension pneumothorax would produce hyperresonance. (Objective 66)

25. B. Closing of the mitral and tricuspid valves as the ventricles contract produces the S_1 sound. The aortic and pulmonic valves are the semilunar valves, and their contraction produces the S_2 sound. (Objective 72)

26. C. Jugular venous distention is best assessed while the patient is sitting upright and at a 45-degree angle. (Objective 64)

27. D. The vital signs are not consistent with predictable changes that occur because of body position.
Sitting up or standing normally will produce a slight increase in heart rate and blood pressure. If a patient is hypovolemic, sitting up or standing will produce a rise in heart rate and a drop in blood pressure. This patient's responses are consistent with neither of these expected sets of changes. (Objective 70)

28. B. He is alert and oriented to person and place only. (Objectives 11, 12)

29. C. Cranial nerve V provides sensation over the face and motor function for the muscles of chewing. (Objective 86)

30. B. The "lub" of the heart sounds represents closing of the mitral and tricuspid valves. (Objective 68)

31. B. Wheezing is best described as high-pitched sounds caused by constriction of the smaller airways.

Disease processes other than asthma can produce wheezing. (Objective 65)

32. C. The S$_3$ heart sound is most commonly associated with congestive heart failure. (Objective 68)

33. B. The sounds of bruits are associated with turbulent blood flow in narrowed blood vessels. (Objectives 61, 62)

34. A. Because a hyphema is present in the anterior chamber, it will be visible without increasing the depth of focus. Lesions such as cataracts and vitreous hemorrhages also are usually visible without increasing the depth of focus. Viewing the retina, the optic blood vessels, and the optic disc requires progressive increases in the depth of focus. (Objective 57)

35. B. Diabetes mellitus produces retinal hemorrhages. (Objective 2)

36. B. A patient who has flat neck veins when lying supine probably is hypovolemic. The neck veins should be slightly distended when the patient is supine. Tension pneumothorax, right-sided heart failure, and cardiac tamponade will produce distended neck veins, even with the patient in a semisitting position. (Objectives 64, 65)

37. A. Battle's sign suggests the presence of a basilar skull fracture. (Objective 54)

38. B. Rales (crackles), increased fremitus, and presence of egophony and bronchophony are consistent with the presence of pus and other fluid in the alveoli and small airways. Presence of fluid in the alveoli and small airways increases the transmission of vibrations to the lung periphery and chest wall, increasing fremitus and producing egophony and bronchophony. Fluid or air in the pleural space will decrease lung sounds and fremitus by separating the lung from the chest wall. (Objectives 66, 68)

39. A. Bronchovesicular breath sounds are most easily heard between the scapulae or at the second or third intercostal space lateral to the sternum. Bronchovesicular sounds represent the transition zone from the bronchial sounds produced by air movement in the larger airways and the vesicular sounds produced by air movement in the alveoli and smaller airways. (Objective 65)

40. C. Vesicular sounds are soft, swishy, and lowest pitched. (Objective 65)

41. C. The sound of the aortic valve is best auscultated at the second intercostal space at the right of the sternum. (Objective 68)

42. C. Kyphosis is exaggerated thoracic concavity, also called hunchback. (Objective 85)

43. D. Scoliosis is lateral spinal curvature. (Objective 85)

44. D. Increased muscle tone when passive movement is applied, especially at the end of the range of motion, is spasticity. (Objective 85)

45. C. Increased resistance to active movement throughout the entire range of motion is rigidity. (Objective 85)

46. A. Loss of muscle tone, causing the limb to be loose, is flaccidity. (Objective 85)

47. B. Sudden changes in muscle tone during passive movement, resulting in either increased or decreased resistance, are paratonia. (Objective 85)

Case Studies

Case one

1. A detailed examination should be performed. (Objectives 40, 41)

2. The mechanism of injury released a large amount of energy that could have produced injuries other than those immediately obvious to the patient. (Objectives 40, 41)

Case two

1. A focused examination should be performed. (Objectives 40, 41)

2. The mechanism of injury released a minimal amount of energy. The patient's injuries are probably limited to the areas where he is experiencing pain. (Objectives 40, 41)

Case three

1. A focused examination of the cardiovascular system should be performed (Objectives 43, 44)

2. The patient is conscious and is able to provide a chief complaint and history that suggest the problem involves his cardiovascular system, specifically the heart. (Objectives 40, 41)

Case four

1. A detailed examination should be performed. (Objectives 40, 41)

2. This patient appears to be suffering from a medical problem, although trauma cannot be entirely ruled out. Because he is unable to provide a chief complaint and history, a detailed examination is necessary to identify signs that will help establish a field diagnosis. (Objectives 40, 41)

Case five

1. Absence of distal pulses and cold, cyanotic skin in the distal extremity suggest that the extremity's arterial blood flow has been interrupted, probably by damage at the fracture site. (Objective 85)

Case six

1. Priorities are support of airway, oxygenation, and ventilation while maintaining manual stabilization of the cervical spine; decompression of a possible tension pneumothorax on the left side of the chest; control of external bleeding from the open femur fracture; application of a cervical collar, long spine board, and cervical immobilization device; and rapid transport with IVs being established in route for volume replacement. (Objectives 24, 25, 35, 36)

2. Problems identified during the initial assessment should be addressed in an A-B-C sequence. A trauma patient with absent or diminished breath sounds on

one side of the chest accompanied by signs of shock should be treated for a tension pneumothorax by performing a pleural decompression. External bleeding should be controlled in the field to avoid worsening the effects of internal blood loss. IV access for volume replacement should take place in route. There is no way to know whether IVs established in the field will be able to keep up with the rate of blood loss. Therefore remaining on the scene to establish IV access delays definitive care in the operating room with no guarantee of adequately replacing the lost blood volume. (Objectives 24, 25, 35, 36)

Case seven

1. The patient probably has pneumonia in the right middle lobe of the lung associated with pleurisy. (Objectives 65)
2. The presence of a fever suggests an infection. The productive cough with infected sputum suggests a pulmonary infection. Pain in the right chest suggests the infection is in the right lung. The presence of crackles, bronchophony, and whispered pectoriloquy in the right middle lobe suggest infectious fluids in the small airways and alveoli (i.e., pneumonia). The presence of a pleural rub suggests inflammation also has spread to the pleura, causing pleurisy. (Objectives 65)

Case eight

1. Congestive heart failure with pulmonary edema and ventilatory failure. (Objectives 63, 65, 68, 69)
2. The presence of a third heart sound suggests congestive heart failure. The presence of distended neck veins and pitting edema of the extremities is consistent with right-sided heart failure. The presence of crackles and wheezing are consistent with pulmonary edema produced by left-sided heart failure. The clinical presentation of paroxysmal nocturnal dyspnea also is characteristic of pulmonary edema secondary to congestive heart failure. The patient's use of her respiratory accessory muscles indicates that she is in ventilatory failure because she cannot maintain an adequate minute volume using her chest wall and diaphragm alone. (Objectives 63, 65, 68, 69)

Case nine

1. The patient has ascites secondary to hepatic cirrhosis. (Objectives 50, 75)
2. The presence of ascites is indicated by abdominal distention, dullness of the abdomen to percussion, and the presence of an abdominal fluid wave. Hepatic cirrhosis can produce ascites by causing hypertension in the hepatic portal circulation. The presence of jaundice, enlarged veins radiating from the umbilicus, tenderness in the right upper abdominal quadrant, and emaciation suggests hepatic cirrhosis. This classic clinical presentation of jaundice, distended abdomen, and emaciated extremities is sometimes referred to as the "lemon on toothpicks" appearance. (Objectives 50, 75)

Case ten

1. The patient has facial neuritis, also known as Bell's palsy. (Objective 87)
2. Bell's palsy is caused by inflammation of cranial nerve VII. (Objective 87)
3. The cranial nerve controls the muscles of facial expression, accounting for the paralysis of one side of her face. Cranial nerve VII also controls taste over the anterior two thirds of the tongue, explaining the alterations in the patient's sense of taste. (Objective 87)

Case eleven

1. Occlusion of the arterial blood supply to the distal left lower extremity secondary to peripheral vascular disease associated with diabetes mellitus. (Objectives 70, 85)
2. Pulselessness, paresthesias, pallor, paralysis, and coolness to touch indicate loss of arterial blood flow to an extremity. The patient reports having experienced pain and cramping in the extremity during exertion for 2 weeks. This phenomenon, called intermittent claudication, suggests narrowing of an artery by peripheral vascular disease. Diabetes mellitus tends to produce rapidly progressing atherosclerotic vascular disease. (Objectives 70, 85)

Case twelve

1. Deep vein thrombophlebitis in the left lower extremity. (Objectives 70, 85)
2. Fever suggests the presence of an infectious or inflammatory process. The dull pain in the distal left lower extremity localizes the problem to this area. The warmth, edema, and purplish-red discoloration suggest something is interfering with the venous return from the affected extremity. Weak pulses and sluggish capillary refill indicate that the arterial circulation is present but is being obstructed by the slow venous return. Pain in the posterior calf when attempting to dorsiflex the foot is Homan's sign. It suggests the presence of deep vein thrombophlebitis. The ropelike structure in the back of the calf is the thrombosed vein. (Objectives 70, 85)

Case thirteen

1. The patient has suffered an injury to cranial nerve III, the oculomotor nerve. (Objectives 56, 86)
2. The oculomotor nerve controls pupillary response. It also controls all extraocular movements except the ability to look outward, which is controlled by the abducens nerve, and the ability to look outward and upward, which is controlled by the trochlear nerve. (Objectives 56, 86)

Case fourteen

1. Compromise of the arterial blood flow to the left forearm secondary to brachial artery injury at the site of the humerus fracture. (Objectives 70, 85)
2. The radial pulse will be absent. Capillary refill will be absent or very sluggish. (Objectives 70, 85)

CHAPTER 18: COMMUNICATION

Short Answer

1. a. Simplex: A simplex communications system uses radios that transmit and receive on the same frequency. This means that only one radio in the system can transmit at a time.

   b. Duplex: A duplex communications system uses radios that transmit and receive on different frequencies. The paired receive and transmit frequencies in a duplex system are referred to as a channel. In a duplex system, radios can transmit and receive simultaneously, allowing communications to take place as if they were going over a telephone line.

   c. Multiplex: A multiplex system has the capability of transmitting two signals, usually voice and ECG, on the same frequency. This capability allows a paramedic to transmit ECG telemetry to a hospital while continuing to talk with the on-line medical control physician.

   d. Trunked systems pool several frequencies and use a computer to route incoming transmissions to the next available frequency. Trunking frees the dispatcher or field unit from having to search for an available frequency. (Objective 16)

2. Verbal. Written. Electronic. (Objective 2)

3. Communication between the party requesting help and the dispatcher. Communication between the dispatcher and the paramedic. Communication between the paramedic, patient, receiving facility, and/or medical direction physician.
   Communication with receiving facility personnel on transfer of care. (Objective 2)

4. A repeater receives a signal on one frequency and retransmits it at a higher power on a different frequency. Repeaters extend the range of mobile and portable radios in a communications system. (Objective 14)

5. An encoder is like a combination lock on a radio. By transmitting a series of tones, a transmitting station can unlock the receiver at a particular radio so it can receive traffic intended for it. The advantage of encoders in an EMS communications system is that they keep hospital personnel from having to listen to communications not intended for their facility. (Objective 14)

6. Cellular telephone. Facsimile. Computer. (Objective 12)

7. Advantages of UHF are the fact that they have high penetrating power, are less susceptible to interference than VHF, and can easily pass through buildings. Disadvantages are that they only travel a short distance and are limited to line of sight. Because of the shorter ranges of UHF and penetrating ability, they are more applicable to urban areas. Advantages of VHF are the distances they can travel; however, these frequencies are susceptible to interference from buildings, electrical equipment, and weather. This frequency range is generally more advantageous for rural areas where there are large distances to cover with minimal physical structures to block the waves. VHF low-band frequencies have the ability to follow the curvature of the earth and have the greatest range of the VHF frequencies. VHF high-band frequencies are limited to line of sight, but are less susceptible to interference than VHF low-band frequencies. (Objective 14)

8. The Federal Communications Commission (FCC) regulates the use of radio frequencies in the United States. (Objective 15)

9. The FCC licenses and allocates radio frequencies, establishes technical standards for radio equipment, licenses and regulates technical personnel who repair and operate radio equipment, monitors frequencies to ensure appropriate use, and conducts spot-checks of base stations and dispatch centers for appropriate licenses and records. (Objective 15)

10. Monitoring the frequency before transmitting helps avoid interrupting someone else who already is talking on the frequency. Interrupting the use of a frequency is referred to as "walking on" the user and is considered to be poor manners. (Objective 5)

11. The microphone should be keyed for about 2 seconds before beginning to transmit to allow the repeaters in the communications time to prepare to receive the signal. The microphone should be left keyed for about 2 seconds after the message ends to avoid cutting off the last few words. (Objectives 20, 21)

12. Prearrival instructions are directions for appropriate initial emergency care read to a caller by a trained dispatcher while EMS personnel are responding. (Objective 19)

13.

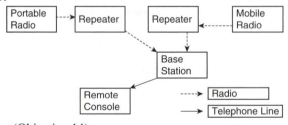

(Objective 14)

Multiple Choice

1. C. Your radio transmission range will be increased by the fact that the radio system has a repeater. You will not be able to transmit ECG data while talking with medical control because the system does not have multiplex capability. You must wait to begin talking after pushing the push to talk button to give the repeater time to prepare to receive the signal. (Objective 14)

2. B. In emergency services communications, the public safety answering point (PSAP) refers to the single location where 9-1-1 calls from a specific geographic area are routed for answering. (Objective 18)

3. A. The purpose of an encoder in an EMS communications system is to allow base stations to share a frequency without having to listen to traffic not intended for them. (Objective 14)

4. B. In a simplex radio system, only one frequency is used and only one unit can transmit at a time. (Objective 16)

5. B. The EMS dispatcher determines the crew and vehicle that will respond to a call. (Objective 17)

6. D. When a radio system has multiplex capability, it can transmit two different signals (e.g., voice and ECG on the same frequency) simultaneously. (Objective 16)

7. B. UHF has better penetration in metropolitan areas. VHF has a greater range than UHF but is more susceptible to interference. (Objective 14)

8. D. Repeaters extend the range of mobile radios by receiving signals and retransmitting them at higher power on a different frequency. (Objective 14)

9. A. The government agency that controls radio frequency allocations and regulates radio use is the Federal Communications Commission. (Objective 15)

10. B. Radio reports to medical facilities always should follow a standard format because significant information is less likely to be omitted and hospital personnel are less likely to miss significant details. (Objective 21)

11. A. The principal transmitter and receiver of a communications system is the base station. (Objective 14)

Case Study

1. Patient identification: We have a 24-year-old male who is awake and responding appropriately to questions.

   Mechanism of injury: He was involved in a single vehicle collision with a concrete retaining wall. There was significant intrusion to the vehicle's passenger compartment. There are no other patients involved.

   Subjective data: He complains of pain in his right chest and of a headache. He has a history of hypertension and thyroid disease and takes hydro-chlorothiazide and L-thyroxine daily.

   Objective data: Vital Signs are: BP—118/70 mm Hg, P—144 beats/min, R—28 breaths/min. There is a hematoma to the left forehead and bruising under both eyes. Pupils are dilated, equal, and reactive. He is able to follow a penlight with his eyes. He responds to requests to open his mouth, stick out his tongue, and swallow. Lung sounds are clear on the left and diminished with wheezes on the right. His abdomen is soft and nontender. He has a possible fracture of the left arm. He is able to move his hands and feet.

   Plan: We have provided full spinal motion restriction. The patient is receiving supplemental oxygen. We have established IV access and have splinted the left arm. We are transporting code 3. (Objective 21)

CHAPTER 19: DOCUMENTATION

Short Answer

1. Medical: Helping to ensure continuity of patient care

   Administrative: Quality improvement, billing

   Research: Evaluation of efficacy of system design, protocols, procedures, equipment

   Legal: Documentation of actions taken during a call that can be presented during court proceedings (Objective 2)

2. Make a single line through the error so it is still readable. Initial and date the error. Then write in the correct information. (Objectives 1, 4)

3. Inform your supervisor that a correction needs to be made. Prepare an addendum to the original report that corrects the error. Date and sign the addendum. Ensure the addendum is attached to the original report, and that the original report is marked with a note to "see addendum." Ensure all holders of copies of the report receive copies of the addendum. (Objective 15)

4. A properly completed EMS run report is accurate, complete, legible, and free of extraneous or unprofessional information. It is completed and filed in a timely manner. (Objectives 8, 15)

5. "The patient was drunk." Without access to blood alcohol levels it is impossible to determine whether a patient is intoxicated. A more appropriate report might state that the patient was confused, had slurred speech, and walked with an ataxic gait without speculating on the cause. The patient may, in fact, have a head injury, be hypoxic, or be suffering from hypoperfusion or hypoglycemia. (Objective 11)

   "The patient was shocky." *Shocky is a* nonspecific term. It would be more appropriate to report that the patient was restless and anxious and had rapid, shallow respirations; cool, pale, moist skin; rapid, weak peripheral pulses; and prolonged capillary refill time. (Objective 11)

   "Vital signs: Pulse—normal; Respirations—normal; BP—120/80." A normal heart rate and respirations can vary significantly with patient age, size, and physical condition. Without numbers for these vital signs, it could be difficult to justify a field diagnosis or therapy provided on the basis of that diagnosis. It also would be difficult to demonstrate that trends in the vital signs were monitored appropriately. (Objective 11)

6. **Subjective:** information obtained from the patient history

   Chief complaint

   History of present illness

   Past history

   Current health status

   Family history

   Psychosocial history

   Review of systems

Objective: information obtained from the physical examination
- Vital signs
- General impression
- Physical exam
- Diagnostic tests

Assessment: a statement of the field diagnosis

Plan: all treatment provided to the patient
- Standing orders
- Physician orders
- Effects of interventions
- Mode of transportation
- Ongoing assessment

(Objective 10)

7. **Chief complaint**

History
- History of present illness
- Past history
- Current health status
- Review of systems

Assessment
- Vital signs
- General impression
- Diagnostic tests
- Field diagnosis

Rx (treatment)
- Standing orders
- Physician orders

Transport
- Effects of interventions
- Mode of transportation
- Ongoing assessment

(Objective 10)

8. A thorough patient assessment. An assessment of the patient's capacity to refuse care. Your recommendations for care and transport. Explanations to the patient about possible consequences of refusing care and transport. Other suggestions for accessing care. Willingness to return if the patient changes his/her mind. The patient's understanding of statements and suggestions and apparent capacity to refuse care based on that understanding. (Objective 13)

9.

Chief complaint	CC
Date of birth	DOB
History	Hx
Signs and symptoms	S/S
Vital signs	VS
Abdominal aortic aneurysm	AAA
Left upper quadrant	LUQ
As needed	prn
Within normal limits	WNL

(Objectives 6, 7)

10.

PERRLA	Pupils equal, round, reactive to light and accommodation
IDDM	Insulin-dependent diabetes mellitus
HPI	History of present illness
EtOH	Ethyl alcohol
CHF	Congestive heart failure
HTN	Hypertension

CABG	Coronary artery bypass graft
npo	Nothing by mouth

(Objectives 6, 7)

Multiple Choice

1. A. "A BP could not be obtained because of massive extremity trauma." This clear documentation of the facts explains why important information was omitted from the report. Stating that a patient was drunk is speculation based on signs that could be caused by other problems. The term *shocky* is vague and nondescriptive of the patient's presentation. The statement that vital signs were normal omits essential information and raises the question of what *normal* means. (Objective 12)

2. C. In the subjective section state that the patient says she ingested six of her prescription Prozac and reports a history of depression. The fact that a bottle of Prozac was found near the patient is an objective observation. The fact that the patient says she took six Prozac is subjective, not objective information. An appropriate assessment would be "possible ingestion of six Prozac." Attempting to infer the patient's intent would not be appropriate. (Objectives 4, 11, 12)

3. C. Jaundice is a sign because it is an objective observation made by the paramedic. Headache, dizziness, and nausea are all symptoms, subjective information that must be reported by the patient. (Objective 11)

4. A. Chest pain is a symptom because it is subjective information that must be reported by the patient. Cyanosis, diaphoresis, and vomiting are all signs and objective observations that can be made by the paramedic. (Objective 11)

5. D. This information should be included in the subjective section of your report because it is based on information told to you by the patient rather than something you can directly observe. (Objective 11)

6. C. If you make an error while writing a run report form, you should draw a single line through the error, write in the correct information, and initial the change. (Objectives 1, 15)

7. C. Writing on a PCR that a patient "probably has AIDS secondary to IV substance abuse" could place you at risk of being sued for libel. Libel is putting untrue information in written form that damages a person's reputation. Slander is saying untrue things about a person that damages a person's reputation. (Objectives 1, 12)

8. C. The prehospital care report becomes documentation of care, a legal record, and a source of information for research and quality improvement. (Objective 2)

9. A. If an error is discovered after a prehospital care report is submitted, you should draw a single line through the error, write a note with the correct information at the end of the report, initial and date all changes, and distribute the corrected report to all appropriate personnel. (Objectives 1, 15)

Case Studies

Case one

1. **Subjective**

    Chief complaint: 24-year-old male complaining of pain in right chest and a headache

    Past history: Hypertension and thyroid disease

    Current health status: Medications—takes hydrochlorothiazide and L-thyroxine daily

    Objective

    General: Driver of vehicle involved in vehicle vs. concrete retaining wall collision

    No other patients

    Significant intrusion of vehicle's passenger compartment

    Patient awake and responds appropriately to questions

    Vital signs: BP—118/70 mm Hg, P—144 beats/min, R—28 breaths/min

    HEENT: Hematoma to left forehead; bruising under both eyes; pupils dilated, equal, and reactive; able to follow penlight with his eyes; able to open mouth, stick out tongue, and swallow

    Chest: Lung sounds clear on left, diminished with wheezes on right

    Abdomen: Soft, nontender

    Extremities: Able to move feet and hands

    Assessment

    Facial trauma, r/o basilar skull fracture, possible chest trauma, r/o right simple pneumothorax, r/o right pulmonary contusion

    Plan

    On-scene: Oxygen provided before beginning rapid trauma assessment

    Spinal motion restriction using back board, cervical collar, head blocks, tape, spider straps

    Transport: Transported code 3 by ground ambulance to community level I trauma center

    IV access established in route

    Left arm splinted in route

    Arrival: Transferred care to nurse Jones

    (Objectives 4, 5, 10, 11, 15)

Case two

1. **Complaint**

    Chief complaint: The patient is a 40-year-old male who denies pain, difficulty breathing, and any other complaints. States he "simply wants to go home."

    History

    Past history: Seizure disorder. Denies any other significant medical history.

    Current health status: Medications—Dilantin for seizures. Patient states he is taking his Dilantin daily, as prescribed. Takes no other medications.

    Assessment

    General: Responded to report of possible seizure patient in parking lot of grocery store. Patient presented sitting on curb. Initially awake and alert, but confused. During examination patient's orientation improved. Patient no longer confused. Patient aware of his name, location, and day of week.

Vital signs: BP—140/88 mm Hg, P—110 beats/min, R—20 breaths/min, skin—warm and sweaty

HEENT: Patient appears to have bitten his tongue. Odor of alcoholic beverage noted on breath.

Neck: No injuries or other abnormalities noted.

Chest: No injuries or other abnormalities noted.

Abdomen: No injuries or other abnormalities noted.

Pelvis: No injuries or other abnormalities noted.

Extremities: No injuries or other abnormalities noted.

Posterior: No injuries or other abnormalities noted.

Labs: Deferred

Possible postictal state from seizure

Rx (Treatment)

No treatment provided

Transport

On-scene: Transportation to the emergency department was offered.

Patient refused transport to hospital and stated he wanted to go home. Patient lives only 3 blocks away.

Patient was advised of suspected possible seizure, that his medications might not longer be adequately controlling his seizure disorders, and that additional seizures possibly could occur, resulting in injury or complications such as aspiration. The patient stated that he understood and continued to refuse treatment. The patient was advised to contact his physician and advise him of the seizure. He also was advised to contact EMS if he changed his mind regarding transport to the emergency department. The patient seemed to understand these suggestions.

(Objectives 3, 4, 10, 11, 13, 15)

CHAPTER 20: HEAD, EAR, EYE, NOSE, AND THROAT DISORDERS

Short Answer

1. Nits are white, shiny clusters near the hair roots that do not fall off readily. Dandruff appears as flakes on the scalp and will fall off readily when the hair is parted. (Objective 1)

2. The patient will complain of pain in the ear that is worsened by gentle traction on the external ear. The lining of the external auditory canal will be red and swollen. An accumulation of moist debris may be present in the external auditory canal. The patient may complain of decreased hearing on the affected side caused by edema closing the auditory canal. (Objective 5)

3. The patient will complain of a sore throat that becomes progressively more severe and more unilateral. Pain may be referred to the neck and ear. The patient also may complain of difficulty swallowing or opening the mouth. Edema of the tissues lateral and superior to the affected tonsil will be present with medial and/or anterior displacement of the involved tonsil. The uvula will be displaced to the opposite side of the pharynx. Fever and tachycardia will be present. The patient may be drooling. (Objective 9)

4. Patients with peritonsillar abscess can gag or choke, rupturing the abscess and aspirating infected materials into their lungs. Smaller children with peritonsillar abscess may be at risk for airway obstruction from associated edema in the pharynx and larynx. (Objective 10)

5. Nasal foreign bodies should not be removed in the prehospital setting. The parent or guardian should be instructed to take the child to a hospital, urgent care center, or physician's office for treatment. (Objective 8)

6. Vertigo is the sensation of spinning or whirling that occurs as a result of a disturbance in equilibrium. A patient who feels as if his or her head is spinning has subjective vertigo. A patient who feels as if objects are spinning around him or her has objective vertigo. (Objective 5)

7. Thrush is an infection with the fungus *Candida albicans* that produces white, scaly patches on the tongue, inside the mouth, and in the throat that can ulcerate if left untreated. Thrush is most common in newborns and very young children but can occur in immunocompromised adults. (Objective 9)

8. The patient should be assessed for injury of the jaw, face, and head. Once the face has been determined to be intact, the tooth and tooth socket should be evaluated.
   If the patient is alert, the tooth should be rinsed gently with clean water and reinserted into the socket. If the tooth cannot be reinserted, it should be placed in milk or an appropriate "tooth saver" solution as quickly as possible and transported with the patient to the hospital. (Objective 10)

9. Tinnitus is a constant buzzing or humming sound. This patient should be asked if she has been taking more aspirin than usual to control the pain of her osteoarthritis. Aspirin toxicity is a common cause of tinnitus. (Objective 5)

10. A patient with epistaxis should lean forward to keep blood from draining into the oropharynx. (Objective 8)

Multiple Choice

1. B. Loss of hearing, itching, discharge, and tenderness when the ear is tugged indicate otitis externa. (Objective 5)

2. A. You should suspect acute glaucoma. A cerebrovascular accident would be associated with more widespread neurologic deficits and would be more likely to cause a headache than eye pain. Digitalis toxicity does not cause pain. Retinal detachment causes painless loss of vision. (Objective 3)

3. B. Painless loss of vision in one eye that occurs rapidly and completely most likely is the result of central retinal artery occlusion. Acute glaucoma causes pain. Retinal detachment causes painless loss of vision but typically produces the sensation of an object floating in the visual field rather than a progressive graying out of vision. A cerebrovascular accident would be expected to produce more widespread neurologic deficits. (Objective 3)

4. A. The patient has Bell's palsy, also known as facial neuritis. (Objective 1)

5. C. Bell's palsy is due to inflammation of cranial nerve VII, the facial nerve. (Objective 1)

6. C. Cluster headaches occur more commonly in males than in females. Cluster headaches typically begin during adulthood. They are felt on one side of the head as a burning or stabbing sensation. (Objective 1)

7. C. Classic migraine headaches involve one side of the head and last for hours to days. (Objective 1)

8. C. Headaches associated with muscle tension produce pain that is throbbing. Tension headaches affect both genders equally. (Objective 1)

9. B. This patient has Ludwig's angina. (Objective 2)

10. A. Ludwig's angina is an immediate life-threatening condition because it can cause loss of the airway. (Objective 2)

11. B. An infection of the oil glands of the eyelid, commonly called a stye, also is known as a hordeolum. (Objective 3)

12. B. Chronic glaucoma produces gradual loss of peripheral vision, creating the sensation of looking down a tunnel. (Objective 3)

13. A. This patient has epiglottitis, which puts him at risk for complete airway obstruction. (Objective 9)

14. A. A honey-colored crust formed from the exudate released as the vesicles rupture characterizes impetigo. The lesions of impetigo are not associated with fever and typically appear on the face and extremities. Poison ivy is more likely to cause lesions on the extremities than on the face. (Objective 1)

Case Study

1. The patient is suffering from acute glaucoma. (Objective 3)

2. Acute glaucoma is caused by a shift in the position of the iris that blocks the canals that drain aqueous humor from the anterior chamber of the eye. This results in a quick, severe, and painful increase in intraocular pressure. (Objective 3)

3. The patient should be transported immediately for evaluation and treatment by an ophthalmologist. (Objective 4)

4. Timolol is a beta-blocker that prevents dilation of the pupil, reducing the chance that the iris will obstruct the outflow of aqueous humor from the anterior chamber. Some patients with acute glaucoma require an iridotomy, a surgical procedure that uses a laser to open a new channel in the iris to improve drainage of aqueous humor. (Objective 4)

CHAPTER 21: PULMONOLOGY

Matching

1. __A__ Air sacs in which gas exchange occurs
   __G__ Double membrane covering lungs
   __D__ Flap covering the windpipe's opening
   __C__ Point where mainstem bronchi branch

331

__B__	Smallest airways in respiratory tract	
__I__	Space between epiglottis and base of tongue	
__E__	Voice box	
__H__	Windpipe	
__F__	Throat (Objectives 3, 7)	

2.   __A__   80% of cases begin before age 30

     __A__   Bronchospasm, excess mucus, bronchial edema

     __B__   Cyanosis present early in course of disease

     __C__   Cyanosis present only late in course of disease

     __B__   Excess bronchial mucus for at least 3 months for 2 successive years

     __C__   Progressive loss of alveolar wall elasticity

     __A__   Reversible obstructive airway disease (Objective 8)

3.   __A__   Fine bubbling sounds caused by fluid in smaller airways and alveoli; do not change with coughing

     __D__   Harsh sound produced by partial obstruction of upper airway by base of tongue

     __E__   High-pitched, crowing sound on inspiration caused by narrowing of upper airway

     __C__   Rattling sound from mucus obstruction of larger airway; disappears or changes location and quality with coughing

     __B__   Sound like two pieces of dry leather moving across each other; associated with inflammation of chest cavity's lining

     __F__   Whistling sound primarily on exhalation as air moves through narrow lower airways (Objectives 4, 5, 6, 8, 9)

Short Answer

1. Complete the following chart contrasting croup (laryngotracheobronchitis) and epiglottitis. (Objective 4)

	Croup	Epiglottitis
Age group	6 months to 6 years	1 to 6 years, adults
Type of organism	Viral	Bacterial
Speed of onset	Gradual (several days)	Rapid (hours)
Fever	Low	High
Drooling	Absent	Present
Sore throat	Mild or absent	Severe

2. The nasal cavity warms, humidifies, and filters inhaled air. (Objective 3)
3. The thyroid cartilage. (Objective 3)
4. The cricoid cartilage. (Objective 3)
5. The cricoid cartilage. (Objective 3)
6. The cricothyroid membrane. (Objective 3)
7. The right mainstem bronchus is shorter and straighter than the left because the left mainstem bronchus must extend past the heart to enter the left lung. (Objective 7)

8. The right lung has three lobes. The left lung has two lobes. The left lung's middle lobe is absent to create a space that the heart occupies. (Objective 7)
9. The pleura. (Objective 7)
10. Bronchioles do not have cartilage in their walls. (Objective 7)
11. Gases move between the alveoli and the pulmonary capillaries by diffusion along concentration gradients. (Objective 7)
12. The phrenic nerve. (Objective 7)
13. The phrenic nerve arises from the spinal cord at the level of the third, fourth, and fifth cervical vertebrae. (Objective 7)
14. When a patient inhales, the diaphragm and intercostal muscles contract. (Objective 6)
15. Contraction of the diaphragm and intercostal muscles increases intrathoracic volume and decreases intrathoracic pressure. (Objective 6)
16. Inhalation is an active process. (Objective 6)
17. When a patient exhales, the diaphragm and intercostal muscles relax. (Objective 6)
18. Relaxation of the diaphragm and the intercostal muscles allows the lungs to recoil to their resting position, pulling the chest wall inward. The intrathoracic volume decreases and the intrathoracic pressure increases. (Objective 6)
19. Exhalation is a passive process. (Objective 6)
20. Respirations normally are stimulated by an increase in the arterial carbon dioxide level. (Objective 6)
21. The hypoxic drive provides the backup to the respiratory drive. (Objective 6)
22. The hypoxic drive is triggered by a decrease in arterial oxygen levels. (Objective 6)
23. Patients with chronic obstructive pulmonary disease have increased arterial carbon dioxide levels. (Objective 6)
24. Because COPD patients have chronically elevated arterial carbon dioxide levels, the respiratory center stops responding to changes in $PaCO_2$. The patient will rely on the hypoxic drive to stimulate respirations. (Objective 6)
25. Giving high-concentration oxygen to a patient who is breathing on his/her hypoxic drive can theoretically result in respiratory depression. However, this is unlikely and oxygen should never be withheld from a patient in respiratory distress. (Objective 6)
26. No. If a patient with COPD needs oxygen to correct hypoxia, oxygen should be given. Oxygen is essential for life processes to continue. (Objective 8)
27. 500 mL/breath × 20 breaths/min = 10,000 mL/min. (Objective 3)
28. The vital capacity is the maximum amount of air that can be exhaled following the deepest possible inhalation. (Objective 8)
29. Elasticity, also called *elastic recoil*. (Objective 3)
30. Emphysema decreases the elasticity of the lungs. (Objective 8)
31. Surfactant is a substance produced by the type II pneumocytes that reduces the surface tension of

the water on the inner surface of the alveoli. This effect helps keep the alveoli from collapsing. (Objective 8)

32. The anatomic dead air space is the portion of the respiratory tract where gas exchange with the blood does not take place. (Objective 2)

33. 35 to 45 mm Hg. (Objective 2)

34. 80 to 100 mm Hg. (Objective 2)

35. Atelectasis is localized collapse of the alveoli. (Objective 8)

36. Because atelectasis will result in blood flowing past alveoli that are not being ventilated, extensive atelectasis will cause the $PaCO_2$ to increase and the PaO_2 to decrease. (Objective 8)

37. If the respiratory rate and tidal volume decrease, the $PaCO_2$ will increase. (Objectives 7, 8)

38. If the respiratory rate and tidal volume increase, the $PaCO_2$ will decrease. (Objectives 7, 8)

39. Most of the oxygen transported by blood is carried in the form of oxyhemoglobin inside the erythrocytes. (Objective 7)

40. Most of the carbon dioxide carried by the blood is transported as bicarbonate in the plasma. (Objective 7)

41. A fall in the PaO_2 to below 60 torr moves the patient onto the "steep" portion of the oxyhemoglobin dissociation curve. This means that hemoglobin will on-load and off-load oxygen more easily. Small changes in PaO_2 will produce large changes in hemoglobin oxygen saturation. (Objective 2)

42. Acidosis and hyperthermia shift the oxyhemoglobin dissociation curve to the right. The affinity of hemoglobin for oxygen will decrease. (Objective 2)

43. Alkalosis and hypothermia will shift the oxyhemoglobin dissociation curve to the left. The affinity of hemoglobin for oxygen will increase. (Objective 2)

44. Pulse rate will increase. Skeletal muscles may display fine tremors. Level of consciousness will increase, causing the patient to feel restless or nervous. (Objective 8)

45. a. Arterial CO_2 concentration will increase. (Objective 7)
    b. Hypoventilation. (Objective 7)
    c. The pH will decrease. (Objective 7)
    d. Respiratory acidosis. (Objective 7)

46. a. Arterial CO_2 concentration will decrease. (Objective 7)
    b. Hyperventilation. (Objective 7)
    c. The pH will increase. (Objective 7)
    d. Respiratory alkalosis. (Objective 7)

47. The patient should be coached to slow his/her ventilations. This will cause retention of CO_2, a decrease in pH, and a reversal of respiratory alkalosis. (Objective 9)

48. The patient should be encouraged to cough and should be transported to the hospital. (Objective 4)

49. Abdominal thrusts should be performed to dislodge the foreign body from the airway unless contraindicated, in which case chest thrusts should be performed. (Objective 4)

50. One of the features of asthma is oversecretion of mucus in the lower airway. Giving nonhumidified oxygen can dry this mucus, causing obstruction to air flow and worsening the asthma attack. (Objective 8)

51. A nonrebreather mask to ensure the highest possible FiO_2. (Objective 8)

52. Status asthmaticus is a severe, prolonged asthma attack that will not respond to repeated doses of beta$_2$-adrenergic agonists. Status asthmaticus should be treated by support of oxygenation and ventilation, continued administration of nebulized bronchodilators, possible administration of epinephrine or terbutaline subcutaneously, infusion of IV fluids to ensure hydration and prevent drying of mucous plugs in the lower airway, and preparation for endotracheal intubation. (Objective 8)

53. First, patients with asthma frequently will abuse their metered dose inhalers during an attack and may be overdosed on beta agonists, producing extreme tachycardia and myocardial irritability. In this situation, the patient should be monitored closely if EMS personnel continue giving beta agents. Second, asthma patients who abuse their inhalers may develop resistance to the bronchodilating effects of their usual medications. In this case, EMS personnel may want to try a different beta$_2$ agent to see if better results will be obtained. (Objective 8)

54. Albuterol is a beta$_2$-adrenergic agonist. Stimulation of beta$_2$-receptor sites in the lower airways causes smooth muscle relaxation, reversing bronchospasm. (Objective 8)

55. Racemic epinephrine is administered using a small-volume nebulizer. (Objective 8)

56. Respiratory distress in croup is produced by inflammatory edema of the tissues of the larynx. The alpha$_1$ effects of racemic epinephrine produce vasoconstriction in the inflamed tissues, decreasing edema and resistance to air flow. (Objective 4)

57. 95% to 99%. (Objective 2)

58. The patient immediately should be placed on supplemental oxygen. If his or her respiratory rate or tidal volume are not adequate, ventilations should be assisted with a bag-mask device and oxygen. (Objective 2)

59. Because the patient was in an environment where carbon monoxide probably was present, the oximeter reading might be inaccurate. (Objective 2)

60. For a pulse oximeter to measure oxygen saturation, blood flow must be present under the oximeter's probe. During cardiac arrest, peripheral perfusion essentially is absent so an oximeter will not provide reliable information. (Objective 2)

Multiple Choice

1. A. The most appropriate initial management would be 0.3 mg of epinephrine Sub-Q. The patient probably is not responding to nebulized bronchodilators

because her tidal volume is insufficient to deliver the medications to her lower airway. Giving epinephrine by the subcutaneous route may produce enough bronchodilation to reverse the asthma attack. Because the patient is perfusing well, giving epinephrine by the IV route is not indicated. Methylprednisolone has a very slow onset of action and is not useful in managing the acute phase of an asthma attack. (Objective 8)

2. B. Epinephrine stimulates beta$_2$ receptors, which cause bronchial smooth muscle relaxation. Epinephrine also will stimulate beta$_1$ receptors, increasing heart rate and myocardial contractility, and alpha$_1$ receptors, causing peripheral vasoconstriction. (Objective 8)

3. C. When blood bypasses alveoli without being oxygenated in the lungs because of malfunctioning alveoli (such as in pulmonary edema or atelectasis), the situation is referred to as a $\dot{V}/\dot{Q}$ *mismatch* or *shunting*. (Objective 6)

4. A. Your first impression of this patient leads you to suspect an acute asthma attack. Diffuse wheezing would be characteristic of asthma. Chronic bronchitis typically occurs in middle-age and older patients with a history of smoking or chronic exposure to irritants in their workplace. Pneumonia would more likely be associated with a productive cough and a localized area of crackles, rhonchi, and wheezing. (Objective 8)

5. C. Shortness of breath, fever, chills, and a productive cough suggest pneumonia. (Objective 9)

6. B. The presence of a productive cough occurring on most days for at least 3 months of the year for at least 2 consecutive years indicates chronic bronchitis. (Objective 8)

7. B. This finding may be referred to as *orthopnea* or *paroxysmal nocturnal dyspnea*. (Objective 9)

8. B. Clubbing of the fingers and peripheral cyanosis are associated with chronic hypoxemia. (Objective 8)

9. A. Cystic fibrosis is a congenital condition that results in abnormal secretion of thick bronchial mucus. (Objective 8)

10. A. The physician's request is correct because IV infusion is an acceptable route for administering terbutaline. Terbutaline also can be given by inhalation or by subcutaneous injection. (Objective 8)

11. C. Neurologic initiation of ventilation begins in the medulla. (Objective 1)

12. A. The *primary* control for ventilation relies on the PaCO$_2$ level. An increase in PaCO$_2$ produces a decrease in the cerebrospinal fluid pH, which stimulates central chemoreceptors and triggers respirations. (Objective 5)

13. A. Based solely on this information, you correctly determine the patient is breathing spontaneously. Use of CPAP requires that the patient be breathing spontaneously. (Objective 10)

14. A. The decreased PaCO$_2$ is a result of the patient's increased respiratory rate causing excessive removal of CO$_2$ from the body. (Objective 9)

15. B. In addition to respiratory symptoms associated with a chronic cough and diffuse wheezing, patients with cystic fibrosis frequently experience pancreatic duct obstruction. Cystic fibrosis is a congenital problem that is diagnosed when the patient is very young. Because cystic fibrosis also affects the sweat glands, patients with this disease do not tolerate hot environments well. (Objective 8)

16. D. The signs and symptoms of hyperventilation syndrome result from a respiratory alkalosis without an underlying pathology. (Objective 8)

17. B. Slow onset, low-grade fever, nocturnal episodes of stridor, and a "seal bark" cough indicate croup. (Objective 4)

18. C. Nausea, headache, and restlessness are typical side effects of Ventolin. (Objective 8)

19. C. The role of the Hering-Breuer reflex in pulmonary function is that it prevents overinflation of the lungs. (Objective 1)

20. C. You would assess this patient for dependent edema by examining the posterior legs, buttocks, and lower back. Because she is bedridden, fluid is more likely to accumulate in these areas than in her ankles and lower legs. (Objective 8)

21. A. Your next step is to assess the patient because this may be impending respiratory failure. A patient with asthma whose respirations are slowing following a severe attack may be developing respiratory failure secondary to fatigue. (Objective 8)

22. D. The next best course of action for you to initiate would be to give terbutaline 0.25 mg Sub-Q. A patient who has not responded to multiple treatments with nebulized bronchodilators may not be moving sufficient amounts of air for the bronchodilator to reach the lower airway. Giving a beta$_2$-specific agent subcutaneously may reverse bronchospasm in these patients. Terbutaline is a safer beta agonist for subcutaneous administration in older patients because it is more beta$_2$ specific than epinephrine and less likely to cause undesirable increases in blood pressure, myocardial oxygen demand, and myocardial irritability. (Objective 8)

23. C. This patient probably has a pulmonary embolism. Myocardial infarction produces pain that is squeezing or crushing. Emphysema typically is found in middle-age and older adults and does not produce chest pain. A spontaneous pneumothorax would produce decreased breath sounds on the affected side. The lack of lower extremity movement associated with prolonged air flights increases the risk of pulmonary embolism. (Objective 8)

24. D. Pleural effusion refers to fluid within the patient's pleural space. (Objective 6)

25. B. The history of hypertension, a previous myocardial infarction, and episodes of paroxysmal nocturnal dyspnea indicate congestive heart failure with pulmonary edema. (Objective 8)

26. A. The patient appears to have hyperventilation syndrome. You should coach her to slow her breathing. (Objective 8)
27. D. You should ventilate the patient's lungs using a bag-mask device and oxygen at 12 to 15 L/min. A patient with emphysema who experiences respiratory arrest should be treated in the same way as any other patient. Maintenance of adequate oxygenation and ventilation is essential. (Objective 8)
28. C. Sudden, sharp chest pain, dyspnea, and decreased breath sounds indicate spontaneous pneumothorax. (Objective 6)
29. C. Chronic bronchitis is characterized by excessive mucus production in the bronchial tree and a recurrent productive cough. (Objective 8)
30. D. Emphysema is characterized by loss of elasticity in the lung tissue and destructive changes in the alveolar walls. (Objective 8)
31. C. Asthma is an obstructive pulmonary disease characterized by episodes of severe bronchospasm, bronchial edema, and hypersecretion of mucus in the lower airways. (Objective 8)
32. B. Cyanosis tends to occur early in the course of chronic bronchitis but late in the course of emphysema. Chronic obstructive pulmonary disease is more common in males who live in urban areas and have a history of smoking. Chronic bronchitis patients cough up large amounts of mucus. Emphysema patients tend to purse their lips as they exhale. (Objective 8)
33. C. Common signs and symptoms of an acute asthma attack include wheezing heard primarily on expiration. (Objective 7)
34. D. Patients with chronic obstructive pulmonary disease may breathe in response to decreased oxygen concentration in the arterial blood. (Objective 6)
35. A. Normally the body's stimulus to breathe is based on the level of carbon dioxide in the arterial blood. (Objective 6)

Case Studies

Case one

1. The patient probably has a pulmonary embolism. (Objective 8)
2. The most likely cause of this problem is a blood clot associated with the recent surgery to the patient's ankle. (Objective 8)
3. Pulmonary embolism also can be caused by amniotic fluid, air, fat particles from long bone fractures, and foreign matter introduced into the circulation by substance abuse. (Objective 8)
4. Three risk factors are associated with an increased risk for pulmonary embolism. Virchow's triad consists of vessel wall injury, venous stasis, and hypercoagulability. (Objective 8)
5. A blood clot has blocked a branch of the pulmonary artery, interrupting blood flow through a portion of the patient's left lung. Gas exchange is no longer

taking place in this part of the lung. As a result of this, the patient cannot remove carbon dioxide rapidly enough to keep up with the body's production of this gas. The excess arterial carbon dioxide is stimulating the respiratory center in the brainstem, creating a sensation of shortness of breath. (Objective 8)
6. Because part of the pulmonary circulation is obstructed by a blood clot, blood cannot flow from the right side of the heart into the lungs as rapidly as normal. This is resulting in a backup of blood into the systemic circulation that is distending the jugular veins. (Objective 8)
7. Partial obstruction of blood flow through the lungs is decreasing the preload of the left ventricle. The decrease in preload has caused a drop in stroke volume, cardiac output, and blood pressure. The increase in heart rate is an attempt to compensate for the decrease in stroke volume. (Objective 8)
8. Surgery can result in vessel wall injury, which can trigger blood clot formation. Also, the immobility that occurs during convalescence from surgery can increase the risk of blood clot formation. (Objective 8)
9. Birth control pills cause blood to clot more easily. This effect increases the risk of pulmonary embolism. (Objective 8)
10. The use of codeine is not significant. None of the effects of codeine increase the risk of clot formation or pulmonary embolism. (Objective 8)

Case two

1. Emphysema. (Objective 8)
2. The most common cause of emphysema is smoking. (Objective 8)
3. The $PaCO_2$ will increase. Emphysema results in a loss of elasticity of the lung tissue and in destruction of alveolar walls, which decreases the amount of gas exchange surface in the lungs. The combination of decreased gas exchange surface and decreased ability to fully exhale causes retention of carbon dioxide. (Objective 8)
4. Loss of lung tissue elasticity prevents the lungs from pulling the chest wall inward and the diaphragm upward. Therefore the ribs tend to move up and out, producing a "barrel chest." A chest radiograph of a patient with emphysema also will show a low, flat diaphragm. (Objective 8)
5. Rapid drops in airway pressure during exhalation can cause the smaller airways of emphysema patients to collapse. By pursing their lips, patients with emphysema prolong exhalation and slow the accompanying pressure drop. (Objective 8)
6. The chest of a patient with emphysema is hyper-resonant because of excess air trapped in the inelastic lungs. (Objective 8)
7. Loss of pulmonary elasticity decreases the amount of air that moves in the lower airway as a patient with emphysema breathes and leads to air-trapping and overexpansion of the lungs. These effects decrease the volume of the breath sounds. (Objective 8)

8. Emphysema normally is not associated with a productive cough. (Objective 8)
9. The presence of a cough that produces of thick, white sputum suggests the presence of chronic bronchitis. (Objective 8)
10. A cough productive of yellow, green, rust-colored, or blood-streaked sputum suggests the presence of pneumonia. (Objective 9)
11. The patient probably has ruptured a bleb in his lung and now has a spontaneous pneumothorax. (Objective 6)

Case three

1. Bronchospasm, bronchial edema, excessive mucus production. (Objective 8)
2. Administration of unhumidified oxygen can dry the excessive mucus being secreted into the lower airway, resulting in formation of mucous plugs. (Objective 8)
3. Status asthmaticus. (Objective 8)
4. A patient with a prolonged asthma attack will develop respiratory acidosis. (Objective 8)
5. Beta-adrenergic compounds work most effectively at normal pH. An acidosis can interfere with the ability of these agents to produce bronchodilation. (Objective 8)
6. The near absence of wheezing indicates the patient is moving very little air. (Objective 8)
7. Dry mucous membranes indicate the patient is becoming dehydrated from a combination of decreased fluid intake and increased respiratory water loss. Dehydration can worsen an asthma attack by causing thick mucous plugs to form in the lower airway. (Objective 8)
8. First, because the patient is moving very little air, medication administered using a small-volume nebulizer is unlikely to be effective. A subcutaneous injection of epinephrine may be more effective. Second, beta-adrenergic agents tend to produce restlessness and irritability, so the patient may become less cooperative after medication is given. (Objective 8)
9. Atrovent blocks the effects of the parasympathetic nervous system on the lower airway. Because parasympathetic stimulation causes bronchoconstriction, use of a parasympathetic blocker can potentiate the bronchodilating effects of a beta$_2$ agent. (Objective 8)
10. Steroids have an anti-inflammatory effect that helps reverse the inflammatory edema present during a asthma attack. (Objective 8)
11. Steroids have a very slow onset of action. Therefore they are of little value during the acute management of an asthma attack. (Objective 8)

Case four

1. The patient has a respiratory alkalosis. (Objective 8)
2. Yes. During the early phases of an asthma attack, respiratory alkalosis is a common acid-base imbalance. (Objective 8)
3. The patient's respiratory rate is increased, resulting in increased elimination of carbon dioxide. (Objective 8)
4. The patient's PaO$_2$ is decreasing, indicating that gas exchange is not improving. The PaCO$_2$ is increasing and the pH is decreasing. These changes suggest the patient no longer can compensate for the asthma attack by increasing her respiratory rate and is in the early stages of ventilatory failure. (Objective 8)

Case five

1. Chronic bronchitis. (Objective 8)
2. Chronic bronchitis most commonly is caused by smoking. Some patients develop chronic bronchitis because of long-term exposure to pulmonary irritants in their workplace. (Objective 8)
3. Chronic bronchitis results in decreased movement of air into and out of the alveoli, causing an increase in PaCO$_2$. (Objective 8)
4. Yes. Patients with chronic bronchitis typically have a cough that produces large amounts of thick, white sputum. (Objective 8)
5. Cyanosis typically occurs early in the progression of chronic bronchitis. Because chronic bronchitis interferes with oxygenation as well as ventilation, patients with this disease attempt to compensate for chronic hypoxia by increasing the number of red cells in the blood. The larger number of red cells results in a larger portion of red cells not carrying oxygen, leading to a chronic state of cyanosis. (Objective 8)
6. The presence of yellow sputum with blood in it suggests the patient has a lower respiratory tract infection, possibly pneumonia. (Objective 9)
7. In the pulmonary circulation, hypoxia and hypercarbia produce vasoconstriction. Vasoconstriction increases the resistance against which the right heart must pump. Over time this can lead to right-sided heart failure. Right-sided heart failure associated with pulmonary pathology is called cor pulmonale. (Objective 8)

CHAPTER 22: CARDIOVASCULAR DISORDERS

Short Answer

1. Epicardium, myocardium, endocardium. (Objective 5)
2. Pericardium. (Objective 5)
3. The visceral pericardium lies against the heart. The parietal pericardium touches the diaphragm and pleura. (Objective 5)
4. Tunica adventitia, tunica media, tunica intima. (Objective 4)
5. Arteries. (Objective 4)
6. No. The pulmonary artery carries unoxygenated blood. (Objective 4)
7. Veins. (Objective 4)
8. No. The pulmonary vein carries oxygenated blood. (Objective 4)
9. Veins contain valves. (Objective 4)
10. The valves prevent backflow of blood within the veins. (Objective 4)

11. The arterioles control the resistance of the cardiovascular system. (Objective 4)

12. The veins control the capacitance of the cardiovascular system. (Objective 4)

13. Capillaries provide the exchange surface between the cardiovascular system and the interstitial space. (Objective 4)

14. On the arterial side of the circulation blood is moved by the pressure generated by the heart's contractions. (Objective 4)

15. The heart valves ensure that blood flow though the heart and the pulmonary circulation occurs only in one direction. (Objective 5)

16. Tricuspid, pulmonic, mitral (bicuspid), aortic. (Objective 5)

17. The tricuspid and mitral valves are the AV valves. (Objective 5)

18. The pulmonic and aortic valves are called the semilunar valves because the leafs of these valves resemble half-moons (semi = half, lunar = moon). (Objective 5)

19. During ventricular systole the AV valves are closed. (Objective 5)

20. During ventricular systole the semilunar valves are open. (Objective 5)

21. During ventricular diastole the AV valves are open. (Objective 5)

22. During ventricular diastole the semilunar valves are closed. (Objective 5)

23. The chordae tendineae attach the leafs of the AV valves to the papillary muscles. They keep the pressure generated by ventricular contractions from turning the valves inside out. (Objective 5)

24. Stenosed means that a valve is narrow or tight. (Objective 5)

25. Valvular regurgitation means that a valve is too loose to prevent backflow of blood. (Objective 5)

26. The coronary arteries, which supply blood and oxygen to the myocardium, arise from the base of the aorta. (Objective 8)

27. The coronary arteries fill with blood during ventricular diastole. (Objective 8)

28. The left anterior descending artery supplies most of the blood flow to the left ventricle's anterior surface. (Objective 8)

29. The left circumflex artery supplies most of the blood flow to the left ventricle's lateral surface. (Objective 8)

30. The right coronary artery supplies most of the blood flow to the right ventricle and to the inferior surface of the left ventricle. (Objective 8)

31. Left dominant coronary circulation means the flow to the inferior wall of the left ventricle is being supplied by the left coronary artery. Left dominant coronary circulation occurs in about 20% of the population. (Objective 8)

32. Right dominant coronary circulation means the flow to the inferior wall of the left ventricle is being supplied by the right coronary artery. Right dominant coronary circulation occurs in about 80% of the population. (Objective 8)

33. The right coronary artery provides most of the blood flow to the SA and AV nodes. (Objective 9)

34. SA node, internodal pathways, AV node, bundle of His, bundle branches, Purkinje fibers. (Objective 20)

35. SA node, 60 to 100 beats/min; AV node, 40 to 60 beats/min; ventricular conduction system, 20 to 40 beats/min. (Objective 21)

36. The SA node normally paces the heart because it has the highest intrinsic rate of firing. Before any of the other pacemaker sites can generate an impulse to depolarize the heart, the SA node fires and depolarizes them. (Objective 21)

37. Stimulation of the vagus nerve slows the firing of the SA node and the rate of conduction through the AV node. (Objective 10)

38. Stimulation of the sympathetic nervous system will increase the firing rate of the SA node, increase the rate of impulse conduction through the AV node, and increase the force of ventricular contraction. (Objective 10)

39. Preload is the amount of blood in the ventricles at the end of diastole. Physiologists usually express preload in terms of the pressure exerted by the blood against the ventricular walls at the end of diastole. (Objective 13)

40. To a point, increasing preload will increase myocardial contractility. Beyond that point, increased preload will no longer increase contractility and may result in a decrease. This phenomenon is known as the Frank-Starling effect. (Objectives 13, 14)

41. Contraction of muscles is a result of cross-bridge formation between overlapping strands of actin and myosin in the sarcomeres. Cross-bridge formation allows the myosin filaments to pull themselves across the actin filaments, shortening the sarcomeres. To a point, stretching the muscle increases the distance the myosin filaments can pull themselves across the actin filaments, increasing contractility. Beyond that point, further stretching of the muscle fibers eliminates the overlap between the actin and myosin filaments necessary for cross-bridge formation and contraction to occur. (Objective 15)

42. Afterload is the resistance the ventricles must overcome to eject blood into the arterial circulation. (Objective 13)

43. Stroke volume is the amount of blood the heart pumps with each contraction. (Objective 12)

44. Increased preload increases stroke volume. (Objective 12)

45. Decreased preload decreases stroke volume. (Objective 12)

46. Increased contractility increases stroke volume. (Objective 12)

47. Decreased contractility decreases stroke volume. (Objective 12)

48. Increased afterload will decrease stroke volume. (Objective 12)

337

49. Decreased afterload will increase stroke volume. (Objective 12)

50. Cardiac output = heart rate × stroke volume. (Objective 12)

51. Increased stroke volume increases cardiac output. (Objective 12)

52. Decreased stroke volume decreases cardiac output. (Objective 12)

53. Generally speaking, increased heart rate should increase cardiac output. (Objective 12)

54. Increases in heart rate are accomplished by shortening diastole, the period between beats. The heart fills during diastole. Therefore, if the heart rate becomes too high, diastolic filling time is shortened to the point where preload, stroke volume, and cardiac output decrease. (Objective 12)

55. Blood pressure = cardiac output × peripheral vascular resistance. (Objective 12)

56. Constricting the arterioles will increase peripheral vascular resistance. (Objective 12)

57. Dilating the arterioles will decrease peripheral vascular resistance. (Objective 12)

58. Increased peripheral vascular resistance will increase blood pressure. (Objective 12)

59. Decreased peripheral vascular resistance will decrease blood pressure. (Objective 12)

60. Increased heart rate or stroke volume will increase myocardial workload and oxygen demand. (Objective 12)

61. Decreased heart rate and stroke volume will decrease myocardial workload and oxygen demand. (Objective 12)

62. Coughing increases intrathoracic pressure. Increased intrathoracic pressure decreases venous return to the heart, causing a drop in preload, stroke volume, and cardiac output. (Objective 12)

63. In congestive heart failure, the heart is unable to pump out blood as quickly as it returns. The heart's inability to keep up with venous return results in pooling of blood in the systemic or pulmonary circulation. Sitting up and dangling the lower extremities uses gravity to slow venous return to the heart, more closely matching the preload to the amount of blood that the ventricles are able to move effectively. (Objective 12)

64. Epinephrine is an adrenergic agonist that stimulates alpha$_1$, beta$_1$, and beta$_2$ receptors. (Objective 10)

65. Epinephrine will increase heart rate, myocardial contractility, peripheral vascular resistance, blood pressure, and myocardial oxygen demand. (Objective 10)

66. The beta$_1$ effects of isoproterenol will increase heart rate, myocardial contractility, and myocardial oxygen demand. The beta$_2$ effects of isoproterenol will cause peripheral vasodilation, which will decrease peripheral resistance. (Objective 10)

67. Isoproterenol will increase cardiac output, which can increase blood pressure. However, it also can decrease peripheral resistance, which can decrease

blood pressure. The effect will depend on whether the cardiac effects or peripheral effects dominate. Therefore changes in blood pressure with administration of isoproterenol are difficult to predict. (Objective 10)

68. Nitroglycerin causes relaxation of smooth muscle in blood vessel walls, causing vasodilation. Dilation of the coronary arteries can result in improved blood flow to the myocardium. Dilation of the peripheral circulation decreases venous return to the heart, lowering preload, stroke volume, myocardial workload, and myocardial oxygen demand. The principal benefit from administration of nitroglycerin to patients with myocardial ischemia results from peripheral dilation and decreased myocardial workload. (Objective 72)

69. Nitroglycerin decreases peripheral resistance and blood pressure. (Objective 12)

70. Because nitroglycerin decreases venous return, preload, and stroke volume, it can produce a compensatory increase in heart rate. Increased heart rate can increase myocardial workload and oxygen demand, worsening myocardial ischemia. (Objective 12)

71. Norepinephrine is an adrenergic agonist that primarily stimulates alpha$_1$ receptors, with lesser stimulation of beta$_1$ and beta$_2$ receptors. (Objective 10)

72. Norepinephrine's beta$_1$ effects will increase heart rate and myocardial contractility, raising cardiac output. Norepinephrine's alpha$_1$ effects will increase peripheral vascular resistance. The increase in heart rate, myocardial contractility, and peripheral resistance will increase blood pressure. Increased heart rate, myocardial contractility, and peripheral resistance also will increase myocardial workload and oxygen demand. (Objective 10)

73. A decreased heart rate decreases myocardial workload and oxygen demand. As long as a patient with an acute myocardial infarction is maintaining adequate cardiac output, blood pressure, and systemic perfusion, a slow heart rate should be left untreated because the decreased myocardial workload and oxygen demand decreases the extension of the infarction. (Objective 72)

74. Increasing the preload of a heart in congestive failure will increase the amount of fluid that the heart is unable to pump, resulting in an increase in pulmonary or peripheral edema. (Objective 13)

75. Inderal is a beta-blocker that blocks both beta$_1$ and beta$_2$ receptors. (Objective 10)

76. Inderal will decrease heart rate, myocardial contractility, cardiac output, blood pressure, and myocardial oxygen demand. (Objective 10)

77. Inderal decreases heart rate and myocardial contractility. Decreasing heart rate and myocardial contractility in a patient with congestive heart failure can result in a decreased cardiac output and a worsening of the backup of fluid into the systemic or pulmonary circulation. (Objective 10)

78. Morphine is a vasodilator. By increasing venous capacitance, morphine decreases venous return, lowering the amount of blood the failing heart must pump. By decreasing afterload, morphine increases stroke volume, allowing the failing heart to move more blood forward. Morphine also decreases anxiety, which decreases sympathetic tone and lowers myocardial workload. (Objective 76)

79. Morphine is an analgesic. Relieving the pain of acute myocardial infarction decreases sympathetic tone, lowering myocardial workload, oxygen demand, and irritability. Morphine is also a vasodilator. Vasodilation decreases preload and afterload, lowering myocardial workload and oxygen demand. (Objective 72)

80. AV conduction defects frequently accompany lesions in the right coronary artery because most of the blood flow to the SA and AV nodes is provided by this vessel. (Objective 9)

81. Pulmonary edema and systemic hypoperfusion frequently accompany lesions in the left anterior descending coronary artery. Blockage of the left anterior descending coronary artery infarcts the anterior wall of the left ventricle, which is responsible for the "power stroke" that pushes blood into the systemic circulation. Loss of left ventricular contractility can lead to pulmonary edema and systemic hypoperfusion. (Objective 8)

82. Yes, but only if the patient has left dominant coronary circulation. In a patient with left dominant coronary circulation, blockage of the left circumflex coronary artery can produce an inferolateral infarction. (Objective 8)

83. Giving a vasodilator to a patient with a right ventricular infarction can decrease cardiac output and blood pressure. Vasodilators increase venous capacitance and reduce the amount of blood returning to the heart; they also decrease systemic vascular resistance. In a normal heart, a drop in preload that is large enough to produce a drop in cardiac output and blood pressure will trigger a compensatory increase in ventricular contractility. However, infarcting myocardium loses its ability to contract, so a drop in right ventricular preload and in systemic vascular resistance in a patient with a right ventricular infarction might not be adequately compensated. (Objective 72)

84. Before morphine or nitroglycerin is given to a patient with a right ventricular infarct, the patient should have isotonic crystalloid solution infused. The additional intravascular volume provided by an infusion of normal saline or Ringer's lactate will help offset the drop in preload and right ventricular output caused by vasodilation. (Objective 72)

85. Mitral stenosis will decrease left ventricular preload and cardiac output. Mitral stenosis will increase the pressure in the pulmonary capillary beds, possibly producing pulmonary edema. (Objective 88)

86. Mitral stenosis will cause dilation of the left atrium over time. An enlarged left atrium manifests itself on the ECG as a "notched" or "double-humped" P wave. (Objective 88)

87. Mitral insufficiency will decrease cardiac output because part of the blood that should be moving into the systemic circulation is pushed backward into the left atrium and the pulmonary circulation. Mitral insufficiency also can produce increased pressure in the pulmonary capillary beds and pulmonary edema. (Objective 88)

88. Aortic stenosis decreases cardiac output. Over time, the additional work created by pumping against a narrow or tight aortic valve will cause hypertrophy of the left ventricular myocardium. (Objective 88)

89. Emphysema and chronic bronchitis increase the afterload of the right ventricle. (Objective 75)

90. Dobutamine is a beta₁-adrenergic agent that increases the contractility of the myocardium. Dobutamine is useful in managing congestive heart failure because it increases stroke volume and cardiac output. Nitroglycerin is a vasodilator that decreases preload and afterload. Less blood enters the heart, and the blood that enters is pushed out more efficiently. (Objective 76)

91. Nipride is a direct vasodilator that decreases blood pressure. The physician has ordered Nipride to decrease the pressure of blood against the wall of the aortic aneurysm. A beta-blocker will decrease the heart rate and force of myocardial contraction. These effects will further lower blood pressure and decrease the stress that is placed on the wall of the aortic aneurysm during ventricular systole. (Objective 87)

92. Nitroglycerin is a vasodilator that increases venous capacitance and decreases peripheral vascular resistance. In this patient, the decreases in preload and peripheral vascular resistance have caused a drop in blood pressure. This decrease in blood pressure accounts for the patient becoming pale, cool, and diaphoretic. The heart rate has increased in an attempt to compensate for decreased preload and peripheral resistance. Because nitroglycerin is a vasodilator, it tends to cause a more significant drop in diastolic pressure than systolic pressure. The coronary arteries fill during diastole; therefore the nitroglycerin has worsened this patient's myocardial ischemia. The patient should be treated by placing her in a supine position and infusing isotonic crystalloid to increase preload, cardiac output, and blood pressure. (Objective 12)

93. Congestive heart failure with pulmonary edema. (Objective 75)

Multiple Choice

1. B. You should place the patient supine, elevate her lower extremities, and infuse NS or LR. The vasodilating effects of nitroglycerin have caused a drop in blood pressure. Filling the dilated vascular space with isotonic crystalloid solution is the quickest, safest way to restore adequate perfusion. (Objective 12)

2. B. You should immediately charge the defibrillator to 360 J and defibrillate. The definitive therapy for ventricular fibrillation is defibrillation. In this case CPR by the first responders should have corrected any hypoxia or acidosis that developed immediately after the arrest, so an immediate shock is indicated. With monophasic defibrillators, all shocks should be delivered at 360 J. With biphasic defibrillators, the shock should be delivered at the energy setting that has been shown to be most effective for the specific type of device being used (typically 120 to 200 J). If the rescuer does not know the effective dose range for the device, the initial shock should be delivered at 200 J. (Objective 43)

3. D. The initial treatment for this patient should be to have the patient do a vagal maneuver to increase her parasympathetic tone. Vagal maneuvers are the first therapy that should be used for stable patients with supraventricular tachycardia. (Objective 34)

4. B. The initial treatment for a stable patient with ventricular tachycardia should be administration of a ventricular antidysrhythmic such as amiodarone, 150 mg infused over 10 minutes, or lidocaine, 1-1.5 mg/kg IV push. (Objective 39)

5. A. The initial management for an unstable patient with supraventricular tachycardia would be to give oxygen, start an IV, give 5 mg of midazolam, and perform synchronized cardioversion at 50-100 J. (Objective 34)

6. A. After giving O$_2$ and starting an IV, you should perform synchronized cardioversion at 100 J. Synchronized cardioversion is the most appropriate treatment for an unstable patient with a tachydysrhythmia. (Objective 39)

7. C. The correct order of treatment is evaluate adequacy of oxygenation and ventilation; atropine 0.5 mg IV push while awaiting application of the pacemaker; transcutaneous pacing; dopamine infusion at 5 mcg/kg/min if pacing is ineffective. (Objective 33)

8. B. This patient should be treated with oxygen, an IV with NS or LR, and nebulized albuterol to help bronchodilate him and decrease his work of breathing. The patient's ECG shows atrial flutter with a rate of 100 beats/min. Because this rhythm has a rate within the normal range, it is unlikely to be the cause of the patient's signs and symptoms and is not increasing the workload of his heart. There is no reason to attempt to slow or convert it. (Objective 34)

9. A. Your goals in managing a patient with congestive heart failure with pulmonary edema are to decrease preload, improve myocardial contractility, and decrease afterload. Decreasing preload will decrease the amount of blood the heart must pump. Improving myocardial contractility will raise stroke volume. Decreasing afterload will increase cardiac output and lower myocardial workload. (Objective 13)

10. D. Initial management for the patient in the previous question should include oxygen, CPAP, nitroglycerin, furosemide, and morphine. Nitroglycerin and morphine will decrease preload and afterload by causing vasodilation. Furosemide will decrease preload by decreasing intravascular volume and by producing vasodilation. Calcium channel blockers decrease myocardial contractility and are not indicated in congestive heart failure. Cardioversion would be ineffective in this case because the patient's rhythm is sinus tachycardia. Dopamine is not indicated because the patient has an adequate blood pressure and adequate perfusion. (Objective 76)

11. D. The dysrhythmia is sinus rhythm with first-degree AV block. (Objective 44)

12. B. The dysrhythmia in the patient in the previous question is most probably being caused by digitalis. Digitalis slows the rate of depolarization of the SA node and slows conduction through the AV junction, predisposing patients to bradycardias and AV blocks. (Objective 44)

13. D. A lesion in the patient's right coronary artery probably has caused his problem. The right coronary artery supplies blood to the right ventricle, the SA node, the AV node, and the inferior wall of the left ventricle. Blockage of the right coronary artery tends to produce bradycardias, AV blocks, and right ventricular infarctions. Hypoperfusion, clear lungs, and jugular vein distention are clinical signs that suggest right-sided heart failure and right ventricular infarction. (Objectives 8, 9)

14. C. You would anticipate seeing ST segment elevation in leads II, III, aV$_F$, and V$_{4R}$ on the 12-lead ECG of the patient in the previous question. These changes would indicate injury to the inferior wall of the left ventricle and to the right ventricle. (Objectives 71, 72)

15. D. The most appropriate action would be to continue CPR and transport immediately while establishing two large-bore IVs with NS or LR en route. This patient has pulseless electrical activity. A pulseless sinus tachycardia in a healthy young person following trauma suggests hypovolemia, tension pneumothorax, or cardiac tamponade. Presence of equal breath sounds bilaterally eliminates tension pneumothorax as a possibility. Flat neck veins associated with bruising over the chest and abdomen suggest hypovolemia. Cardiac tamponade usually produces distended neck veins. However, concurrent injuries that have caused hypovolemia may result in flat neck veins in the presence of cardiac tamponade. The patient's electrical rhythm is sinus tachycardia. Adenosine and cardioversion are not indicated. (Objectives 81, 82, 83)

16. D. Your best course of action would be to provide supplemental oxygen to maintain an oxygen saturation of 94%, start an IV, and initiate

transcutaneous pacing. Pacing is the preferred therapy for second-degree, type II AV block and complete AV block because it is more likely to be successful than atropine. Lidocaine is contraindicated in AV blocks because it reduces the possibility of an effective ventricular escape rhythm if the patient develops a complete block. Morphine lowers blood pressure and should be avoided if a patient is hypotensive. (Objective 44)

17. D. This rhythm is p wave asystole (primary ventricular standstill). It is a form of PEA in which the SA node and atria are depolarizing normally, yet the ventricles are not responding. As it is a form of PEA it is treated as such. After ensuring high quality CPR initiate an IV and administer 1 mg of epinephrine 1:10,000 every 3-5 minutes while searching for treating reversible causes of the arrest. (Objectives 81, 82, 83)

18. C. The patient should be given high-concentration oxygen, an IV should be started, and synchronized cardioversion should be performed at 120-200 J. The patient is in atrial fibrillation with a rapid ventricular response. The treatment for a tachydysrhythmia in an unstable patient is synchronized cardioversion. (Objective 34)

19. A. This patient should be treated with oxygen and a dopamine infusion at 5 mcg/g/min titrated to her blood pressure and perfusion. The patient's rhythm is atrial fibrillation with a controlled rate. The patient does not have a tachydysrhythmia, so cardioversion is not indicated. Verapamil and diltiazem also are not indicated because the rate is controlled and these drugs could worsen the hypotension that is present. Nitroglycerin, furosemide, and morphine are contraindicated in hypotensive patients. Dopamine will improve myocardial contractility and increase cardiac output and blood pressure. Improving cardiac output also will help clear fluid from the patient's lungs. (Objective 80)

20. B. Continue CPR while attempting to obtain vascular access and defibrillate after 2 minutes of CPR. (Objectives 81, 82, 83)

21. A. A 45-year-old female diagnosed with type 1 diabetes 22 years ago would be most likely to present with atypical, unusual, or vague signs and symptoms. Patients with diabetes develop peripheral neuropathies that decrease their ability to feel pain, increasing their risk of silent myocardial infarction. (Objective 72)

22. D. Sodium bicarbonate therapy would be most likely to be effective in a patient with documented tricyclic antidepressant toxicity. Sodium bicarbonate antagonizes the cardiotoxic effects of tricyclic antidepressants. Sodium bicarbonate produces a metabolic alkalosis, which can lower serum potassium levels. Therefore it is contraindicated in hypokalemia. The treatment for respiratory acidosis resulting from a tension pneumothorax or a cardiac arrest of short duration is assisted ventilation. (Objective 81)

23. B. The defibrillator will not deliver a shock because it is attempting to synchronize the shock with an R wave, and no R waves are present in ventricular fibrillation. If a defibrillator that has been used for synchronized cardioversion refuses to shock ventricular fibrillation, the first step should be to check the synchronizer to ensure it turned off after the synchronized shock was delivered. (Objective 43)

24. A. After giving oxygen and starting an IV, the next treatment should be atropine to increase cardiac output and blood pressure by increasing heart rate. Bradycardias can result in ventricular ectopy by unmasking irritable foci in the ventricles that normally are kept from firing by the higher rate of the SA node. Increasing the heart rate can suppress these ectopic foci by depolarizing them before they can generate beats. At the same time, increasing the heart rate can improve cardiac output. (Objectives 33, 39)

25. D. Runs of ventricular tachycardia in a patient with myocardial ischemia may be a forerunner of ventricular tachycardia or ventricular fibrillation. (Objective 39)

26. D. Management of the patient should include oxygen, aspirin, an IV, nitroglycerine, and morphine if the pain continues. The patient is in a sinus rhythm at a rate of 70 without evidence of hypotension, but rather presents with adequate perfusion. As issues with the rate and blood pressure do not exist there is no indication for a fluid bolus or the administration of atropine to increase the rate. Atropine would increase the myocardial workload and oxygen demand without providing any benefits. (Objective 72)

27. C. The rhythm is a ventricular pacemaker with failure to capture. (Objectives 45, 46)

28. C. The most appropriate treatment for this patient would be IV diltiazem to slow ventricular response. The patient is hemodynamically stable. However, the high heart rate produced by uncontrolled atrial fibrillation is increasing myocardial oxygen demand. A calcium channel blocker can be used to slow impulse conduction through the AV node and lower the response of the ventricles to the fibrillating atria into a more reasonable range. (Objective 34)

29. B. The dysrhythmia is atrial flutter. (Objective 34)

30. C. Management of the patient in the previous question should include nitroglycerine and furosemide. The patient's heart rate is within an acceptable range and is unlikely to be the cause of her signs and symptoms. Therefore use of adenosine, cardioversion, or diltiazem is not indicated. The patient should be treated for congestive heart failure with pulmonary edema using oxygen, nitroglycerin, furosemide, and morphine. (Objective 76)

31. D. The patient is experiencing angina pectoris that has changed in its presentation from earlier episodes. You should suspect unstable angina pectoris. Unstable angina is angina that is triggered by less physiologic stress than previous episodes, that requires more nitroglycerin or longer periods of rest for relief, or that is accompanied by signs and symptoms not present during previous episodes. (Objective 71)

32. B. This patient has deep vein thrombosis. Occlusion of venous return from an extremity by clot formation causes the extremity to become swollen, warm, and bluish-red. Obstruction of arterial flow to an extremity causes the limb to become cool and pale with absent pulses. (Objective 96)

33. D. The patient in the previous question should be transported because she has an increased risk of pulmonary embolism. (Objective 96)

34. C. This patient has peripheral arterial insufficiency with intermittent claudication. Intermittent claudication is pain in the muscles of the lower extremities that results from inadequate blood flow during periods of increased activity. Intermittent claudication is the peripheral circulation's analog to angina pectoris in the heart. (Objective 96)

35. A. You suspect the patient may have suffered acute arterial occlusion. Acute arterial occlusion is characterized by severe pain, pulselessness, pallor, paresthesias, and paralysis in the affected extremity. (Objective 96)

36. C. Cor pulmonale is right-sided heart failure produced by pulmonary disease. You would expect the patient to have distended neck veins and pedal edema produced by blood backing up into the peripheral circulation behind the failing right ventricle. Crackles and dyspnea would be associated with left-sided heart failure. (Objective 75)

37. A. This patient is most likely to be suffering from acute myocardial infarction. Silent myocardial infarction should be suspected whenever a patient with diabetes presents with any clinical syndrome characterized by vague signs and symptoms that include weakness, nausea, vomiting, shortness of breath, pallor, or diaphoresis. It is reasonable to assume that any "sick" diabetic patient possibly is having an acute myocardial infarction until proven otherwise. (Objective 71)

38. D. Increasing the heart rate shortens systole and diastole. Most of the increase comes by decreasing the length of diastole and the amount of time available for the heart to fill between beats. (Objectives 12, 13)

39. B. The major modifiable risk factors for developing atherosclerosis include hypertension, smoking, and elevated serum lipid levels. Gender, age, and family history are not modifiable risk factors. (Objective 71)

40. B. Increasing the preload of a heart that is in congestive failure will worsen the congestive failure. By definition, a heart in congestive failure cannot pump blood out as rapidly as it is entering. Increasing the amount of blood entering the heart will increase the severity of congestive failure. (Objective 13)

41. C. Management of this patient should include norepinephrine. This patient is in cardiogenic shock with severe hypotension. Norepinephrine is indicated to rapidly improve the perfusion of the brain, heart, and lungs to prevent cardiac arrest. Morphine and nitroglycerin would lower the patient's blood pressure. Aspirin cannot be given because a patient with altered mental status cannot take medications by mouth. (Objective 80)

42. C. The most appropriate action at this point would be to check the placement of the ECG leads. The ECG rhythm is ventricular fibrillation, which cannot produce a pulse. If the patient has a pulse, he cannot be in ventricular fibrillation. (Objectives 81, 82)

Case Studies

Case one

1. Atrial flutter. (Objective 34)
2. Congestive heart failure with pulmonary edema. (Objective 75)
3. Failure of the right ventricle is resulting in a backup of blood into the jugular veins. (Objective 75)
4. The patient's respiratory distress is being caused by failure of the left ventricle. As the contractility of the left ventricle decreases, blood backs up into the pulmonary circulation. The pressure in the pulmonary circulation increases and fluid is squeezed out of the capillary beds into the interstitial spaces of the lung and into the alveoli. The fluid in and around the alveoli increases the work of breathing and interferes with gas diffusion, causing shortness of breath. (Objective 75)
5. Assess the patient's airway, breathing, and circulation. Place the patient in a sitting position with his legs dangling to slow venous return to the heart. Administer high-concentration oxygen using a nonrebreather mask. Because the patient's respirations are shallow and gasping, consider assisting his ventilations with a bag-mask device using CPAP, if available. If adequate oxygenation and ventilation cannot be maintained with a bag-mask device and oxygen, the patient may have to be endotracheally intubated, using a benzodiazepine and a neuromuscular blocker to facilitate the process. Establish a keep-open IV. Limit the amount of fluid infused to avoid worsening volume overload. Ask the patient about use of erectile dysfunction drugs during the past 48 hours. Administer 0.4 mg of nitroglycerin sublingually to produce vasodilation that will decrease preload and afterload. Administer 40 mg of furosemide IV push to produce preload reduction through vasodilation and diuresis. Administer 2 mg of morphine sulfate IV push to reduce preload and afterload through vasodilation and to help calm the patient. Obtain a 12-lead ECG to help exclude silent myocardial infarction as a cause of the congestive failure. If the ECG indicates myocardial ischemia or

injury is present, give 325 mg of aspirin by mouth. (Objective 76)

Case two

1. Diabetes mellitus increases the risk of developing atherosclerosis and its complications, including acute myocardial infarction. Patients with diabetes develop peripheral neuropathies that result in their experiencing silent myocardial infarctions. (Objective 71)
2. Inferior myocardial infarction. (Objective 31)
3. The right coronary artery. (Objective 8)
4. You should acquire right-sided precordial leads (V_{3R}, V_{4R}, V_{5R}, V_{6R}) to determine whether a right ventricular infarction is present. Because the right coronary artery supplies blood to the right ventricle and the inferior wall of the left ventricle in 80% of the population, patients with inferior myocardial infarction have a high probability of also having a right ventricular infarction. This patient's clear lung fields, distended neck veins, and low blood pressure suggest that a right ventricular infarction may be present. (Objectives 71, 72)
5. Assess the patient's airway, breathing, and circulation. Place the patient physically and psychologically at rest. Administer high-concentration oxygen using a nonrebreather mask. After asking about medication allergies give 325 mg of aspirin by mouth. Monitor the ECG. Establish an IV. Obtain a 12-lead ECG and right-sided precordial leads. If a right ventricular infarction is present, infuse 1 L of isotonic crystalloid while monitoring respirations, lung sounds, and oxygen saturation carefully. Ask the patient about use of erectile dysfunction drugs during the previous 48 hours. Administer 0.4 mg of nitroglycerin sublingually while monitoring the patient's blood pressure. If the patient becomes hypotensive, place him supine, elevate his lower extremities, and infuse isotonic crystalloid solution. Transport to a facility capable of performing reperfusion therapy for acute myocardial infarction. (Objectives 71, 72)

Case three

1. The patient's 12-lead ECG indicates the presence of an anteroseptal acute myocardial infarction. (Objective 31)
2. The decrease in nerve conduction velocity that occurs with the aging process decreases pain sensation. Older patients are at increased risk of having silent myocardial infarctions. (Objective 71)
3. The left anterior descending coronary artery. (Objective 8)
4. Place the patient physically and psychologically at rest. Administer high-concentration oxygen using a nonrebreather mask. After asking about medication allergies give 325 mg of aspirin by mouth. Monitor the ECG. Establish an IV at a keep-open rate. Limit the amount of fluid infused. Obtain a 12-lead ECG. Ask the patient about use of erectile dysfunction drugs during the previous 48 hours. (Yes, ask about these drugs even with older patients and females. The results of giving nitroglycerin to a patient who recently has taken erectile dysfunction drugs are too catastrophic to ever risk making this error.) Administer 0.4 mg of nitroglycerin sublingually while monitoring the patient's blood pressure. Transport to a facility capable of performing reperfusion therapy for acute myocardial infarction. (Objective 72)

Case four

1. The patient has a left bundle branch block. (Objective 31)
2. Left bundle branch block is a myocardial infarction imitator that makes it difficult to read a 12-lead ECG for ST segment changes suggesting acute myocardial infarction. However, this patient's clinical presentation suggests he is having an acute myocardial infarction. Additionally, a new-onset left bundle branch block strongly suggests the presence of an anteroseptal acute myocardial infarction. (Objective 31)

Case five

1. Ventricular pacemaker rhythm. (Objective 45)
2. Ventricular pacemaker rhythm is a myocardial infarction imitator that makes it difficult to read a 12-lead ECG for ST segment changes suggesting acute myocardial infarction. However, this patient's clinical presentation suggests he is having an acute myocardial infarction. In fact, his altered mental status; pale, cool skin; and low blood pressure suggest he is in cardiogenic shock. This patient "normally" is hypertensive, so a blood pressure of 98/50 mm Hg may be hypotensive for him. (Objective 31)
3. Assess the patient's airway, breathing, and circulation. Place the patient physically and psychologi-cally at rest. Administer high-concentra-tion oxygen using a nonrebreather mask. After asking about medication allergies give 325 mg of aspirin by mouth. Monitor the ECG. Establish an IV at a keep-open rate. Limit the amount of fluid infused. Obtain a 12-lead ECG. Establish a continuous infusion with dopamine at 5 mcg/kg/min. Titrate the infusion using the patient's blood pressure and other indicators of adequacy of perfusion. When the patient is perfusing adequately, ask about use of erectile dysfunction drugs during the previous 48 hours. (Yes, ask about these drugs even with older patients and females. The results of giving nitroglycerin to a patient who recently has taken erectile dysfunction drugs are too catastrophic to ever risk making this error.) Administer 0.4 mg of nitroglycerin sublingually while monitoring the patient's blood pressure. Because the patient is experiencing pain, consider administration of 2 mg of morphine sulfate repeated as needed to control pain. Transport to a facility capable of performing reperfusion therapy for acute myocardial infarction. (Objectives 72, 80)

Case six

1. The 12-lead ECG shows an inferolateral pattern of injury. Assuming only one vascular lesion is present, the patient must have left dominant coronary circulation with blood flow to the lateral and inferior walls of the left ventricle being supplied by the left coronary artery. (Objectives 8, 31)

Case seven

1. The ECG shows a second-degree, type II AV block. However, because the patient has no pulse he has pulseless electrical activity. (Objectives 42, 44)
2. Continue cardiopulmonary resuscitation. Secure the airway with an endotracheal tube. Obtain vascular access. Administer 1.0 mg of epinephrine 1:10,000 IV push every 3 to 5 minutes. Because the heart rate is less than 60 beats/minute, administer 1 mg of atropine every 3 to 5 minutes to a maximum of 0.04 mg/kg (3 mg for the average adult). Attempt to identify the underlying cause of the pulseless electrical activity. (Objectives 81, 82)
3. Hypovolemia, hypoxia, hydrogen ions (acidosis), hypo/hyperkalemia, hypoglycemia, hypothermia, toxins, tamponade, tension pneumothorax, thrombosis (pulmonary or coronary), trauma. (Objectives 81, 82)

CHAPTER 23: DISORDERS OF THE NERVOUS SYSTEM

Short Answer

1. The neuron is the basic unit of the nervous system. (Objective 1)
2. Dendrites are extensions of a neuron that carry nerve impulses toward the cell body. (Objective 1)
3. Axons are extensions of a neuron that carry impulses away from the cell body. (Objective 1)
4. The myelin sheath is coating that surrounds the axons, insulating them and speeding nerve impulse conduction. (Objective 1)
5. The nodes of Ranvier are gaps in the myelin sheath that occur at regular intervals along the axon. The nodes of Ranvier increase the rate of nerve impulse conduction by allowing impulses to move along the axon by skipping the myelinated areas and leaping from node to node. (Objective 1)
6. Nerve impulses move on neurons as action potentials created by opening of sodium channels in the neuron's plasma membrane. When the sodium channels open, sodium rapidly enters the neuron, causing it to depolarize. Movement of potassium out of the neuron though potassium channels repolarizes the neuron and prepares it to conduct another action potential. (Objective 1)
7. The gaps between neurons are called synapses. (Objective 1)

8. Impulses cross synapses through the release and diffusion of chemicals called neurotransmitters. (Objective 1)
9. GABA is an inhibitory neurotransmitter that decreases the ability of neurons to depolarize. (Objective 1)
10. The central nervous system consists of the brain and the spinal cord. (Objective 1)
11. The dura mater, the arachnoid membrane, and the pia mater surround the central nervous system. Collectively these membranes are referred to as the meninges. (Objective 1)
12. CSF cushions and supports the brain. It also transports nutrients, waste products, and chemical messengers. The CSF normally is located in the subarachnoid space between the pia mater and the arachnoid membrane. (Objective 1)
13. The medulla oblongata of the brainstem controls breathing, heart rate, and vasomotor tone. (Objective 1)
14. Body temperature is controlled in the hypothalamus. (Objective 1)
15. The reticular activating system, located in the portion of the brainstem known as the mid-brain, stimulates the cerebral cortex to promote attention and wakefulness. (Objective 1)
16. If the connection is lost between the cerebral cortex and the RAS, the patient becomes unresponsive. (Objective 1)
17. Posture, balance, and equilibrium are controlled in the cerebellum. (Objective 1)
18. The cerebrum controls conscious perception, action, thought, and personality. (Objective 1)
19. The frontal lobe controls personality and abstract intellectual functions such as ability to predict future consequences of events or actions. The frontal lobe also controls skeletal muscle movements. (Objective 1)
20. The parietal lobe receives and processes sensations of touch, pressure, heat, cold, and pain from the body surface. (Objective 1)
21. The temporal lobe is the location of centers responsible for hearing and speech. (Objective 1)
22. The occipital lobe is responsible for sight. (Objective 1)
23. The sensory and motor centers in the brain's right side control sensation and movement for the left side of the body and vice versa. (Objective 1)
24. The speech center is located in the temporal lobe. In right-handed persons, the speech center typically is located in the left temporal lobe. In left-handed persons, the speech center may be located either in the right temporal lobe or in the left temporal lobe. (Objective 1)
25. Thiamine (vitamin B_1) is essential to the metabolism of glucose. Patients who are thiamine deficient may develop Wernicke's syndrome or Korsakoff's psychosis. Wernicke's syndrome is characterized by ataxia, eye muscle weakness or paralysis, loss of memory, and disorientation. Korsakoff's psychosis is

characterized by disorientation, muttering delirium, insomnia, delusions, and hallucinations. (Objective 1)

26. A cranial nerve is a nerve that connects directly to the brain without passing through the spinal cord. (Objective 1)

27.

Nerve	Name	Function
I	Olfactory	Sensory: smell
II	Optic	Sensory: sight
III	Oculomotor	Motor: pupil constriction, superior rectus and inferior oblique muscle of eye
IV	Trochlear	Motor: superior oblique muscle of eye
V	Trigeminal	Sensory: orbital structures, nasal cavity, skin of forehead, upper eyelid, eyebrows, nose, lips, gums, teeth, cheek, palate Motor: chewing muscles (temporalis, masseter, pterygoids)
VI	Abducens	Motor: lateral rectus muscle of eye
VII	Facial	Sensory: taste from anterior two thirds of tongue Motor: muscles of facial expression, lacrimal gland, submandibular and sublingual salivary glands
VIII	Acoustic	Sensory: hearing, balance
IX	Glossopharyngeal	Sensory: taste from posterior one third of tongue; portions of pharynx and palate Motor: pharyngeal muscles and parotid salivary gland
X	Vagus	Sensory: pharynx; external ear, diaphragm; thoracic and abdominal viscera Motor: palatal and pharyngeal muscles; thoracic and abdominal viscera
XI	Spinal accessory	Motor: voluntary muscles of palate, pharynx, larynx; sternocleidomastoid and trapezius muscles
XII	Hypoglossal	Motor: tongue muscles

(Objective 1)

28. The spinal cord carries sensory impulses to the brain and motor impulses from the brain. It controls spinal reflexes. (Objective 1)

29. C3: Base of neck
T4: Nipple line
T10: Umbilicus
L1: Groin (Objective 1)

30. The autonomic nervous system controls functions that take place below the level of consciousness. (Objective 1)

31. The sympathetic nervous system controls responses to stress. (Objective 1)

32. Norepinephrine is the sympathetic nervous system's postganglionic neurotransmitter. (Objective 1)

33. The parasympathetic nervous system controls vegetative or routine housekeeping functions. (Objective 1)

34. The vagus nerve (cranial nerve X) mediates most of the body's parasympathetic activity. (Objective 1)

35. Acetylcholine is the parasympathetic nervous system's postganglionic neurotransmitter. (Objective 1)

36. Muscarinic receptors are the sites to which acetylcholine released by the parasympathetic nervous system binds. (Objective 1)

37. Acetylcholine is the neurotransmitter released by motor neurons to activate skeletal muscles. (Objective 1)

38. Nicotinic receptors are the sites to which acetylcholine released by motor neurons binds. (Objective 1)

39. A = Alcohol, acidosis
E = Epilepsy
I = Insulin (hypoglycemia or hyperglycemia)
O = Overdose
U = Uremia
T = Trauma, tumor, toxin
I = Infection
P = Psychosis, poison
S = Seizure, stroke
(Objective 4)

40. Support of airway, breathing, and circulation is the initial priority in the management of all patients with coma of unknown cause. (Objective 5)

41. Alcohol abusers frequently are thiamine deficient. Because thiamine is required from cells to completely metabolize glucose, administration of glucose to a thiamine-deficient patient can result in incomplete metabolism of glucose to toxic intermediate compounds, causing neurologic signs and symptoms that can include seizures. (Objective 5)

42. Thrombus, embolus, hemorrhage. (Objective 4)

43. Hypertension, chronic atrial fibrillation, cigarette smoking, diabetes mellitus, hyperlipidemia, cardiovascular disease, sickle cell disease,

345

polycythemia, hypercoagulability, birth control pill use, stimulant abuse. (Objective 4)

44. A transient ischemic attack is an episode of impaired neurologic function resulting from temporary interference with the brain's blood supply that resolves itself with no residual deficit. (Objective 4)

45. Transient ischemic attacks are associated with a high probability of having a stroke. (Objective 4)

46. An aura is a subjective sensation that precedes a seizure. Auras can include olfactory, visual, auditory, or taste hallucinations. (Objective 4)

47. The nature of the aura can provide a neurologist with clues to the location of the irritable focus in the brain that triggered the seizure. (Objective 4)

48. Aura, tonic phase, clonic phase, postictal phase. (Objective 4)

49. A patient who makes asymmetrical or purposeful movements or who can recall things done or said to him during a seizure is faking the seizure activity. Faked seizure activity is referred to as a pseudoseizure or hysterical seizure. (Objective 4)

50. Focal motor seizures (simple partial seizures) are characterized by tonic-clonic movements of a body part. (Objective 4)

51. Complex partial seizures, also called psychomotor seizures, are characterized by loss of consciousness and apparently purposeful movements such as lip-smacking and repetitive movements. (Objective 4)

52. Status epilepticus is a series of two or more generalized motor seizures without an intervening period of consciousness. (Objective 4)

53. Benzodiazepines, such as diazepam or lorazepam, are the agents of choice for prehospital management of status epilepticus. (Objective 5)

54. Hypoxia resulting from loss of airway is the most common cause of death from seizures. (Objective 4)

Multiple Choice

1. C. Unequal pupils, as may be seen in a patient with increased ICP, indicate the possibility of pressure on cranial nerve III. Unequal pupils are associated with hemorrhagic stroke. (Objective 3)

2. B. The postictal phase of a generalized seizure is characterized by fatigue, confusion, and a possible headache. (Objective 4)

3. D. A significant characteristic differentiating hemorrhagic stroke from ischemic stroke is the rapid onset of severe symptoms seen in hemorrhagic stroke. (Objective 4)

4. A. Cushing's triad consists of abnormal breathing pattern, bradycardia, and hypertension. (Objective 4)

5. A. Petit mal seizures are most common in children. Petit mal seizures also are called *absence seizures*. (Objective 4)

6. C. The patient probably has had a seizure from a CVA. The patient's vital signs are consistent with increased intracranial pressure from a cerebral hemorrhage. The deviation of his eyes to the left suggests some type of continuing neurologic problem.

A patient seizing from a drug overdose or alcohol withdrawal probably would have shown other signs before collapsing. (Objective 4)

7. A. The patient probably fainted because of excess vagal tone produced by straining to have a bowel movement. (Objective 4)

8. D. Tonic-clonic activity isolated to one part of the body is a simple partial seizure. This type of seizure also is called a focal motor seizure. (Objective 4)

9. B. A patient who is actively seizing should be gently supported and guided to keep him from injuring himself. Attempting to place something in the patient's mouth can result in injury. Restraining the patient can cause musculoskeletal trauma. Placing a patient in a prone position can make monitoring the airway difficult and interfere with ventilations. (Objective 5)

10. D. Focal motor seizures (simple partial seizures) are characterized by tonic-clonic movements of one part of the body. (Objective 4)

11. D. Status epilepticus is two or more seizures without an intervening period of consciousness. (Objective 4)

12. C. A type of seizure characterized by brief loss of consciousness without loss of postural tone is a petit mal or absence seizure. (Objective 4)

13. B. During the postictal phase of a seizure, a patient most probably will complain of a headache and wish to sleep. (Objective 4)

14. D. A cerebrovascular accident may be caused by rupture of an artery in the brain or blockage of a cerebral artery by a thrombus or embolus. (Objective 4)

Case Studies

Case one

1. The patient is having a cerebrovascular accident. (Objective 4)

2. Cerebrovascular accidents are caused by hemorrhage, emboli, or thrombus formation. (Objective 4)

3. Severe, rapid onset of signs and symptoms, unequal pupils, and the presence of Cushing's triad suggest a hemorrhagic stroke. (Objective 4)

4. Dilation of the right pupil and loss of motor and sensory function in the left arm and leg indicate the stroke is occurring on the right side of the brain. (Objective 4)

5. The patient's vital signs indicate increased intracranial pressure. (Objective 4)

6. The patient's airway should be intubated. Controlled hyperventilation with high-concentration oxygen should be used to control the rise in intracranial pressure. An IV should be established using an isotonic crystalloid solution. The ECG should be monitored. Because neurologic signs are present, the blood glucose level should be evaluated. The patient should be transported rapidly to a facility with neurosurgical capabilities. (Objective 5)

Case two

1. Yes, the seizure activity probably is related to the patient's diabetes. There is no history of a seizure disorder. However, the patient has recently been diagnosed with diabetes mellitus. Patients with new-onset diabetes, and in particular adolescents, frequently have difficulty regulating their insulin dose, food intake, and activity levels to maintain stable blood glucose levels. (Objective 4)

Case three

1. The patient is having a cerebrovascular accident. (Objective 4)
2. Cerebrovascular accidents are caused by hemorrhage, emboli, or thrombus formation. (Objective 4)
3. This patient probably has formed a thrombus in a cerebral artery. (Objective 4)
4. The motor deficit in the left side suggests a stroke involving the brain's right side. (Objective 4)
5. In patients who are right-hand dominant, the speech center is located on the left side of the brain. (Objective 4)
6. Hypertension causes damage to the tunica intima of blood vessels that promotes formation of atheromatous plaques. Rupture of plaques and creation of turbulence by narrowing of the vessel increase the risk for clot formation. (Objective 4)
7. A cerebrovascular accident involving the right cerebral hemisphere can cause a patient to develop "neglect" of the extremities controlled by that hemisphere. The patient will see the weak or paralyzed extremities but not acknowledge they are part of his/her body. (Objective 4)
8. When a patient displays signs of a stroke on awakening, the onset of the stroke must be assumed to have occurred shortly after the patient went to sleep. If more than 3 hours have elapsed since the patient laid down for his nap, he may no longer be a candidate for thrombolytic therapy. (Objective 5)
9. Assess airway, breathing, and circulation. Administer high-concentration oxygen using a nonrebreather mask. Keep the patient supine or in the recovery position to help ensure adequate blood flow to the brain. Determine the blood glucose level. Start an IV with an isotonic crystalloid. Monitor the cardiac rhythm. Protect the patient's paralyzed extremities. Transport rapidly to a facility with capabilities to manage an ischemic stroke. (Objective 5)

CHAPTER 24: ENDOCRINE EMERGENCIES AND NUTRITIONAL DISORDERS

Short Answer

1. An endocrine gland is a ductless gland that distributes its products by secreting them into the bloodstream. (Objective 2)
2. Hormones. (Objective 2)
3. The target cells, or target organ(s). (Objective 2)
4. The hypothalamus produces "releasing factors" that control secretion of hormones from the anterior pituitary. The hypothalamus also produces antidiuretic hormone and oxytocin, which then are released from the posterior pituitary gland. (Objective 2)
5. Diabetes insipidus is caused by inadequate production of antidiuretic hormone, leading to production of massive amounts of dilute urine. Patients with diabetes insipidus may produce 20 L of urine per day. (Objective 14)
6. The pituitary gland is called the *master gland* because it produces hormones that control the functions of other endocrine glands. (Objective 2)
7. Growth hormone—stimulates body growth in childhood: Adrenocorticotropic hormone—stimulates hormone release from adrenal cortex. Thyroid-stimulating hormone—stimulates release of hormones from thyroid gland. Follicle-stimulating hormone—stimulates development of ova or sperm. Luteinizing hormone—stimulates release of hormones from ovaries or testes. Prolactin—stimulates production of breast milk. (Objective 2)
8. Antidiuretic hormone—stimulates reabsorption of water by kidneys. Oxytocin—stimulates uterine contractions and release of milk from breast. (Objective 2)
9. Excess thyroid hormone will cause a high metabolic rate. (Objective 17)
10. Agitation, insomnia, poor heat tolerance, weight loss, elevated body temperature, tachycardia, new-onset atrial fibrillation. (Objective 18)
11. Hypothyroidism. (Objective 17)
12. Lethargy, fatigue, cold intolerance, decreased appetite with weight gain, thickened skin that is pale and cool, hypothermia, bradycardia, slow respirations. (Objective 18)
13. The thyroid. (Objective 2)
14. Calcitonin lowers blood calcium levels by stimulating calcium uptake by bones. (Objective 2)
15. The parathyroid glands are located on the posterior surface of the thyroid gland. (Objective 2)
16. Parathyroid hormone (PTH). (Objective 2)
17. PTH stimulates calcium release from bone, calcium uptake from the GI tract, and calcium reabsorption from the kidney. Excess PTH will cause hypercalcemia and loss of bone density, leading to pathologic fractures. (Objective 20)
18. Hypoparathyroidism will cause hypocalcemia. (Objective 20)
19. The adrenal medulla releases epinephrine. (Objective 2)
20. Aldosterone is produced in the adrenal cortex. (Objective 2)
21. Aldosterone promotes reabsorption of sodium and water by the kidney and excretion of potassium. (Objective 2)
22. The glucocorticosteroids are produced in the adrenal cortex. (Objective 2)
23. The glucocorticosteroids raise the blood glucose level by promoting conversion of protein to sugar. They also

suppress the inflammatory and immune responses. (Objective 2)

24. Addison's disease is insufficient production of hormones by the adrenal cortex. (Objective 23)

25. Decreased aldosterone levels cause increased loss of sodium and water in the urine, leading to hypovolemia and hypotension. Decreased aldos-terone levels cause potassium retention, leading to hyperkalemia. Decreased glucocorticoid levels can cause hypoglycemia. (Objective 24)

26. Restore intravascular volume using normal saline solution. (Ringer's lactate contains potassium.) Monitor blood glucose levels and administer $D_{50}W$ if the patient becomes hypoglycemic. Monitor the ECG for dysrhythmias produced by hyperkalemia and other electrolyte imbalances. (Objective 25)

27. Islets of Langerhans. (Objective 2)

28. Beta cells of the islets of Langerhans. (Objective 2)

29. Insulin lowers blood glucose levels by promoting transport of sugar into the cells. (Objective 3)

30. Alpha cells of the islets of Langerhans. (Objective 2)

31. Glucagon raises blood glucose levels by promoting breakdown of liver glycogen. (Objective 3)

32. Insulin. (Objective 5)

33. Type 1 diabetes is an autoimmune disease resulting from destruction of the beta cells of the islets of Langerhans. In type 1 diabetes there is no insulin produced. Insulin is required to manage type 1 diabetes. Most patients with type 1 diabetes develop the disease as children or young adults. Type 2 diabetes is a familial disease resulting from decreased insulin production and increased resistance of body tissues to insulin's effects. Most patient's with type 2 diabetes develop the disease during middle age. Because type 2 diabetes involves a relative insulin deficiency, it can be managed initially with weight loss, diet, and oral medications that lower blood glucose levels or promote insulin release. Some patients with type 2 diabetes eventually must take insulin by injection to manage their disease. (Objective 4)

34. The pH of a patient with diabetic ketoacidosis falls, resulting in a metabolic acidosis. (Objective 10)

35. Polyuria, polydipsia, and polyphagia. (Objective 10)

36. A silent myocardial infarction is a myocardial infarction that occurs without pain. Diabetic patients tend to develop impaired nerve function (peripheral neuropathies) as their disease progresses. As a result they may not feel the pain of a myocardial infarction. Diabetes also results in an increased risk for atherosclerosis, cerebrovascular accident, and myocardial infarction. (Objective 5)

37. Patients with HHNC do not use fat as an alternative metabolic fuel to glucose. Therefore they do not develop the ketoacidosis that is present in DKA. (Objective 4)

38. Patients with type 2 diabetes are prone to HHNC. Because they still produce small amounts of insulin, patients with HHNC are able to move enough sugar into their cells to avoid using fat as a metabolic fuel and developing ketoacidosis. (Objective 4)

39. Gestational diabetes is a tendency toward elevated blood glucose levels that develops during pregnancy. Gestational diabetes results from the tendency of progesterone to antagonize the action of insulin. (Objective 5)

Multiple Choice

1. D. The body attempts to compensate for the acidosis associated with diabetic ketoacidosis by increasing the rate and depth of ventilations. (Objective 10)

2. D. The islets of Langerhans secrete insulin from the beta cells, which decreases the blood glucose levels. (Objective 2)

3. C. He is experiencing HHNC. Diabetes of recent onset in a 45-year-old man is more likely to be type 2 diabetes. Patients with type 2 diabetes are more likely to develop HHNC than DKA. Type 2 diabetes frequently does not require insulin injection therapy. (Objective 12)

4. A. Because the kidneys can only concentrate urine to a certain osmotic pressure, they must excrete more water than usual. (Objectives 10, 12)

5. A. The body system that has the most significant interaction with the endocrine system's functions is the autonomic nervous system. (Objective 2)

6. C. The presence of a thyroid goiter, tachycardia, fever, and weight loss are typically associated with Graves' disease. (Objective 18)

7. A. Addisonian crisis. Myxedema and Graves' disease involve the thyroid gland. Cushing's disease involves the adrenal gland, but is more likely to produce hypertension. The patient shows signs and symptoms of volume loss, which are consistent with an addisonian crisis. (Objective 24)

8. D. Establish an IV and give 25 g of $D_{50}W$. The patient is hypoglycemic, so the preferred treatment is intravenous administration of glucose. Because her mental status is altered, placing anything in her mouth creates the risk of aspiration. Glucagon is given IM in situations where vascular access cannot be obtained. (Objective 7)

9. B. This woman has the classic signs and symptoms of Cushing's syndrome. (Objective 24)

10. C. Type 1 diabetes is associated with an autoimmune origin. (Objective 4)

11. A. Calcitonin is responsible for decreasing the amount of calcium in the blood by inhibiting breakdown of bone. (Objective 2)

12. B. Myxedema coma would be expected to cause bradycardia and hypotension. (Objective 18)

Case Studies

Case one

1. New-onset diabetes mellitus. (Objective 10)

2. This patient probably has type 1 diabetes because she is an adolescent and is exhibiting signs and symptoms of diabetic ketoacidosis. (Objective 4)

348

3. Type 1 diabetes is an autoimmune disease that produces an absolute insulin deficiency. Its onset typically occurs in children or young adults, and it must be managed with insulin injections. Type 2 diabetes is a familial disease that produces relative insulin deficiency. Its onset typically occurs in middle-aged adults. Type 2 diabetes often can be managed with weight loss, diet, and oral medications, but may progress to requiring insulin therapy. (Objective 4)
4. Diabetic ketoacidosis. (Objective 10)
5. The patient is increasing the rate at which she is removing carbon dioxide from her body to compensate for a metabolic acidosis. (Objective 10)
6. Kussmaul respirations. (Objective 10)
7. Ketone bodies present in the exhaled air. (Objective 10)
8. The patient is using fat as a metabolic fuel because her lack of insulin prevents her from transporting glucose into her cells. Ketone bodies are the products of fat metabolism. (Objective 10)
9. Too high. Her pancreas is not producing insulin; therefore she cannot move glucose from the blood into the cells. (Objective 10)
10. Her blood pH will be decreased, because ketone bodies are acids. (Objective 10)
11. Metabolic acidosis. (Objective 10)
12. The hyperglycemia associated with diabetes produces an osmotic diuresis that increases urine output and leads to hypovolemic shock. (Objective 10)
13. Administer high-concentration oxygen. Establish an IV with normal saline and begin volume replacement. Monitor the ECG. Transport to the hospital for insulin therapy. (Objective 11)
14. An isotonic crystalloid is needed to treat volume loss. Normal saline would be preferred over Ringer's lactate because Ringer's lactate contains potassium. Acidotic states can cause a shift of potassium from the intracellular space to the extracellular space, producing hyperkalemia. IV fluids that contain potassium can worsen this problem. (Objective 11)
15. Tall, peaked T waves suggest hyperkalemia secondary to acidosis. (Objective 11)
16. Sodium bicarbonate can be used to promote movement of potassium back into the intracellular space. However, it is important to remember that this therapy should be reserved for suspected hyperkalemia, and not used solely in an effort to treat acidosis. (Objective 11)
17. The hyperkalemia present in ketoacidosis results from a shift of potassium from the intracellular space to the extracellular space. Because patients with diabetic ketoacidosis have ongoing extracellular fluid loss, they may significantly reduce their total body potassium. As the acidosis associated with DKA is corrected, potassium will shift back to the intracellular space, producing hypokalemia. (Objective 11)

Case two

1. This patient probably has type 2 diabetes. (Objective 4)

2. Hyperglycemic hyperosmolar nonketotic coma (HHNC). (Objective 12)
3. Patients with HHNC do not develop a ketoacidosis. Therefore they do not display Kussmaul respirations. (Objective 12)
4. Patients with HHNC continue to metabolize glucose rather than using fat as an alternative fuel. Therefore they do not produce ketone bodies and do not have a fruity breath odor. (Objective 12)
5. Because type 2 diabetes is caused by a relative insulin deficiency, patients with this disease process continue to use glucose as a metabolic fuel rather than shifting to use of fats. As a result, they continue to raise their blood glucose levels in an attempt to provide adequate fuel for their cells. (Objective 12)
6. Hypovolemic. (Objective 12)
7. The elevated blood glucose levels in HHNC produce an osmotic diuresis that causes hypovolemia. (Objective 12)
8. Very high blood glucose levels can produce in increase in blood viscosity that can interfere with blood flow in smaller vessels, leading to tissue hypoxia. (Objective 12)
9. Since the patient is hypovolemic, over time she will develop lactic acidosis secondary to hypoperfusion. This will cause a drop in the pH. (Objective 12)
10. Metabolic (lactic) acidosis secondary to hypovolemia. (Objective 12)
11. Secure the airway, assist ventilations with high-concentration oxygen, establish an IV using normal saline and begin to correct volume loss, monitor ECG, acquire a 12-lead ECG to evaluate for possible acute myocardial infarction, transport. (Objective 13)

Case three

1. Hypoglycemia. (Objective 6)
2. The brain does not require insulin to move glucose from the blood into its cells. However, the brain requires a continuous supply of glucose to function properly. (Objective 6)
3. When the blood glucose level falls, the adrenal glands release epinephrine to mobilize the glycogen stores in the liver. Epinephrine causes tachycardia, pallor, and diaphoresis. (Objective 6)
4. If the patient is able to swallow and protect his own airway, administer oral glucose. If the patient cannot safely take glucose by the oral route, establish an IV and give 25 g of $D_{50}W$. (Objective 7)

Case four

1. Gestational diabetes. (Objective 3)
2. Progesterone antagonizes the effects of insulin, raising blood glucose levels during pregnancy. (Objective 3)
3. This effect normally is useful because it increases the amount of glucose available to the developing fetus. (Objective 3)
4. Because oral contraceptives also contain progesterone, some women taking birth control pills

349

also may develop symptoms of gestational diabetes. (Objective 3)

Case five

1. The patient is having a silent myocardial infarction. (Objective 5)
2. Diabetic patients tend to develop peripheral neuropathies that interfere with their ability to feel pain, including the pain of a heart attack. (Objective 5)
3. The elderly also are prone to silent myocardial infarction because of deterioration of nerve function with age. (Objective 5)

Case six

1. Alcohol inhibits the function of the liver enzyme systems that carry out gluconeogenesis—conversion of protein into sugar. Consuming alcohol after not having eaten for several hours can result in a hypoglycemic state that can mimic intoxication. (Objectives 3, 6)

Case seven

1. The patient is suffering from a thyrotoxic crisis (thyroid storm). (Objective 18)
2. Thyrotoxic crisis can result in hyperthermia, severe tachycardia, cardiac dysrhythmias, heart failure, shock. (Objective 17)
3. Airway/ventilation/oxygen, ECG monitor, IV access—cautious IV fluids, control hyperthermia, active cooling, acetaminophen, beta-blockers, consider benzodiazepines for anxiety. (Objective 19)

Case eight

1. Myxedema coma. (Objective 18)
2. Secure the airway, support ventilations, monitor ECG, establish an IV but limit fluids, monitor pulmonary and cardiac function, transport. (Objective 19)

Case nine

1. The adrenal cortex. (Objective 24)
2. The blood glucose levels probably will be elevated. Her adrenal cortex is secreting excessive amounts of glucocorticoids, which will raise her blood glucose levels. (Objective 24)
3. She probably will be hypertensive. (Objective 24)
4. The adrenal cortex is secreting excessive amounts of aldosterone. This will cause her to retain sodium and water, which will produce hypertension. (Objective 23)
5. She probably will be hypokalemic. Increased aldosterone secretion will cause increased potassium loss in the urine. (Objective 24)
6. The adrenal cortex produces small amounts of male sex hormones. Hyperadrenalism in a female can stimulate beard growth. (Objective 23)

Case ten

1. The patient has an addisonian crisis caused by failure to properly taper his dose of oral steroids. Steroid therapy suppresses the release of ACTH from the anterior pituitary, which results in an absence of hormone release from the adrenal cortex. Failure to gradually taper the dose of steroids does not allow the pituitary time to become active again and can result in hypoadrenalism. (Objective 24)
2. He is hypovolemic because his adrenal cortex is not secreting aldosterone. (Objective 23)
3. It would have been increased. (Objective 24)
4. His blood glucose levels would be low because he is not secreting glucocorticoid hormones from his adrenal cortex. (Objective 24)
5. His serum potassium levels will be elevated because his aldosterone levels are decreased and aldosterone normally promotes excretion of potassium in the urine. (Objective 24)
6. Administer high-concentration oxygen, establish an IV with normal saline and begin volume replacement, check the blood glucose levels and administer $D_{50}W$ if hypoglycemia is present, monitor the ECG for dysrhythmias associated with hyperkalemia. (Objective 25)

CHAPTER 25: IMMUNE SYSTEM DISORDERS

Short Answer

1. IgE. (Objective 16)
2. Histamine. (Objective 16)
3. Vasodilation, increased capillary permeability, contrac-tion of nonvascular smooth muscle. (Objective 16)
4. An isotonic crystalloid such as normal saline or Ringer's lactate. Hypoperfusion in anaphylaxis is caused by a combination of vasodilation and loss of intravascular fluid into the interstitial space. An isotonic solution will help fill the dilated vascular space and replace volume lost from increased capillary permeability. (Objective 24)
5. Epinephrine and diphenhydramine. (Objective 24)
6. Diphenhydramine is an antihistamine. (Objective 24)
7. Intravenous or intramuscular. (Objective 24)
8. Intravenous. Patients suffering from anaphylaxis have poor peripheral perfusion. Drugs given by the intramuscular or subcutaneous routes will not be absorbed and distributed quickly enough. (Objective 22)
9. The alpha effects of epinephrine cause peripheral vasoconstriction, which helps to reverse the vasodilation produced by histamine. (Objective 24)
10. Epinephrine's beta$_2$ effects produce relaxation of bronchial smooth muscle, reversing the bronchospasm caused by histamine. Epinephrine's beta$_1$ effects improve myocardial contractility, helping to support cardiac output and blood pressure. (Objective 24)
11. Epinephrine should be given first to begin reversing life-threatening vasodilation and bronchoconstric-tion produced by histamine release. Diphenhydra-mine blocks histamine receptors. Therefore it is not effective in relieving the immediate effects of

histamine release, only in keeping them from continuing. (Objective 24)

12. Corticosteroids suppress inflammatory response. Therefore they are useful in providing long-term protection against reoccurrence of an allergic reaction. However, because the onset of their action is very slow, they are of little value in managing the immediate life threats present in anaphylaxis. (Objective 24)

13. B-lymphocytes. (Objective 3)

14. The thymus. (Objective 3)

15. The helper T-cell coordinates the activities of the immune system's other components. (Objective 3)

16. Macrophages ingest and destroy pathogens. They then present surface antigens from pathogens to the helper T-cells to aid them in identifying the specific pathogen and coordinating a response to it. (Objective 3)

17. Mild allergic reactions are characterized by cutaneous signs and symptoms such as itching and the presence of a rash or urticaria (hives). Difficulty breathing or hypoperfusion is not present. (Objective 20)

18. A moderate allergic reaction is characterized by the presence of difficulty breathing. The patient's perfusion is not affected. (Objective 20)

19. Anaphylaxis is an allergic reaction that produces hypotension and cardiovascular collapse. It may also be associated with respiratory distress and failure. (Objective 20)

20. Systemic lupus erythematosis is an autoimmune disease caused by production of an antibody that attacks the patient's nucleic acid, producing widespread damage to the body's tissues. (Objective 9)

21. Serositis (pleurisy, pericarditis). Renal injury/failure. CNS involvement with seizures/psychosis. Peripheral vasculitis/gangrene. (Objective 9)

Multiple Choice

1. A. Administration of epinephrine can correct urticaria associated with anaphylaxis. This can best be explained by epinephrine's effect on alpha-receptor sites, which produces vasoconstriction in the periphery. (Objective 22)

2. D. The release of histamine causes increased vascular membrane permeability and bronchospasm. (Objective 16)

3. C. Management of this patient should include oxygen followed by 50 mg of diphenhydramine IM to treat a mild allergic reaction. Use of albuterol or subcutaneous epinephrine is not indicated because there are no respiratory symptoms. Methylprednisolone's onset of action is too slow to make its administration immediately useful. (Objective 22)

4. C. Antibodies or immunoglobulins are a component of humoral immunity and are produced by B-lymphocytes. (Objective 3)

5. D. IgE-type antibodies are primarily bound to mast cells in the tissues. (Objective 6)

6. A. The T-lymphocytes that coordinate the activities of the immune system's other components are the helper T-cells. (Objective 3)

7. B. A 20-year-old man is experiencing an anaphylactic reaction. After administration of oxygen, the first drug that should be administered to this patient is epinephrine. Epinephrine will reverse the vasodilation and bronchoconstriction caused by histamine. IV fluids given to patients with anaphylaxis should be isotonic. Diphenhydramine and Solu-Medrol are useful in keeping an allergic reaction from continuing, but do not reverse the immediately life-threatening problems present in anaphylaxis. (Objective 22)

8. C. You suspect this patient is experiencing an anaphylactic reaction. The fact that the patient has a positive orthostatic test indicates that she is not perfusing adequately. (Objective 21)

9. A. In a type I hypersensitivity reaction, the IgE antibody is bound to basophils or mast cells. (Objective 19)

10. B. Mast cells release histamine, heparin, and leukotrienes. Macrophages are another type of leukocyte involved in the immune response. (Objective 19)

11. A. Crohn's disease involves the immune system through an unknown mechanism. Historically this condition was thought to be an autoimmune disorder, but contemporary thought is that the disorder occurs secondary to an overreaction of the immune system to environmental, infectious, or dietary agents. Diverticulitis also affects the GI system, but it is not an autoimmune disease. (Objective 9)

12. C. Type 1 diabetes mellitus has an autoimmune origin. (Objective 9)

13. B. Use of diphenhydramine should be avoided in patients with a history of asthma. (Objective 22)

14. A. Abdominal pain associated with an allergic reaction occurs because of smooth muscle spasm. (Objective 19)

15. B. Oxygen should be given to a patient who is having an allergic reaction by nonrebreather mask at 15 L/min. (Objective 22)

16. D. When a nebulized bronchodilator is given to a patient, tremors and an increased pulse rate should be anticipated. Nebulized bronchodilators also will cause nervousness and restlessness. (Objective 22)

17. D. The classic signs and symptoms of anaphylaxis include tachycardia and hypotension. (Objective 20)

Case Study

1. Securing the airway by placing an endotracheal tube. The presence of stridor indicates edema of the larynx and upper airway that could progress to complete obstruction. (Objective 24)

2. Yes. As long as the stinger remains in the patient, it will continue to introduce antigen. The stinger should be removed by scraping it off. Using tweezers is not appropriate because grasping the venom sac can squeeze more antigen into the patient. (Objective 24)

351

3. Histamine released from the mast cells is causing vasodilation and loss of fluid from the vascular space secondary to increased capillary permeability. (Objective 19)

4. An isotonic crystalloid should be used because it will remain in the vascular space. This will help fill the dilated vascular compartment and replace fluid lost into the interstitial space. (Objective 24)

5. Medications should be given by the intravenous route. The patient is hypoperfusing. Therefore medications given by the intramuscular or subcutaneous routes will not be absorbed rapidly enough. (Objective 24)

6. The first-line drug for the management of anaphylaxis is epinephrine. Epinephrine will reverse the vasodilation and bronchospasm caused by histamine release during anaphylaxis. (Objective 24)

7. Diphenhydramine. (Objective 24)

8. Diphenhydramine blocks histamine receptor sites and prevents allergic reaction from continuing. (Objective 24)

9. Corticosteroids such as Solu-Medrol inhibit the inflammatory response and are useful for long-term prevention of allergic reactions. (Objective 24)

10. The onset of Solu-Medrol's effects is very slow. Therefore it has little immediate value in the management of anaphylaxis. (Objective 24)

CHAPTER 26: GASTROINTESTINAL DISORDERS

Short Answer

1.

RLQ	Hollow	Appendix
RUQ	Solid	Liver
LUQ	Hollow	Stomach
LUQ	Solid	Spleen
RUQ	Hollow	Gallbladder
RUQ/LUQ	Solid	Pancreas
LLQ	Hollow	Sigmoid colon
RUQ	Solid	Right kidney

(Objective 3)

2. The peritoneum is a double-sided serous membrane that lines the abdominal cavity. The visceral peritoneum is the side of the peritoneum that surrounds and covers the abdominal organs. (Objective 3)

3. The peritoneum is a double-sided serous membrane that lines the abdominal cavity. The parietal peritoneum is the side of the peritoneum that lies against the body wall. (Objective 3)

4. Visceral pain is dull, poorly localized pain that results from inflammation, distention, or ischemia of a hollow organ. (Objective 6)

5. Somatic pain is sharp, localized pain that originates from inflammation of the parietal peritoneum and the structures of the body wall. (Objective 5)

6. Referred pain is pain that originates from a structure that is in a region other than where the pain is felt. (Objective 7)

7. The heart, lungs, and male genitalia can refer pain to the abdomen. Diseases such as acute myocardial infarction, pneumonia (particularly in the lower lobes), and testicular torsion may present with abdominal pain. (Objective 7)

8. A dark, tarry, foul-smelling stool is called *melena*. (Objective 102)

9. Melena is produced by the digestion of blood that has entered the gastrointestinal tract. Therefore melena is a sign of gastrointestinal bleeding, usually from the upper gastrointestinal tract. (Objective 102)

10. Bright red blood in the stool usually indicates bleeding from a site in the lower gastrointestinal tract. However, rapid loss of a large amount of blood into the upper GI tract can result in bright red blood in the stool. (Objective 107)

11. The abdomen should be palpated after auscultating. Palpation can stimulate the gastrointestinal tract and produce falsely hyperactive bowel sounds. (Objective 14)

12. Esophageal varices are dilated veins in the esophagus. Varices can produce massive upper gastrointestinal bleeding with a mortality higher than 35%. (Objective 55)

13. Chronic alcohol abuse produces scar tissue formation (cirrhosis) in the liver. Hepatic cirrhosis increases resistance to blood flow entering the liver from the hepatic portal circulation, producing portal hypertension. The blood in the hepatic portal circulation seeks other paths by which it can return to the central circulation and reroutes itself through veins in the distal esophagus, causing them to dilate. Portal hypertension also results in dilation of the venous plexus in the rectum, increasing the tendency of patients with alcoholism to rectal hemorrhage. (Objective 56)

14. Mallory-Weiss syndrome is bleeding associated with a tear in the lining of the esophagus near the gastroesophageal junction. Mallory-Weiss tears usually result from forceful vomiting. (Objective 46)

15. Abdominal distention, nausea, vomiting, cramping pain, and high-pitched "tinkling" bowel sounds indicate the presence of a bowel obstruction. (Objective 117)

16. If a patient has perforated the gastrointestinal tract, materials given by mouth could leak from the GI tract into the peritoneal cavity, worsening inflammation. Also, acute abdominal disorders result in decreased motility in the gastrointestinal tract and an increased risk of vomiting. Giving the patient anything by mouth increases the risk of vomiting and aspiration, particularly if the patient must go to the operating room. (Objectives 145, 148)

17. Acute myocardial infarction can refer pain to the upper abdomen, mimicking an acute condition of the abdomen. (Objective 7)

18. IVs for patients with acute abdominal pain should be started with an isotonic crystalloid. Patients with an acute condition of the abdomen are at risk for hypovolemia, either from bleeding into the gastrointestinal tract or from fluid loss into the abdominal cavity from an inflamed peritoneum or

into an obstructed bowel. An isotonic crystalloid will remain in the vascular space, replacing lost blood volume. (Objectives 145, 148)

19. McBurney's point is the location where pain from appendicitis tends to localize. It is located 1½ to 2 inches above the anterior iliac crest along a direct line from the iliac crest to the umbilicus. (Objective 122)

20. Murphy's sign is an abrupt cessation of inhalation secondary to pain when palpating under the right costal margin. (Objective 77)

Multiple Choice

1. D. This patient's pain is most characteristic of pancreatitis. Epigastric pain radiating directly through to the mid-back in a patient with a history of significant alcohol consumption indicates pancreatitis. (Objective 82)

2. B. Because this patient has abdominal pain associated with signs of blood loss, it would be most important to ask about the chronic use of aspirin, anticoagulants, and NSAIDs. Use of these medications can predispose a patient to gastrointestinal bleeding. (Objective 100)

3. B. The pain of acute appendicitis most often begins as nonspecific periumbilical pain. As appendicitis progresses, the pain localizes to the right lower quadrant. Pain after eating a fatty meal is characteristic of cholecystitis. (Objective 122)

4. A. The single most likely diagnosis for this patient is abdominal aortic aneurysm. The pain of appendicitis begins in the peri-umbilical area and shifts to the right lower quadrant. Renal calculus causes pain that radiates from the costovertebral angle around the flank to the groin, but not typically into the leg. Diverticulitis usually causes pain in the left lower quadrant that does not radiate to the leg. Pain radiating to the right leg associated with numbness of the extremity suggests vascular involvement and the probably presence of an abdominal aortic aneurysm. (Objectives 12, 137)

5. A. Uniform inflammation of the mucosal lining of the colon and rectum resulting in bloody diarrhea and abdominal pain is most likely the result of colitis. Crohn's disease tends to involve the small bowel more frequently than other portions of the gastrointestinal tract and produces inflamed segments interspersed with unaffected areas. (Objective 127)

6. B. Severe burning pain in the upper abdomen during periods of stress, epigastric tenderness, and signs of bleeding into the gastrointestinal tract suggest a bleeding duodenal ulcer. Kidney stones produce cramping pain that radiates around the flank to the groin and are not associated with GI bleeding. An abdominal aortic aneurysm is more likely to produce back pain, hypovolemic shock, and signs of poor perfusion to the lower extremities. Gallbladder disease produces right upper quadrant pain that radiates to the right shoulder or the tip of the right scapula; this pain typically occurs following consumption of fatty foods. (Objective 97)

7. C. Severe, constant abdominal pain worsened by movement; a distended, rigid, diffusely tender abdomen; warm, moist skin; and absent bowel sounds suggest peritonitis. A ruptured aortic aneurysm would produce more severe signs and symptoms of hypovolemic shock. Appendicitis produces localized tenderness in the right lower quadrant following a period of discomfort surrounding the umbilicus. Patients with kidney stones experience intense, cramping pain that makes it difficult for them to remain still. (Objective 90)

8. B. You should avoid giving the patient anything by mouth. Patients with abdominal pain should not be given anything by mouth because of the probability they will need to go to the operating room. (Objectives 145, 148)

9. A. Pain and tenderness that begin around the umbilicus and move to the right lower abdominal quadrant are characteristic of appendicitis. (Objective 122)

10. C. The most common cause of cholecystitis is gallstones. (Objective 76)

11. D. An overweight 42-year-old female with 5 children would be most likely to develop cholecystitis. (Objective 76)

12. A. Duodenal ulcers are more common in persons under stress. The pain from gastric ulcers is worse when the stomach is full. Pain from duodenal ulcers is more common at night. (Objective 97)

13. D. Low-fiber diets and advanced age are risk factors for developing diverticulitis. (Objective 136)

14. C. The most common causes of pancreatitis are gallstones and alcohol abuse. (Objective 81)

15. C. Somatic pain is caused by stimulation of nerve fibers in the parietal peritoneum. (Objective 5)

16. D. Visceral pain is caused by distention of a hollow organ. (Objective 6)

17. A. Abdominal pain radiating from the right upper quadrant around the right side to the angle of the scapula is most likely caused by cholecystitis. (Objective 77)

18. A. Hematochezia is bright red blood in the stool. (Objective 107)

19. C. Melena means that the stool was dark and tarry. (Objective 102)

Case Studies

Case one

1. This patient has appendicitis. (Objective 122)

2. Appendicitis is usually caused by obstruction of the opening that connects the appendix with the cecum, usually with a hard piece of fecal matter called a fecalith. Accumulation of secretions from glands in the wall of the appendix that are unable to drain into the cecum distends the appendix, reducing blood flow

353

through its walls and causing ischemia, which triggers an inflammatory response. (Objective 121)

3. The embryonic structure that eventually develops into the appendix forms near the location of the appendix, and then migrates downward into the right lower abdominal quadrant and the intestinal tract forms. As the appendix moves into the right lower quadrant of the developing embryo, it pulls its nerve supply with it. When the appendix becomes inflamed, the initial pain is referred to the periumbilical area where the embryonic appendix and its nerve supply originated. (Objective 121)

4. Inflammation from appendicitis frequently spreads to the iliopsoas muscle, which connects from the lower back through the pelvis to the femur. Lying on the right side with the knee flexed reduces stress on the inflamed iliopsoas muscle and relieves part of the pain of appendicitis. (Objective 122)

5. The sudden relief of pain is the result of the appendix rupturing. The patient needs to go to the hospital immediately for emergency surgery to reduce the risk of developing peritonitis. (Objective 124)

6. Administer high-concentration oxygen by nonrebreather mask. Establish an IV with an isotonic crystalloid. Allow the patient to assume a comfortable position. Administer nothing by mouth. (Objective 124)

Case two

1. The patient probably has a duodenal ulcer that is bleeding into the gastrointestinal tract. (Objective 97)

2. No, a patient with blood loss would be expected to have a tachycardia. However, this patient just experienced an episode of vomiting. Vomiting is a vagal stimulus, which can result in a temporary decrease in the heart rate. (Objective 145)

3. Melana is a dark, tarry stool that results from blood being digested as it passes through the gastrointestinal tract. If the patient has only recently begun bleeding or is losing only a small amount of blood into the GI tract, melena might not be present. (Objectives 101, 102)

4. The changes in the patient's vital signs and mental status when he is moved to a sitting position indicate he is hypovolemic. (Objective 102)

5. Keep the patient in a supine position with his lower extremities elevated. Give high-concentration oxygen using a nonrebreather mask. Establish an IV with an isotonic crystalloid. Give nothing by mouth. Transport. (Objectives 99, 104)

Case three

1. Cramping pain, abdominal distention, and inability to have a bowel movement indicate the presence of a bowel obstruction. (Objective 117)

2. Abdominal surgery can result in the formation of adhesions that can predispose a patient to bowel obstruction. (Objective 116)

3. The patient's vital signs indicate she is in shock. Patient's with bowel obstruction lose fluid into the lumen of the bowel that cannot be reabsorbed because they never reach the colon, which is

responsible for recovering body fluids lost into the gastrointestinal tract. This loss of fluid volume into the obstructed bowel results in hypovolemia. (Objective 116)

4. The obstruction probably is in the distal portion of the small bowel. The materials accumulating in the bowel have not been able to back up to the point where the patient begins to vomit. (Objective 117)

5. When the patient begins to vomit, the vomitus is likely to contain fecal matter. (Objective 117)

6. Administer high-concentration oxygen using a nonrebreather mask. Establish an IV with an isotonic crystalloid. Allow the patient to assume a comfortable position. Give nothing by mouth. Transport. (Objective 119)

CHAPTER 27: RENAL AND UROGENITAL DISORDERS

Short Answer

1. Regulating water and electrolytes. Regulating acid-base balance. Excreting waste products and foreign chemicals. Regulating arterial blood pressure. Promoting production of red blood cells. Producing new sugar (gluconeogenesis). (Objective 1)

2. The nephron is the basic functional unit of the kidney. (Objective 1)

3. The adrenal cortex secretes aldosterone. (Objective 1)

4. Aldosterone promotes reabsorption of sodium, chloride, and water and secretion of potassium in the distal tubule and collecting duct, leading to decreased urine output. (Objective 1)

5. The posterior pituitary gland secretes antidiuretic hormone. Antidiuretic hormone is produced in the hypothalamus and moves to the posterior pituitary for storage and release. (Objective 1)

6. Antidiuretic hormone promotes reabsorption of water from the distal tubule and collecting duct, leading to decreased urine output. (Objective 1)

7. Atrial natriuretic hormone is secreted by the atria of the heart. (Objective 1)

8. Atrial natriuretic hormone causes a decrease in reabsorption of sodium and chloride in the distal tubule and collecting duct, leading to increased urine output. (Objective 1)

9. Mannitol increases the osmolality of the urine, inhibiting water and sodium reabsorption in the proximal tubule. Lasix reduces sodium, potassium, and chloride reabsorption in the loop of Henle. Hydrochlorothiazide inhibits sodium and chloride reabsorption in the distal tubule. (Objective 1)

10. Decreased renal blood flow causes the kidney to secrete renin into the bloodstream. Renin acts on angiotensinogen to convert it to angiotensin I. The angiotensin-converting enzyme then converts angiotensin I to angiotensin II. Angiotensin II is a potent vasoconstrictor. It also promotes release of aldosterone from the adrenal cortex and acts directly on the proximal tubule to promote reabsorption of

sodium, chloride, and water. The intravascular fluid volume increases and the size of the vascular compartment decreases, leading to an increase in blood pressure. (Objective 1)

11. The kidneys secrete 90% of the body's erythropoietin, a hormone that stimulates production of red blood cells by the bone marrow. Loss of renal erythropoietin leads to a drop in red cell production, causing severe anemia. (Objective 1)

12. In acute renal failure the kidneys suddenly stop functioning either partially or completely. However, they eventually recover full or nearly full functioning. Chronic renal failure is characterized by a structural or functional abnormality that produces irreversible loss of a large number of nephrons. (Objectives 5, 7)

13. End-stage renal disease is characterized by an almost total loss of functioning nephrons that results in renal function that is less than 10% of baseline. End-stage renal function cannot be reversed and must be treated with dialysis or transplantation. (Objective 7)

14. Prerenal, intrarenal, postrenal. (Objective 5)

15. Prerenal acute renal failure is caused by a reduction in blood supply to the kidneys. Common causes include hypovolemia; cardiac problems; stenosis, embolism, or thrombosis of the renal artery; blockage of prostaglandin synthesis by excessive aspirin intake; and hypotension secondary to peripheral vasodilation. (Objective 5)

16. Intrarenal acute renal failure is caused by disease processes that directly damage the kidney's small blood vessels or glomerulus, the renal tubules, or the renal interstitial tissue. Causes include atherosclerosis of the kidney's small blood vessels, malignant hypertension, acute glomerulonephritis, ischemic necrosis of the tubules, toxic damage to the tubules, or acute pyelonephritis. (Objective 5)

17. Postrenal acute renal failure is caused by conditions that block the flow of urine from the kidney. Causes include blockage of the renal pelvis or ureters by large kidney stones or blood clots, obstruction of the urinary bladder, and urethral obstruction. (Objective 5)

18. Edema results from fluid retention that expands the extracellular fluid volume. Dysrhythmias result from electrolyte imbalances, particularly hyperkalemia. Jaundice results from retention in the bloodstream of yellow pigments normally excreted in the urine. Hypertension results from expansion of the intravascular fluid volume. If renal failure is a result of decreased blood flow to the kidney, the renin-angiotensin-aldosterone system also contributes to the increase in blood pressure. (Objectives 5, 7)

19. Renal failure produces hyperkalemia. The principal route used by the body to eliminate excess potassium is the urinary tract. If urinary removal of potassium decreases, the amount of potassium in the extracellular fluid will rise. (Objective 1)

20. Renal failure produces metabolic acidosis. The kidneys are the body's route for eliminating sulfuric and phosphoric acids produced by protein metabolism. Renal failure results in retention of these acids in the extracellular fluid and an increase in hydrogen ion concentration. (Objectives 5, 7)

21. Do not take the patient's blood pressure in the right arm. Do not apply firm, direct pressure to the right arm. Loosen tight or restrictive clothing on the right arm. Do not use the fistula to give drugs or fluids except in a life-threatening emergency when no other route is available. (Objective 9)

22. Sodium bicarbonate and calcium chloride will be administered early in the management of this patient. A patient receiving dialysis who is in cardiac arrest probably is hyperkalemic. Calcium antagonizes the cardiotoxic effects of excess potassium. Sodium bicarbonate helps correct the metabolic acidosis present in renal failure. Sodium bicarbonate also produces an alkalotic state that causes an intracellular shift of potassium that corrects hyperkalemia. (Objective 10)

23. Gently palpate the graft or fistula for the vibration, referred to as a *thrill*, that is produced by blood flow. (Objective 9)

24. Disequilibrium syndrome is a complication of dialysis that develops when the extracellular fluid becomes hypotonic relative to the intracellular fluid. Water shifts to the intracellular space. This fluid shift produces cerebral edema that manifests itself though headache, restlessness, and nausea. Severe disequilibrium syndrome can cause confusion, seizures, and coma. (Objective 10)

25. Females are more prone to developing urinary tract infections. The female urethra is shorter than the male urethra. This anatomic difference favors colonization of the female urinary tract by bacteria. (Objective 15)

26. Priapism is a prolonged, painful erection of the penis. (Objective 25)

27. (1) Disorders of the blood such as sickle cell anemia, myeloma, and leukemia. (2) Accidental or surgical trauma. (3) Nervous system damage caused by multiple sclerosis or diabetes mellitus. (4) Erectile dysfunction drugs such as Viagra, Levitra, or Cialis. (5) Drugs injected to enhance sexual performance. (6) Psychotropic medications such as trazodone and chlorpromazine. (Objective 25)

28. Benign prostatic hypertrophy is a noncancerous enlargement of the prostate gland that tends to occur as males age. (Objective 27)

29. Benign prostatic hypertrophy predisposes patients to urinary retention, urinary tract infections, renal calculi, and renal failure caused by obstruction. (Objective 27)

Multiple Choice

1. B. Signs and symptoms of renal failure include edema, low urine output, and signs of heart failure. (Objectives 5, 7)

2. A. This patient is suffering from epididymitis, which resulted from a urethral infection that migrated

355

through the vas deferens to the epididymis. (Objective 21)

3. A. Based upon this information, you are concerned that this patient may be experiencing cardiac ischemia. During dialysis, a portion of the patient's blood volume leaves the vascular space to enter the dialysis machine. This external shift of blood can produce hypotension and increase the heart's workload and oxygen demand, causing myocardial ischemia. (Objective 10)

4. D. Hyperkalemia is associated with peaked T waves. Hyperkalemia also causes the P-R interval to lengthen. As hyperkalemia worsens, the P waves become smaller and disappear. (Objective 10)

5. C. Flank pain, dysuria, urinary frequency, fever, and chills suggest pyelonephritis. (Objective 15)

6. B. The most common causes of chronic renal failure are hypertension and diabetes. (Objective 7)

7. B. Cardiac arrest in a patient with chronic renal failure usually is associated with hyperkalemia. (Objective 18)

8. A. A patient with chronic renal failure would be most likely to develop congestive heart failure secondary to volume overload. Patients with chronic renal failure tend to become hypertensive because of increased intravascular fluid volume. They develop metabolic acidosis secondary to inability to excrete hydrogen ion through the kidney. Chronic renal failure tends to result in tissue resistance to insulin, producing glucose intolerance and hyperglycemia. (Objective 7)

9. D. Urinary calculus (kidney stone) produces severe flank pain that radiates to the groin. Patients with kidney stones typically are very restless and are unable to sit and lie still. One of the risk factors for developing kidney stones is concentration of the urine that results from increased sweating and inadequate fluid intake. (Objective 11)

10. C. Hypovolemia results in prerenal acute renal failure by causing decreased blood flow through the kidney. (Objective 5)

11. A. Acute pyelonephritis results in intrarenal acute renal failure. (Objective 5)

12. B. Obstruction of the urethra by prostate cancer would produce postrenal acute renal failure. (Objective 5)

13. C. Restlessness, confusion, headache, nausea, loss of consciousness, and seizures in a patient receiving dialysis suggest disequilibrium syndrome. (Objective 10)

Case Studies

Case one

1. Pulseless ventricular tachycardia with rounded QRS complexes and T waves that are difficult to distinguish from each other is called a *sine wave*. The sine wave pattern is characteristic of cardiac arrest secondary to hyperkalemia. (Objective 7)

2. This patient would have metabolic acidosis. The kidneys serve as the body's primary route for excreting sulfuric and phosphoric acids generated by protein metabolism. Renal failure causes these acids to accumulate in the extracellular fluid, producing an acidosis. (Objective 7)

3. Calcium chloride and sodium bicarbonate. (Objective 10)

4. Calcium is given to antagonize the effects of excess potassium on the heart. Sodium bicarbonate is given to correct metabolic acidosis and to create a mild alkalosis that shifts potassium into the intracellular space, correcting hyperkalemia. (Objective 5)

5. A patient in chronic renal failure who has missed dialysis is unable to remove excess water from the body. He will be in volume overload. (Objectives 7,8)

6. Generally dialysis fistulas should not be used for vascular access. First, the blood passing though the fistula is under high pressure, making it difficult to maintain an adequately flowing, patent IV. Second, an attempt to establish the fistula could damage the site, creating problems with providing dialysis for the patient. Generally, a dialysis access site should not be used for vascular access except in a life-threatening situation in which no other vascular access is available. (Objective 9)

7. This is a life-threatening situation in which no other vascular access is available. The fistula should be used to administer medications. During cardiac arrest there is no pressure on the arterial side of the fistula, creating fewer problems maintaining the site and administering medications. (Objective 9)

Case two

1. Renal calculus (kidney stone). (Objective 11)

2. A renal calculus can obstruct the ureter, blocking the flow of urine through the ureter from the kidney to the bladder, producing postrenal acute renal failure. (Objective 11)

3. The patient's skin is pale, cool, and moist because of increased sympathetic tone secondary to pain. (Objective 11)

4. Hot, humid climates tend to promote excessive loss of body water as sweat, particularly by persons who work outside for extended periods of time. Excessive body water loss causes the kidneys to increase their reabsorption of water, making the urine more concentrated. Concentrated urine is more likely to form kidney stones. (Objective 11)

5. These foods are rich in calcium, the amino acid purine, or oxalic acid. Increased concentrations of these substances in the urine increase the probability of kidney stone formation. (Objective 11)

6. Establish an IV and administer narcotic analgesics to control the patient's pain. Transport to the hospital. (Objective 12)

7. The patient should be encouraged to increase his fluid intake when he is working hard in hot weather.

He also should be encouraged to discuss with his physician dietary habits and medication use that may increase his risk of kidney stones. (Objective 12)

Case three

1. Testicular torsion. (Objective 30)
2. The testis is surrounded by the tunic vaginalis, a double-walled membrane that attaches to the posterolateral surface of the testis, anchoring it within the scrotum. In some patients the attachment of the tunica vaginalis to the testis is too high to adequately secure it, allowing the testis to rotate on the spermatic cord within the tunica vaginalis. This occludes the blood flow to the testis, causing ischemia and infarction. (Objective 30)
3. If testicular torsion has not occurred by the time a male reaches his early 20s, the anatomic defect that allows torsion to occur probably is not present. (Objective 30)
4. Although the patient has the elevated respiratory rate and blood pressure that are consistent with severe pain and anxiety, his heart rate is much lower than would be expected. (Objective 30)
5. The patient should be asked about his participation in sports and other physical activities. If he is an athlete, particularly an endurance athlete, he would be expected to have a lower than normal heart rate. For this patient, a heart rate of 88 beats/min may be elevated. (Objective 30)

CHAPTER 28: MUSCULOSKELETAL DISORDERS

Matching

1. Match the bones with the correct classification.
   - __D__ Carpals, metacarpals, tarsals, metatarsals, phalanges
   - __C__ Humerus, radius, ulna, femur, tibia, fibula
   - __A__ Sternum, ribs, bones of cranium
   - __B__ Vertebrae, bones of face (Objective 1)

Short Answer

1. Protecting vital structures. Supporting the body. Providing a mechanical basis for movement. Producing blood cells. Storing elements such as calcium, phosphorus, and magnesium. (Objective 1)
2. Skull, vertebral column, sternum, ribs. (Objective 1)
3. Clavicle, scapula, pelvis, bones of upper and lower extremities. (Objective 1)
4. Sesamoid bone. (Objective 1)
5. Periosteum. (Objective 1)
6. Ligament. (Objective 1)
7. Tendon. (Objective 1)
8. A muscle's origin is its point of attachment that does not move when the muscle contracts. (Objective 1)
9. A muscle's insertion is its point of attachment that moves when the muscle contracts. (Objective 1)
10. A strain is a stretching injury of a muscle or its associated tendon, sometimes resulting in a partial or complete tear. A sprain is an injury to a ligament that occurs when the ligament is overstretched, leading to a tear or complete disruption of the ligament. (Objective 5)
11. Rheumatoid arthritis. (Objective 7)
12. Septic arthritis. (Objective 7)
13. The patient relaxes while the examiner moves the affected area. (Objective 2)
14. The patient moves the affected area using his/her own muscles. (Objective 2)
15. Discrepancies between passive and active range of motion may indicate muscle weakness or a joint disorder. (Objective 2)
16. Pain in the lower back and leg resulting from impingement and irritation of the sciatic nerve, usually from a herniated disk. (Objective 3)
17. A group of symptoms associated with compression of the peripheral nerves still within the spinal canal below the level of the first lumbar vertebra characterized by lower back pain, motor and sensory deficits, and incontinence of bladder and bowel. (Objective 3)
18. Sciatica typically involves only pain and is unilateral. Cauda equina syndrome produces both decreased sensation and weakness and is bilateral. (Objective 3)
19. Myocardial ischemia, pancreatitis, pneumonia, aortic dissection. (Objective 3)
20. Cervical strain, cervical spondylosis, cervical disk herniation. (Objective 4)
21. Frequent use of the wrist, particularly with repeated flexion or constant pressure on the volar wrist joint, causes thickening of the ligament that overlies the tunnel between the carpal bones through which the medial nerve travels to the hand. The thickened ligament presses on the medial nerve, producing the symptoms of carpal tunnel syndrome. (Objective 5)
22. Numbness and weakness of the first three fingers of the hand, pain that radiates to the elbow or neck, weakness of thumb abduction, pain in the distribution of the medial nerve with hyperflexion of the wrist for 60 seconds, paresthesia in the medial nerve distribution while tapping the volar wrist over the medial nerve. (Objective 5)
23. Injury to skeletal muscle producing necrosis and release of intracellular contents. (Objective 6)
24. Rhabdomyolysis causes release of myoglobin into the bloodstream. When myoglobin is filtered from the bloodstream by the kidney and enters the acidic environment within the nephron, it precipitates and clogs the kidney's filtering system. (Objective 6)
25. A condition in which increased pressure within a fixed anatomic compartment results in compromised blood flow, producing tissue death. (Objective 6)
26. Severe resting pain, pain on palpation of the affected area, a tense or firm extremity, pain on active or passive flexion of the involved muscles. (Objective 6)

27. Osteoarthritis, rheumatoid arthritis, gouty arthritis. (Objective 7)
28. An infection of a bone. (Objective 8)
29. History of intravenous drug abuse, sexually transmitted diseases, or immunosuppression; sickle cell disease; recent orthopedic surgery; vascular disease; chronic steroid use. (Objective 8)
30. A fracture that results from an underlying disease process that weakens the mechanical properties of a bone. (Objective 9)

Multiple Choice

1. D. The sternum is part of the axial skeleton. (Objective 1)
2. C. The scapula is part of the appendicular skeleton. (Objective 1)
3. C. The patella is a sesamoid bone. (Objective 1)
4. C. The pain associated with a herniated lumbar disk is most likely to be described as shooting and radiating down the posterior aspect of one leg. (Objective 3)
5. D. Cauda equina syndrome is characterized by weakness of the muscles of the buttocks and posterior thighs, sensory deficits, and loss of bladder and bowel continence. (Objective 3)
6. A. The principal risk factor for developing osteoarthritis is age. (Objective 7)
7. C. The disease process most likely to be the cause of her signs and symptoms is rheumatoid arthritis. (Objective 7)
8. B. The first metatarsophalangeal joint (big toe) is most commonly affected by gout. (Objective 7)
9. D. Fever associated with a tenderness, swelling, and redness of a single joint indicates the presence of septic arthritis. (Objective 8)

Case Studies

Case one

1. The patient has developed rhabdomyolysis secondary to a crush injury of his left arm and leg. (Objective 6)
2. The patient had been lying on his left side for an extended time, compressing the soft tissues of his arm and leg. The pressure interfered with blood flow, resulting in ischemic tissue injury. Potassium, creatinine, and myoglobin are leaking from damaged skeletal muscles into the circulation. Fluid is moving from the extracellular to the intracellular space, producing edema and hypovolemia. The discoloration of the urine is being produced by myoglobin, which is being filtered from the bloodstream into the urine. The patient is at risk for renal failure from precipitation of myoglobin in the filtering system of the kidney. (Objective 6)
3. An IV should be established in the patient's right arm using normal saline solution. Normal saline is preferred over Ringer's lactate because saline does not contain potassium, which can worsen the hyperkalemia that develops following a crush injury.

IV fluid should be infused at 500 mL per hour to maintain a urine output of 200 to 300 mL per hour. Sodium bicarbonate can be administered to alkalinize the urine and prevent precipitation of myoglobin. Mannitol can be administered to promote diuresis. An osmotic diuretic such as mannitol is preferred to furosemide, a loop diuretic. Loop diuretics can acidify the urine and produce precipitation of myoglobin. (Objective 6)

Case two

1. The patient probably has an abdominal aortic aneurysm that has extended to the right iliac artery, compromising blood flow to the right lower extremity. (Objective 3)
2. A musculoskeletal problem could produce pain, numbness, and possibly even weakness in the lower extremities. However, it would not be expected to cause signs and symptoms of decreased circulation such as pallor, mottling, or weak pulses. (Objective 3)
3. Assess airway, breathing, and circulation. Give high-concentration oxygen using a nonrebreather mask. Establish two large-bore IVs with an isotonic crystalloid solution at a keep-open rate. Monitor the ECG. Place the patient in an uninflated pneumatic anti-shock garment. Transport rapidly to a facility with the capability of managing an abdominal aortic aneurysm. If the patient becomes increasingly hypotensive, inflate the pneumatic anti-shock garment and rapidly infuse IV solution to support blood pressure and perfusion. (Objective 3)

CHAPTER 29: CUTANEOUS DISORDERS

Matching

1.
B	A flat, circumscribed, discolored lesion
H	A firm, rounded elevation of the skin that is evanescent and pruritic
F	A lesion that contains purulent material
A	A localized, fluid-filled lesion greater than 0.5 cm in diameter
G	An elevated lesion that contains clear fluid
C	An elevated, solid lesion greater than 0.5 cm in diameter in the deep skin or subcutaneous tissues
E	An elevated, solid lesion greater than 0.5 cm in diameter that lacks a deep component
D	An elevated, solid lesion less than 0.5 in diameter (Objective 2)

2.
A	A collection of cellular debris or dried blood
F	A collection of new collective tissue resulting from dermoepidermal damage
G	A full-thickness crater that involves the dermis and epidermis with loss of the surface epithelium
C	A linear erosion caused by scratching
B	Partial focal loss of epidermis that usually heals without scarring

    ___E___ Thick stratum corneum resulting from hyperproliferation or increased cohesion of keratinocytes

    ___D___ A vertical loss of epidermis and dermis with sharply defined walls forming a crack in the skin (Objective 3)

3.   ___F___ Tinea capitis
    ___A___ Tinea corporis
    ___C___ Tinea cruris
    ___D___ Tinea manuum
    ___B___ Tinea pedis
    ___E___ Tinea unguium
    ___G___ Tinea versicolor (Objective 14)

Short Answer

1. Providing a protective barrier against the environment; regulating body temperature; storing water, fat, and vitamin D; providing sensations of heat, cold, touch, pressure, and pain. (Objective 1)
2. Epidermis, dermis, subcutaneous layer. (Objective 1)
3. The dermis. (Objective 1)
4. Nonmelanoma skin cancer and malignant melanoma. (Objective 4)
5. Malignant melanoma. (Objective 5)
6. A localized area of tissue necrosis that tends to develop when soft tissue is compressed between a body prominence and an external surface for a prolonged time. (Objective 6)
7. Breaks in the skin's integrity, pressure-induced changes, contamination producing bacterial infection. (Objective 6)
8. A chronic inflammatory skin disease that is familial with allergic features and characterized by an itch that erupts when scratched. (Objective 7)
9. Pruritis; typical morphology and distribution; chronic or relapsing course; personal or family history of asthma, allergic rhinitis, or atopic dermatitis. (Objective 7)
10. Inflammation of the skin resulting from direct skin exposure to a substance. (Objective 8)
11. Allergins and irritants. (Objective 8)
12. Red, discrete flat-topped persistent plaques and papules with silvery scales. (Objective 9)
13. *Staphylococcus aureus*. (Objective 10)
14. A combination of vesicles and pustules that rupture and form a crust with a honey-like appearance. (Objective 10)
15. A painful inflammatory nodule that involves a hair follicle and usually drains pus. (Objective 12)
16. A series of subcutaneous abscesses that drain through the hair follicles. (Objective 12)
17. *Staphylococcus aureus*. (Objective 12)
18. Small, wingless insects that are ectoparasites. (Objective 16)
19. Body lice (*Pediculus humanus corporis*), head lice (*Pediculus humanus capitis*), pubic lice (*Phthirus pubis*). (Objective 16)
20. Sexual abuse. (Objective 16)
21. A mite (*Sarcoptes scabiei*). (Objective 17)
22. Between the fingers, sides of the hands, wrists, elbows, axillae, groin, breasts, and feet. (Objective 17)
23. Human papillomavirus. (Objective 18)
24. An itchy vesicular rash found mostly on the trunk that includes a mixture of macules, papules, vesicles, and crusting lesions at any point during the infection. (Objective 19)
25. The herpes simplex virus. (Objective 20)
26. Painful indurated erythema followed by grouped vesicles that become pustules, and then rupture and drain. (Objective 20)
27. Shingles is a skin eruption that follows a particular nerve distribution (dermatome) caused by the varicella zoster virus. (Objective 21)
28. The skin lesions of shingles typically follow a particular nerve distribution on one side of the trunk. Shingles can occur on the head and face. Shingles rarely is seen on the extremities or bilaterally. (Objective 21)
29. Urticaria are hives. (Objective 22)
30. Erythema multiforme is an immunologic reaction in the skin that is characterized by a "target" lesion with three zones of color. The epidermis may be normal, blistered, or necrotic. The variety of presentations of this condition leads to the name *multiforme*. (Objective 23)
31. Allergic reactions to drugs, particularly penicillins, barbiturates, hydantoid, and sulfonamides. (Objective 23)
32. The skin lesions are petechiae. The patient probably has meningitis. (Objective 2)
33. These lesions are called telangiectasia. They are produced by chronic dilation of the arterioles and capillary beds, in this case from the vasodilating effects of alcohol. (Objective 2)
34. This lesion is an ulcer. (Objective 2)
35. These lesions are vesicles. (Objective 2)
36. These lesions are macules produced by an infection with the measles virus. (Objective 2)
37. This lesion is a paronychia. (Objective 2)
38. This lesion is called a *keloid*. (Objective 3)

Multiple Choice

1. B. A primary skin lesion has not been altered by scratching, scrubbing, or other trauma. (Objective 2)
2. A. Most cancerous skin lesions are caused by exposure to ultraviolet light. (Objective 4)
3. A. The most common form of skin cancer is basal cell carcinoma. (Objective 4)
4. D. Atopic dermatitis often coincides with asthma and allergic rhinitis. Atopic dermatitis is most common in urban areas of developed countries. It typically appears by age 5 to 7 and seems to have a genetic component. (Objective 7)
5. C. Contact dermatitis most commonly is caused by exposure to irritants. Contact dermatitis is more common in females than in males. (Objective 8)
6. A. The typical lesion produced by psoriasis is erythematous papules and plaques with a silver scale. (Objective 9)

359

7. C. The majority of bacterial skin infections are caused by *Staphylococcus aureus* and group A beta-hemolytic streptococci. (Objective 10)

8. A. In impetigo a thick golden crust tends to form as the primary lesions rupture. Impetigo is caused by *Staphylococcus aureus*. It is more common in warm, moist environments. The lesions tend to occur on the face, particularly around the mouth and nose. (Objective 10)

9. B. The organisms that most commonly cause folliculitis are *Pseudomonas aeruginosa* and *Staphylococcus aureus*. *P. aeruginosa* infection typically results from exposure to swimming pools, whirlpools, and hot tubs with inadequate chlorination. (Objective 11)

10. C. A painful inflammatory nodule that involves a hair follicle and drains pus is a furuncle. (Objective 12)

11. D. A dermatophyte infection on the trunk that produces pink, tan, or white patches with fine desquamating scale is called *Tinea versicolor*. (Objective 14)

12. C. Head lice occur commonly among school children. Pubic lice can be found in the areolar hair, axillary hair, beard, scalp margins, eyebrows, and eyelashes. Head lice are very rare among African Americans. Body lice primarily live in clothing and lay their eggs there. (Objective 16)

13. D. Transmission of scabies usually is from person to person by direct contact. Scabies is caused by a mite, not an insect. The lesions typically do not occur on the head. Scabies is characterized by intense itching. (Objective 17)

14. A. Cauliflower-like lesions that form on and around the rectum, perineum, inguinal folds, and external genitalia are condylomata acuminatum, also known as venereal warts. (Objective 18)

15. C. Chickenpox is characterized by a rash that occurs primarily on the trunk and consists of a mixture of macules, papules, vesicles, and crusting lesions. (Objective 19)

16. B. HSV-1 causes oral infection. HSV-2 causes genital infection. Both HSV-1 and HSV-2 cause recurrent infections. (Objective 20)

17. A. Acyclovir is used to treat herpes simplex virus infections. (Objective 20)

18. C. The lesions of herpes zoster (shingles) are vesicles that follow a particular nerve distribution on the trunk or face on one side of the body. (Objective 21)

19. D. The medical term used for hives is urticaria. (Objective 22)

20. A. The most common cause of erythema multiforme is allergic reactions to drugs. (Objective 23)

21. D. Large areas of reddish-purple blotches on the skin associated with specific disease states are called purpura (Objective 2).

CHAPTER 30: TOXICOLOGY

Short Answer

1. Initial management of any poisoning or overdose should focus on support of the airway, breathing, and circulation. There are few specific antidotes for toxins. In most cases, the only way to manage the toxin is to support the patient's cardiopulmonary function, allowing time for the patient's liver and kidneys to remove the toxin. (Objective 7)

2. The eyes should be irrigated with water or saline solution to remove the toxin. No substance other than water or an isotonic crystalloid solution should ever be introduced into a patient's eyes. (Objectives 8, 13)

3. 1. What was taken?
   2. How much was taken?
   3. How long ago was it taken?
   4. Has any attempt been made to treat the poisoning?
   5. Is the patient under psychiatric care? Why?
   6. Was any alcohol ingested?
   7. What is the patient's weight?
   (Objective 6)

4. Because the end products of methanol and ethylene glycol metabolism are acids, poisoning with these compounds produces metabolic acidosis. Sodium bicarbonate might be considered to correct this imbalance. (Objective 13)

5. Carbon monoxide is colorless, odorless, and tasteless. (Objective 13)

6. Carbon monoxide binds to hemoglobin, occupying the sites on which oxygen normally is transported to the tissues. This reduces the blood's oxygen-carrying capacity and produces tissue hypoxia. (Objective 13)

7. This patient is poisoned with cyanide. Cyanide is present in a variety of plant materials including peach seeds, apple seeds, pear seeds, and apricots. Cyanide blocks the use of oxygen as the final acceptor of electrons on the electron transport chain. This blocks electron transport and shuts down cellular production of ATP. In cyanide toxicity, the venous blood is bright red because oxygen is not being removed from the bloodstream by cellular respiration. (Objective 13)

8. Amyl nitrite, sodium nitrite, and sodium thiosulfate. (Objective 13)

9. Organophosphates and carbamates produce these symptoms by inhibiting the action of the enzyme acetylcholinesterase, leading to an excess of the neuro-transmitter acetylcholine in the synapses of the parasympathetic nervous system and at the neuromuscular junction. (Objective 13)

10. Atropine is used to immediately reverse the effects of excess acetylcholine in organophosphate or carbamate toxicity. 2-PAM (pralidoxime) is used to reactivate acetylcholinesterase by uncoupling the

organophosphate molecule from it. Pralidoxime is not used in the management of carbamate toxicity. (Objective 13)

11. Hydrocarbons sensitize the myocardium to the effects of catecholamines. Administration of catecholamines to a patient who has been poisoned with a hydrocarbon can cause increased ventricular irritability, leading to ventricular tachycardia or ventricular fibrillation. (Objective 13)

12. Calcium will reverse the bradycardia, hypotension, and decreased myocardial contractility present in calcium channel blocker toxicity. (Objective 12)

13. Freon and other inhaled hydrocarbon compounds sensitize the myocardium to the effects of catecholamines. This effect places the patient at risk of increased myocardial irritability that can lead to ventricular fibrillation. (Objective 13)

Multiple Choice

1. C. *N*-Acetylcysteine is the antidote for acetaminophen overdose. (Objective 12)

2. B. Bag-mask ventilation, IV access, Narcan 2 mg × 2, check glucose, intubate, ventilate. Because the patient has presented with a decreased level of consciousness and slow respirations, Narcan is indicated. Because Narcan may reverse the effects of an opiate overdose and produce a sudden return of consciousness, it is prudent to delay endotracheal intubation until after Narcan has been given unless adequate oxygenation and ventilation cannot be maintained without an endotracheal tube. Any patient with a decreased level of consciousness also should have a blood glucose level checked because hypoglycemia can cause altered mental status. (Objective 12)

3. B. Blurred vision is an early sign of most tricyclic antidepressant overdoses along with other signs of anticholinergic drug effects such as dry mouth, absence of sweating, dilated pupils, and flushed skin. Widening of the QRS complex, ventricular dysrhythmias, and respiratory arrest are later signs of tricyclic antidepressant toxicity. (Objective 12)

4. B. Verapamil is a calcium channel blocker and would be most likely to produce hypotension and bradycardia. Movement of calcium into the pacemaker cells of the SA node is responsible for the spontaneous diastolic depolarization that accounts for cardiac automaticity. Blockage of the calcium channels in the SA node decreases automaticity and slows heart rate. Calcium also couples the electrical event of depolarization to the mechanical event of contraction. Blocking calcium channels in the membranes of cardiac muscle cells produces decreased contractility and lower cardiac output. Blocking calcium channels in the smooth muscle cells located in the walls of blood vessels causes vasodilation and a drop in peripheral resistance. (Objective 12)

5. A. Calcium chloride can be used to reverse the effects of calcium channel blocker toxicity. Increasing the serum calcium levels allows calcium ions to out-compete the calcium channel blocker molecules for access to the calcium channels. (Objective 12)

6. A. Amphetamines, cocaine, and phencyclidine will produce hypertension and tachycardia. Sedative-hypnotics, digoxin, parasympathomimetics, organophos-phates, beta-blockers, and calcium channel blockers all can either slow the heart rate or produce hypotension. (Objective 12)

7. D. The time of ingestion of a drug in a suspected overdose or poisoning is important because treatment decisions will be affected by the amount of time that has passed since ingestion. For example, activated charcoal is often not administered if more than one hour has passed since the ingestion. (Objective 6)

8. D. Signs and symptoms of organophosphate poisoning include urinary incontinence, wheezing, and paralysis. The excess acetylcholine that accumulates in organophosphate toxicity produces constricted pupils and bradycardia. Although the classic SLUDGE syndrome provides a way to quickly recognize cholinesterase inhibitor toxicity, the most significant danger associated with these poisons is weakness and paralysis resulting from an excess of acetylcholine at the neuromuscular junction. (Objective 13)

9. B. While this patient may indeed be intoxicated, his presentation is not consistent with isolated ethanol intoxication. Intoxication may depress respirations, but it is also likely to cause hypotension rather than hypertension (as this patient is presenting). Also tachycardia would be a more common response in intoxication (compensating for the hypotension), whereas this patient is bradycardic. These findings indicate the need to search for another/additional cause of his unresponsiveness. As you will learn in later chapters this patient exhibits the classic pattern of altered mental status, hypertension, bradycardia, and altered respiratory pattern associated with increased intracranial pressure. Chronic abusers of alcohol are at a high risk for intracranial hemorrhages which can lead to increased intracranial pressure.

10. C. Narcan is administered in doses sufficient to improve respirations to an acceptable rate and tidal volume without awakening the patient. Narcotic abusers who are awakened with Narcan frequently are very combative and uncooperative. (Objective 12)

11. A. An internal combustion engine running in an enclosed area can generate toxic concentrations of carbon monoxide. Carbon monoxide binds to hemoglobin and interferes with oxygen transport. (Objective 13)

12. C. You should disregard the oximeter because carbon monoxide may cause inaccurate readings. A pulse oximeter indicates the percentage of hemoglobin that is saturated by binding to another substance. However, it does not indicate what that substance is. Since carbon monoxide occupies locations on the hemoglobin molecule to which oxygen normally binds, it can create falsely high oxygen saturation readings. (Objective 13)

13. C. The administration of sodium nitrite and amyl nitrite to a cyanide-poisoned patient results in hemoglobin converting to methemoglobin. The ferric iron in methemoglobin has a high affinity for cyanide. Cyanide leaves the cells and binds to the methemoglobin in the red cells, reactivating the electron transport system in the cells. (Objective 13)

14. B. Dilated pupils caused by the anticholinergic effects of Elavil, a tricyclic antidepressant, probably will be present. Tricyclics inhibit sweating and salivation. They also suppress urinary bladder contractility and can produce urinary retention. (Objective 12)

15. C. Naloxone (Narcan) works by competing against opiate molecules for the opiate receptors in the CNS. (Objective 12)

16. C. The antidote works because it inhibits metabolism of the toxin. Windshield washer fluid contains methanol. In the body methanol is converted (metabolized) to formaldehyde by the enzyme alcohol dehydrogenase. The formaldehyde is later converted to formic acid which is very toxic to the body. The antidotes (ethanol or fomepizole) for methanol poisoning, as well as ethylene glycol poisoning, are competitive inhibitors of alcohol dehydrogenase. This does not allow the alcohol dehydrogenase to convert methanol to formaldehyde and stops the cascading reaction before it starts, and therefore formic acid is never created. This allows the methanol to circulate unchanged until it can be excreted by the body, or removed by hemodialysis. (Objective 13)

17. A. The acid-base imbalance most likely to develop in a patient poisoned with methanol (or ethylene glycol) is metabolic acidosis. This is because methanol and ethylene glycol are metabolized to acids. Sodium bicarbonate is often administered in the emergency department when treating these patients. It can be considered in the field in the setting of prolonged transport times, however it is not routinely used in the prehospital setting as the patients pH level is not known. (Objective 13)

18. D. Tinnitus (ringing or buzzing in the ears) is a common symptom of toxicity from salicylates such as aspirin. (Objective 12)

19. B. Benzodiazepines affect the CNS by binding to the GABA receptors. Gamma-aminobutyric acid (GABA) is the inhibitory neurotransmitter. GABA binds to receptor sites on cell membrane chloride channels, causing the channels to open and admit larger amounts of negatively-charge chloride ions into the cell. The increase in the number of cations within the cell hyperpolarizes the cell membrane and slows nerve impulse transmission. Benzodiazepines bind to receptor sites on chloride channels and enhance the CNS-depressing effect of this neurotransmitter. (Objective 12)

20. C. This patient's signs and symptoms are a result of increased parasympathetic tone caused by excessive amounts of acetylcholine. The mechanism of injury and the clinical presentation suggest exposure to an organophosphate insecticide. Organophosphates inhibit the action of acetylcholinesterase, leading to an excess of acetylcholine. (Objective 13)

21. C. Flumazenil is a benzodiazepine antagonist that competes with benzodiazepine molecules for their receptor site on the chloride channels. Flumazenil will reverse the effects of benzodiazepine toxicity. However, if a patient is toxic with another substance that can cause over stimulation of the CNS, administration of flumazenil can trigger seizures that cannot be stopped by giving a benzodiazepine. Since it frequently is difficult to identify all substances taken in a mixed overdose, use of flumazenil in an emergency care setting can be very dangerous. Therefore this medication is often not administered in the pre-hospital setting. (Objective 12)

22. D. The most dramatic form of alcohol withdrawal is referred to as delirium tremens. (Objective 17)

23. C. Toxicity results from sodium channel inhibition. (Objective 12)

24. A. A black widow spider probably bit the patient. Black widow spider envenomization is characterized by severe muscle spasms in the bitten extremity. The brown recluse spider's venom produces extensive tissue necrosis at the bite site. The sting of most scorpions found in the United States produces instantaneous severe pain and swelling. A coral snake's venom produces neurotoxic effects that result in respiratory arrest. (Objective 14)

25. D. Narcotic overdose is characterized by decreased level of consciousness, depressed respirations, and pinpoint pupils. (Objective 12)

26. C. The patient should be decontaminated by removing her clothing and washing her with large amounts of water. (Objective 8)

27. D. Open the airway, insert an oral airway, assist ventilation with a BVM and oxygen, and transport. Because the patient's respirations are depressed, administration of oxygen by facemask would not be adequate. (Objective 12)

28. B. When you are managing a patient who has ingested an unknown poison, particular attention should be paid to the patient's airway, breathing, and circulation. Few specific antidotes for toxins exist. In most cases of poisoning and overdose, the only treatment is to support the patient's cardiopulmonary function to allow the liver and kidneys time to deal with the toxin. (Objective 4)

29. C. The most immediate indication a patient has been bitten by a pit viper is local pain and swelling. As the effects of pit viper venom progress, hematuria may appear. Drooping eyelids and respiratory arrest would be more typical of coral snake envenomization. (Objective 14)

30. A. Delirium tremens results from alcohol withdrawal. (Objective 17)

31. C. The venom is heat labile, meaning it is destroyed by heat. Therefore pouring warm (110-113 F) water over the area will destroy the venom. Pouring vinegar over the area will deactivate any nematocysts that have not yet discharged, but it will not have any effect on those that have, or any venom that is already in the patient. Despite urban legend, studies have failed to show that the application of human urine to the area has any effect on the venom or on nematocycts that have not discharged. (Objective 14)

32. C. These medications are narcotics, as are pentazozine (Talwin), hydromorphone (Dilaudid), and propoxyphene (Darvon). (Objective 12)

33. C. Contraindications to administration of activated charcoal include ingestion of acids and alkalis or inability to swallow. Ingestion of diazepam (Valium), aspirin, and digitalis is not a contraindication to activated charcoal administration if the patient is awake and able to swallow. (Objective 10)

34. C. The dose range for adult administration of activated charcoal is 50 to 100 grams. (Objective 10)

35. C. Inhaled poisons such as carbon monoxide are best treated by removing the patient to fresh air and administering either supplemental oxygen or assisted ventilation. (Objective 13)

36. A. The coral snake has fixed (non erectile) fangs and must chew to inject its venom. Coral snakes are not related to pit vipers. (Objective 14)

Case Studies

Case one

1. Support of airway, breathing, and circulation. The airway should be opened and respirations should be assisted with a bag-mask device and oxygen. Chest compressions should be started at a rate of 100 per minute. (Objective 12)

2. A 2-year-old child should be intubated with a 4.5 mm endotracheal tube $[2(age)/4] + 4 = 4.5$. (Objective 12)

3. Yes, chest compressions should be started because the heart rate is less than 60 beats/min with signs of poor perfusion. (Objective 12)

4. Verapamil slows the firing rate of the SA node. (Objective 12)

5. Verapamil decreases ventricular contractility. (Objective 12)

6. Verapamil causes peripheral vasodilation. (Objective 12)

7. Yes. Verapamil slows conduction through the AV junction, so complete AV block can be caused by verapamil toxicity. (Objective 12)

8. In addition to supporting cardiopulmonary function with chest compressions and ventilation, an IV should be started. Calcium should be given to antagonize the effects of the calcium channel blocker and improve heart rate, myocardial conductivity and contractility, and vascular tone. An isotonic crystalloid can be infused to help fill the dilated vascular space and support the blood pressure. However, because verapamil depresses myocardial contractility, fluid should be administered in 5 to 10 mL/kg boluses rather than the standard 20 mL/kg, and the patient should be monitored carefully for signs of pulmonary edema. (Objective 12)

Case two

1. The patient probably has ingested cyanide. Cyanide is present in apple seeds. (Objective 13)

2. Cyanide binds to the iron atom in cytochrome a_3, the terminal carrier in the electron transport chain. This prevents cytochrome a_3 from accepting electrons and transferring them to oxygen, blocking use of oxygen in cellular respiration. Interruption of electron transport shuts down aerobic metabolism and production of ATP. (Objective 13)

3. The patient's blood is bright red because the cells cannot use oxygen. Therefore oxygen is remaining on the hemoglobin molecules in the red cells. (Objective 13)

4. Amyl nitrite, sodium nitrite, and sodium thiosulfate. (Objective 13)

5. Amyl nitrite and sodium nitrite oxidize the iron in hemoglobin from the 2+ state to the 3+ state, forming a compound called methemoglobin. Because cyanide has a high affinity for iron in the 3+ state, it leaves the cells and binds to the 3+ iron in the red blood cells, reactivating electron transport and ATP production. Sodium thiosulfate provides sulfide anion to rhodonese, a naturally occurring enzyme that detoxifies cyanide by converting it to thiocyanate. (Objective 13)

Case three

1. The combination of decreased level of consciousness, depressed respirations, and pinpoint pupils is characteristic of opiate toxicity. (Objective 12)

2. Narcotics have a sympatholytic effect. When the effects of the sympathetic nervous system are blocked, an excess of parasympathetic tone causes the pupils to constrict. (Objective 12)

3. The patient should be given Narcan (naloxone). (Objective 12)

4. Narcan competes with the opiate by binding to the same receptor sites and blocking the opiate's effects. (Objective 12)

5. Naloxone is only effective on narcotics, it will not reverse the effects of other medications. Acute withdrawal may occur in the patient who is addicted to apiods. Naloxone has a shorter half life than many narcotics, therefore the patient must be closely

monitored for the return of signs and symptoms of overdose. (Objective 12)

6. The half-life of naloxone is shorter than those of the opiates it antagonizes. The patient's naloxone levels have fallen to a subtherapeutic level, and signs of opiate toxicity are returning. (Objective 12)

7. Administer another dose of naloxone (Narcan) titrated to improve the patient's respirations. (Objective 12)

Case four

1. Amitriptyline (Elavil) is a tricyclic antidepressant. (Objective 12)

2. Tricyclic antidepressants have an anticholinergic effect that results in tachycardia, decreased sweating, decreased salivation, and dilated pupils. (Objective 12)

3. Tricyclic antidepressants have a sodium channel blocking effect similar to Vaughn-Williams Class Ia agents. This effect slows impulse conduction within the myocardium and can lead to ventricular irritability. (Objective 12)

4. Sodium bicarbonate will reverse the cardiotoxic effects of tricyclic antidepressants. (Objective 12)

Case five

1. Ethylene glycol. (Objective 13)

2. Ethylene glycol is metabolized to oxalic acid. (Objective 13)

3. Ethanol is the antidote used for methanol or ethylene glycol toxicity. (Objective 13)

4. Ethanol competes with ethylene glycol for the enzyme alcohol dehydrogenase. By saturating alcohol dehydrogenase, ethanol blocks metabolism of methanol and ethylene glycol to formic acid and oxalic acid, respectively. A newer antidote, fomepizole, has the same action as ethanol with the advantage of not intoxicating the patient. (Objective 13)

5. Metabolic acidosis caused by formation of formic acid and oxalic acid. (Objective 13)

6. The patient is attempting to compensate for metabolic acidosis by increasing the rate at which he is removing carbon dioxide from his bloodstream. (Objective 13)

7. Sodium bicarbonate to correct metabolic acidosis by buffering hydrogen ions released by formic acid and oxalic acid. (Objective 13)

CHAPTER 31: INFECTIOUS AND COMMUNICABLE DISEASES

Short Answer

1. Standard precautions, formerly called universal precautions, is a strategy for infection control that is based on the assumption that all patients have a blood-borne communicable disease and that every body fluid is capable of transmitting that disease. (Objective 5)

2. Attempting to recap needles. Needles should be placed in an approved sharps container without attempting to recap them. (Objective 15)

3. Hand-washing immediately after patient contact. (Objective 5)

4. Meningococcal meningitis. (Objective 24)

5. By contact with respiratory tract secretions. (Objective 24)

6. Wear a mask, consider masking the patient, avoid close contact with respiratory tract secretions, use particular caution during intubation and suctioning. Receive appropriate post-exposure prophylaxis with rifampin, ciprofloxacin, or ceftriaxone. (Objective 24)

7. Hepatitis. (Objectives 17, 18, 20, 21, 22)

8. Fecal-oral contact. (Objective 17)

9. Direct contact with contaminated body fluids (blood, semen, vaginal fluid, saliva). (Objective 18)

10. Needle stick and sexual contact. (Objective 20)

11. Hepatitis D can only reproduce itself if the hepatitis B virus is present. Preventing hepatitis B infection effectively prevents hepatitis D infection. (Objective 21)

12. Airborne respiratory droplets. (Objective 23)

13. If they have not had a PPD skin test during the previous year, they should receive an immediate baseline test followed by a second test 4 weeks later. A reaction to the second test suggests they have been exposed to tuberculosis, and they should receive prophylaxis with isoniazid. (Objective 23)

14. If a pregnant woman had active herpes simplex lesions, her baby should be delivered by cesarean section to avoid infection of the infant. (Objective 43)

15. AIDS is an immunocompromised state that results from infection with the human immunodeficiency virus (HIV). HIV targets and destroys helper T-cells with the CD4 marker. The destruction of the helper T-cells disables the patient's immune system and leaves the patient open to infection by a variety of pathogens that do not infect persons with healthy immune systems. (Objective 16)

16. AIDS is caused by the human immunodeficiency virus (HIV). (Objective 16)

17. The HIV virus is transmitted through contact with infected blood, blood products, semen, vaginal secretions, and breast milk. Infection has been documented as a result of sexual intercourse (anal, vaginal, oral), contaminated blood and blood products, shared injection equipment, prenatal or perinatal transmission across the placenta, and breast-feeding after birth. Healthcare providers also may be at risk from exposure to cerebrospinal fluid, synovial fluid, and amniotic fluid. There have been no documented cases of transmission via saliva, tears, urine, or bronchial secretions. (Objective 16)

18. AIDS is present when the helper T-cell count drops below $250/mm^3$ in a patient who is HIV positive. This is generally when the patient begins to acquire life-threatening opportunistic infections. (Objective 16)

19. Use standard precautions. Treat all sharp objects as potentially infective. Do NOT recap needles. Clean blood spills with bleach solution. Wash hands

between patients. Consider wearing a mask to prevent exposure of the patient to opportunistic pathogens carried by the paramedic. Pregnant paramedics should avoid contact with AIDS patients because of the risk for cytomegalovirus exposure. Cytomegalovirus has been demonstrated to cause birth defects. (Objective 16)

20. *Pneumocystis carinii* is an opportunistic pathogen that produces pneumonia in patients with AIDS. (Objective 16)

21. Pneumocystic pneumonia is the most common life-threatening opportunistic infection in patients with AIDS. (Objective 16)

22. The rubella virus can cause prenatal infections that produce severe birth defects. Unvaccinated female paramedics who are pregnant place their unborn child at risk. Unvaccinated male paramedics risk acquiring the virus and carrying it home to a pregnant spouse. (Objective 32)

23. Gonorrhea is transmitted through direct contact with exudates from the mucous membranes of an infected individual, primarily through sexual contact. (Objective 40)

24. In males, painful urination and mucopurulent urethral discharge. In females, urinary frequency, vaginal discharge, fever, abdominal pain, signs and symptoms of pelvic inflammatory disease. (A significant portion of infected females are asymptomatic.) Gonorrhea also can produce septic arthritis, meningitis, and sepsis. (Objective 40)

Multiple Choice

1. D. The greatest risk of hepatitis C infection would be posed by performing hemodialysis or any other procedure that possibly could result in exposure to the patient's blood. Hepatitis C is not transmitted by the fecal-oral route, and there is no evidence that it can be transmitted through saliva or by casual contact. (Objective 20)

2. A. Acyclovir is commonly used to treat symptoms of herpes simplex virus (HSV). (Objective 43)

3. D. The hepatitis B virus (HBV) may survive outside a human host on an inanimate surface for as long as approximately 1 week. (Objective 18)

4. C. The drug of choice in the prophylactic treatment of tuberculosis is isoniazid. (Objective 23)

5. A. The form of hepatitis transmitted by the fecal-oral route is hepatitis A. (Objective 17)

6. A. The most common sign of syphilis in the *primary stage* is a chancre, a painless lesion that forms at the site where the spirochete entered the body. (Objective 39)

7. C. For an EMS provider, the best method of minimizing his or her risk of disease transmission is to assume all body fluids and secretions are infectious. While wearing gloves provides protection against exposure through contact between the rescuer's hands and infected body fluids, it does not safeguard against exposure through other routes and does not protect against needle stick. (Objective 5)

8. A. The lesions associated with Lyme disease initially appear as large and circular lesions called *erythema migrans*. (Objective 46)

9. D. Stretcher side rails of an ambulance are a vehicle for transmission of a communicable disease. A vehicle is an inanimate object that can transfer a pathogen from one person to another. A needle would be another example of a vehicle. Insects and other living organisms that transmit disease are vectors. (Objective 2)

10. B. Nausea, vomiting, weakness, loss of appetite, yellow sclerae, fever, and right upper quadrant tenderness are signs and symptoms of hepatitis. (Objectives 17, 18, 20, 21, 22)

11. C. Altered mental status, severe headache, nausea, vomiting, stiff neck, and a rash consisting of pinpoint areas of hemorrhage under the skin are signs and symptoms of meningitis. (Objective 24)

12. A. Hepatitis A can be transmitted by fecal-oral contamination. (Objective 17)

13. C. Hepatitis B is a blood-borne pathogen that can be transmitted by needle stick and sexual intercourse. (Objective 18)

14. B. EMS personnel should observe standard precautions when caring for any patient. The basic principle of standard precautions is to assume that every patient has an infectious disease and that any of the patient's body fluids could transmit the disease. (Objective 5)

15. B. The most common mode of transmission for meningitis is inhalation of infected airborne droplets. (Objective 24)

16. A. Human immunodeficiency virus is transmitted through blood, semen, and vaginal secretions. HIV cannot be transmitted through urine. (Objective 16)

17. D. Ticks transmit Lyme disease. (Objective 46)

Case Studies

Case one

1. Meningitis. (Objective 24)
2. Wear a facemask. Consider placing a facemask on the patient if she will tolerate it. Avoid contact with the patient's respiratory tract secretions. Use particular caution during airway management procedures. Ensure follow-up for appropriate antibiotic prophylaxis. (Objective 24)

Case two

1. Tuberculosis. (Objective 23)
2. You should advise the first responders to immediately place facemasks on themselves. If the patient will tolerate a facemask, one also should be placed on him. Availability of a baseline TB skin test within the last year should be verified for all personnel caring for the patient. Those who cannot document a baseline skin test should have one done as soon as possible.

All personnel should have skin tests performed in 4 weeks. Positive reactors should be referred for prophylaxis with isoniazid. Personnel who are positive reactors to the PPD test should be screened with chest radiographs. Administration of the PPD test to a known positive reactor can cause a severe inflammatory reaction. (Objective 23)

CHAPTER 32: PSYCHIATRIC DISORDERS AND SUBSTANCE ABUSE

Matching

1. __I__ Acute discomfort with close relationships, eccentric behavior, cognitive distortions
   __H__ Detachment from social relationships
   __A__ Disregard for the rights of others
   __G__ Distrust and suspiciousness
   __E__ Excessive emotions and attention seeking
   __J__ Grandiosity, need for admiration, lack of empathy
   __C__ Instability in interpersonal relationships, self-image, and impulsivity
   __F__ Preoccupation with orderliness, perfectionism, control
   __B__ Social inhibition, feelings of inadequacy, hypersensitivity to criticism
   __D__ Submissive or clinging behavior, excessive need to receive care (Objective 11)

Short Answer

1. A behavioral emergency is a situation in which a patient's behavior has become alarming to himself or herself or to others and requires intervention. Behavioral emergencies include conditions that interfere with essential life functions, that pose a threat to the safety of the patient or others, or that significantly deviate from society's expectations. (Objective 2)
2. Affect consists of the outward signs that indicate a person's inward mood. (Objective 7)
3. Delirium is a cognitive disorder characterized by relatively rapid onset of widespread disorganized thought. Patients with delirium suffer from confusion, inattention, memory impairment, disorientation, and general clouding of consciousness. Vivid visual hallucinations may be present. Delirium frequently is due to underlying physiologic causes and reverses itself when the underlying cause is treated.
4. Paranoid: the patient suffers auditory hallucinations and is preoccupied with a feeling of persecution. Disorganized: the patient displays disordered or bizarre behavior, dress, and speech. Catatonic: the patient becomes immobile and rigid. Undifferentiated: the patient meets the criteria for a diagnosis of schizophrenia but does not readily fit one of the other categories. (Objective 11)
5. Bipolar disorder is a mood disorder characterized by manic episodes that alternate with periods of depression or of normal mood. During the manic

phase of bipolar disorder, a patient has inflated self-esteem, experiences a decreased need for sleep, is talkative, has the feeling his or her thoughts are racing, is easily distracted, has an increase in goal-directed behavior, may participate in highly risky pleasurable activities, and may experience delusional thoughts. (Objective 11)
6. Lithium commonly is used to treat bipolar disorder. (Objective 15)
7. Patients with anorexia nervosa have an intense fear of obesity and complain of being fat even though their body weight is low. They fast excessively. Patients with bulimia nervosa engage in binge eating followed by self-induced vomiting or diarrhea, excessive exercise, or dieting. They are fully aware of the abnormality of their behavior. (Objectives 11, 14)
8. You should leave the scene immediately and request a response by law enforcement officers. (Objective 5)
9. You should leave the restraints in place until the patient reaches the hospital. A violent patient may become calm when restrained but become violent again when the restraints are removed. Removing restraints in the patient compartment of a moving ambulance creates a significant risk of injury to the patient and the paramedic. (Objective 5)
10. You should tell the patient that everything she needs will be provided at the hospital. If she continues to insist on going to the bedroom, you and your partner should accompany her. If she leaves your sight, there is a possibility she will attempt to injure herself. (Objectives 5, 19)
11. You should make contact with the patient and attempt to engage him in conversation. A patient who is threatening suicide should be kept talking; this is an important strategy for keeping him from following through with an action to kill himself. (Objectives 17, 18, 19)
12. Hypoxia, hypoglycemia, hypoperfusion, head injury or cerebrovascular accident, drug toxicity. (Objective 4)
13. Have you thought about killing yourself? (Objective 19)
14. Previous attempts
   History of depression
   Male gender (females attempt suicide more frequently, but males are more likely to succeed)
   Age: 15 to 24 or older than 60 years
   History of substance abuse
   Divorced or widowed
   Living alone or in increased isolation
   Homosexuality
   Recent loss of a mate, loved one, job, significant possession
   Major physical stresses
   Disabling illness or other loss of independence
   Suicide of the same-sexed parent
   Lack of goals and plans for the future
   Giving away personal belongings

Expression of detailed suicide plans, particularly ones that are highly lethal

Possession of a means for committing suicide, particularly one that is highly lethal

(Objective 18)

15. Ideally, the interview should take place in the patient's presence with his/her permission. Leaving the room with a relative or bystander or conducting a conversation in hushed tones just out of earshot of the patient might be perceived by the patient as plotting against him/her. (Objective 9)

Multiple Choice

1. A. This patient may be suffering from conversion hysteria. Conversion hysteria occurs when a patient takes a psychological conflict and manifests it in a physiologic disturbance that resolves the conflict. For example, a person faced with the choice of preserving their own life or risking their life to safe another may become blind or paralyzed. (Objective 11)

2. A. Characteristics of depression may include helpless or hopeless feelings, increased risk of suicide, and loss of interest in hobbies. Paranoia usually does not characterize depression. (Objective 11)

3. D. This patient is suffering from paranoid schizophrenia. Patients with paranoid schizophrenia have auditory and visual hallucinations that convince them they are being watched or others are conspiring against them. Paranoia is distinguished from paranoid schizophrenia by the absence of hallucinations and by the content of the delusions of persecution. Patients with paranoia believe persons who are part of their everyday life—for example, supervisors, spouses, and acquaintances—are plotting against them. Patients with paranoid schizophrenia believe they are the focus of bizarre plots involving the government, aliens, or organized professional groups, for example. (Objective 11)

4. B. The most appropriate response to this question would be, "I think it is important for you to go to the hospital." Agreeing with a patient's delusions is unethical and potentially harmful. Giving a patient a choice that does not lead them in the direction of the outcome you desire is not a good strategy because they may choose the option you do not want them to select—for example, not going to the hospital or going to jail. (Objectives 9, 20)

5. D. The first action you should take is to make contact with the patient and try to get her to talk to you. The patient does not represent a threat to you; so waiting for the police is not appropriate. Daring a suicidal patient to act or challenging his/her commitment to committing suicide is very dangerous and can result in the patient following through with an action that results in serious injury or death. (Objective 9)

6. C. After applying restraints to a combative patient, you should not loosen the straps until the patient reaches a medical facility. Removing restraints from a patient during transport could result in the patient being able to injure you or themself. (Objectives 5, 21)

7. B. The best option available if you cannot calm a hostile, aggressive patient is to obtain appropriate assistance from law enforcement. Attempting to disarm, subdue, or restrain a hostile patient without appropriate training and manpower can result in serious injury. (Objective 5)

8. D. Schizophrenia, depression, hypoglycemia, and cerebrovascular accident may produce behavioral changes. (Objective 4)

9. A. The most appropriate action in handling a noncombative emotionally disturbed patient would be to allow the patient adequate time to discuss his feelings. (Objectives 9, 15)

10. C. You should encourage the patient to think about alternatives and the effects her suicide might have on others. A patient who is threatening suicide always should be transported for evaluation by a psychiatrist. Daring a patient to commit suicide or challenging his/her intentions may result in the patient following through with a suicide attempt. (Objectives 9, 15)

11. A. Chronic substance abuse indicates the greatest risk for successful suicide of the factors listed. Males successfully kill themselves more frequently than females. Detailed plans indicate the greatest risk of suicide. Persons with strong ties to family and friends have a low risk of killing themselves. (Objective 18)

12. C. The word that best describes a patient with paranoia is *suspicious*. (Objective 11)

13. D. The most effective technique for managing a patient with paranoia is being truthful with the patient. Excessive concern and warmth could be interpreted by a patient with paranoia as an attempt to trick the patient. Agreeing with delusional statements to gain a patient's confidence is unethical and can lead to unexpected reactions by the patient. Discussions with bystanders and family members should take place in his or her presence with his or her consent. Leaving the patient's presence to talk with someone else or holding a hushed conversation in the patient's presence might be interpreted as "plotting" against him or her. (Objectives 9, 15)

14. D. A patient who presents with dizziness, tremors, tachycardia, dyspnea, and sweating may have either a physiologic problem or a psychological problem, but should be assessed and treated for the physiologic problem first. (Objectives 4, 6)

15. C. Because there is a potential threat to your safety, you should keep the woman and her children in a safe place and request a response by the police. (Objective 5)

16. D. Purchase of a gun by a person with a history of clinical depression may indicate suicidal intentions and indicates a need for therapeutic intervention. Suicide usually is preceded by warning signs and can prevented if appropriate interventions occur. (Objectives 18, 19)

17. D. "When did you being feeling like you want to die?" is an example of an open-ended question

because it requires more than a "yes" or "no" answer. (Objective 9)

18. D. Given the preceding scenario, your most appropriate initial action would be to remove the supervisor from the room. Removing the supervisor will eliminate a distraction that can interfere with your ability to interact with the patient. Attempting to restrain the patient or stepping between the patient and the supervisor could result in you being injured. (Objective 8)

19. B. Acknowledging the patient's anger and asking him to describe the situation that led to it is a way to open communication and begin defusing the situation. Making demands or issuing threats is likely to cause the situation to escalate. (Objectives 9, 15)

20. A. Identifying yourself and stating you are here to help keeps options for resolving the situation open. Telling the patient you are going to take him to the hospital could upset him further. Saying you are here at the request of his "friends" could convince him you are part of the plot to "get him." (Objectives 9, 15)

21. A. Asking the patient to put down the letter opener so you can talk with him indicates you are willing to work with him to find a solution. If the patient complies with your request to put down the letter opener, you have taken a positive step toward controlling the situation. Telling a patient with paranoia to trust you or playing along with his delusions invites mistrust and can have unexpected consequences. Telling an upset person to "calm down" is likely to make them more upset. Threatening the patient or taking away his options probably will inflame the situation. (Objectives 9, 15)

22. D. Telling the patient you understand he feels he is right and you respect his point of view, even though you may not always agree with him, avoids either creating the impression you are allied with the patient against those who are "out to get him" or giving the patient the idea you are working with his enemies. Telling a patient with paranoia that you "don't take sides" may be interpreted as your saying you are avoiding admitting you are siding with his enemies. (Objectives 9, 15)

23. B. Saying "I think a doctor could help you if you will go with us to the hospital" would be the best way to ask the patient to go to the hospital. The patient probably would react negatively to being told he is "mentally ill." Asking him if he would like to go to the hospital gives him the opportunity to say, "no." Giving him the opportunity to go with EMS or with the police may anger him or may lead to a decision to go with the police. (Objectives 9, 15)

24. A. You should acknowledge that he might feel angry and wonder why he should trust you; then repeat your offer to help. Ignoring the patient is likely to anger him. Attempting to justify your competence surrenders control of the situation to the patient. (Objectives 9, 15)

25. C. If the patient refuses to go to the hospital, you should remain calm and continue to talk to him while waiting for police assistance. Leaving an emotionally disturbed patient without ensuring his safety would constitute abandonment if he injured himself. Tricking a patient into taking medication by providing false information about its effects is unethical. (Objectives 9, 15)

Case Studies

Case one

1. The patient has agoraphobia, fear of open spaces. (Objective 11)
2. Stress to the patient the importance of receiving care for the myocardial infarction. Talk her through the process of preparing her for transport, moving her to the ambulance, and transporting her to the hospital. Minimize the amount of time outside of the patient's home before placing her in the ambulance. In addition to standard therapy for an acute myocardial infarction, consult with medical control about administration of a benzodiazepine to decrease the patient's anxiety during transport. (Objectives |9, 15)

Case two

1. The patient is experiencing a conversion reaction, also called *conversion hysteria*. (Objective 11)
2. Patients experience conversion reactions because they are presented with a psychological conflict that they are unable to resolve. By developing a loss of function, the patient resolves the conflict by limiting the actions he or she is able to take. In this case the patient was faced with the choice of saving the persons in the wrecked vehicle at the risk of losing his own life. By becoming blind, he resolved his dilemma because he would have helped them if he could have, but the blindness stopped him. (Objective 4)
3. Patients with conversion reactions often are much calmer than would be expected because the loss of function they have developed has helped resolve an overwhelming psychological conflict. (Objective 4)
4. The patient should be treated as though his blindness was caused by a physiologic problem and transported for evaluation. There is the possibility of an underlying physiologic cause. Even if the patient's blindness is psychogenic, he will require evaluation and treatment by a psychiatrist. (Objective 15)

Case three

1. The patient is disoriented to place and time. (Objective 11)
2. Disorientation is a common problem among geriatric patients who are acutely ill or injured because it provides a way for them to escape the stresses of their current situation by placing themselves in a time and place when they felt more secure and in control of their lives. Disorientation also can result from chronic

disease processes, such as Alzheimer's disease. (Objective 4)

3. Acute disorientation can be a result of physiologic causes such as hypoglycemia, hypoxia, hypoperfusion, cerebrovascular accident, head injury, drug toxicity, or electrolyte imbalance. (Objective 3)

4. Attempt to identify and treat an underlying cause while continuing to reorient the patient to his/her surroundings. (Objective 15)

5. Attempting to reorient a patient who is chronically disoriented can create additional stress and confusion for the patient. You should acknowledge the patient's comments about his/her location in place and time without challenging them or embellishing them. (Objective 15)

CHAPTER 33: HEMATOLOGIC DISORDERS

Short Answer

1. The formed elements found in blood are erythrocytes (red cells), leukocytes (white cells), and thrombocytes (platelets). (Objective 2)

2. The erythrocytes transport oxygen to the tissues. (Objective 4)

3. Type A—antigen A
Type B—antigen B
Type AB—antigens A and B
Type O—no antigens
(Objective 18)

4. Type A—B antibodies
Type B—A antibodies
Type AB—no antibodies
Type O—A and B antibodies
(Objective 18)

5. Type O is the universal donor. Because there are no antigens on the red cells of patients with type O blood, their red cells will not be attacked by the antibodies present in the plasma of patients with types A, B, or O. (Objective 18)

6. Type AB is the universal recipient. Because persons with type AB blood carry both A and B antigens on their erythrocytes, they cannot have the antibody for either antigen in their plasma. Therefore they can safely be given any type of blood. (Objective 18)

7. Thrombocytes help control bleeding by forming plugs at sites of bleeding and secreting factors that help promote clot formation. (Objective 14)

8. The extrinsic clotting pathway is triggered by exposure of blood to collagen in damaged areas of the blood vessel wall. The intrinsic clotting pathway is triggered by damage to the platelets caused by turbulent blood flow. (Objectives 13, 14, 15)

9. Plasmin breaks down (lyses) blood clots. (Objectives 13, 16)

10. Persons with one gene for normal hemoglobin and one gene for sickle hemoglobin have higher resistance to the malaria parasite than persons with two genes for normal hemoglobin. This gives them a higher chance of surviving in areas where malaria is endemic and causes the gene for sickle hemoglobin to persist in these areas. (Objective 20)

11. Sickle cell thrombo-occlusive crisis is treated with high-concentration oxygen to reduce the tendency of red cells to sickle, IV fluid to correct dehydration that may have triggered the crisis, and pain control using narcotic analgesics. (Objective 20)

12. Sickled red cells clump together and obstruct blood flow through blood vessels in the brain. (Objective 20)

13. The most common cause of death in patients with hemophilia is increased intracranial pressure from intracranial bleeding. (Objective 21)

14. The most common site of hemorrhages in patients with hemophilia is into the joints. (Objective 21)

15. The bleeding should be controlled using the standard techniques of hemorrhage control. The normal hemostatic mechanisms still function. They just take longer. Supplemental oxygen and IV fluid should be used to treat the effects of hypoperfusion. Splinting of injured joints will help slow bleeding and control pain. Caution should be taken to avoid causing other injuries that would result in additional bleeding. (Objective 21)

16. Leukopenia is a reduction in the number of leukocytes. (Objectives 9, 10)

17. Patients with leukopenia have an increased risk of infection. (Objectives 9, 10)

18. Leukemia is a cancer of the blood-forming tissues in which the precursors of white blood cells replicate abnormally within the bone marrow and then spread to the peripheral circulation. (Objective 22)

19. The abnormal white cells formed in leukemia are ineffective in fighting infection. (Objective 22)

20. As the blood-forming tissues shift to production of increased numbers of white cells, the number of platelets decreases. A drop in the platelet count increases the patient's tendency to bleed. (Objective 22)

21. Disseminated intravascular coagulation is triggered by widespread tissue damage or by extensive blood loss that triggers activation of the clotting cascade on a large scale. The level of clotting factors in the blood drops to the point where the patient can no longer form clots. Additionally, as the clots formed in response to the problem triggering DIC begin to lyse, they release split fibrin products into the bloodstream that inhibit further clotting. (Objective 21)

22. In pregnancy DIC may be triggered by massive hemorrhage from a placental abruption or placenta previa, or it may result from exposure of the blood to dead fetal tissue from an incomplete abortion. (Objective 21)

23. If a female with Rh-negative blood is exposed to Rh-positive blood, her immune system will produce antibodies to the Rh antigen. If she subsequently becomes pregnant with an Rh-positive fetus, the Rh antibodies in her bloodstream can cross the placenta and attack the red cells of the Rh-positive fetus. (Objective 18)

369

Multiple Choice

1. D. Type O is the "universal donor." (Objective 18)
2. B. Type AB is the "universal recipient." (Objective 18)
3. B. Eosinophils release chemicals that inactivate the chemical mediators of allergic reactions and release chemicals that fight parasitic infections. Basophils release histamine. (Objective 10)
4. A. The principal function of neutrophils is to ingest and destroy invading microorganisms. (Objective 10)
5. B. Humoral immunity is mediated by B-lymphocytes and involves production of antibodies. (Objective 11)
6. A. T-lymphocytes are responsible for cellular immunity through direct attacks on cells carrying specific antigens. (Objective 10)
7. C. If Rh-positive blood is given to a female with Rh-negative blood, the patient may produce antibodies that could attack the red cells of an Rh-positive fetus during a future pregnancy. (Objective 18)
8. C. Antibodies or immunoglobulins are a component of humoral immunity and produced by the B-lymphocytes. (Objective 10)
9. C. The type of leukocyte responsible for recognizing foreign antigens, producing antibodies, and developing memory is the lymphocyte. (Objective 10)
10. A. One of the functions of the inflammatory response is walling off an infected area. The inflammatory response is a nonspecific response to tissue damage that involves the same responses regardless of the cause of the damage. (Objective 8)
11. B. If a person has type AB blood, the erythrocyte's cell membrane contains both A and B antigens. The plasma of a person with type AB blood will contain neither A nor B antibodies. (Objective 18)
12. D. The extrinsic pathway of hemostasis is activated by trauma to blood vessel walls. (Objective 14)
13. C. The most common cause of death in a patient with hemophilia is intracranial bleeding that produces increased intracranial pressure. (Objective 21)
14. A. Disseminated intravascular coagulation in pregnancy is most likely to result from activation of the clotting mechanism by dead fetal tissue or hemorrhage associated with the pregnancy. (Objective 21)
15. D. Hemophilia is inherited as an X-linked recessive disorder. (Objective 21)
16. B. Problems that can develop in patients with multiple myeloma include anemia, increased risk of infection, and pathologic fractures. (Objective 22)
17. A. Patients with thrombocytopenia are at increased risk of bleeding. (Objective 21)
18. D. The most common presenting sign of non-Hodgkin's lymphoma is swelling of the lymph nodes. (Objective 22)
19. A. von Willebrand disease involves both a clotting factor dysfunction and abnormal platelet function. von Willebrand disease is inherited as an autosomal recessive disease that affects males and females with equal frequency. The associated bleeding is less severe than the bleeding caused by hemophilia A. (Objective 21)

Case Study

1. DIC is an inability to clot triggered by widespread activation of the clotting cascade. (Objective)
2. DIC is caused by an event that produces systemic activation of the clotting cascade. Events causing DIC can include sepsis, burns, obstetric complications, massive hemorrhage, cancer, and hemolytic transfusion reactions. As the clotting cascade attempts to respond to widespread tissue damage or massive loss of blood, the body's supply of clotting factors drops to a critically low level. Additionally, the clots formed begin to release split fibrin products into the circulation, inhibiting further clotting. Overactivity of the clotting mechanism produces a state in which the patient no longer is able to form clots. (Objective)
3. Abruptio placentae can trigger DIC because attempts to control the massive bleeding taking place within the uterus consume the body's supply of clotting factors. (Objective)
4. DIC is characterized by oozing blood at venipuncture and wound sites and the appearance of petechiae and purpura under the skin. DIC can result in internal hemorrhage and produce hemodynamic instability. (Objective)
5. The patient should receive high-concentration oxygen and IV fluid to help counter the effects of hypoperfusion caused by blood loss. Definitive treatment of DIC involves correcting the underlying cause and administering fresh frozen plasma and platelets to restore normal clotting. (Objective)

CHAPTER 34: SHOCK AND RESUSCITATION

Matching

1. __B__ 23 y.o. h/o vomiting & diarrhea × 4 days; BP—98/76 mm Hg, P—120 beats/min, R—22 breaths/min

   __D__ 27 y.o. c/o abdominal pain following an incomplete abortion 3 days ago; skin warm, flushed; BP—96/56 mm Hg, P—136 beats/min, R—26 breaths/min shallow, T—103° F

   __C__ 30 y.o. c/o loss of lower extremity motor function following a motor vehicle collision; BP—96/40 mm Hg, P—72 beats/min, R—24 breaths/min shallow

   __A__ 77 y.o. c/o substernal chest pain and SOB; BP—70/56 mm Hg, P—130 beats/min irregular, R—36 breaths/min (Objectives 3 to 11)

Short Answer

1. Adequate blood volume, adequate cardiac function, adequate vascular resistance. (Objective 1)
2. Inability of the cardiovascular system to deliver sufficient oxygen and nutrients to the tissues to

support aerobic metabolism. Shock is metabolic failure caused by inadequate tissue perfusion. (Objective 2)

3. A falling blood pressure is a late sign of shock. In early shock, the body adjusts peripheral resistance and cardiac output to compensate for inadequate perfusion. These compensatory responses can result in a near-normal blood pressure even though a patient's cardiovascular system cannot maintain adequate perfusion of all body tissues. A falling blood pressure in shock indicates that the body's compensatory mechanisms have failed. (Objective 2)

4. Inadequate delivery of oxygen to the tissues results in anaerobic metabolism with a significant decrease in cellular production of ATP. Lactic acid and pyruvic acid are produced as byproducts of anaerobic metabolism, resulting in metabolic acidosis. Acidosis causes a shift of potassium from the intracellular space to the extracellular space, causing hyperkalemia. (Objective 2)

5. Because shock results from failure of tissue oxygenation, the most important treatment that can be given to any patient who is in shock is oxygen. (Objectives 3 to 11)

6. Spinal cord injury can interrupt the output of the sympathetic nervous system, which arises from the thoracic and lumbar portions of the spinal cord. A drop in sympathetic tone causes the peripheral blood vessels below the level of the injury to dilate, decreasing peripheral vascular resistance. The drop n peripheral resistance causes a drop in blood pressure, resulting in inadequate perfusion. Sweating is stimulated by increased sympathetic tone; therefore patients in neurogenic shock have dry skin. The decrease in sympathetic nervous system output that can result from a spinal cord injury causes unopposed action by the parasympathetic nervous system on the heart, slowing the heart rate. (Objectives 7, 8)

7. Hypovolemia should be treated with an isotonic solution. Hypovolemic shock results from inadequate intravascular volume. An isotonic solution will tend to remain in the vascular space, replacing lost intravascular volume and helping to support adequate tissue perfusion. (Objective 4)

8. If a large amount of fluid is infused rapidly into a patient with inadequate cardiac function, the heart may be unable to circulate all of the fluid. The excess fluid can accumulate in the lungs, resulting in pulmonary edema. (Objective 6)

9. A significant portion of the elderly population suffers from chronic hypertension. Patients with hypertension become dependent on their elevated blood pressures to maintain adequate tissue perfusion. In a chronically hypertensive patient, a drop in blood pressures to "normal" levels can reduce oxygen and nutrient delivery to a level where

cellular metabolism fails and shock develops. (Objective 4)

10. Because children generally have healthy cardiovascular systems, they have a rapid, strong compensatory response to hypoperfusion. Children typically are able to compensate for hypoperfusion much more quickly than adults and for longer time periods. However, when the compensatory mechanisms fail, children decompensate much more rapidly than adults. (Objective 4)

11. Increased resistance to blood flow in the abdomen and lower extremities, resulting in increased blood volumes and blood flow in the head and chest. Direct pressure to the lower extremities and abdomen, slowing external and internal bleeding. Splinting of fractures of the pelvis and lower extremities. (Objective 4)

12. PASG should never be applied to a patient in heart failure with pulmonary edema. Increasing the volume of blood circulating in the upper body by compressing the abdomen and lower extremities would further overload the failing heart and worsen the pulmonary edema. (Objective 4)

13. During early shock, decreased delivery of oxygen to the brain and increased blood levels of epinephrine and norepinephrine make patients restless and anxious. (Objective 2)

14. During early shock, a patient's respirations will be rapid. Hypoperfusion produces a state of inadequate tissue oxygenation, resulting in anaerobic metabolism. Two of the products of anaerobic metabolism are lactic acid and pyruvic acid. Their presence results in a metabolic acidosis. The body's buffering of the hydrogen ions released by lactic acid and pyruvic acid causes increased blood carbon dioxide levels. The excess carbon dioxide stimulates the respiratory center in the medulla oblongata, resulting in an increased respiratory rate. (Objective 2)

15. Because the PASG is compressing the patient's lower body, the tissues there have been ischemic. Rapid deflation of the PASG can result in a rapid release of lactic acid and potassium into the central circulation, causing dysrhythmias and depressed myocardial function. Also, the PASG is supporting the perfusion of the heart, lungs, and brain by limiting blood flow to the lower body. Sudden deflation of the PASG without first taking steps to restore adequate circulating blood volume can cause severe hypotension. (Objective 4)

16. An adult cannot lose enough blood into the cranial cavity to cause hypovolemic shock. Therefore the patient is losing blood somewhere in his body other than his head. (Objective 3)

17. Yes a PASG can be applied to this patient. Cerebral perfusion pressure is the difference between the average arterial blood pressure pushing blood into the brain and the intracranial pressure resisting blood flow.

371

If a patient has increased intracranial pressure from a head injury and decreased blood pressure from bleeding elsewhere, hypoperfusion of the brain will occur much more quickly than it would with an isolated head injury or isolated blood loss. Application of a PASG will help support the blood pressure so the patient can continue to maintain cerebral perfusion. (Objective 4)

18. Histamine, released during an allergic reaction, causes peripheral vasodilation, increased capillary permeability, and contraction of the smooth muscle in the lower airway and GI tract. Epinephrine can be given to produce peripheral vasoconstriction and bronchodilation. Diphenhydramine (Benadryl) can be administered to block the effects of histamine at its receptor sites. Solu-Medrol, a steroid, can be given to produce long-term inhibition of inflammation. (Objective 7)

19. The underlying causes of hypovolemic and cardiogenic shock do not involve problems with the peripheral blood vessels. In hypovolemic and cardiogenic shock, peripheral vasoconstriction can be used as a mechanism to compensate for decreased intravascular volume or cardiac output. Therefore in both of these conditions, the skin will become pale and cool. In anaphylactic and neurogenic shock, hypoperfusion results from peripheral vasodilation and loss of vascular resistance to blood flow. Because peripheral vasoconstriction cannot occur, the skin has a flushed appearance. (Objectives 3, 4, 5, 6, 7)

20. In shock, cerebral hypoxia and release of large amounts of epinephrine and norepinephrine cause restlessness and anxiety. (Objective 2)

21. In early hypovolemic shock, peripheral vasoconstriction will cause an increase in the diastolic blood pressure. The rise in diastolic blood pressure accompanied by the absence of change or a slight drop in the systolic blood pressure narrows the pulse pressure. (Objective 3)

22. Shock results in a shift at the cellular level from aerobic to anaerobic metabolism. Anaerobic metabolism produces significantly less heat than aerobic metabolism. Therefore the body temperature of hypoperfused patients tends to fall and they frequently complain of feeling cold. (Objective 2)

23. By decreasing blood flow to the lower body, PASG causes an increase in circulating blood volume and blood pressure in the head and chest. If a patient is hemorrhaging in the thoracic cavity, these changes can increase the rate of blood loss. Additionally, the PASG pushes the abdominal organs against the lower surface of the diaphragm. This can interfere with the patient's ability to ventilate, particularly if a thoracic injury is present. (Objective 4)

24. The body compensates for hypovolemia by releasing epinephrine and norepinephrine, which constrict blood vessels in the skin, kidneys, and digestive tract and shunt blood to the heart, lungs, and brain. A patient who is compensating for hypovolemia has very little blood flow in the vessels of the kidneys and gastrointestinal tract. Administration of a vasopressor such as dopamine or norepinephrine before adequate blood volume has been restored can increase the vasoconstriction in these areas, causing renal and bowel infarctions. (Objective 4)

25. Hypovolemic shock. (Objective 3)

26. A patient who hypoperfuses will adjust his or her heart rate and peripheral vascular resistance to compensate for the problem causing the hypoperfusion. These compensatory responses will maintain the blood pressure at a near-normal level. Blood pressure will not begin to fall until the compensatory responses fail. (Objective 3)

Multiple Choice

1. A. A patient cannot lose enough blood inside his skull to cause shock. Therefore the patient must be bleeding elsewhere. Hypovolemic shock produces tachycardia and cool, moist skin. Neurogenic shock produces bradycardia and flushed, dry skin. Shock associated with closed head injury will produce a more rapid decrease in cerebral perfusion pressure than occurs with an isolated head injury. (Objectives 3, 4)

2. A. The patient is suffering from anaphylactic shock, caused by an allergic reaction to wasp venom. (Objective 7)

3. C. The patient is suffering from neurogenic shock caused by a spinal cord injury. The combination of hypotension, slow pulse rate, and neurologic deficits following an event that could have produced a spinal injury suggests neurogenic shock. (Objective 7)

4. D. Restlessness; anxiety; dizziness; thirst; weak, rapid pulses; rapid respirations; and a sensation of being cold suggest hypovolemic shock in a trauma patient. (Objective 3)

5. B. The combination of a rising pulse rate and a falling blood pressure in a trauma patient suggests hypovolemic shock from internal blood loss. If the patient was experiencing the effects of anxiety, the heart rate would be expected to slow over time. An adult cannot lose enough blood into the cranial cavity to produce hypovolemia, so the patient must be bleeding elsewhere. (Objective 3)

6. C. Neurogenic shock is indicated by a slow heart rate and a low blood pressure. (Objective 7)

7. If you suspect that a patient is in hypovolemic shock, you should place the patient in the supine position. Oxygen should be administered at high concentrations using a nonrebreather mask at 10 to 15 L/min. The patient should be kept from losing body heat, but you should not attempt to raise the body temperature. Attempting to replace lost volume using oral fluids can lead to vomiting and aspiration. (Objective 4)

8. C. The PASG can be useful in prehospital care because it will immobilize pelvic and lower extremity fractures, reduce internal blood loss, and compress lower extremity bleeding. (Objective 4)

9. C. Shock can be caused by inadequate blood volume, dilation of the blood vessels, or pump failure. (Objective 2)

10. B. Shock may be produced by spinal cord injury because the blood vessels below the injury become dilated and there is no longer enough blood to fill them. (Objective 7)

11. D. Shock may be produced by a systemic infection (sepsis) because toxins released by bacteria dilate blood vessels, enlarging the vascular space and causing "relative" hypovolemia. (Objective 7)

12. A. If signs of shock are present, use of the PASG would be indicated for a pelvic injury with signs of intraabdominal bleeding. The PASG helps stabilize a pelvic fracture and support adequate perfusion. PASG is not indicated with chest trauma because it can increase bleeding within the thoracic cavity and interfere with adequate ventilation. PASG is also not indicated in hypo-volemic shock caused by injuries above the level of the garment because it can worsen bleeding. (Objective 4)

13. B. Damage to the sympathetic nervous system caused by a spinal fracture can produce peripheral vasodilation leading to a drop in blood pressure and hypothermia because of increased heat loss through dilated peripheral vessels. Decreased sympathetic tone from a spinal cord injury will cause a fall in the heart rate. (Objective 7)

14. C. The shock that follows spinal cord injury is due to loss of peripheral resistance. (Objective 7)

Case Studies

Case one

1. Hypovolemia. (Objective 3)
2. An isotonic crystalloid because it will remain in the patient's vascular space and support adequate perfusion. (Objective 4)

Case two

1. Overhydrated. (Objective 5)
2. Because this patient has poor cardiac output, rapid infusion of an isotonic crystalloid would overload the pump and cause additional fluid to accumulate in the lungs, worsening the pulmonary edema that already is present. (Objectives 5, 6)
3. A hypotonic fluid should be used because it will leave the vascular space rapidly and not worsen the volume overload. If a hypotonic fluid is not available, then an isotonic fluid infused at a very slow rate should be used to maintain a drug administration route. (Objective 6)

4. Fluid should be infused only at the rate necessary to keep the IV open as a route for giving medications. Rapid infusion of fluid will overload the patient's failing heart and produce pulmonary edema as excess fluid accumulates in the lungs. (Objective 6)

Case three

1. Hypovolemic. (Objective 3)
2. An isotonic solution should be used because it will remain in the vascular space to help replace the blood volume being lost from internal bleeding. (Objective 4)
3. A 10 or 15 gtt/mL set should be used rather than a 60 gtt/mL set to ensure that fluid can be infused rapidly enough to keep up with the volume loss from bleeding. A large-bore (14- or 16-gauge) IV catheter should be used so adequate amounts of fluid can be infused rapidly. (Objective 4)
4. Because the patient is bleeding into his abdominal cavity, application of the PASG should be considered. The PASG will help support an adequate circulating blood volume in the head and chest and will apply direct pressure that will slow bleeding within the abdominal cavity. (Objective 4)

Case four

1. Neurogenic shock. The mechanism of injury, chief complaint, and presence of neurologic deficits suggest a spinal cord injury. In the presence of a spinal cord injury, a slow heart rate and low blood pressure indicate neurogenic shock. (Objective 7)
2. An isotonic solution should be infused to fill the dilated vascular space and restore adequate perfusion. An isotonic solution is indicated because it will remain in the blood vessels and help fill the oversized vascular container that has resulted from a loss of sympathetic tone. (Objective 8)
3. Diaphoresis and tachycardia in shock result from increased sympathetic tone. Spinal injuries that cause neurogenic shock result in decreased sympathetic tone. Therefore patients who are in neurogenic shock have slow heart rates and do not sweat heavily. (Objective 7)
4. A vasopressor such as norepinephrine, phenylephrine, or high-dose dopamine can be infused to decrease the size of the vascular space through vasoconstriction. Also, application of a PASG may be useful in severe neurogenic shock because it increases peripheral vascular resistance by squeezing the vascular compartment. (Objective 8)

Glossary

800 MHz A type of radio signal in the ultra-high-frequency range that allows splitting a frequency into individual talk groups used as communication links with other system users.

9-1-1/E9-1-1 A set of three numbers that automatically sends the call to the emergency dispatch center. E9-1-1 is enhanced 9-1-1, which gives the dispatcher the ability to determine the caller's location by routing the call through several CAD systems.

Abandonment Terminating care when it is still needed and desired by the patient and without ensuring that appropriate care continues to be provided by another qualified health care professional.

Abbreviation A shorter way of writing something.

Abdominal compartment syndrome Syndrome caused by diffuse intestinal edema, a result of fluid accumulation in the bowel wall. It may be caused by overresuscitation with crystalloids and results in shock and renal failure.

Abdominal evisceration An injury in which a severe laceration or incision of the abdomen breaches through all layers of muscle to allow abdominal contents, most often the intestines, to protrude above the surface of the skin.

Aberrant Abnormal.

Abortion The ending of a pregnancy for any reason before 20 weeks' gestation; the lay term miscarriage is referred to as a *spontaneous abortion.*

Abruptio placentae Separation of the placenta from the uterine wall after the twentieth week of gestation.

Abscess A collection of pus.

Absence seizure A generalized seizure characterized by a blank stare and an alteration of consciousness.

Absolute refractory period Corresponds with the onset of the QRS complex to approximately the peak of the T wave; cardiac cells cannot be stimulated to conduct an electrical impulse. no matter how strong the stimulus.

Absorption Movement of small organic molecules, electrolytes, vitamins, and water across the digestive tract and into the circulatory system. Also the movement of a drug from the site of input into the circulation.

Abuse Use of a substance for other than its approved, accepted purpose or in a greater amount than prescribed.

Acalculus cholecystitis Inflammation of the gallbladder in the absence of gallstones.

Acceptance A grief stage in which the individual has come to terms with the reality of his or her (or a loved one's) imminent death.

Accessory muscles Muscles of the neck, chest, and abdomen that become active during labored breathing.

Accessory pathway An extra bundle of working myocardial tissue that forms a connection between the atria and ventricles outside the normal conduction system.

Accreditation Recognition given to an EMD center by an independent auditing agency for achieving a consistently high level of performance based on industry best practice standards.

Acetylation A mechanism in which a drug is processed by enzymes.

Acetylcholinesterase A body chemical that stops the action of acetylcholine (a neurotransmitter involved in the stimulation of nerves).

Acid Fluid produced in the stomach; breaks down the food material within the stomach into chyme.

Acid-base balance Delicate balance between the body's acidity and alkalinity.

Acidic pH less than 7.0.

Acids Materials that have a pH value less than 7.0 (e.g., hydrochloric acid, sulfuric acid).

Acquired immunity Specific immunity directed at a particular pathogen that develops after the body has been exposed to it once (e.g., immunity to chickenpox after first exposure).

Acquired immunodeficiency syndrome (AIDS) An acquired immunodeficiency disease that can develop after infection with HIV.

Acrocyanosis A condition in which the core of a newborn is pink and the extremities are cyanotic.

Action potential A five-phase cycle that reflects the difference in the concentration of charged particles across the cell membrane at any given time.

Activated charcoal An adsorbent made from charred wood that effectively binds many poisons in the stomach; most effective when administered within 1 hour of intake.

Activation phase In phases of immunity, the stage at which a single lymphocyte activates many other lymphocytes and significantly expands the scope of immune response in a process known as amplification.

Active immunity Induced immunity in which the body can continue to mount specific immune response when exposed to the agent (e.g., vaccination).

Active listening Listening to the words that the patient is saying as well as paying attention to the significance of those words to the patient.

Active range of motion The degree of movement at a joint as determined by the patient's own voluntary movements.

Active transport A process used to move substances against the concentration gradient or toward the side that has a higher concentration; requires the use of energy by the cell but is faster than diffusion.

Acute arterial occlusion A sudden blockage of arterial blood flow that occurs because of a thrombus, embolus, tumor, direct trauma to an artery, or an unknown cause.

Acute care Short-term medical treatment usually provided in a hospital for patients who have an illness or injury or who are recovering from surgery.

Acute coronary syndrome (ACS) A term used to refer to patients presenting with ischemic chest discomfort. Acute coronary syndromes consist of three major syndromes: unstable angina, non–ST-segment elevation myocardial infarction and ST-segment elevation myocardial infarction.

Acute exposure An exposure that occurs over a short timeframe (less than 24 hours); usually occurs at a spill or release.

Acute renal failure (ARF) When the kidneys suddenly stop functioning, either partially or completely, but eventually recover full or nearly full functioning over time.

Acute respiratory distress syndrome (ARDS) Collection of fluid in the alveoli of the lung, usually as a result of trauma or serious illness.

Addiction The involvement in a repetitive behavior (gambling, substance abuse, etc.). In physical addiction the individual has become dependent on an external substance and develops physical withdrawal symptoms if the substance is unavailable.

Addictive behavior The involvement in repetitive behavior such as gambling or substance abuse.

Additive effect The combined effect of two drugs given at the same time that have similar effects.

Adenosine triphosphate (ATP) Formed from metabolism of nutrients in the cell; serves as an energy source throughout the body.

Adipocyte A fat cell; a connective tissue cell that has differentiated and become specialized in the synthesis (manufacture) and storage of fat.

Adipose (fat) connective tissue Tissue that stores lipids; acts as an insulator and protector of the organs of the body.

Administrative law A branch of law that deals with rules, regulations, orders, and decisions created by governmental agencies.

Adrenergic Having the characteristics of the sympathetic division of the autonomic nervous system.

Adrenocortical steroids Hormones released by the adrenal cortex essential for life; assist in the regulation of blood glucose levels, promote peripheral use of lipids, stimulate the kidneys to reabsorb sodium, and have antiinflammatory effects.

Adsorb To gather or stick to a surface in a condensed layer.

Acute respiratory distress syndrome (ARDS) A life-threatening condition that causes lung swelling and fluid buildup in the air sacs.

Advance directive A document in which a competent person gives instructions to be followed regarding his or her health care in the event the person later becomes incapacitated and unable to make or communicate those decisions to others.

Advanced emergency medical technician (AEMT) An EMS professional who provides basic and limited advanced skills to patients who access the EMS system.

Adverse effect (reaction) An unintentional, undesirable, and often unpredictable effect of a drug used at therapeutic doses to prevent, diagnose, or treat disease.

Advocate A person who assists another person in carrying out desired wishes; a paramedic should function as a patient's advocate in all aspects of prehospital care.

Aerosol A collection of particles dispersed in a gas.

Affect Description of the patient's visible emotional state.

Afferent division Nerve fibers that send impulses from the periphery to the central nervous system.

Affinity The intensity or strength of the attraction between a drug and its receptor.

Afterload Pressure or resistance against which the ventricles must pump to eject blood.

Ageism Stereotypical and often negative bias against older adults.

Agonal respirations Slow, shallow, irregular respirations resulting from anoxic brain injury.

Agonist A drug that causes a physiologic response in the receptor to which it binds.

Agonist-antagonist A drug that blocks a receptor. It may provide a partial agonist activity, but it also prevents an agonist from exerting its full effects.

Agoraphobia Consistent anxiety and avoidance of places and situations where escape during a panic attack would be difficult or embarrassing.

Air emboli Bubble of air that has entered the vasculature. Emboli can result in damage similar to a clot in the vasculature, typically resulting in brain injury or pulmonary emboli when neck vessels are damaged.

Air embolism Introduction of air into venous circulation, which can ultimately enter the right ventricle, closing off circulation to the pulmonary artery and leading to death.

Air trapping A respiratory pattern associated with an obstruction in the pulmonary tree; the breathing rate increases to overcome resistance in getting air out, the respiratory effort becomes more shallow, the volume of trapped air increases, and the lungs inflate.

Airbag identification The various shapes, sizes, colors, and styles of visual identification labels indicating that an airbag is present.

Airbags Inflatable nylon bags designed to supplement the protection of occupants during crashes; one of the most common new technology items confronting responders at crash scenes; also known as *supplemental restraint systems*.

Air-reactive materials Materials that react with atmospheric moisture and rapidly decompose.

Alarm reaction The body's autonomic, sympathetic nervous system response to stimuli designed to prepare the individual to fight or flee.

Alcoholic ketoacidosis (AKA) Condition found in patients who chronically abuse alcohol accompanied by vomiting, a built-up of ketones in the blood, and little or no food intake.

Alcoholism Addiction and dependence on ethanol; often develops over many years.

Aldosterone A hormone responsible for the reabsorption of sodium and water from the kidney tubules.

Alkali A substance with a pH above 7.0; also known as a *base* or *caustic.*

Alkaline pH greater than 7.0.

Alkaloids A group of plant-based substances containing nitrogen and found in nature.

Allergen A substance that can provoke an allergic reaction.

Allergic reaction An abnormal immune response, mediated by immunoglobulin E antibodies, to an allergen that should not cause such a response and to which the patient has already been exposed; usually involves excessive release of immune agents, especially histamines.

All-hazards emergency preparedness A cross-cutting approach in which all forms of emergencies, including manmade and natural disasters, epidemics, and physical or biologic terrorism, are managed from a common template that uses consistent language and structure.

Allografting Transplanting organs or tissues from genetically nonidentical members of the same species.

All-terrain vehicle (ATV) Any of a number of models of small open motorized vehicles designed for off-road and wilderness use; three-wheeled (all-terrain cycles) and four-wheeled (quads) versions are most often used for personnel insertion; six- and eight-wheeled models exist for specialized applications.

Alpha particle A positively charged particle emitted by certain radioactive materials.

Altered mental status Disruption of a person's emotional and intellectual functioning.

Altitude illness A syndrome associated with the relatively low partial pressure of oxygen in the atmosphere at altitudes encountered during mountain climbing or travel in unpressurized aircraft.

Alveolar air volume In contrast to dead air space, alveolar volume is the amount of air that does reach the alveoli for gas exchange (approximately 350 mL in the adult male). It is the difference between tidal volume and dead-space volume.

Alveoli Functional units of the respiratory system; area in the lungs where the majority of gas exchange takes place; singular form is *alveolus.*

Alzheimer's disease Progressive dementia seen mostly in the elderly and marked by decline of memory and cognitive function.

Amniotic sac (bag of waters) The fluid-filled protective sac that surrounds the fetus inside the uterus.

Amplitude Height (voltage) of a waveform on the ECG.

Ampule A sealed sterile container that holds a single dose of liquid or powdered medication.

Amygdala Almond-shaped structure at the end of each hippocampus that attaches emotional significance to incoming stimuli; has a large role in the fear response; plural form is *amygdale.*

Amylase Enzyme in pancreatic juice.

Amyotrophic lateral sclerosis (ALS) Autoimmune disorder affecting the motor roots of the spinal nerves, causing progressive muscle weakness and eventually paralysis.

Anal canal Area between the rectum and the anus.

Analgesia A state in which pain is controlled or not perceived.

Anaphylactic reaction An unusual or exaggerated allergic reaction to a foreign substance.

Anaphylactoid reaction Reaction that clinically mimics an allergic reaction but is not mediated by immunoglobulin E antibodies, so not a true allergic reaction.

Anaphylaxis Life-threatening allergic reaction.

Anasarca Massive generalized body edema.

Anatomic plane The relation of internal body structures to the surface of the body; imaginary straight line divisions of the body.

Anatomic position The position of a person standing erect with his or her feet and palms facing the examiner.

Anatomy Study of the body's structure and organization.

Anchor point A single secure connection for an anchor.

Anchors The means of securing the ropes and other elements of the high-angle system.

Anemia Deficiency in red blood cells or hemoglobin; most common form is iron-deficiency anemia.

Anesthesia A process in which pain is prevented during a procedure.

Aneurysm Localized dilation or bulging of a blood vessel wall or wall of a heart chamber.

Anger A stage in the grieving process in which the individual is upset by the stated future loss of life.

Angina pectoris Chest discomfort or other related symptoms of sudden onset that may occur because the increased oxygen demand of the heart temporarily exceeds the blood supply.

Anginal equivalents Symptoms of myocardial ischemia other than chest pain or discomfort.

Angioedema Swelling of the tissues, including the dermal layer; often found in and around the mouth, tongue, and lips.

Angle of Louis An angulation of the sternum that indicates the point where the second rib joins the sternum; also called the *manubriosternal junction.*

Anhedonia Lack of enjoyment in activities one used to find pleasurable.

Anion A negatively charged ion.

Anorexia nervosa Eating disorder characterized by a preoccupation that one is obese; drastic, intentional weight loss; and bizarre attitudes and rituals associated with food and exercise.

Anoxia A total lack of oxygen availability to the tissues.

Antagonist A drug that does not cause a physiologic response when it binds with a receptor.

Antegrade amnesia The inability to remember short-term memory information after an event during which the head was struck.

Antepartum The period before childbirth.

Anterior The front, or ventral, surface.

Anterior cord syndrome Collection of symptoms seen after the compression, death, or transection of the anterior portion of the spinal cord.

Anthrax An acute bacterial infection caused by inhalation, contact, or ingestion of *Bacillus anthracis* organisms. Three forms of anthrax disease may occur depending on the route of exposure. Inhalational anthrax disease occurs after the inhalation of anthrax spores. Cutaneous anthrax disease is the most common form and occurs after the exposure of compromised skin to anthrax spores. Gastrointestinal anthrax disease occurs after the ingestion of live *B. anthracis* in contaminated meat.

Antiarrhythmic Medications used to correct irregular heartbeats and slow hearts that beat too fast.

Antibacterial Medication that kills or limits bacteria.

Antibiotic In common medical terms, a drug that kills bacteria.

Antibody Agents produced by B lymphocytes that bind to antigens, thus killing or controlling them and slowing or stopping an infection; also called *immunoglobulin.*

Antidiuretic hormone (ADH) A hormone released in response to detected loss of body water; prevents further loss of water through the urinary tract by promoting the reabsorption of water into the blood.

Antidote A substance that can reverse the adverse effects of a poison.

Antifungal Agent that kills fungi.

Antigen A marker on a cell that identifies the cell as "self" or "not self"; antigens are used by antibodies to identify cells that should be attacked as not self.

Antihistamine Medication that reduces the effects of histamine.

Antiinflammatory mediators Protein entities, often produced in the liver, that act as modulators of the immune response to the proinflammatory response to injury; also called *cytokines.*

Antipyretic medication A medication that reduces or eliminates a fever.

Antisepsis Prevention of sepsis by preventing or inhibiting the growth of causative microorganisms; in the field, the process used to cleanse local skin areas before needle puncture with products that are alcohol or iodine based.

Antivenin A substance that can reverse the adverse effects of a venom by binding to it and inactivating it.

Antiviral Medication that kills or impedes a virus.

Antonym A root word, prefix, or suffix that has the *opposite* meaning of another word.

Anucleated Cells of the body that do not have a central nucleus, such as those in cardiac muscle.

Anus The end of the anal canal.

Anxiety The sometimes vague feeling of apprehension, uneasiness, dread, or worry that often occurs without a specific source or cause identified. It is also a normal response to a perceived threat.

Aorta Delivers blood from the left ventricle of the heart to the body.

Aortic valve Semilunar valve on the left of the heart; separates the left ventricle from the aorta.

Apex Tip.

Apex of the heart Lower portion of the heart, tip of the ventricles (approximately the level of the fifth left intercostal space); points leftward, downward, and forward.

Apgar score A scoring system applied to an infant after delivery; key components include appearance, pulse, grimace, activity, and respiration.

Aphasia Loss of speech.

Apnea Respiratory arrest.

Apnea monitor A technologic aid used to warn of cessation of breathing in a premature infant; also may warn of bradycardia and tachycardia.

Apocrine glands Sweat glands that open into hair follicles, including in and around the genitalia, axillae, and anus; secrete an organic substance (which is odorless until acted upon by surface bacteria) into the hair follicles.

Appendicitis A tubular process that extends from the colon.

Appendicular region Area that includes the extremities (e.g., arms, pelvis, and legs).

Appendicular skeleton Consists of all the bones not within the axial skeleton: upper and lower extremities, the girdles, and their attachments.

Appendix Accessory structure of the cecum.

Application of principles The step at which the paramedic applies critical thinking in a clinical sense and arrives at a field impression or a working diagnosis.

Aqueous humor Fluid that fills the anterior chamber of the eye; maintains intraocular pressure.

Arachnoid mater Second layer of the meninges.

Arachnoid membrane Weblike middle layer of the meninges.

Areolar connective tissue A loose tissue found in most organs of the body; consists of weblike collagen, reticulum, and elastin fibers.

Arnold-Chiari malformation A complication of spina bifida in which the brainstem and cerebellum extend down through the foramen magnum into the cervical portion of the vertebrae.

Arrector pili Smooth muscle that surrounds each follicle; responsible for "goose bumps," which pull the hair upwards.

Arrhythmia Term often used interchangeably with dysrhythmia; any disturbance or abnormality in a normal rhythmic pattern; any cardiac rhythm other than a sinus rhythm.

Arterial puncture Accidental puncture into an artery instead of a vein.

Arterioles Small arterial vessels; supply oxygenated blood to the capillaries.

Arteriosclerosis A chronic disease of the arterial system characterized by abnormal thickening and hardening of the vessel walls.

Arthritis Inflammation of a joint that results in pain, stiffness, swelling, and redness.

Artifact Distortion of an ECG tracing by electrical activity that is noncardiac in origin (e.g., electrical interference, poor electrical conduction, patient movement).

Artificial anchors The use of specially designed hardware to create anchors where good natural anchors do not exist.

Arytenoid cartilages Six paired cartilages stacked on top of each other in the larynx.

Ascending colon Part of the large intestine.

Ascites Marked abdominal swelling from a buildup of fluid in the peritoneal cavity.

Asepsis Sterile; free from germs, infection, and any form of life.

Asphyxiants Chemicals that impair the body's ability to either get or use oxygen.

Aspiration Inhalation of foreign contents into the lungs.

Aspiration pneumonitis Inflammation of the bronchi and alveoli caused by inhaled foreign objects, usually acids such as stomach acid.

Assault A threat of imminent bodily harm to another person by someone with the obvious ability to carry out the threat.

Assay A test of a substance to determine its components.

Assessment-based management Taking the information you obtain from your assessment and using it to treat the patient.

Asthma Allergic response of the airways causing wheezing and dyspnea.

Asynchronous pacemaker Fixed-rate pacemaker that continuously discharges at a preset rate regardless of the patient's intrinsic activity.

Asystole A total absence of ventricular electrical activity.

Ataxia Inability to control voluntary muscle movements; unsteady movements and staggering gait.

Atelectasis An abnormal condition characterized by the collapse of alveoli, preventing the respiratory exchange of carbon dioxide and oxygen in a part of the lungs.

Atherosclerosis A form of arteriosclerosis in which the thickening and hardening of the vessel walls are caused by a buildup of fatty deposits in the inner lining of large and middle-sized muscular arteries (from *athero*, meaning gruel or paste, and *sclerosis*, meaning hardness).

Atlas First cervical vertebra.

Atopic A genetic disposition to an allergic reaction that is different from developing an allergy after one or more exposures to a drug or substance.

Atresia Absence of a normal opening.

Atria Two receiving chambers of the heart; singular form is *atrium*.

Atrial kick Remaining 20% to 30% of blood forced into the right ventricle during atrial contraction.

Atrioventricular junction The atrioventricular node and the nonbranching portion of the bundle of His.

Atrioventricular node A group of cells that conduct an electrical impulse through the heart; located in the floor of the right atrium immediately behind the tricuspid valve and near the opening of the coronary sinus.

Atrioventricular sequential pacemaker Type of dual-chamber pacemaker that stimulates first the atrium, then the ventricle, mimicking normal cardiac physiology.

Atrioventricular valve Valve located between each atrium and ventricle; the tricuspid separates the right atrium from the right ventricle, and the mitral (bicuspid) separates the left atrium from the left ventricle.

Atrophy Decrease in cell size that negatively affects function.

Attenuated vaccine A vaccine prepared from a live virus or bacteria that has been physically or chemically weakened to produce an immune response without causing the severe effects of the disease.

Attributes Qualities or characteristics of a person.

Auditory ossicles Three small bones (malleus, incus, and stapes) that articulate with each other to transmit sounds waves to the cochlea.

Augmented limb lead Leads aVR, aVL, and aVF; these leads record the difference in electrical potential at one location relative to zero potential rather than relative to the electrical potential of another extremity, as in the bipolar leads.

Aura Sensory disturbances caused by a partial seizure; may precede a generalized seizure.

Auricle Outer ear; also called the *pinna*.

Auscultation The process of listening to body noises with a stethoscope.

Authority having jurisdiction The local agency having legal authority for the type of rescue and the location at which it occurs.

Autoantibodies Antibodies produced by B cells that mistakenly attack and destroy "self" cells belonging to the patient; autoantibodies are the pathophysiologic agent of most autoimmune disorders.

Autografting Transplanting organs or tissues within the same person.

Autoignition point The temperature at which a material ignites and burns without an ignition source.

Autologous skin grafting The transplantation of skin of one patient from its original location to that of a wound on the same patient, such as a burn. Autologous means "derived from the same individual."

Automatic location identification Telephone technology used to identify the location of a caller immediately.

Automatic number identification Telephone technology that provides immediate identification of the caller's 10-digit telephone number.

Automaticity Ability of cardiac pacemaker cells to initiate an electrical impulse spontaneously without being stimulated from another source (such as a nerve).

Autonomic dysreflexia Massive sympathetic stimulation unbalanced by the parasympathetic nervous system because of spinal cord injury, usually at or above T6.

Autonomic dysreflexia syndrome A condition characterized by hypertension superior to an SCI site caused by overstimulation of the sympathetic nervous system.

Autonomic nervous system Provides unconscious control of smooth muscle organ and glands.

AVPU Mnemonic for *a*wake, *v*erbal, *p*ain, *u*nresponsive; used to evaluate a patient's mental status.

Axial compression (loading) The application of a force of energy along the axis of the spine, often resulting in compression fractures of the vertebrae.

Axial loading Application of excessive pressure or weight along the vertical axis of the spine.

Axial region Area that includes the head, neck, thorax, and abdomen.

Axial skeleton Part of the skeleton composed of the skull, hyoid bone, vertebral column, and thoracic cage.

Axis Imaginary line joining the positive and negative electrodes of a lead.

Axon Branching extensions of the neuron where impulses exit the cell.

Azotemia The increase in nitrogen-containing waste products in the blood secondary to renal failure.

B lymphocytes Cells present in the lymphatic system that mediate humoral immunity (also known as *B cells*).

B pillar The structural roof support member on a vehicle located at the rear edge of the front door; also referred to as the *B post*.

Babinski's sign An abnormal finding indicated by the presence of great toe extension with the fanning of all other toes on stimulation of the sole of the foot when it is stroked with a semi-sharp object from the heel to the ball of the foot.

Bacillus anthracis A gram-positive, spore-forming bacterium that causes anthrax disease in human beings and animals.

Bacteremia The presence of bacteria in the blood. This condition could progress to septic shock. Fever, chills, tachycardia, and tachypnea are common manifestations of bacteremia.

Bacteria Prokaryotic microorganisms capable of infecting and injuring patients; however, some bacteria, as part of the normal flora, assist in the processes of the human body.

Bacterial tracheitis A potentially serious bacterial infection of the lower portions of the upper airway: larynx, trachea, and bronchi.

Band A range of radio frequencies.

Bargaining A stage of the grieving process. The individual may attempt to "cut a deal" with a higher power to accomplish a specific goal or task.

Bariatric ambulance Ambulance designed to transport morbidly obese patients.

Barotrauma An injury resulting from rapid or extreme changes in pressure.

Barrier device A thin film of material placed on the patient's face used to prevent direct contact with the patient's mouth during positive-pressure ventilation.

Base of the heart Top of the heart; located at approximately the level of the second intercostal space.

Baseline Straight line recorded on ECG graph paper when no electrical activity is detected.

Bases Materials with a pH value greater than 7.0 (e.g., sodium hydroxide, potassium hydroxide).

Basilar skull fracture Loss of integrity to the bony structures of the base of the skull.

Basophils Type of granulocyte (white blood cell or leukocyte) that releases histamine.

Battery Touching or contact with another person without that person's consent.

Battle's sign Significant bruising around the mastoid process (behind the ears).

Beck's triad Classic signs of cardiac tamponade that include jugular venous distention, hypotension, and muffled heart sounds.

Behavior The conduct and activity of a person that is observable by others.

Behavioral emergency Actions or ideations by the patient that are harmful or potentially harmful to the patient or others.

Belay A safety technique used to safeguard personnel exposed to the risk of falling; the belayer is the person responsible for operation of the belay.

Bell's palsy An inflammation of the facial nerve (cranial nerve VII) that often is preceded by a viral upper respiratory tract infection.

Benchmarking Comparison of operating policies, procedures, protocols, and performance with those of other agencies in an effort to improve results.

Benzodiazepine Any of a group of minor tranquilizers with a common molecular structure and similar pharmacologic activity, including antianxiety, sedative, hypnotic, amnestic, anticonvulsant, and muscle-relaxing effects.

Beriberi Disease caused by a deficiency of thiamine and characterized by neurologic symptoms, cardiovascular abnormalities, and edema.

Beta particle A negatively charged particle emitted by certain radioactive materials.

Bevel The slanted tip at the end of the needle.

Bicuspid valve Left atrioventricular valve in the heart; also called the *mitral valve*.

Bile salts Manufactured in the liver; composed of electrolytes and iron recovered from red blood cells when they die.

Bilevel positive airway pressure (BiPAP) The delivery of two (bi) levels of positive-pressure ventilation; one during inspiration (to keep the airway open as the patient inhales) and the other (lower) pressure during expiration to reduce the work of exhalation.

Bilevel positive airway pressure (BiPAP) device Breathing device that can be set at one pressure for inhaling and a different pressure for exhaling.

Bioassay A test that determines the effects of a substance on an organism and compares the result with some agreed standard.

Bioavailability The speed with which and how much of a drug reaches its intended site of action.

Bioburden Accumulation of bacteria in a wound; does not necessarily imply an infection is present.

Biologic agent A disease-causing pathogen or a toxin that may be used as a weapon to cause disease or injury to people.

Biot respirations Irregular respirations varying in rate and depth and interrupted by periods of apnea; associated with increased intracranial pressure, brain damage at the level of the medulla, and respiratory compromise from drug poisoning.

Biphasic Waveform that is partly positive and partly negative.

Bipolar disorder An illness of extremes of mood, alternating between periods of depression and episodes of mania (type I) or hypomania (type II).

Bipolar limb lead ECG lead consisting of a positive and negative electrode; a pacing lead with two electrical poles that are external from the pulse generator; the negative pole is located at the extreme distal tip of the pacing lead, and the positive pole is located several millimeters proximal to the negative electrode. The stimulating pulse is delivered through the negative electrode.

Birth canal Part of the female reproductive tract through which the fetus is delivered; includes the lower part of the uterus, the cervix, and the vagina.

Blast lung syndrome Injuries to the body from an explosion, characterized by anatomic and physiologic changes from the force generated by the blast wave hitting the body's surface and affecting primarily gas-containing structures (lungs, gastrointestinal tract, and ears).

Bleeding Escape of blood from a blood vessel.

Blister agent A chemical used as a weapon designed specifically to injure the body tissue internally and externally of those exposed to its vapors or liquid; the method of injury is to cause painful skin blisters or tissue destruction of the exposed surface area (e.g., mustard, lewisite).

Blocked premature atrial complex Premature atrial contraction not followed by a QRS complex.

Blocking A position that places the emergency vehicle at an angle to the approaching traffic, across several lanes of traffic if necessary; this position begins to shield the work area and protects the crash scene from some of the approaching traffic.

Blood Liquid connective tissue; allows transport of nutrients, oxygen, and waste products.

Blood agents Chemicals absorbed into the body through the action of breathing, skin absorption, or ingestion (e.g., hydrogen cyanide, cyanogen chloride).

Blood alcohol content Milligrams of ethanol per deciliter of blood divided by 100; a fairly standard measure of how intoxicated a person is.

Blood-brain barrier A layer of tightly adhered cells that protects the brain and spinal cord from exposure to medications, toxins, and infectious particles.

Blood pressure Force exerted by the blood against the walls of the arteries as the ventricles of the heart contract and relax.

Bloody show Passage of the protective blood and mucus plug from the cervix; often is an early sign of labor.

Body mass index A calculation strongly associated with subcutaneous and total body fat and with skinfold thickness measurements.

Body surface area (BSA) Area of the body covered by skin; measured in square meters.

Boiling liquid expanding vapor explosion An explosion that can occur when a vessel containing a pressurized liquid ruptures.

Boiling point The temperature at which the vapor pressure of the material being heated equals atmospheric pressure (760 mm Hg); water boils to steam at $100°$ C ($212°$ F).

Bone Hard connective tissue; consists of living cells and a matrix made of minerals.

Borborygmi Hyperactivity of bowel sounds.

Borderline personality disorder Cluster B disorder marked by unstable emotions, relationships, and attitudes.

Botulism A severe neurologic illness caused by a potent toxin produced by *Clostridium botulinum* organisms; the three forms are food borne, wound, and infant (also called intestinal) botulism.

Bowel sounds The noises made by the intestinal smooth muscles as they squeeze fluids and food products through the digestive tract.

Bowman's capsule Located in the renal corpuscle.

Boyle's law Gas law that demonstrates that as pressure increases, volume decreases; explains the pain that can occur in flight in the teeth and ears and barotrauma in the gastrointestinal tract.

Bradycardia Heart rate slower than 60 beats/min (from *brady,* meaning "slow").

Bradykinesia Abnormal slowness of muscular movement.

Bradypnea A respiratory rate that is persistently slower than normal for age; in adults, a rate slower than 12 breaths/min.

Brain injury A traumatic insult to the brain capable of producing physical, intellectual, emotional, social, and vocational changes.

Brainstem Part of the brain that connects it to the spinal cord; responsible for many of the autonomic functions the body requires to survive (also called *vegetative functions*).

Brake bar rack A descending device consisting of a U-shaped metal bar to which several metal bars are attached that create friction on the rope. Some racks are limited to use in personal rappelling, whereas others also may be used for lowering rescue loads.

Braxton-Hicks contractions (false labor) Benign and painless contractions that usually occur after the third month of pregnancy.

Breach of duty Violation by the defendant of the standard of care applicable to the circumstances.

Breech presentation Presentation of the buttocks or feet of the fetus as the first part of the infant's body to enter the birth canal.

Bronchioles Smallest of the air passages.

Bronchiolitis An acute, infectious, inflammatory disease of the upper and lower respiratory tracts that results in obstruction of the small airways.

Bronchitis Inflammation of the lower airways, usually with mucus production. Often chronic and related to tobacco abuse.

Bronchopulmonary dysplasia (BPD) Respiratory condition in infants usually arising from preterm birth.

Bronchospasm Wheezing.

Brown-Séquard syndrome Group of symptoms that develop after the herniation or transection of half of the spinal cord manifested with unilateral damage.

Bruit The blowing or swishing sound created by the turbulence within a blood vessel.

Bubonic Relating to an inflamed, enlarged lymph gland.

Buccal An administration route in which medication is placed in the mouth between the gum and the mucous membrane of the cheek and absorbed into the bloodstream.

Buffer systems Compensatory mechanisms that act together to control pH.

Bulbourethral glands Pair of small glands that manufacture a mucous-type secretion that unites with the prostate fluid and spermatozoa to form sperm.

Bulimia nervosa Eating disorder consisting of a pattern of eating large amounts of food in one sitting (binging) and then forcing oneself to regurgitate (purging), with associated guilt and depression.

Bulk containers Large containers and tanks used to transport large quantities of hazardous materials.

Bulla A localized, fluid-filled lesion usually greater than 0.5 cm.

Bundle branch block (BBB) Abnormal conduction of an electrical impulse through either the right or left bundle branches.

Bundle of His Fibers located in the upper portion of the interventricular septum that conduct an electrical impulse through the heart.

Burnout Exhaustion to the point of not being able to perform one's job effectively.

Bursitis Chronic or acute inflammation of the small synovial sacs known as bursa.

Burst Three or more sequential ectopic beats; also referred to as a *salvo* or *run*.

Cadaveric transplantation Transplantation of organs from an already deceased person to a living person.

Calibration Regulation of an ECG machine's stylus sensitivity so that a 1-mV electrical signal will produce a deflection measuring exactly 10 mm.

Call processing time The elapsed time from the moment a call is received by the communications center to the time the responding unit is alerted.

Cancer A group of diseases that allow unrestrained growth of cells in one or more of the body organs or tissues.

Capacitance vessels Venules that have the capability of holding large amounts of volume.

Capillaries Tiny vessels that connect arterioles to venules; deliver blood to each cell in the body.

Capillary leak Loss of intravascular fluid (plasma, water) from a loss of capillary integrity or an opening of gap junctions between the cells of the capillaries.

May be caused by thermal injury to capillaries or the intense inflammatory reaction to burn injury, infection, or physical trauma.

Caplet A tablet with an oblong shape and a film-coated covering.

Capnograph A device that provides a numerical reading of exhaled CO_2 concentrations and a waveform (tracing).

Capnography Continuous analysis and recording of CO_2 concentrations in respiratory gases.

Capnometer A device used to measure the concentration of CO_2 at the end of exhalation.

Capnometry A numeric reading of exhaled CO_2 concentrations without a continuous written record or waveform.

Capsid Layer of protein enveloping the genome of a virion; composed of structural units called the capsomeres.

Capsule A membranous shell surrounding certain microorganisms, such as the pneumococcus bacterium.

Capture Ability of a pacing stimulus to depolarize successfully the cardiac chamber being paced; with one-to-one capture, each pacing stimulus results in depolarization of the appropriate chamber.

Carbamate A pesticide that inhibits acetylcholinesterase.

Carbon dioxide narcosis Condition mostly seen in patients with chronic obstructive pulmonary disease, in whom carbon dioxide is excessively retained, causing mental status changes and decreased respirations.

Carboys Glass or plastic bottles commonly used to transport corrosive products.

Carbuncle A series of abscesses in the subcutaneous tissues that drain through hair follicles.

Cardiac arrest Absence of cardiac mechanical activity confirmed by the absence of a detectable pulse, unresponsiveness, and apnea or agonal, gasping respirations.

Cardiac cycle Period from the beginning of one heartbeat to the beginning of the next; normally consisting of PQRST waves, complexes, and intervals.

Cardiac output Amount of blood pumped into the aorta each minute by the heart.

Cardiac rupture An acute traumatic perforation of the ventricles or atria.

Cardiac sphincter Circular muscle that controls the movement of material into the stomach.

Cardiogenic shock A condition in which heart muscle function is severely impaired, leading to decreased cardiac output and inadequate tissue perfusion.

Cardiomyopathy A disease of the heart muscle.

Cardiovascular disorders A collection of diseases and conditions that involve the heart (cardio) and blood vessels (vascular).

Carina Area in the bronchial tree that separates into the right and left mainstem bronchi.

Carotid bruit The noise made when blood in the carotid arteries passes over plaque buildups.

Carpal tunnel syndrome A medical condition in which the median nerve is compressed at the wrist (within the carpal tunnel), resulting in pain and numbness of the hand.

Carpopedal spasm Spasm of the muscles of the hand when a blood pressure cuff is inflated. Can occur in the feet if the cuff is placed on the leg. A result of hyperventilation.

Cartilage Connective tissue composed of chondrocytes; exact makeup depends on the location and function in the body.

Cartilaginous joint Unites two bones with hyaline cartilage or fibrocartilage.

Case law Interpretations of constitutional, statutory, or administrative law made by the courts; also known as *common law* or *judge-made law.*

Catabolic Refers to the metabolic breakdown of proteins, lipids, and carbohydrates by the body to produce energy.

Catabolism Process of breaking down complex substances into more simple ones.

Catalepsy Abnormal state characterized by a trancelike level of consciousness and postural rigidity; occurs in hypnosis and in certain organic and psychological disorders such as schizophrenia, epilepsy, and hysteria.

Cataract A partial or complete opacity on or in the lens or lens capsule of the eye, especially one impairing vision or causing blindness.

Catatonia A state of psychologically induced immobility with muscular rigidity, at times interrupted by agitation.

Catatonic schizophrenia A form of schizophrenia characterized by alternating periods of extreme withdrawal and extreme excitement. During the withdrawal stage stupor, waxy flexibility, muscular rigidity, mutism, blocking, negativism, and catalepsy may be seen; during the period of excitement, purposeless and impulsive activity may range from mild agitation to violence. See *Catatonia.*

Cathartics Substances that decrease the time a poison spends in the gastrointestinal tract by increasing bowel motility.

Catheter shear/catheter fragment embolism Breaking off the tip of the intravenous catheter inside the vein, which then travels through the venous system; it can lodge in pulmonary circulation as a pulmonary embolism.

Cation A positively charged ion.

Cauda equina Peripheral nerve bundles descending through the spinal column distal to the conus medullaris. Cauda equina are not spinal nerves.

Cauda equina syndrome A group of symptoms associated with the compression of the peripheral nerves still within the spinal canal below the level of the first lumbar vertebra, characterized by lumbar back pain, motor and sensory deficits, and bowel or bladder incontinence.

Caudal A position toward the distal end of the body; usually inferior.

Causation In a negligence case, the negligence of the defendant must have caused or created the harm sustained by the plaintiff; also referred to as *proximate cause.*

Caustic A substance with a pH above 7.0; also known as a *base* or *alkali.*

Cecum First segment of the large intestine; the appendix is its accessory structure.

Cell body Portion of the neuron containing the organelles, where essential cellular functions are performed.

Cell-mediated immunity Form of acquired immunity; results from activation of T lymphocytes that were previously sensitized to a specific antigen.

Cellular swelling Swelling of cellular tissues, usually from injury.

Cellulitis An inflammation of the skin.

Cementum A layer of tough tissue that anchors the root of a tooth to the periodontal membrane/ligament.

Central cord syndrome Collection of symptoms seen after the death of the central portion of the spinal cord.

Central nervous system The brain and spinal cord.

Central neurogenic hyperventilation Similar to Kussmaul respirations; characterized as deep, rapid breathing; associated with increased intracranial pressure.

Central retinal artery occlusion A condition in which the blood supply to the retina is blocked because of a clot or embolus in the central retinal artery or one of its branches.

Central vein A major vein of the chest, neck, or abdomen.

Central venous catheter A catheter through a vein to end in the superior vena cava or right atrium of the heart for medication or fluid administration.

Centrioles Paired, rodlike structures that exist in a specialized area of the cytoplasm known as the centrosome.

Centrosome Specialized area of the cytoplasm; plays an important role in the process of cell division.

Cephalic A position toward the head; usually superior.

Cerebellum Area of the brain involved in fine and gross coordination; responsible for interpretation of actual movement and correction of any movements that interfere with coordination and the body's position.

Cerebral contusion A brain injury in which brain tissue is bruised in a local area but does not puncture the pia mater.

Cerebral palsy Neuromuscular condition in which the patient has difficulty controlling the voluntary muscles because of damage to a portion of the brain.

Cerebral perfusion pressure Pressure inside the cerebral arteries and an indicator of brain perfusion; calculated by subtracting intracranial pressure from mean arterial pressure (CPP = MAP − ICP).

Cerebrospinal fluid (CSF) Fluid that bathes, protects, and nourishes the central nervous system.

Cerebrovascular accident (CVA) Blockage or hemorrhage of the blood vessels in the brain, usually causing focal neurologic deficits; also known as a *stroke.*

Cerebrum Largest part of the brain, divided into right and left hemispheres.

Certification An external verification of the competencies that an individual has achieved and typically involves an examination process; in healthcare these processes are typically designed to verify that an individual has achieved minimal competency to ensure safe and effective patient care.

Certified Flight Paramedic (FP-C) A certification obtained by paramedics on successful completion of the Flight Paramedic Examination.

Certified Flight Registered Nurse (CFRN) A nurse who has completed education, training, and certification beyond a registered nurse with a focus on air medical transport of potentially critically ill or injured patients.

Cerumen Earwax.

Ceruminous glands Glands lining the external auditory canal; produce cerumen or earwax.

Cervical spondylosis Degeneration of two or more cervical vertebrae, usually resulting in a narrowing of the space between the vertebrae.

Cervical vertebrae First seven vertebrae in descending order from the base of the skull.

Cervix Inferior portion of the uterus.

Chalazion A small bump on the eyelid caused by a blocked oil gland.

Charles' law Law stating that oxygen cylinders can have variations in pressure readings in different ambient temperatures.

Chelating agent A substance that can bind metals; used as an antidote to many heavy metal poisonings.

Chemical Abstracts Services (CAS) number Unique identification number of chemicals, much like a person's Social Security number.

Chemical asphyxiants Chemicals that prevent the transportation of oxygen to the cells or the use of oxygen at the cellular level.

Chemical name A precise description of a drug's chemical composition and molecular structure.

Chemical restraints Agents such as sedatives that can suppress a patient's neurologic and/or motor capabilities and reduce the threat to the paramedic; also known as *pharmacologic restraints.*

Cheyne-Stokes respirations A pattern of gradually increasing rate and depth of breathing that tapers to slower and shallower breathing with a period of apnea before the cycle repeats itself; often described as a crescendo-decrescendo pattern or periodic breathing.

Chief complaint The reason the patient has sought medical attention.

Child maltreatment An all-encompassing term for all types of child abuse and neglect, including physical abuse, emotional abuse, sexual abuse, and neglect.

Chloracetophenone Tear gas; commercially known as *Mace.*

Choanal atresia Narrowing or blockage of one or both nares by membranous or bony tissue.

Choking agent An industrial chemical used as a weapon to kill those who inhale the vapors or gases; the method of injury is asphyxiation resulting from lung damage from hydrochloric acid burns (e.g., chlorine, phosgene); also known as a pulmonary agent.

Cholangitis Inflammation of the bile duct.

Cholecystitis Inflammation of the gallbladder.

Choledocholithiasis The presence of gallstones in the common bile duct.

Cholelithiasis The presence of stones in the gallbladder.

Cholinergic Having the characteristics of the parasympathetic division of the autonomic nervous system.

Cholinesterase inhibitor A chemical that blocks the action of acetylcholinesterase; thus the neurotransmitter acetylcholine is allowed to send its signals continuously to innervate nerve endings.

Chordae tendineae Fibrous bands of tissue in the valves that attach to each part or cusp of the valve.

Chorioamnionitis Infection of the amniotic sac and its contents.

Choroid Vascular layer of the eyeball.

Choroid plexus Group of specialized cells in the ventricles of the brain; filters blood through cerebral capillaries to create the cerebrospinal fluid.

Chromatin Material within a cell nucleus from which the chromosomes are formed.

Chromosomes Any of the threadlike structures in the nucleus of a cell that function in the transmission of genetic information; each consists of a double strand of DNA attached to proteins called histones.

Chronic Long, drawn out; applied to a disease that is not acute.

Chronic exposure An exposure to low concentrations over a long period.

Chronic obstructive pulmonary disease (COPD) A progressive and irreversible condition characterized by diminished inspiratory and expiratory capacity of the lungs.

Chronic renal failure The gradual, long-term deterioration of kidney function.

Chronology The arrangement of events in time.

Chronotropism A change in heart rate.

Chute time The time required to get a unit en route to a call from dispatch.

Chyme Semifluid mass of partly digested food expelled by the stomach into the duodenum.

Ciliary body Consists of muscles that change the shape of the lens in the eye; includes a network of capillaries that produce aqueous humor.

Circadian A daily rhythmic activity cycle based on 24-hour intervals or events that occur at approximately 24-hour intervals, such as certain physiologic occurrences.

Circadian rhythm The 24-hour cycle that relates to work and rest time.

Circumflex artery Division of the left coronary artery.

Circumoral paresthesia A feeling of tingling around the lips and mouth caused by hyperventilation.

Circumstantial thinking Adding detours and extra details to conversations but eventually returning to the main topic.

Cirrhosis A chronic degenerative disease of the liver.

Civil law A branch of law that deals with torts (civil wrongs) committed by one individual, organization, or group against another.

Clarification Asking to speaker to help you understand.

Classic heat stroke Heat stroke caused by environmental exposure that results in core hyperthermia greater than 40°C. (104°F).

Clean To wash with soap and water.

Cleft lip Incomplete closure of the upper lip.

Cleft palate Incomplete closure of the hard and/or soft palate of the mouth.

Clinical performance indicator A definable, measurable, skilled task completed by the dispatcher that has a significant impact on the delivery of patient care.

Clitoris Small, erectile structure at the entrance to the vagina.

Closed-ended questions A form of interview question that limits a patient's response to simple, brief words or phrases (e.g., "yes or no," "sharp or dull").

Closed fracture Fracture of the bone tissue that has not broken the skin tissue.

Clostridium botulinum A bacterium that produces a powerful toxin that causes botulism disease in human beings, waterfowl, and cattle.

Cluster A personality disorders Odd and eccentric type of personality disorders, including paranoid, schizoid, and schizotypal; characterized by social isolation and odd thought processes.

Cluster B personality disorders Emotional and dramatic type of personality disorders, including histrionic, borderline, antisocial, and narcissistic; characterized by impulsive, unpredictable behavior, and manipulation of others.

Cluster C personality disorders Anxious and fearful type of personality disorders, including avoidant, dependent, and compulsive; marked by anxiety, shyness, and avoidance of conflict.

Cluster headache A migraine-like condition characterized by attacks of intense unilateral pain. The pain occurs most often over the eye and forehead and is accompanied by flushing and watering of the eyes and nose. The attacks occur in groups, with a duration of several hours.

CNS-PAD An acronym for *c*entral *n*ervous *s*ystem padding: *p*ia matter, *a*rachnid matter, *d*ura matter.

Coagulation Formation of blood clots with the associated increase in blood viscosity.

Coagulation cascade A set of interactions of the circulating clotting factors.

Coagulation necrosis Dead or dying tissue that forms a scar or eschar.

Cocaine hydrochloride Fine, white powdered form of cocaine, a powerful central nervous system stimulant; typically snorted intranasally.

Coccyx (coccygeal vertebrae) Terminal end of the spinal column; a tail-like bone composed of three to five vertebra. No nerve roots travel through the coccyx.

Cochlea Bony structure in the inner ear resembling a tiny snail shell.

Code of ethics A guide for interactions between members of a specific profession (such as physicians) and the public.

Codependence A psychological concept defined as exhibiting too much and often inappropriate caring behavior.

Cognition Operation of the mind by which one becomes aware of objects of thought or perception; includes all aspects of perceiving, thinking, and remembering.

cognitive disability An impairment that affects an individual's awareness and memory as well as his or her ability to learn, process information, communicate, and make decisions.

Cognitive phase In the phases of immune response, the stage at which a foreign antigen is recognized to be present.

Cold diuresis The occurrence of increased urine production on exposure to cold.

Cold protective response The mechanism associated with cold water in which individuals can survive extended periods of submersion.

Cold zone A safe area isolated from the area of contamination; also called the *support zone*. This zone has safe and easy access. It contains the command post and staging areas for personnel, vehicles, and equipment. EMS personnel are stationed in the cold zone.

Collagen A fibrous protein that provides elasticity and strength to skin and the body's connective tissue.

Collapsed lung See *Pneumothorax.*

Colostomy Incision in the colon for the purpose of making a temporary or permanent opening between the bowel and the abdominal wall.

Combination deployment Using a mix of geographic coverage and demand posts to best serve the community given the number of ambulances available at any one time.

Combining form A word root followed by a vowel.

Combining vowel A vowel that is added to a word root before a suffix.

Comfort care Medical care intended to provide relief from pain and discomfort, such as the control of pain with medications.

Command post The location from which incident operations are directed.

Comminuted skull fracture Breakage of a bone or bones of the skull into multiple fragments.

Communicable period The period after infection during which the diease may be transmitted to another host.

Communication The exchange of thoughts, messages, and information.

Compartment syndrome (CS) A condition in which compartment pressures increase in an injured extremity to the point that capillary circulation is stopped; often only correctable through surgical opening of the compartment.

Compensatory pause Pause for which the normal beat after a premature complex occurs when expected; also called a *complete pause.*

Complete abortion Passage of all fetal tissue before 20 weeks of gestation.

Complex Several waveforms.

Complex partial seizure A seizure affecting only one part of the brain that does alter consciousness.

Compliance The resistance of the patient's lung tissue to ventilation.

Compound presentation Presentation of an extremity beside the major presenting fetal part.

Compound skull fracture Open skull fracture.

Compound word Word that contains more than one root.

Computer-aided dispatch (CAD) A computer-aided system that automates dispatching by enhanced data collection, rapid recall of information, dispatch mapping, as well as unit tracking and the ability to track and dispatch resources.

Concealment To hide or put out of site; provides no ballistic protection.

Concept formation The initial formation of an overall concept of care for a particular patient begins when the paramedic arrives on location of the incident.

Conception The act or process of fertilization; beginning of pregnancy.

Concurrent medical direction Consultation with a physician or other advanced health care professional by telephone, radio, or other electronic means, permitting the physician and paramedic to decide together on the best course of action in the delivery of patient care.

Concussion A brain injury with a transient impairment of consciousness followed by a rapid recovery to baseline neurologic activity.

Conducting arteries Large arteries of the body (e.g., aorta and the pulmonary trunk); have more elastic tissue and less smooth muscle; stretch under great pressures and then quickly return back to their original shapes.

Conduction system A system of pathways in the heart composed of specialized electrical (pacemaker) cells.

Conductive hearing loss Type of deafness that occurs where there is a problem with the transfer of sound from the outer to the inner ear.

Conductivity Ability of a cardiac cell to receive an electrical stimulus and conduct that impulse to an adjacent cardiac cell.

Confidentiality Protection of patient information in any form and the disclosure of that information only as needed for patient care or as otherwise permitted by law.

Confined space By Occupational Safety and Health Administration (OSHA) definition, a space large enough and configured so that an employee can enter and perform assigned work but has limited or restricted means for entry or exit (e.g., tanks, vessels, silos, storage bins, hoppers, vaults, and pits are spaces that may have limited means of entry); not designed for continuous employee occupancy.

Confrontation Focusing on a particular point made during the interview.

Congenital Present at or before birth.

Conjunctiva Thin, transparent mucous membrane that covers the inner surface of the eyelids and the outer surface of the sclera.

Conjunctivitis Inflammation of the conjunctiva.

Connective tissue Most abundant type of tissue in the body; composed of cells that are separated by a matrix.

Conscious sedation A medication or combination of medications that allows a patient to undergo what could be an unpleasant experience by producing an altered level of consciousness but not complete anesthesia. The goal is for the patient to breathe spontaneously and maintain his or her own airway.

Consensus formula Formula used to calculate the volume of fluid needed to properly resuscitate a burn patient. The formula is 2 to 4 mL/kg/% total body surface area burned. This is the formula currently regarded by the American Burn Association as the standard of care in adult burn patients. Several other, similar formulas exist that also may be used.

Consent Permission.

Constricted affect Emotion shown in degrees less than expected.

Contamination The deposition or absorption of chemical, biologic, or radiologic materials onto personnel or other materials.

Contamination reduction zone See *Warm zone.*

Continuing education (CE) Lifelong learning.

Continuous positive airway pressure (CPAP) The delivery of slight positive pressure throughout the respiratory cycle to prevent airway collapse, reduce the work of breathing, and improve alveolar ventilation.

Continuous positive airway pressure (CPAP) device Breathing device that allows delivery of slight positive pressure to prevent airway collapse and improve oxygenation and ventilation in spontaneously breathing patients.

Continuous quality improvement (CQI) Programs designed to improve the level of care; commonly driven by quality assurance.

Contractility Ability to shorten in length actively.

Contraction Rhythmic tightening of the muscular uterine wall that occurs during normal labor and leads to expulsion of the fetus and placenta from the uterus.

Contraction interval The time from the beginning of one contraction to the beginning of the next contraction.

Contraction time The time from the beginning to the end of a single uterine contraction.

Contraindication Use of a drug for a condition when it is not advisable.

Contrecoup injury An injury at another site, usually opposite the point of impact.

Contributory negligence An injured plaintiff's failure to exercise due care that, along with the defendant's negligence, contributed to the injury.

Conus medullaris Terminal end of the spinal cord.

Conus medullaris syndrome Complications resulting from injury to the conus medullaris.

Conventional silo A vertical structure used to store ensiled plant material in a aerobic environment.

Cor pulmonale Right-sided heart failure caused by pulmonary disease.

Core body temperature The measured body temperature within the core of the body; generally measured with an esophageal probe; normal is 98.6° F.

Cornea Avascular, transparent structure that permits light through to the interior of the eye.

Coronary artery disease Disease of the arteries that supply the heart muscle with blood.

Coronary heart disease Disease of the coronary arteries and their resulting complications, such as angina pectoris or acute myocardial infarction.

Coronary sinus Venous drain for the coronary circulation into the right atrium.

Corrosive A substance able to corrode tissue or metal (e.g., acids and bases).

Corticosteroids See *Adrenocortical steroids*.

Cosmesis Of or referring to the improvement of physical appearance.

Costal angle The angle formed by the margins of the ribs at the sternum.

Costochondritis Inflammation of the cartilage in the anterior chest that causes chest pain.

Coughing A protective mechanism usually induced by mucosal irritation; the forceful, spastic expiration experienced during coughing aids in the clearance of the bronchi and bronchioles.

Coup contrecoup An injury most often associated with a blow to the skull in which the force of the impact is transmitted through the skull bones to the opposite side of the head, where the bruise, fracture, or other sign of injury appears.

Coup injury An injury directly below the point of impact.

Couplet Two consecutive premature complexes.

Cover A type of concealment that hides the body and offers ballistic protection.

Crack cocaine Solid, brownish-white crystal form of cocaine, a powerful central nervous system stimulant; typically smoked.

Crackles (rales) As the name implies, when fluid accumulates in the smaller airway passages, air passing through the fluid creates a moist crackling or popping sound heard on inspiration.

Cranial nerve Twelve pairs of nerves that exit the brain and innervate the head and face; some also are part of the visceral portion of the peripheral nervous system.

Cranium The vaultlike portion of the skull, behind and above the face.

Creatinine End product of creatine metabolism; released during anaerobic metabolism. Elevated levels of creatinine are common in advanced stages of renal failure.

Creatine kinase An enzyme in skeletal and cardiac muscles that is released into circulation as a result of tissue damage. Can be used as a laboratory indicator of muscle damage.

Credentialing A local process by which an individual is permitted by a specific entity (e.g., medical director) to practice in a specific setting (e.g., EMS agency).

Crepitation A crackling sound indicative of bone ends grinding together.

Crepitus The grating, crackling, or popping sounds and sensations experienced under skin and joints.

Cricoid cartilage Most inferior cartilage of the larynx; only complete ring in the larynx.

Cricothyroid membrane A fibrous membrane located between the cricoid and thyroid cartilages.

Cricothyrotomy An emergency procedure performed to allow rapid entrance to the airway (by the cricothyroid membrane) for temporary oxygenation and ventilation.

Crime scene A location where any part of a criminal act has occurred or where evidence relating to a crime may be found.

Criminal law A branch of law in which the federal, state, or local government prosecutes individuals on behalf of society for violating laws designed to safeguard society.

Cross tolerance Decreasing responsiveness to the effects of a drug in a drug classification (such as narcotics) and the likelihood of development of decreased responsiveness to another drug in that classification.

Crossmatch The process by which blood compatibility is determined by mixing blood samples from the donor and recipient.

Croup A viral infection of the upper airway that is notorious for causing a "seal bark" cough.

Crown The visible part of a tooth.

Crowning The appearance of the first part of the infant at the vaginal opening during delivery.

Crush points Formed when two objects are moving toward each other or when one object is moving toward a stationary object and the gap between the two is decreasing.

Crush syndrome Renal failure and shock after crush injuries.

Crust A collection of cellular debris or dried blood; often called a *scab*.

Cryogenic Pertaining to extremely low temperatures.

CSM A mnemonic for *c*irculation, *s*ensation, and *m*ovement.

Cullen's sign Yellow-blue ecchymosis surrounding the umbilicus.

Cultural beliefs Values and perspectives common to a racial, religious, or social group of people.

Cultural imposition The tendency to impose your beliefs, values, and patterns of behavior on an individual from another culture.

Cumulative action Increased intensity of drug action evident after administration of several doses.

Current Flow of electrical charge from one point to another.

Current health status Focus on the environmental and personal habits of the patient that may influence the patient's general state of health.

Cushing syndrome Disorder caused by the overproduction of corticosteroids; characterized by a "moon face," obesity, fat accumulation on the upper back, increased facial hair, acne, diabetes, and hypertension.

Cushing's triad Characteristic pattern of vital signs during rising intracranial pressure, presenting as rising hypertension, bradycardia, and abnormal respirations.

Customs A practice or set of practices followed by a group of people.

Cyanogen chloride A highly toxic blood agent.

Cyanosis A bluish coloration of the skin as a result of hypoxemia, or deoxygenation of hemoglobin.

Cyclohexyl methyl phosphonofluoridate G nerve agent. The G agents tend to be nonpersistent, volatile agents.

Cyclothymia A less-severe form of bipolar disorder marked by more frequently alternating periods of a dysphoric mood that does not meet the criteria for depression and hypomania.

Cylinders Nonbulk containers that normally contain liquefied gases, nonliquified gases, or mixtures under pressure; cylinders also may contain liquids or solids.

Cyst A walled cavity that contains fluid or purulent material.

Cystic fibrosis (CF) Genetic disease marked by hypersecretion of glands, including mucus glands in the lungs.

Cystic medial degeneration A connective tissue disease in which the elastic tissue and smooth muscle fibers of the middle arterial layer degenerate.

Cystitis Infection isolated in the bladder.

Cytokines Protein molecules produced by white blood cells that act as chemical messengers between cells.

Cytoplasm Fluid-like material in which the organelles are suspended; lies between the plasma membrane and the nucleus.

Cytoplasmic membrane Encloses the cytoplasm and its organelles; forms the outer border of the cell.

Cytosol Liquid medium of the cytoplasm.

Dalton's law (law of partial pressure) Law relating to the partial pressure of oxygen during transport; defines that it is more difficult for oxygen to transfer from air to blood at lower pressures.

Damages Compensable harm or other losses incurred by an injured party (plaintiff) because of the negligence of the defendant.

Data interpretation The step that uses all the data gathered in the concept formation stage with the paramedic's knowledge of anatomy, physiology, and pathophysiology to continue the decision-making process.

Daughter cells Two cells that result from mitosis.

Dead air space Not all the air inspired during a breath participates in gas exchange and can be further classified as anatomic or physiologic dead space. In the average adult male this equates to approximately 150 mL. Anatomic dead space includes airway passages such as the trachea and bronchi, which are incapable of participating in gas exchange. Alveoli that have the potential to participate in gas exchange but do not because of disease or obstruction, as in chronic obstructive pulmonary disease (COPD) or atelectasis, are referred to as physiologic dead space.

Deafness A complete or partial inability to hear.

Debridement Removal of foreign material or dead tissue from a wound (pronounced *da brēd'*).

Decannulation Removal of a tracheostomy tube.

Decompensated shock A clinical state of tissue perfusion that is inadequate to meet the body's metabolic demands; accompanied by hypotension; also called *progressive* or *late shock.*

Decompression sickness An illness occurring during or after a diving ascent that results when nitrogen in compressed air converts back from solution to gas, forming bubbles in tissues and blood.

Decontamination The process of removing dangerous substances from the patient; may involve removing substances from the skin (external decontamination) and/or removing substances from the gastrointestinal tract (internal decontamination).

Deep fascia Fibrous, nonelastic connective tissue that forms the boundaries of muscle compartments.

Deep partial-thickness burn A burn in which the mid- or deeper dermis is injured. Results in injury to the deeper hair follicle, glandular, nerve, and blood vessel structures.

Deep venous thrombosis (DVT) A blood clot that forms in the deep venous system of the pelvis or legs; may progress to a pulmonary embolism.

Defamation The publication of false information about a person that tends to blacken the person's character or injure his or her reputation.

Defendant The person or institution being sued; also called the *respondent.*

Defibrillation Therapeutic use of electric current to terminate lethal cardiac dysrhythmias.

Degenerative joint disease See *Osteoarthritis.*

Dehydration A state in which the body has an excessive water loss from the tissues.

Delayed reaction A delay between exposure and onset of action.

Delirium Short-term and temporary mental confusion and fluctuating level of consciousness, often caused by intoxication from various substances, hypoglycemia, or acute psychiatric episodes.

Delirium tremens (DT) The most severe form of ethanol withdrawal, including hallucinations, delusions, confusion, and seizures.

Delta wave Slurring of the beginning portion of the QRS complex caused by preexcitation.

Delusion False perception and interpretation of situations and events that a person believes to be true no matter how convincing evidence is to the contrary.

Delusions of reference A belief that ordinary events have a special, often dangerous, meaning to the self.

Demand pacemaker Synchronous pacemaker that discharges only when the patient's heart rate drops below the preset rate for the pacemaker.

Dementia Long-term decline in mental faculties such as memory, concentration, and judgment; often seen with degenerative neurologic disorders such as Alzheimer's disease.

Dendrite Branchlike projections from a neuron that receive impulses or sensory information.

Denial A common defense mechanism that presents with feelings of disbelief, such as "no, that can't be right" when a life-threatening or terminal diagnosis is received; one of the stages of the grief response.

Denominator The number or mathematic expression below the line in a fraction; the denominator is the sum of the parts.

Dentin A hard but porous tissue found under the enamel and cementum of a tooth.

Deoxyribonucleic acid (DNA) Specialized structure within the cell that carries genetic material for reproduction.

Depersonalization A sudden sense of the loss of one's identity.

Deployment Matching production capacity of an ambulance system to the changing patterns of call demand.

Depolarization Movement of ions across a cell membrane, causing the inside of the cell to become more positive; an electrical event expected to result in contraction.

Depressed skull fracture A fracture of the skull with inward displacement of bone fragments.

Depression Sorrow and lack of interest in the things that previously produced pleasure.

Derealization A sudden feeling that one's surroundings are not real, as if one is watching a movie or television, not reality.

Dermatomes Areas of the body innervated by specific sensory spinal nerves; also a device used to remove healthy skin from somewhere on the body of the burn patient for the purpose of transplanting (grafting) at another site, such as an excised burn wound or other open wound.

Dermis Located below the epidermis and consists mainly of connective tissue containing both collagen and elastin fibers; contains specialized nervous tissue that provides sensory information, pain, pressure, touch, and temperature, to the central nervous system; also contains hair follicles, sweat and sebaceous glands, and a large network of blood vessels.

Descending colon Part of the large intestine.

Desired action The intended beneficial effect of a drug.

Developmental disabilities Disabilities that involve some degree of impaired adaptation in learning, social adjustment, or maturation.

Diabetes insipidus (DI) Disorder caused by insufficient production of ADH in the posterior pituitary gland, causing a larger than normal increase in the secretion of free water in the urine and poor absorption of water into the bloodstream.

Diabetic ketoacidosis (DKA) Condition found in diabetic patients caused by the lack or absence of insulin, leading to an increase of ketone bodies and acidosis in the blood.

Dialysis The process of diffusing blood across a semipermeable membrane to remove substances that the kidney would normally eliminate.

Dialysis shunt Shunt composed of two plastic tubes (one inserted into an artery, the other into a vein) that stick out of the skin to allow easy access and attachment to a dialysis machine for filtering waste products from the blood.

Diapedesis Migration of phagocytes through the endothelial wall of the vasculature into surrounding tissues.

Diaphragm Muscle that separates the thoracic cavity from the abdominal cavity.

Diaphragmatic hernia Protrusion of the abdominal contents into the chest cavity through a opening in the diaphragm.

Diaphysis Shaft of the bone where marrow is found that forms red and white blood cells.

Diastole Phase of the cardiac cycle in which the atria and ventricles relax between contractions and blood enters these chambers; when the term is used without reference to a specific chamber of the heart, the term implies ventricular diastole.

Diastolic blood pressure The pressure exerted against the walls of the large arteries during ventricular relaxation.

Diencephalon Portion of the brain between the brainstem and cerebrum; contains the thalamus and hypothalamus and the temperature regulatory centers for the body.

Differential diagnosis The list of problems that could produce the patient's chief complaint.

Differentiation Process of cell maturation; the cell becomes specialized for a specific purpose, such as a cardiac cell versus a bone cell.

Diffuse axonal injury (DAI) A type of brain injury caused by shearing forces that occur between different parts of the brain as a result of rotational acceleration.

Diffusion Spreading out of molecules from an area of higher concentration to an area of lower concentration.

Digestion Chemical breakdown of food material into smaller fragments that can be absorbed into the circulatory system.

Digestive tract Series of muscular tubes designed to move food and liquid.

Digoxin A medication derived from digitalis that acts by increasing the force of myocardial contraction and the refractory period and decreasing the conduction rate of the atrioventricular node; used to treat heart failure, most supraventricular tachycardias, and cardiogenic shock.

Dilation Spontaneous opening of the cervix that occurs as part of labor.

Diplomacy Tact and skill in dealing with people.

Direct (closed-ended) questions Questions that can be answered with short responses such as "yes" or "no."

Direct communication Method of intercellular communication in which one cell communicates with the cell adjacent to it by using minerals and ions.

Dirty bomb A conventional explosive device used as a radiologic agent dispersal device.

Disaster An incident involving 100 or more persons.

Disaster Medical Assistance Team (DMAT) Field-deployable hospital teams that include physicians, nurses, emergency medical technicians, and other medical and nonmedical support personnel.

Disaster Mortuary Operations Teams Teams composed of forensic and mortuary professionals trained to deal with human remains after disaster situations.

Discrimination Treatment or consideration based on class or category rather than individual merit.

Disease period The interval between the first appearance of symptoms and resolution.

Disinfect To clean with an agent that should kill many of, or most, surface organisms.

Disinfection Process of cleaning the ambulance, the cot, and equipment; disinfectant substances are toxic to body tissues.

Disorganized schizophrenia A subtype of schizophrenia characterized by an earlier age of onset, usually at puberty, and a more severe disintegration of personality than occurs in other forms of the disease; symptoms include incoherence, loose associations, gross disorganization or behavior, and flat or inappropriate affect.

Dispatch A central location that receives information and collects, disseminates, and transmits the information to the proper resources.

Dispatch factors Training and education of communications personnel, rapid call taking, call prioritization (selecting the most appropriate resources to respond), managing out-of-chute times (getting crews on the road quickly), and providing crews with route selection assistance.

Dispatch life support The provision of clinically approved, scripted instructions by telephone by a trained and certified emergency medical dispatcher.

Disseminated intravascular coagulation (DIC) A complex, systemic, thrombohemorrhagic disorder involving the generation of intravascular fibrin and the consumption of procoagulants and platelets.

Dissociatives Substances that cause feelings of detachment (dissociation) from one's surroundings and self; includes PCP, ketamine, and dextromethorphan.

Distal A position farthest away from a limb to the trunk.

Distracting injury An injury that occupies the patient's attention and focus. The injury causes significant enough pain that the patient may not feel pain from other injuries, particular spine injuries.

Distraction A self-defense measure that creates diversion in a person's attention.

Distress Stress that is perceived as negative; it may be seen as physical or mental pain or suffering.

Distributing arteries Blood vessels that have well-defined adventitia layers and larger amounts of smooth muscle; capable of altering blood flow.

Distribution The movement of drugs from the bloodstream to target organs.

Distributive shock Inadequate tissue perfusion as a result of fluid shifts between body compartments. Burn shock is a distributive shock in which plasma and water are lost from the vascular tree into the surrounding tissues. This shock also is seen in the setting of sepsis, in which a similar fluid redistribution occurs.

Diuretic An agent that promotes the excretion of urine.

Diversity Differences of any kind such as race, class, religion, gender, sexual preference, personal habitat, and physical ability.

Diverticulitis Inflammation of a diverticulum, especially of the small pockets in the wall of the colon that fill with stagnant fecal material and become inflamed.

Diverticulosis A condition of the colon in which outpouches develop.

Documentation Written information to support actions that lead to conclusive information; written evidence.

Donor skin site A site on the body from which healthy skin is removed for the purpose of grafting a burn or other open wound.

Do not resuscitate (DNR) orders Orders limiting cardiopulmonary resuscitation or advanced life support treatment in the case of a cardiac arrest. These orders may be individualized in that they may allow for differing levels of interventions. When individualized, they usually grant or deny permission for chest compressions, intubation or ventilation, and life-saving medications.

Dorsal Referring to the back of the body; posterior.

Dosage The amount of medication that can be safely given for the average person for a specified condition. Also the administration of a therapeutic agent in prescribed amounts.

Dose The exact amount of medication to be given or taken at one time.

Down syndrome A genetic syndrome characterized by varying degrees of mental retardation and multiple physical defects.

Downregulation The process by which a cell decreases the number of receptors exposed to a given substance to reduce its sensitivity to that substance.

Dromotropism The speed of conduction through the atrioventricular junction.

Drop (or drip) factor The number of drops per milliliter that an intravenous administration set delivers.

Drowning The process of experiencing respiratory impairment from immersion or submersion in a liquid.

Drug Any substance (other than a food or device) intended for use in the diagnosis, cure, relief, treatment, or prevention of disease or intended to affect the structure or function of the body of human beings or animals.

Drug allergy The reaction to a medication with an adverse outcome.

Drug antagonism The interaction between two drugs in which one partially or completely inhibits the effects of the other.

Drug dependence A physical need or adaptation to the drug without the psychological need to take the drug.

Drug interaction The manner in which one drug and a second drug (or food) act on each other.

Drug overdose Internalization of more than the safe amount of a medication or drug; often associated with illegal drugs when a user administers too great an amount of substance; may be used to commit suicide.

Drug-food interaction Changes in a drug's effects caused by food or beverages ingested during the same period.

Dual-chamber pacemaker Pacemaker that stimulates the atrium and ventricle.

Dual-stage airbags An airbag with two inflation charges inside; only one of the two charges may deploy during the initial crash, causing the bag to inflate; the second charge of the dual-stage airbag may remain.

Ductus arteriosus Blood vessel that connects the pulmonary trunk to the aorta in a fetus.

Ductus deferens Also known as *vas deferens;* tubes that extend from the end of the epididymis and through the seminal vesicles.

Ductus venosus Fetal blood vessel that conects the umbilical vein and the inferior vena cava.

Due process The constitutional guarantee that laws and legal proceedings must be fair regarding an individual's legal rights.

Due regard Principle used when driving an emergency vehicle of ensuring that all other vehicles and citizens in the area see and grant the emergency vehicle the right of way.

Duodenum First part of the small intestine; has important accessory structures that help digest various types of nutrients.

Duplex A radio system that allows transmitting and receiving at the same time through two different frequencies.

Dura mater Toughest layer of the meninges; top layer.

Durable power of attorney for health care A type of advanced directive that allows an individual to appoint someone to make health care decisions for him or her if the person's ability to make these decisions or communicate wishes is lost.

Duty to act A legal obligation (created by statute, contract, or voluntarily) to provide services.

Dysarthria An articulation disorder in which the patient is not able to produce speech sounds.

Dyspareunia Pain during sexual intercourse.

Dyspepsia Epigastric discomfort often occurring after meals.

Dysphagia Difficulty swallowing.

Dysphoric mood (dysphoria) An unpleasant emotional state characterized by sadness, irritability, or depression.

Dysplasia Abnormal cell growth; cells take on an abnormal size, shape, and organization as a result of ongoing irritation or inflammation.

Dyspnea An uncomfortable awareness of one's breathing that may be associated with a change in the breathing rate, effort, or pattern.

Dysrhythmia An abnormal heart rhythm.

Dysthymia A constant, chronic, low-grade form of depression.

Dystonia Impairment of muscle tone, particularly involuntary muscle contractions of the face, neck, and tongue; often caused by a reaction to certain antipsychotic medications.

Ebola A viral hemorrhagic fever illness caused by the Ebola virus (Filovirus family); seen mostly in Africa; transmitted by person-to-person contact with body fluids of infected individuals; no specific treatment is available, and it often is fatal within several days.

Ecchymosis Collection of blood within the skin that appears blue-black, eventually fading to a greenish-brown and yellow. Commonly called a *bruise.*

Eclampsia A life-threatening condition of pregnancy and the postpartum period characterized by hypertension, edema, and seizures.

Economic abuse Preventing others from having or keeping a job; forcing control of another's paycheck; restricting access or forcing conditions on others to receive an allowance; stealing money; not allowing others to know about or have access to economic assets.

Ecstasy (MDMA) A synthetic, hallucinogenic stimulant drug similar to both methamphetamine and mescaline.

Ectopic Impulse(s) originating from a source other than the sinoatrial node.

Ectopic pregnancy A pregnancy that implants outside the uterus, usually in the fallopian tube.

Eczema A disorder of the skin characterized by inflammation, itching, blisters, and scales.

Edema A collection of water in the interstitial space.

Effector The muscle, gland, or organ on which the autonomic nervous system exerts an effect; target organ.

Effector phase In phases of immunity, the stage at which the infection is eradicated.

Efferent division Nerve fibers that send impulses from the central nervous system to the periphery.

Efficacy The ability of a drug to produce a physiologic response after attaching to a receptor.

Efflux Flowing out of.

Ejection fraction Fraction (expressed as a percentage) of blood ejected from the ventricle of the heart with each contraction. Generally at least 60% of the blood entering the ventricle should be forced to the lungs or systemic circulation.

Elasticity Ability of muscle to rebound toward its original length after contraction.

Electrical alternans A beat-to-beat change in waveform amplitude on the ECG.

Electrodes Adhesive pads that contain a conductive gel and are applied at specific locations on the patient's chest wall and extremities and connected by cables to an ECG machine.

Electrolytes Elements or compounds that break into charged particles (ions) when melted or dissolved in water or another solvent.

Elevated mood (euphoria) Exaggerated sense of happiness and joy; a feeling of being on top of the world.

Elimination The process of removing a drug from the body.

Elixir A clear, oral solution that contains the drug, water, and some alcohol.

Emancipated minor A self-supporting minor. This status often depends on the minor receiving an actual court order of emancipation.

Embryo The developing egg from approximately 2 weeks after fertilization until approximately 8 weeks of pregnancy.

Emergency decontamination The process of decontaminating people exposed to and potentially contaminated with hazardous materials by rapidly removing most of the contamination to reduce exposure and save lives, with secondary regard for completeness of decontamination.

Emergency medical dispatching (EMD) The science and skills associated with the tasks of an emergency medical dispatcher.

Emergency medical responder (EMR) An EMS professional who provides initial basic life-support care to patients who access the EMS system; formerly called *first responder.*

Emergency Medical Treatment and Active Labor Act (EMTALA) A federal law that requires a hospital to provide a medical screening examination to anyone who comes to that hospital and to provide stabilizing treatment to anyone with an emergency medical condition without considering the patient's ability to pay.

Emergency operations center A gathering point for strategic policymakers during an emergency incident.

Emergency service function (ESF) A grouping of government and certain private sector capabilities into an organizational structure to provide the support, resources, program implementation, and services most likely to be needed to save lives, protect property and the environment, restore essential services and critical infrastructure, and help victims and communities return to normal, when feasible, after domestic incidents.

Emesis Vomiting.

Emotional/mental impairment Impaired intellectual functioning (such as mental retardation), which results in an inability to cope with normal responsibilities of life.

Empathy Identification with and understanding of another's situation, feelings, and motives.

Emphysema Lung disease in which destruction of the alveoli creates dyspnea; often associated with tobacco abuse.

Empyema A collection of pus in the pleural cavity.

EMS Emergency medical services.

EMS system A network of resources that provides emergency care and transportation to victims of sudden illness or injury.

Emulsification The breakdown of fats on the skin surface by alkaloids, creating a soapy substance; penetrates deeply.

Emulsion A water and oil mixture containing medication.

Enabling behavior Behavior that allows another individual to continue to stay ill.

Enamel Hard, white outer surface of a tooth.

Encephalitis Inflammation and usually infection of brain tissue.

Encephalopathy A condition of disturbances of consciousness and possible progression to coma.

Endocardium Innermost layer of the heart that lines the inside of the myocardium and covers the heart valves.

Endocrine communication Method of intercellular communication in which one cell communicates with target cells throughout the body by using hormones.

Endocrine gland Where hormones are manufactured.

Endogenous Produced within the organism.

Endolymph Fluid that fills the labyrinth.

Endometriosis Growth of endometrial tissue outside the uterus, often causing pain.

Endometritis Infection of the endometrium.

Endometrium Innermost tissue lining of the uterus that is shed during menstruation.

Endoplasmic reticulum (ER) Chain of canals or sacs that wind through the cytoplasm.

Endorphins Neurotransmitters that function in the transmission of signals within the nervous system.

Endothelial cells A thin layer of flat epithelial cells that lines serous cavities, lymph vessels, and blood vessels.

Endotoxin A substance contained in the cell wall of gram-negative bacteria, generally released during the destruction of the bacteria by either the host organism's defense mechanisms or by treatment with medications.

Endotracheal (ET) Within or through the trachea.

Endotracheal intubation An advanced airway procedure in which a tube is placed directly into the trachea.

End-stage renal disease (ESRD) When the kidneys function at 10% to 15% of normal and dialysis or transplantation is the only option for the patient's survival.

Enlargement Implies the presence of dilation or hypertrophy or both.

Enteral A drug given for its systemic effects that passes through the digestive tract.

Enteric-coated tablets Tablets that have a special coating so they break down in the intestines instead of the stomach.

Enteral drug One that is given and passed through any portion of the digestive tract.

Entrapment A state of being pinned or entrapped.

Envenomation The process of injecting venom into a wound; venomous animals include snakes, insects, and marine creatures.

Environmental emergency A medical condition caused or exacerbated by weather, terrain, atmospheric pressure, or other local environmental factors.

Environmental hazards Hazards related to the weather and time of day, including extremes of heat, cold, wetness, dryness, and darkness, that increase risks to crews and patients.

Enzyme A large molecule (protein) that performs a biochemical reaction in the cell.

Eosinophils Type of granulocyte (white blood cell, or leukocyte) involved in immune response to parasites as well as in allergic responses.

Epicardium Also known as the *visceral pericardium;* the external layer of the heart wall that covers the heart muscle.

Epidemiologist Medical professional who studies the causes, distribution, and control of disease in populations.

Epidemiology The study of the causes, patterns, prevalence, and control of disease in groups of people.

Epidermis The outermost layer of the skin; made of tightly packed epithelial cells.

Epididymis Convoluted series of tubes located in the posterior portion of the scrotum; final maturation of sperm occurs here.

Epidural hematoma A collection of blood between the skull and dura mater.

Epidural space Potential area above the dura mater; contains arterial vessels.

Epiglottitis An inflammation of the epiglottis.

Epilepsy Group of neurologic disorders characterized by recurrent seizures, often of unknown cause.

Epiphyseal plate Found in children who are still generating bone growth; also known as the *growth plate.*

Epiphysis Either end of the bone where bone growth occurs during the developmental years.

Epistaxis Bloody nose.

Epithelial tissue Covers most of the internal and external surfaces of the body.

Epithelialization Migration of basal cells across a wound and the growth of skin over a wound.

Eponym A word that derives its name from the specific person (or place or thing) for whom (or which) it is named.

Erosion A partial focal loss of epidermis. This lesion is depressed, moist, and does not bleed; usually heals without scarring.

Erythema multiforme An internal (immunologic) reaction in the skin characterized by a variety of lesions.

Erythrocytes Red blood cells.

Erythropoiesis The development and differentiation of red blood cells; typically occurs in the bone marrow.

Erythropoietin A hormone that stimulates peripheral stem cells in the bone marrow to produce red blood cells.

Escape Term used when the sinus node slows or fails to initiate depolarization and a lower pacemaker site spontaneously produces electrical impulses, assuming responsibility for pacing the heart.

Eschar A thick wound covering that consists of necrotic or otherwise devitalized tissue or cellular components. In a burn wound, this is the burned tissue or skin of the wound.

Esophageal atresia (EA) A condition in which the section of the esophagus from the mouth and the section of the esophagus from the stomach end as a blind pouch without connecting to each other.

Esophagitis Inflammation of the esophagus.

Esophagoduodenoscopy Medical procedure in which an endoscope is used to look at the esophagus, stomach, and duodenum.

Esophagus Tube surrounded by smooth muscle that propels material into the stomach.

Essential hypertension High blood pressure for which no cause is identifiable; also called *primary hypertension.*

Estimated date of confinement The due date of the fetus.

Estrogen A female hormone produced mainly by the ovaries from puberty to menopause that is responsible for the development of secondary sexual characteristics and cyclic changes in the thickness of the uterine lining during the first half of the menstrual cycle.

Ethanol (ETOH) Colorless, odorless alcohol found in alcoholic beverages such as beer, wine, and liquor.

Ethics Expectations established by the community at large reflecting their views of the conduct of a profession.

Ethnocentrism Viewing your life as the most desirable, acceptable, or best and to act in a superior manner to another culture's way of life.

Eukaryotes One of the two major classes of cells found in higher life forms (more complex in structure).

Eustachian tube A small tube connecting the middle ear to the posterior nasopharynx; allows the ear to adjust to atmospheric pressure.

Eustress Stress that occurs from events, people, or influences that are perceived as good or positive. Eustress can increase productivity and performance.

Euthymic mood A normal, baseline emotional state.

Evaluation of treatment A reassessment of the patient overall and specifically the body system(s) affected by that treatment to answer two critical questions: Did the treatment work as intended? What is the clinical condition of the patient after the treatment?

Evasive tactic A self-defense measure in which the moves and actions of an aggressor are anticipated and unconventional pathways are used during retreat for personal safety.

Excision In reference to burn surgery, this is the sharp, surgical removal of burned tissue that will never regain function. Excision is carried out before skin grafting.

Excitability Ability to respond to a stimulus.

Excited delirium Acute and sudden agitation, paranoia, aggression, hyperthermia, dramatically increased strength, and decreased sensitivity to pain related to long-term use of stimulant drugs; often ends in sudden death.

Excoriation A linear erosion created by scratching. It is a hollowed out area that is sometimes crusted.

Excretion Removal of waste products from the body.

Exertional heat stroke A condition primarily affecting younger, active persons characterized by rapid onset (developing in hours) and frequently associated with high core temperatures.

Exhaled CO_2 detector A capnometer that provides a noninvasive estimate of alveolar ventilation, the concentration of exhaled CO_2 from the lungs, and arterial carbon dioxide content; also called an *end-tidal CO$_2$ detector.*

Exhaustion The last stage of the stress response and the body's inability to respond appropriately to subsequent stressors.

Exhaustion stage Occurs when the body's resistance to a stressor (decreased reaction to the stress, tolerance) and the ability to adapt fail; the ability to respond appropriately to other stressors may then fail; the immune system can be affected, and the individual may be at risk physically or emotionally.

Exogenous Produced outside the organism.

Exotoxin Proteins released during the growth phase of the bacteria that may cause systemic effects.

Expiratory reserve volume Amount of gas that can be forcefully expired at the end of a normal expiration.

Explanation Sharing objective information related to a message.

Explosive Any chemical compound, mixture, or device, the primary or common purpose of which is to function by detonation or rapid combustion (i.e., with substantial instantaneous release of gas and heat); found in liquid or solid forms (e.g., dynamite, TNT, black powder, fireworks, ammunition).

Exposure When blood or body fluids come in contact with eyes, mucous membranes, nonintact skin, or through a needlestick; it also can occur through inhalation and ingestion.

Expressed consent Permission given by a patient or his or her responsible decision maker either verbally or through some physical expression of consent.

Exsanguinate Near complete loss of blood; not conducive with life.

Exsanguination Bleeding to death.

Extensibility Ability to continue to contract over a range of lengths.

Extension posturing (decerebrate) Occurs as a result of an injury to the brainstem; presents as the patient's arms at the side with wrists turned outward.

External anal sphincter Muscle under voluntary control that allows a controlled bowel movement.

External auditory canal Tube from the external ear to the middle ear; lined with hair and ceruminous glands.

External bleeding Observable blood loss.

External ear Includes the auricle and external auditory canal.

External respiration The exchange of gases between the alveoli of the lungs and the blood cells traveling through the pulmonary capillaries.

External urinary sphincter Ring of smooth muscle in the urethra under voluntary control.

Extracellular Outside the cell or cytoplasmic membrane.

Extracellular fluid (ECF) The fluid found outside of the cells.

Extubation Removal of an endotracheal tube from the trachea.

Exudate Drainage from a vesicle or pustule.

Eyebrows Protect the eyes by providing shade and preventing foreign material (sweat, dust, etc.) from entering the eyes from above.

Eyelids Protect the eyes from foreign objects.

Facilitated diffusion Movement of substances across a membrane by binding to a helper protein integrated into the cell wall and highly selective about the chemicals allowed to cross the membrane.

Facilitated transport The transport of substances through a protein channel carrier with no energy input.

Facilitation Encouraging the patient to provide more information.

Factitious disorder Condition in which patients intentionally produce signs and symptoms of illness to assume the sick role.

Fainting (syncope) A brief loss of consciousness caused by a temporary decrease in blood flow to the brain.

Fallopian tube Paired structures extending from each side of the uterus to each ovary; they provide a way for the egg to reach the uterus.

False imprisonment Confinement or restraint of a person against his or her will or without appropriate legal justification.

False motion Abnormal movement of a bone or joint typically associated with a fracture or dislocation.

Fascia Anatomically, the tough connective tissue covering of the muscles of the body. Fascia contains the muscles within a compartment.

Fascicle Small bundle of nerve fibers.

Fasciotomy A surgical incision into the muscle fascia to relieve intracompartmental pressures; the emergency treatment for compartment syndrome.

Fear Physical and emotional reaction to a real or perceived threat.

Febrile seizure Seizure caused by too rapid of a rise in body temperature; rarely seen after age 2 years.

Fecalith A hard impacted mass of feces in the colon.

Feces Undigested food material that has been processed in the colon.

Federal Communication Commission (FCC) An independent U.S. government agency, directly responsible to Congress, established by the Communications Act of 1934; it regulates interstate and international communications by radio, television, wire, satellite, and cable. The FCC's jurisdiction covers the 50 states, the District of Columbia, and U.S. possessions.

Fetus The term used for an infant from approximately 8 weeks of pregnancy until birth.

Fibrin A threadlike protein formed during the clotting process that crisscrosses the wound opening and forms a matrix that traps blood cells and platelets, thereby creating a clot. Fibrin is formed by the action of thrombin and fibrinogen.

Fibrinolysis The breakdown of fibrin, the main component of blood clots.

Fibrinolytic agent Clot-busting drug; used in very early treatment of acute myocardial infarction, stroke, deep vein thrombosis, pulmonary embolism, and peripheral arterial occlusion.

Fibroblasts A cell that gives rise to connective tissue.

Fibrous connective tissue Composed of bundles of strong, white collagenous fibers (protein) in parallel rows; tendons and ligaments are composed of this type of tissue; relatively strong and inelastic.

Fibrous joints Two bones united by fibrous tissue that have little or no movement.

Fibrous tunic Layer of the eye that contains the sclera and the cornea.

Fick principle Describes the components needed for the oxygenation of the body's cells.

Finance officer The person responsible for providing a cost analysis of an incident.

Fine ventricular fibrillation Ventricular fibrillation with fibrillatory waves less than 3 mm in height.

FiO$_2$ Fraction of inspired oxygen.

"First on the Scene" program An educational program that teaches people what to do and what not to do when they come upon an injury emergency.

First-degree burn Superficial burn involving only the epidermis, such as a minor sunburn.

First-pass effect The breakdown of a drug in the liver and walls of the intestines before it reaches the systemic circulation.

First responder unit The closest trained persons and vehicle assigned to respond to a call; often the closest available fire department vehicle.

Fissure A vertical loss of epidermis and dermis with sharply defined walls (sometimes called a *crack*).

Fistula An abnormal tunnel that has formed from within the body to the skin.

Fixed positioning Establishing a single location in a central point to station an emergency vehicle, such as a fire station.

Fixed-rate pacemaker Asynchronous pacemaker that continuously discharges at a preset rate regardless of the patient's heart rate.

Fixed-station deployment Deployment method of using only geographically based stations.

Fixed-wing aircraft Airplanes used for longer distance medical flights; they can travel higher and faster than rotor-wing aircraft.

Flail segment A free-floating section of the chest wall that results when two or more adjacent ribs are fractured in two or more places or when the sternum is detached.

Flammable The capacity of a substance to ignite.

Flammable gases Any compressed gas that meets requirements for lower flammability limit, flammability limit range, flame projection, or flame propagation as specified in CFR Title 49, Sec. 173.300(b) (e.g., acetylene, butane, hydrogen, propane).

Flammable range The concentration of fuel and air between the lower flammable limit or lower explosive limit and the upper flammable limit or upper explosive limit; the mixture of fuel and air in the flammable range supports combustion.

Flammable solid A solid material other than an explosive that is liable to cause fires through friction or retained heat from manufacturing or processing or that can be ignited readily; when ignited, it burns so vigorously and persistently that it creates a serious transportation hazard (e.g., phosphorus, lithium, magnesium, titanium, calcium resinate).

Flash electrical burn A burn resulting from indirect contact with an electrical explosion.

Flashpoint The minimal temperature at which a substance evaporates fast enough to form an ignitable mixture with air near the surface of the substance.

Flat affect A complete or near-complete lack of emotion.

Flat bones Specialized bones that protect vital anatomic structures (e.g., ribs and bones of the skull).

Flexible deployment See *System status management.*

Flexion posturing (decorticate) Occurs from an injury to the cerebrum; presents as a bending of the arms at the elbow, the patient's arms pulled upwards to the chest, and the hands turned downward at the wrists.

Flight of ideas Moving quickly from topic to topic during conversation but without any connection or transition.

Flow rate The number of drops per minute an intravenous administration set will deliver.

Fluctuance A wavelike motion felt between two fingertips when palpating a fluid-filled structure such as a subcutaneous abscess.

Fluctuant nodule A movable and compressible mass; typically a pocket of pus or fluid within the dermis.

Focal atrial tachycardia Atrial tachycardia that begins in a small area (focus) within the heart.

Focal deficit Alteration or lack of strength or sensation in the body caused by a neurologic problem.

Focal injury An injury limited to a particular area of the brain.

Follicle Small, tubelike structure in which hair grows; contains a small cluster of cells known as the hair papilla.

Follicles Vesicles within the cortex of the ovary.

Folliculitis Inflammation of the follicle; localized to hair follicles and is more common in immunocompromised patients; usually are multiple and measure 5 mm or less in diameter; erythematous, pruritic, and frequently have a central pustule on top of a raised lesion, often with a central hair.

Fontanelles Membranous spaces at the juncture of an infant's cranial bones that later ossify.

Foramen Open passage.

Foramen magnum Opening in the floor of the cranium where the spinal cord exits the skull.

Foramen ovale The opening in the interatrial septum in a fetal heart.

Foreign body Any object or substance found in a organ or tissue where it does not belong under normal circumstances.

Form of thought Ability to compose thoughts in a logical manner.

Formed elements Located in the bloodstream; erythrocytes, leukocytes, and thrombocytes, or platelets.

Formulary A book that contains a list of medicinal substances with their formulas, uses, and methods of preparation.

Fractile response time Method used to determine the time at which 90% all requests for service receive a response; considered a more definitive measure of performance than averages.

Francisella tularensis A hardy, slow-growing, highly infectious, aerobic organism; human infection may result in tularemia, also known as *rabbit fever* or *deer fly fever.*

Free nerve endings Most common type of dermal nerve ending; responsible for sensing pain, temperature, and pressure.

Free radical A molecule containing an extra electron, which allows it to form potentially harmful bonds with other molecules.

Frontal lobe Section of cerebrum important in voluntary motor function and the emotions of aggression, motivation, and mood.

Frontal plane Imaginary straight line that divides the body into anterior (ventral) and posterior (dorsal) sections.

Frostbite A condition in which the skin and underlying tissue freeze.

Frostnip Reversible freezing of superficial skin layer marked by numbness and whiteness of the skin.

Fully deployed Assigning ambulances to a street corner post.

Fulminant Sudden, intense occurrence.

Functional reserve capacity At the end of a normal expiration, the volume of air remaining in the lungs.

Fundus Superior aspect of the uterus.

Fungi Plantlike organisms that do not contain chlorophyll; the two classes of fungi are yeasts and molds.

Furuncles Inflammatory nodules that involve the hair follicle (e. g., boils).

Gag reflex A normal neural reflex elicited by touching the soft palate or posterior pharynx; the responses are symmetric elevation of the palate, retraction of the tongue, and contraction of the pharyngeal muscles.

Gagging A reflex caused by irritation of the posterior pharynx that can result in vomiting.

Gamma A type of electromagnetic radiation.

Gamma-hydroxybutyrate (GHB) A drug structurally related to the neurotransmitter gamma-aminobutyric acid, usually dissolved in liquid, that causes profound central nervous system depression.

Gamma rays A type of electromagnetic radiation that can travel great distances; can be stopped by heavy shielding, such as lead.

Gamow bag Portable hyperbaric chamber that can help with altitude sickness emergencies.

Ganglion The junction between the preganglionic and postganglionic nerves.

Gangrenous necrosis Tissue death over a large area.

Gases Substances inhaled and absorbed through the respiratory tract.

Gasoline and electric hybrid vehicle Vehicle designed to produce low emissions by combining a smaller than normal internal combustion gasoline engine with a special electric motor to power the vehicle.

Gasping Inhaling and exhaling with quick, difficult breaths.

Gastric The route used when a tube is placed into the digestive tract, such as a nasogastric, orogastric, or gastrostomy tube.

Gastric distention Swelling of the abdomen caused by an influx of air or fluid.

Gastric lavage A procedure commonly known as "stomach pumping" in which the stomach is flushed with water; typically used to treat overdose or poisoning.

Gastritis Inflammation of the stomach.

Gastroenteritis Inflammation of the stomach and the intestines.

Gastrostomy tube A tube placed in a person's stomach that allows continuous feeding for an extended time.

Gay-Lussac's law A gas law sometimes combined with Charles' law that deals with the relation between pressure and temperature; in an oxygen cylinder, as the ambient temperature decreases, so does the pressure reading.

Gel cap Soft gelatin shell filled with liquid medication.

Gene The biologic unit of inheritance, consisting of a particular nucleotide sequence within a DNA molecule that occupies a precise locus on a chromosome and codes for a specific polypeptide chain.

Generalized anxiety disorder Condition characterized by excessive worries about everyday life.

Generalized seizure Excessive electrical activity in both hemispheres of the brain at the same time.

Generic name The name proposed by the first manufacturer when a drug is submitted to the FDA for approval; often an abbreviated form of the drug's chemical name, structure, or formula.

Geospatial demand analysis Understanding the different locations of demand within a community.

Germ theory Controversial theory developed in the 1600s in which microorganisms were first identified as the possible cause of some disease processes.

Germinativum Basal layer of the epidermis where the epidermal cells are formed.

Gestation or gestational age The number of completed weeks of pregnancy from the last menstrual period.

Glasgow Coma Scale (GCS) Neurologic assessment of a patient's best verbal response, eye opening, and motor function.

Glaucoma Increased intraocular pressure caused by a disruption in the normal production and drainage of aqueous humor; causes often are unknown.

Global positioning system (GPS) A satellite-based geographic locating system often placed on an ambulance to track its exact location.

Glomerulus Network of capillaries in the renal corpuscle.

Glottis The true vocal cords and the space between them.

Gluconeogenesis Creation of new glucose in the body by using noncarbohydrate sources such as fats and proteins.

Glycogenolysis Breakdown of glycogen to glucose in the liver.

Glycolysis Process by which glucose and other sugars are broken down to yield lactic acid (anaerobic glycolysis) or pyruvic acid (aerobic glycolysis). The breakdown releases energy in the form of adenosine triphosphate.

Glycoside A compound that yields a sugar and one or more other products when its parts are separated.

Golgi apparatus Substance that concentrates and packages material for secretion out of the cell.

Gomphoses Joint in which a peg fits into a socket.

Gout A metabolic disease in which uric acid crystals are deposited onto the cartilaginous surfaces of a joint, resulting in pain, swelling, and inflammation.

Graft Connection by a surgeon of a piece of the patient's saphenous vein to an artery and vein; in lieu of using the patient's own blood vessel, a cow's artery or a synthetic graft may be used.

Graham's law Law stating that gases move from a higher pressure or concentration to an area of lower pressure or concentration; takes into consideration the effect of simple diffusion at a cellular level.

Gram-negative bacteria Bacteria that do not retain the crystal violet stain used in Gram's stain and that take the color of the red counterstain.

Gram-positive bacteria Bacteria that retain the crystal violet stain used in Gram's stain.

Grandiose delusions Dramatically inflated perceptions of one's own worth, power, or knowledge.

Granulocyte A form of leukocyte that attacks foreign material in the wound.

Gravida Number of pregnancies.

Gravidity The number of times a patient has been pregnant.

Great vessels Large vessels that carry blood to and from the heart; superior and inferior venae cavae, pulmonary veins, aorta, and pulmonary trunk.

greenstick fracture The incomplete fracturing of an immature bone.

Grey-Turner's sign Bruising along the flanks that may indicate pancreatitis or intraabdominal hemorrhage.

Ground effect The cushion of air created by downdraft when a helicopter is in a low hover. Ground effect benefits the helicopter flight because it increases lift capacity, meaning less power is required for the helicopter to hover. When the helicopter has ground effect, it is said to be in ground effect. If a helicopter does not have ground effect, it is said to be operating out of ground effect.

Ground electrode Third ECG electrode (the first and second are the positive and negative electrodes), which minimizes electrical activity from other sources.

Grunting A short, low-pitched sound heard at the end of exhalation that represents an attempt to generate positive end-expiratory pressure by exhaling against a closed glottis, prolonging the period of oxygen and carbon dioxide exchange across the alveolar-capillary membrane; a compensatory mechanism to help maintain patency of small airways and prevent atelectasis.

Guarding The contraction of abdominal muscles in the anticipation of a painful stimulus.

Guidelines For emergency medical dispatchers, an unstructured, subjective, unscripted method of telephone assessment and treatment; a less-effective process than protocols.

Guillain-Barré syndrome Autoimmune neurologic disorder marked by weakness and paresthesia that usually travel up the legs.

Gum Plant residue used for medicinal or recreational purposes.

Gurgling Abnormal respiratory sound associated with collection of liquid or semisolid material in the patient's upper airway.

Gurney Stretcher or cot used to transport patients.

Gustation Sense of taste.

Hair papilla Small cluster of cells within a follicle; growth of hair starts in this cluster of cells, which is hidden in the follicle.

Half duplex A radio system that use two frequencies: one to transmit and one to receive; however, like a simplex system, only one person can transmit at a time.

Half-life The time required to eliminate half of a substance from the body.

Hallucination A false sensory perception originating inside the brain, such as hearing the voices of people who are not present.

Hallucinogen Substance that cause hallucinations and intense distortions and perceptions of reality; includes LSD, psilocybin mushrooms, peyote, and mescaline.

Hamman's sign A crunching sound occasionally heard on auscultation of the heart when air is in the mediastinum.

Hangman's fracture A fracture of the axis, the second cervical vertebra. This may occur with or without axis dislocation.

Hazard Communication Standard (HAZCOM) Occupational Safety and Health Administration standard regarding worker protection when handling chemicals.

Hazardous materials A substance (solid, liquid, or gas) capable of posing an unreasonable risk to health, safety, environment, or property.

Hazardous Waste Operations and Emergency Response (HAZWOPER) Occupational Safety and Health Administration and Environmental Protection Agency regulations regarding worker safety when responding to hazardous materials emergencies.

Head bobbing Indicator of increased work of breathing in infants; the head falls forward with exhalation and comes up with expansion of the chest on inhalation.

Head injury A traumatic insult to the head that may result in injury to the soft tissue or bony structures of the head and/or brain injury.

Headache A pain in the head from any cause.

Health A state of complete physical, mental, and social well-being, not merely the absence of disease or infirmity.

Health Insurance Portability and Accountability Act (HIPAA) Rules governing the protection of a patient's identifiable information.

Healthcare professional An individual who has special skills and knowledge in medicine and adheres to the standards of conduct and performance of that medical profession.

Healthcare A business associated with the provision of medical care to individuals.

Heart disease A broad term referring to conditions affecting the heart.

Heart failure A condition in which the heart is unable to pump enough blood to meet the metabolic needs of the body.

Heartbeat Organized mechanical action of the heart.

Heat emergencies Conditions in which the body's thermoregulation mechanisms begin to fail in response to ambient heat, causing illness.

Hematemesis Vomiting of bright red blood.

Hematochezia Bright red blood in the stool.

Hematocrit A measure of the relative percentage of blood cells (mainly erythrocytes) in a given volume of whole blood; also called *volume of packed red cells* or *packed cell volume.*

Hematoma Collection of blood beneath the skin or within a body compartment.

Hematuria Blood found in the urine.

Hemiparesis Muscle weakness of one half of the body.

Hemiplegia Paralysis of one side of the body.

Hemoglobin A protein found on red blood cells that is rich in iron.

Hemolytic anemia Anemia that results from the destruction of red blood cells.

Hemopoietic tissue Connective tissue found in the marrow cavities of bones (mainly long bones).

Hemoptysis The coughing up of blood.

Hemorrhage Heavy bleeding.

Hemorrhagic anemia Anemia caused by hemorrhage.

Hemorrhagic stroke Rupture of a blood vessel in the brain causing decreased perfusion and potentially leading to rising intracranial pressure.

Hemorrhoids Swollen, distended veins in the anorectal area.

Hemostasis Stopping a hemorrhage.

Hemothorax Blood within the thoracic cavity, a potentially life-threatening injury.

Henry's law Law associated with decompression sickness that deals with the solubility of gases in liquids at equilibrium.

Hepatic artery The artery that supplies the liver with blood and nutrients from the circulatory system.

Hepatic duct Connects the gallbladder to the liver; secretes bile into the gallbladder.

Hepatitis Inflammation of the liver.

Hering-Breuer reflex A reflex that limits inspiration to prevent overinflation of the lungs in a conscious, spontaneously breathing person; also called the *inhibito-inspiratory reflex.*

Hernia Protrusion of any organ through an abdominal opening in the muscle wall of the cavity that surrounds it.

Herniated disc A condition in which an intervertebral disc weakens and protrudes out of position, often affecting adjacent nerve roots.

Herniation Protrusion of the brain through an abnormal opening, often the foramen magnum.

Heroin (diacetylmorphine) The most popular, powerful, and addictive member of the opioids.

Herpes simplex A skin eruption caused by the herpes simplex virus, divided into two types; HSV-1 causes oral infection and HSV-2 causes genital infections.

Herpes zoster A skin eruption that follows a particular nerve distribution (dermatome); caused by the varicella zoster virus in persons who have had varicella sometime in their lives (also called *shingles*).

Hiatus A gap or a cleft.

Hiccup (hiccoughing) Intermittent spasm of the diaphragm resulting in sudden inspiration with spastic closure of the glottis; usually annoying and serves no known physiologic purpose.

High angle An environment in which the load is predominately supported by the rope rescue system.

High voltage Greater than 1000 V.

High-altitude cerebral edema The most severe high-altitude illness, characterized by increased intracranial pressure.

High-altitude pulmonary edema A high-altitude illness characterized by increased pulmonary artery pressure and edema, leading to cough and fluid in the lungs (pulmonary edema).

High-angle terrain (vertical terrain) A steep environment such as a cliff or building side where hands must be used for balance when ascending.

Hilum Point of entry for bronchial vessels, bronchi, and nerves in each lung.

Hilus Indentation through which the renal artery, vein, lymphatic vessels, and nerves enter and leave the kidney.

Hippocampi Structures within the limbic system that filter incoming information, determine what stimuli is important, and commit the experiences to memory.

His-Purkinje system Portion of the conduction system consisting of the bundle of His, bundle branches, and Purkinje fibers.

Histamine A substance released by mast cells that promotes inflammation.

History of present illness A narrative detail of the symptoms the patient is experiencing.

Hollow organ An organ (a part of the body or group of tissues that performs a specific function) that contains a channel or cavity within it, such as the large and small intestines.

Homan's sign Pain and tenderness in the calf muscle on dorsiflexion of the foot.

Home care The provision of health services by formal and informal caregivers in the home to promote, restore, and maintain a person's maximal level of comfort, function, and health, including care toward a dignified death.

Homeostasis A state of equilibrium in the body with respect to functions and composition of fluids and tissues.

Homeotherm Organism with a stable independent body temperature; an organism whose stable body temperature generally is independent of the surrounding environment.

Homonyms Terms that sound alike but are spelled differently and have different meanings.

Honeymoon phase A period of remorse by the abuser characterized by the abuser's denial and apologies.

Hordeolum A common acute infection of the glands of the eyelids.

Hormones Chemicals within the body that reach every cell through the circulatory system.

Hospice A care program that provides for the dying and their special needs.

Hospital Incident Command System An emergency management system that uses a logical management structure, defined responsibilities, clear reporting channels, and a common nomenclature to help unify hospitals with other emergency responders.

Hospital off-load time The time necessary for a crew to become available once they arrive at a hospital.

Hot load Loading a patient into a helicopter while the rotors are spinning.

Hot zone The primary danger zone around a crash scene that typically extends approximately 50 feet in all directions from the wreckage.

Hover The condition in which a helicopter remains fairly stationary over a given point, moving neither vertically nor horizontally.

Hub The plastic piece that houses a needle and fits onto a syringe.

Human immunodeficiency virus (HIV) The virus that can cause AIDS.

Human leukocyte antigen Leukocyte antigen that transplant surgeons attempt to match to prevent incompatibility.

Humoral immunity Immunity from antibodies in the blood.

Humoral Pertaining to elements in the blood or other body fluids.

Huntington's disease Programmed cell death of certain neurons in the brain, leading to behavioral abnormalities, movement disorders, and a decline in cognitive function.

Hydration Process of taking in fluids with the normal daily output.

Hydraulic A water hazard caused when water moves over a uniform obstruction to flow.

Hydraulic injection injuries High-pressure fluid that leaks from hydraulic hoses and is injected into the body.

Hydrocarbon A member of a large class of chemicals belonging to the petroleum derivative family; they have a variety of uses, such as solvents, oils, reagents, and fuels.

Hydrocele Collection of fluid in the scrotum or along the spermatic cord.

Hydrocephalus An excessive amount of cerebrospinal fluid.

Hydrogen cyanide A highly toxic blood agent.

Hydrogen ion concentration Concentration of hydrogen ions in a given solution, such as water or blood; used to calculate the pH of a substance.

Hydrogen sulfide A hazardous gas produced by the decomposition of organic material prevalent when manure is stored in a liquid form for an extended period.

Hydrophilic Attracts water molecules.

Hydrophobic Repels water molecules.

Hydrostatic pressure Pressure exerted by a fluid from its weight.

Hydroxylysine An amino acid found in collagen.

Hymen Thin of layer of tissue that covers the vaginal orifice in virgins.

Hypercalcemia A state in which the body has an abnormally high level of calcium.

Hypercapnia An increased amount of carbon dioxide in the blood; may be a result of hypoventilation.

Hypercarbia An excess of CO_2 in the blood.

Hyperdynamic Excessively forceful or energetic. Term is used to describe shock states in which the heart is pumping aggressively to make up for fluid losses, such as in burn or septic shock.

Hyperextension Extension beyond a joint's normal range of motion.

Hyperflexion Flexion beyond a joint's normal range of motion.

Hyperkalemia A state in which the body has an abnormally elevated potassium level.

Hypermagnesemia A state in which the body has an abnormally elevated concentration of magnesium in the blood.

Hypermetabolic A state or condition of the body characterized by excessive production and utilization of energy molecules such as protein.

Hyperopia Farsightedness; difficulty seeing objects close to the person.

Hyperosmolar hyperglycemic nonketotic coma (HHNC) Condition caused by a relative insulin insufficiency that leads to extremely high blood sugar levels while still allowing for normal glucose metabolism and an absence of ketone bodies.

Hyperplasia Abnormal cell division that increases the number or a specific type of cell.

Hyperpnea Increased respiratory rate or deeper than normal breathing.

Hyperresonant A high-pitched sound.

Hypersensitivity disorder A disorder in which the immune system responds inappropriately and excessively to an antigen (in this response, known as allergens).

Hypersensitivity pneumonitis Inflammation in and around the tiny air sacs (alveoli) and smallest airways (bronchioles) of the lung caused by an allergic reaction to inhaled organic dusts or, less commonly, chemicals; also called *extrinsic allergic alveolitis, allergic interstitial pneumonitis,* or *organic dust pneumoconiosis.*

Hypersensitivity reaction An immune response that is excessive beyond the bounds of normalcy to a point that it leads to damage (as with endotoxins) or is potentially damaging to the individual.

Hypersensitivity An altered reactivity to a medication that occurs after prior sensitization; response is independent of the dose.

Hypertension Elevated blood pressure.

Hypertensive emergencies Situations that require rapid (within 1 hour) lowering of blood pressure to prevent or limit organ damage.

Hypertensive urgencies Significant elevations in blood pressure with nonspecific symptoms that should be corrected within 24 hours.

Hyperthermia A core body temperature greater than 98.6° F.

Hypertonic In a membrane, the side with the higher concentration in an imbalance in the ionic concentration from one side to the other.

Hypertrophic scar Scar that forms with excessive amounts of scar tissue. The scar remains contained by the wound boundaries but may be slightly raised and can impair function.

Hypertrophy Enlargement or increase in the size of a cell(s) or tissue.

Hyperventilation Blowing off too much carbon dioxide.

Hyphema Blood in the anterior chamber of the eye.

Hypocalcemia A state in which the body has an abnormally low calcium level.

Hypocarbia An inadequate amount of carbon dioxide in the blood.

Hypokalemia A state in which the level of potassium in the serum falls below 3.5 mEq/L.

Hypomagnesemia A state in which the body has an abnormally low serum concentration of magnesium.

Hypomania An episode of a lesser form of mania that may transition into mania or alternate with depression.

Hypoperfusion The inadequate circulation of blood through an organ or a part of the body; shock.

Hypotension Low blood pressure significant enough to cause inadequate perfusion.

Hypothalamus Interface between the brain and the endocrine system; provides control for many autonomic functions.

Hypothermia A core body temperature below 95° F (35° C).

Hypotonic In a membrane, the side with the lower concentration when an imbalance exists in the ionic concentration from one side to the other.

Hypoventilation Occurs when the volume of air that enters the alveoli and takes part in gas exchange is not adequate for the body's metabolic needs.

Hypovolemic shock Inadequate tissue perfusion caused by inadequate vascular volume.

Hypoxemia An abnormal deficiency in the concentration of oxygen in arterial blood.

Hypoxia Inadequate oxygenation of the cells.

Iatrogenic drug response An unintentional disease or drug effect produced by a physician's prescribed therapy; *iatros* means "physician," and *-genic* is a word root meaning "produce."

Icterus Jaundice.

Idiosyncrasy The unexpected and usually individual (genetic) adverse response to a drug.

Ileostomy Surgical creation of a passage through the abdominal wall into the ileum.

Ileum Last segment of the small intestine; area of decreased absorption where is prepared for entry into the large intestine.

Ileus Decreased peristaltic movement of the colon.

Immediately dangerous to life or health concentrations (IDHLs) Maximal environmental air concentration of a substance from which a person could escape within 30 minutes without symptoms of impairment or irreversible health effects.

Immersion Covering of the face and airway in water or other fluid.

Immunity Protection from legal liability in accordance with applicable laws.

Immunodeficiency Deficit in the immune system and its response to infection or injury.

Immunoglobulin See *Antibody.*

Impetigo A highly contagious infection caused by staphylococcal or streptococcal bacteria. A superficial vesicopustular skin infection that primarily occurs on exposed areas of the face and extremities from scratching infected lesions; usually begins at a traumatized region of the skin, where a combination of vesicles and pustules develops; the pustules rupture and crust, leaving a characteristic thick, golden or honeylike appearance.

Implied consent The presumption that a patient who is ill or injured and unable to give consent for any reason would agree to the delivery of emergency health care necessitated by his or her condition.

Incarcerated hernia Hernia of intestine that cannot be returned or reduced by manipulation; it may or may not become strangulated.

Incendiary device A device designed to ignite a fire.

Incidence The rate at which a certain event occurs, such as the number of new cases of a specific disease occurring during a certain period in a population at risk.

Incidence rate The rate of contraction of a disease versus how many are currently sick with the disease.

Incident commander The person responsible for the overall management of an emergency scene.

Incident scene hazards Hazards directly related to the specific incident scene, including control of crowds, traffic, the danger of downed electrical wires, the presence of hazardous materials, and the location of an emergency.

Incomplete abortion An abortion in which the uterus retains part of the products of the pregnancy.

Incomplete cord transaction A partial cutting (severing) of the spinal cord in which some cord function remains distal to the injury site.

Incontinence Inability to control excretory functions; usually refers to the involuntary passage of urinary or fecal matter.

Incubation period The time between exposure to a disease pathogen and the appearance of the first signs or symptoms.

Incus The anvil-shaped bone located between the malleus and stapes in the middle ear.

Index of suspicion The expectation that certain injuries or patterns of injuries have resulted to a body part, organ, or system based on the mechanism of injury and the force of impact to the patient.

Indication The appropriate use of a drug when treating a disease or condition.

Indicative change ECG changes seen in leads looking directly at the wall of the heart in an infarction.

Induration Hardened mass within the tissue typically associated with inflammation.

Infarction Death of tissue because of an inadequate blood supply.

Inferior Toward the feet; below a point of reference in the anatomic position.

Inferior vena cava Vessels that return venous blood from the lower part of the body to the right atrium.

Infiltration Complication of intravenous therapy when the catheter tip is outside the vein and the intravenous solution is dispersed into the surrounding tissues.

Inflammation A tissue reaction in an injury, infection, or insult.

Influx Flowing into.

Ingestion Process of bringing food into the digestive tract.

Inhalants Substances such as aerosols, fuels, paints, and other chemicals that produce fumes at room temperature; they are breathed in, producing a high.

Inhalation A route in which the medication is aerosolized and delivered directly to the lung tissue.

Injury Intentional or unintentional damage to a person resulting from acute exposure to thermal, mechanical, electrical, or chemical energy or from the absence of such essentials as heat or oxygen.

Injury risk A real or potential hazardous situation that puts individuals at risk for sustaining an injury.

Injury surveillance An ongoing systematic collection, analysis, and interpretation of injury data essential to the planning, implementation, and evaluation of public health practice, closely integrated with the timely dissemination of the data to those who need to know.

Inner ear Location of the sensory organs for hearing and balance.

Inotropic Relating to the force of cardiac contraction.

Inotropism A change in myocardial contractility.

Inspiratory reserve volume Amount of gas that can be forcefully inspired in addition to a normal breath's tidal volume.

Integrity Doing the right thing even when no one is looking.

Integumentary system The largest organ system in the body, consisting of the skin and accessory structures (e.g., hair, nails, glands).

Intense affect Heated and passionate emotional responses.

Intentional injury Injuries and deaths self-inflicted or perpetrated by another person, usually involving some type of violence.

Intentional tort A wrong in which the defendant meant to cause the harmful action.

Interatrial septum Septum dividing the atria in the heart.

Intercalated discs The cell-to-cell connection with gap junctions between cardiac muscle cells.

Interference The ability of one drug to limit the physiologic function of another drug.

Intermittent claudication Pain, cramping, muscle tightness, fatigue, or weakness of the legs when walking or during exercise.

Internal anal sphincter Muscle under autonomic control; has stretch receptors that provide the sensation of the need to defecate.

Internal bleeding Escape of blood from blood vessels into tissues and spaces within the body.

Internal respiration The exchange of gases between blood cells and tissues.

Internal urinary sphincter Ring of smooth muscle in the urethra that is under autonomic control.

International medical surgical response teams Specialty surgical teams that can respond both in the United States and internationally.

Interoperability Describes a radio system that can use the components of several different systems; it can use specialized equipment to connect several different radio systems and components together and have them communicate with each other.

Interpretation Stating the conclusions you have drawn from the information.

Interstitial compartment Area consisting of fluid outside cells and outside the circulatory system.

Interstitium Extravascular and extracellular milieu; also known as the *third space.*

Interval Waveform and a segment; in pacing, the period, measured in milliseconds, between any two designated cardiac events.

Interventricular septum Septum dividing the ventricles in the heart.

Intimal In reference to blood vessels, the innermost lining of an artery; composed of a single layer of cells.

Intimate partner violence and abuse Formerly called *domestic violence,* this is a learned pattern of assaultive and controlling behavior, including physical, sexual, and psychological attacks as well as economic control, which adults or adolescents use against their intimate partners to gain power and control.

Intimate space The area within 1.5 feet of a person.

Intoxication Being under the effect of a toxin or drug; common terminology (nonmedical) refers to intoxication as being under the effect of alcohol or illegal drugs.

Intracardiac The injection of a drug directly into a ventricle of the heart during cardiac arrest.

Intracellular Inside of the cell or cytoplasmic membrane.

Intracellular fluid (ICF) Fluid found within cells.

Intracerebral hematoma Bleeding within the brain tissue itself.

Intracerebral hemorrhage Bleeding within the brain tissue, often from smaller blood vessels.

Intracranial pressure (ICP) Pressure inside the brain cavity; should be very low, usually less than 15 mm Hg.

Intradermal Route of the injection of medication between the dermal layers of skin.

Intralingual Direct injection into the underside of the tongue with a small volume of medication.

Intramuscular (IM) An injection of medication directly into the muscle.

Intranasal The route that offers direct delivery of medications into the nasal passages and sinuses.

Intraosseous An administration route used in emergency situations when peripheral venous access is not established; a needle is passed through the cortex of the bone and the medication is infused into the capillary network within the bone matrix.

Intraosseous infusion The process of infusing medications, fluids, and blood products into the bone marrow cavity for subsequent delivery to the venous circulation.

Intraperitoneal Abdominopelvic organs surrounded by the peritoneum.

Intrathecal The direct deposition of medication into the spinal canal.

Intravascular compartment Area consisting of fluid outside cells but inside the circulatory system; the majority of intravascular fluid is plasma, which is the fluid component of blood.

Intravenous (IV) Administration route offering instantaneous and nearly complete absorption through peripheral or central venous access.

Intravenous (IV) bolus The delivery of a drug directly into an infusion port on the administration set using a syringe.

Intravenous cannulation Placement of a catheter into a vein to gain access to the body's venous circulation.

Intravenous therapy Administration of a fluid into a vein.

Intrinsic rate Rate at which a pacemaker of the heart normally generates impulses.

Intussusception Invagination of a part of the colon into another part of the colon; also referred to as *telescoping*.

Invasion of privacy Disclosure or publication of personal or private facts about a person to a person or persons not authorized to receive such information.

Invasive wound infection An infection involving the deeper tissues of a wound that may be destructive to blood vessels and other structures of the skin and soft tissues.

Investigational drug A drug not yet approved by the Food and Drug Administration.

Involuntary consent The rendering of care to a person under specific legal authority, even if the patient does not consent to the care.

Ion Electrically charged particle.

Ionizing radiation Particles or pure energy that produces changes in matter by creating ion pairs.

Iris Colored part of the eye; ring of smooth muscle that surrounds the pupil; controls the size (diameter) of the pupil.

Irregular bones Unique bones with specialized functions not easily classified into the other types of bone (e.g., vertebrae).

Ischemia Decreased supply of oxygenated blood to a body part or organ.

Ischemic phase Vascular response to shock when precapillary and postcapillary sphincters constrict, halting blood to distal tissues.

Ischemic stroke Lack of perfusion to an area of brain tissue; caused by a thrombus or embolus.

Islets of Langerhans Groups of cells located in the pancreas that produce insulin, glucagon, somatostatin, and pancreatic polypeptide.

Isoelectric line Absence of electrical activity; observed on the ECG as a straight line.

Isografting Transplanting tissue from a genetically identical person (i.e., identical twin).

Isolation The seclusion of individuals with an illness to prevent transmission to others.

Isotonic A balance in the ionic concentration from one side of the membrane to the other.

Jacking the dash Making cuts into the front pillar and A pillar and lifting the dash, instrument panel, steering wheel, column, and even the pedals off a trapped driver or front seat passenger.

Jejunum Second part of the small intestine; major site of nutrient absorption.

Joint dislocation Disruption of articulating bones from their normal location.

Joints Point where two or more bones make contact to allow movement and provide mechanical support.

J-point Point where the QRS complex and ST segment meet.

Jugular venous distension (JVD) The presence of visually enlarged external jugular neck veins.

Jump kit A hard- or soft-sided bag used by paramedics to carry supplies and medications to the patient's side.

Junctional bradycardia A rhythm that begins in the atrioventricular junction with a rate of less than 40 beats/min.

Jurisprudence The theory and philosophy of law.

Kehr's sign Acute left shoulder pain caused by the presence of blood or other irritants in the peritoneal cavity.

Keloid An excessive accumulation of scar tissue that extends beyond the original wound margins.

Keratinized Accumulation of the protein keratin within the cytoplasm of skin cells. These cells comprise the epidermis of the skin. These dead cells function as the first defense against invaders and minor trauma.

Keratinocytes Epidermal cells.

Keratitis Inflammation and swelling of the cornea.

Kernicterus Excessive fetal bilirubin; associated with hemolytic disease.

Ketonemia The presence of ketones in the blood.

Kinetic energy M [mass] × $\frac{1}{2}$ V [velocity]^2; also called the *energy of motion.*

Knee bags Airbags mounted low on the instrument panel designed to deploy against the driver's and front seat passenger's knees in a frontal collision.

Korotkoff sounds The noise made by blood under pressure tumbling through the arteries.

Kussmaul respirations An abnormal respiratory pattern characterized by deep, gasping respirations that may be slow or rapid.

Kwashiorkor A form of malnutrition caused by inadequate protein intake compared with the total needed or required calorie intake.

Kyphosis Abnormally increased convexity in the curvature of the thoracic spine as viewed from the side; also called *hunchback.*

Labeling The application of a derogatory term to a patient on the basis of an event, habit, or personality trait that may not be accurate about the underlying condition.

Labia majora Rounded folds of external adipose tissue of the external female genitalia.

Labia minora Thinner, pinkish folds of skin that extend anteriorly to form the prepuce of the external female genitalia.

Labile Affect that changes frequently and rapidly.

Labor The process by which the fetus and placenta are expelled from the uterus. Usually divided into three stages, starting with the first contraction and ending with delivery of the placenta.

Labyrinth Series of bony tunnels inside the inner ear.

Labyrinthitis An inflammation of the structures in the inner ear.

Lacrimal ducts Small openings at the medial edge of the eye; drain holes for water from the surface of the eye.

Lacrimal fluid Watery, slightly alkaline secretion that consists of tears and saline that moisten the conjunctiva.

Lacrimal gland One of a pair of glands situated superior and lateral to the eye bulb; secretes lacrimal fluid.

Lacrimation Tearing of the eyes.

Lactic acid Byproduct of anaerobic metabolism.

Landing zone An area used to land a helicopter that is 100 feet × 100 feet and free of overhead wires.

Large intestine Organ where a large amount of water and electrolytes is absorbed and where undigested food is concentrated into feces.

Laryngoscope An instrument used to examine the interior of the larynx; during endotracheal intubation the device is used to visualize the glottic opening.

Laryngotracheobronchitis Croup.

Larynx Lies between the pharynx and the lungs; outer case of nine cartilages that protect and support the vocal cords.

Lassa fever A viral hemorrhagic fever illness caused by the Lassa virus (Arenavirus family).

Latent period Period during and after infection in which the disease is no longer transmissable.

Lateral A position away from the midline of the body.

Lateral recumbent Lying on either the right or left side.

Lead Electrical connection attached to the body to record electrical activity.

Left A position toward the left side of the body.

Left coronary artery Vessel that supplies oxygenated blood to the left side of the heart muscle.

Legally blind Less than 20/200 vision in at least one eye or a extremely limited field of vision (such as 20 degrees at its widest point).

Lens Transparent, biconvex elastic disc suspended by ligaments.

Leptomeningitis Inflammation of the inner brain coverings.

Lesions A wound, injury, or pathologic change in body tissue; any visible, local abnormality of the tissues of the skin, such as a wound, sore, rash, or boil.

Lethal concentration 50% (LC50) The air concentration of a substance that kills 50% of the exposed animal population; also commonly noted as LCt50; this denotes the concentration and the length of exposure time that results in 50% fatality in the exposed animal population.

Lethal dose 50% (LD50) The oral or dermal exposure dose that kills 50% of the exposed animal population in 2 weeks.

Leukocytes White blood cells.

Leukocytosis An increase in the number of white blood cells in the blood; typically results from infection, hemorrhage, fever, inflammation, or other factors.

Leukopenia A decrease in the total number of white blood cells in the blood.

Liability The legal responsibility of a party for the consequences of his or her acts or omissions.

Libel False statements about a person made in writing that blacken the person's character or injure his or her reputation.

Lice Wingless insects that live in human hair.

Licensure Permission granted to an individual by a governmental authority, such as a state, to perform certain restricted activities.

Life-threatening conditions A problem to the circulatory, respiratory, or nervous system that will kill a patient within minutes if not properly managed.

Ligaments Fibrous connective tissue that connects bones to bones, forming joint capsules.

Limbic system The part of the brain involved in mood, emotions, and the sensation of pain and pleasure.

Linear laceration Laceration that generally has smooth margins, although not as precise as those of an incision.

Linear skull fracture A line crack in the skull.

Lipid accumulation Accumulation of lipids in cells, usually as a result of the failure or inadequate performance of the enzyme that metabolizes fats.

Lipid peroxidation Process of cellular membrane destruction from exposure of the membrane to oxygen free radicals.

Lipophilic Substances that tend to seek out and bind to fatty substances.

Liquefaction necrosis Dead or dying tissue in which the necrotic material becomes softened and liquefied.

Liver Largest internal organ in the body; serves as a major detoxifier in the body.

Living will A type of advanced directive with written and signed specific instructions to health care providers about the individual's wishes regarding what types of health care measures or treatments should be undertaken to prolong life.

Loaded airbag An airbag that has not deployed during the initial crash.

Local damage Damage present at the point of chemical contact.

Local effect The effects of a drug at the site where the drug is applied or in the surrounding tissues.

Lock out, tag out An industrial workplace safety term describing actions taken to shut off power to a device, appliance, machine, or vehicle and to ensure that power remains off until work is completed.

Logistics officer The person responsible for assembling supplies used during an incident.

Long bones Bones that are longer than they are wide, have attachments for muscles to allow movement, and are found in limbs (e.g., the femur).

Looseness of associations (LOA) Going off track during conversation to varying degrees.

Low-angle terrain An environment in flat or mildly sloping areas in which rescuers primarily support themselves with their feet on the terrain surface.

Low vision Level of visual impairment in which an individual is unable to read a newspaper at the usual viewing distance even if wearing glasses or contact lenses. It is not limited to distance vision and can be a severe visual impairment.

Low voltage Less than 1000 V.

Lower airway Portion of the respiratory tract below the glottis.

Lower airway inhalation injury Injury to the anatomic portion of the respiratory tree below the level of the glottis. Generally caused by the inhalation of the toxic by products of combustion.

Lower flammable limit The minimal concentration of fuel in the air that will ignite; below this point too much oxygen and not enough fuel are present to burn (too lean); also called the *lower explosive limit*.

Ludwig's angina A bacterial infection of the floor of the mouth resulting from an infection in the root of the teeth, an abscessed tooth, or an injury to the mouth.

Lumbar vertebrae Vertebrae of the lower back that do not attach to any ribs and are superior to the pelvis.

Lumen An opening in the bevel of a needle.

Lungs Organs that allow the mechanical movement of air to and from the respiratory membrane.

Lymph Fluid within the lymphatic system.

Lymph nodes Filter out foreign materials and collect infection-fighting cells that kill pathogens.

Lymphadenopathy Swelling of lymph nodes.

Lymphatic system The network of vessels, ducts, nodes, valves, and organs involved in protecting and maintaining the internal fluid environment of the body; part of the circulatory system.

Lymphatic vessels Unidirectional tubes that carry fluid or lymph within the lymphatic system.

Lymphedema Edema that follows when lymphatic pathways are blocked and fluid accumulates in the interstitial space.

Lymphocyte A form of leukocyte.

Lyse To destroy a cell.

Lysergic acid diethylamide (LSD) A powerful synthetic hallucinogen, often called *acid* and found on small squares of blotter paper.

Lysosomes Membrane-walled structures that contain enzymes.

Macrophages A monocyte that has matured and localized in one particular type of tissue; active in the immune system by activating agents that kill pathogens, absorbing foreign materials, and slowing infections and infectious agents.

Macule A flat, circumscribed, discolored lesion (e.g., freckle) measuring less than 1 cm.

Mainstem bronchi Each of two main breathing tubes that lead from the trachea into the lungs. There is one right mainstem bronchus and one left mainstem bronchus.

Malaise General feeling of illness without any specific symptoms.

Malfeasance Performing a wrongful act.

Malignant Highly dangerous or virulent; often used to describe a deadly form of cancer or a spreading of cancer.

Malignant hypertension Severe hypertension with signs of acute and progressive damage to end organs such as the heart, brain, and kidneys.

Malingering Faking illness for a tangible gain (missing work, avoiding incarceration, etc.).

Malleus Hammer-shaped bone located at the front of the middle ear; receives vibrations from the tympanic membrane.

Malocclusion The condition in which the teeth of the upper and lower jaws do not line up.

Mammary glands Female organs of milk production; located within the breast tissue.

Mania An excessively intense enthusiasm, interest, or desire; a craze.

Manure gas A name used for several different gases formed by decomposition of manure (methane, carbon dioxide, ammonia, hydrogen sulfide, and hydrogen disulfide); in certain concentrations all are toxic to animals and human beings.

Marasmus A form of nutritional deficiency from an overall lack of calories that results in wasting.

Marburg A viral hemorrhagic fever illness caused by the Marburg virus (Filovirus family).

Margination Process of phagocytes adhering to capillary and venule walls in the early phases of inflammation.

Marijuana Dried mixture of shredded leaves, stems, and seeds of the hemp plant that usually are smoked and contain many psychoactive compounds, most notably tetrahydrocannabinol (THC).

Mark 1 antidote kit Self-injected nerve agent antidote kit consisting of atropine and 2-pralidoxime (2-PAM).

Mast cells Connective tissue cell that contains histamine; important in initiating the inflammatory response.

Material safety data sheet (MSDS) A document that contains information about the specific identity of a hazardous chemical; information includes exact name and synonyms, health effects, first aid, chemical and physical properties, and emergency telephone numbers.

Matrix Nonliving material that separates cells in the connective tissue.

Mechanical processing Physical manipulation and breakdown of food.

Mechanism of action The manner in which a drug works to produce its intended effect.

Mechanism of injury The way an injury occurs on the body.

Meconium A dark green substance that represents the infant's first bowel movement.

Medial A position toward the midline of the body.

Median lethal dose The dose that kills 50% of the drug-tested population.

Mediastinitis Infection of the mediastinum; a serious medical condition.

Mediastinoscopy Surgical procedure of looking into the mediastinum with an endoscope.

Mediastinum Area that includes the trachea, esophagus, thymus gland, heart, and great vessels.

Medical asepsis Medically clean, not sterile; the goal in prehospital care because complete asepsis is not always possible.

Medical direction Physician oversight of paramedic practice; also called *medical control.*

Medical director A physician responsible for the oversight of the EMS system and the actions of the paramedics; also known as a *physician advisor.*

Medical ethics A field of study that evaluates the decisions, conduct, policies, and social concerns of medical activities.

Medical practice act Legislation that governs the practice of medicine; may prescribe how and to what extent a physician may delegate authority to a paramedic to perform medical acts; varies from state to state.

Medical terminology Greek- and Latin-based words (typically) that function as a common language for the medical community.

Medically clean Disinfected.

Medulla Most inferior part of the brainstem; responsible for some vegetative functions.

Medulla oblongata Lowest portion of brain tissue and the interface between the brain and the spinal cord; responsible for maintenance of basic life functions such as heart rate and respirations.

Meissner corpuscle Encapsulated nerve endings in the superficial dermis responsible for sensing vibrations and light touch.

Melancholy An episode of dysphoric mood with disruptions of homeostasis, including alterations in appetite, activities, and sleep patterns; also called *major* or *severe depression.*

Melena Foul-smelling, dark, and tarry stools stained with blood pigments or with digested blood, often indicating gastrointestinal bleeding.

Melting point The temperature at which a solid changes to a liquid (e.g., ice melting to water at $0°C$ ($32°F$).

Membrane potential Difference in electrical charge across the cell membrane.

Menarche A girl's first menstruation.

Meninges Covering of the brain and spinal cord; layers include the dura mater, arachnoid, and pia mater.

Meningitis Irritation of the connective tissue covering the central nervous system, often from infection or hemorrhage.

Meningocele A type of spina bifida in which the spinal cord develops normally but a saclike cyst that contains the meninges and cerebrospinal fluid protrudes from an opening in the spine, usually in the lumbosacral area.

Meningomyelocele The severest form of spina bifida in which the meninges, cerebrospinal fluid, and a portion of the spinal cord protrude from an opening in the spine and are encased in a sac covered by a thin membrane; also called *myelomeningocele.*

Menopause Cessation of menstruation in the human female.

Menstruation Shedding of endometrial lining.

Mental illness Any form of psychiatric disorder.

Mental retardation Developmental disability characterized by a lower than normal IQ.

Merocrine glands Sweat glands that open directly to the surface of the body; produce a fluid (mainly water) when the temperature rises that allows the body to dispel large amounts of heat through the evaporation process.

Mesentery Layers of connective tissue found in the peritoneal cavity.

Metabolism Sum of all physical and chemical changes that occur within an organism.

Metabolites The smaller molecules from the breakdown that occurs during metabolism.

Metaplasia The transformation of one type of mature differentiated cell into another type of mature differentiated cell.

Metastatic Spread of cancerous cells to a distant site.

Metered-dose inhaler (MDI) A handheld device that disperses a measured dose of medication in the form of a fine spray directly into the airway.

Methamphetamine A powerful, highly addictive central nervous system stimulant found in either a white powder form or a clear crystal form ("crystal meth").

Methemoglobinemia The oxidation of hemoglobin from the ferrous iron to the ferric iron state.

Methicillin-resistant Staphylococcus aureus Any of several bacterial strains of *S. aureus* resistant to methicillin (a penicillin) and related drugs; typically acquired in the hospital.

Micturition Urination.

Midbrain Lies below the diencephalon and above the pons; works with the pons to route information from higher within the brain to the spinal cord and vice versa.

Middle ear Air-filled chamber within the temporal bone; contains the auditory ossicles.

Migraine headache A recurring vascular headache characterized by unilateral onset, severe pain, sensitivity to light, and autonomic disturbances during the acute phase, which may last for hours or days.

Milliampere (mA) Unit of measure of electrical current needed to elicit depolarization of the myocardium.

Millivolt (mV) Difference in electrical charge between two points in a circuit.

Minor In most states, a person younger than 18 years.

Minute volume Amount of gas moved in and out of the respiratory tract per minute. Tidal volume multiplied by ventilatory rate equals minute volume. The minute volume is the true measurement of a patient's ventilatory status and is vital in assessing pulmonary function. It ascertains the ventilatory rate and the depth of each inhalation.

Miosis Pinpoint pupils.

Miscarriage (spontaneous abortion) Loss of the products of conception before the fetus can survive on its own.

Misfeasance Performing a legal act in a harmful manner.

Mitochondria Power plant of the cell and body; site of aerobic oxidation.

Mitosis Process of division and multiplication in which one cell divides into two cells.

Mitral valve Left atrioventricular valve in the heart; also called the *bicuspid valve.*

Mittelschmerz Pain occurring at time of ovulation.

Mixed episode A period of manic-like energy and agitation coupled with the pessimism and dysphoria of severe depression.

Mobile data computer A device used in an ambulance or first responder vehicle to retrieve and send call information; has its own memory storage and processing capability.

Mobile data terminal A device used like a mobile data computer but without its own memory storage and processing capability.

Mobile radio A radio installed in an emergency vehicle; usually transmits by higher wattage than a portable radio.

Modern deployment Deployment that considers workload and how available resources can achieve a balance among coverage, response times, and crew satisfaction.

Mold A multicellular type of fungus that grows hyphae.

Monoblasts Immature monocytes.

Monocytes Type of white blood cell (leukocyte) designed to consume foreign material and fight pathogens; generally become macrophages within a few days after release into the bloodstream.

Monomorphic Having the same shape.

Mons pubis A hair-covered fat pad overlying the symphysis pubis.

Mood The dominant and sustained emotional state of a patient; the emotional lens through which a patient views the world.

Morals Social standards that help a person define right (what a person ought to do) versus wrong (what a person ought not to do).

Morbid obesity Having a body mass index of 40 or more; equates to approximately 100 lb more than ideal weight.

Morbidity A disease state.

Mortality Death.

Mortality rate The number of patients who have died from a disease in a given period.

Motor cortex Area of brain tissue on the frontal lobe that controls voluntary movements.

Mucosa Layer of cells lining body cavities or organs (e.g., the lining of the mouth and digestive tract); generally implies a moist surface.

Multiformed atrial rhythm Cardiac dysrhythmia that occurs because of impulses originating from various sites, including the sinoatrial node, the atria, and/or the atrioventricular junction; requires at least three different P waves seen in the same lead for proper diagnosis.

Multipara A woman who has given birth multiple times.

Multiple-casualty incident An incident involving 26 to 99 persons.

Multiple organ dysfunction syndrome Altered organ function in an acutely ill person in whom homeostasis cannot be maintained without intervention.

Multiple-patient incident An incident involving two to 25 persons.

Multiple sclerosis (MS) Autoimmune disorder in which the immune system attacks the myelin sheath surrounding neurons, causing widespread motor problems and pain.

Multiplex This system allows the crew to transmit voice and data at the same time, enabling the crew to call in a patient report while transmitting an ECG strip to the hospital.

Murphy's sign An inspiratory pause when the right upper quadrant is palpated.

Muscle tissue Contractile tissue that is the basis of movement.

Muscular dystrophy (MD) Hereditary condition causing malformation of muscle tissue and leading to malformation of the musculoskeletal system and physical disability.

Mutate To change in an unusual way.

Mutism A condition in which a person will not speak.

Myasthenia gravis Autoimmune disorder affecting acetylcholine receptors throughout the body, causing widespread muscle weakness.

Mycoses Diseases caused by fungi.

Mydriasis Dilation of the pupils.

Myelomeningocele Developmental anomaly of the central nervous system in which a hernial sac containing a portion of the spinal cord, the meninges, and cerebrospinal fluid protrudes through a congenital cleft in the vertebral column; occurs in approximately two of every 1000 live births, is readily apparent, and is easily diagnosed at birth.

Myocardial cells Working cells of the myocardium that contain contractile filaments and form the muscular layer of the atrial walls and the thicker muscular layer of the ventricular walls.

Myocardial depressant factor An inflammatory mediator (cytokine) produced as a result of significant burn injury; known to affect the contractile function of the cardiac ventricles.

Myocardial infarction (MI) Necrosis of some mass of the heart muscle caused by an inadequate blood supply.

Myocarditis Inflammation of the middle and thickest layer of the heart, the myocardium.

Myocardium Middle and thickest layer of the heart; contains the cardiac muscle fibers that cause contraction of the heart as well as the conduction system and blood supply.

Myoglobin A pigment in muscle tissue that serves as an oxygen carrier (also known as *myohemoglobin*).

Myoglobinuria Presence of myoglobin in the urine; almost always a result of a pathologic (disease) state such as widespread muscle injury.

Myometrium Muscular region of the uterus.

Myopia Nearsightedness; difficulty seeing objects at a distance.

Myositis A rare muscle disease in which the body's immune system is activated, resulting in inflammation and pain of muscle tissue.

Myotomes Areas of the body controlled by specific motor spinal nerves.

Myxedema Severe form of hypothyroidism characterized by hypothermia and unresponsiveness.

N-95 particulate mask (medical) A facial mask worn over the nose and mouth that removes particulates from the inspired and expired air.

Nasal flaring Widening of the nostrils on inhalation; an attempt to increase the size of the airway and increase the amount of available oxygen.

Nasal polyps Small, saclike growths consisting of inflamed nasal mucosa.

Nasogastric The administration route used when a nasogastric tube is in place; bypasses the voluntary swallowing reflex.

Nasogastric tube A tube placed by way of the nose into the stomach.

Nasolacrimal duct Opening at the medial corner of the eye that drains excess fluid into the nasal cavity.

Natal Connected with birth.

National Disaster Medical System An organized response to an event that includes field units, coordination of patient transportation, and provision of hospital beds. The field component is composed of many volunteer teams of medical professionals.

National Fire Protection Association (NFPA) International voluntary membership organization that promotes improved fire protection and prevention and establishes safeguards against loss of life and property by fire; writes and publishes national voluntary consensus standards.

National Flight Paramedics Association (NFPA) Association established in 1984 to differentiate the critical care paramedic from the flight paramedic; has developed a position statement recommending the training considered necessary to perform the duties of a flight paramedic.

National Highway Traffic Safety Administration (NHTSA) An agency within the U.S. Department of Transportation that was first given the authority to develop EMS systems, including the development of curriculum.

National Medical Response Team Quick response specialty teams trained and equipped to provide mass casualty decontamination and patient care after the release of a chemical, biologic, or radiologic agent.

National Registry of EMTs (NREMT) A national organization developed to ensure that graduates of EMS training programs have met minimal standards by measuring competency through a uniform testing process.

National Standard Curriculum (NSC) Document providing information or course planning and structure, objectives, and detailed lesson plans. It also suggests hours of instruction for the EMT-A.

Natural immunity Nonspecific immunity that mounts a generalized response to any foreign material or pathogen (e.g., inflammation).

Natural killer cells Specialized lymphocytes capable of killing infected or malignant cells.

Nebulizer A machine that turns liquid medication into fine droplets in aerosol or mist form.

Necrosis Death of an area of tissue.

Necrotizing Causing the death (necrosis) of tissue.

Negative battery cable An electrical power cable that allows the vehicle's electrical system to be grounded or neutral as an electrical circuit.

Negative pressure Pressure that acts as a vacuum, pulling more fluid from the vascular space at a faster rate than before, further depleting the intravascular volume; also known as *inhibition pressure*.

Neglect Failure of a parent or other person with responsibility for the child to provide needed food, clothing, shelter, medical care, or supervision such that the child's health, safety, and well-being are threatened with harm.

Negligence The failure to act as a reasonably prudent and careful person would under similar circumstances.

Negligence per se Conduct that may be declared and treated as negligent without having to prove what would be reasonable and prudent under similar circumstances, usually because the conduct violates a law or regulation.

Nematocyst The stinging cells many marine creatures use to envenomate and immobilize prey.

Neonatal abstinence syndrome Withdrawal symptoms that occur in newborns born to opioid-addicted mothers.

Neonate An infant from birth to 1 month of age, also called a newborn infant.

Neoplasm Cancerous growth; a tumor that may be malignant or benign.

Neovascularization New blood vessel growth to support healing tissue.

Nephron Functional unit of the kidney.

Nephrotoxic Chemicals, medications, or other substances that can be toxic to the kidneys.

Nerve Neurons and blood vessels wrapped together with connective tissue; the body's information highways.

Nervous tissue Tissue that can conduct electrical impulses.

Neural tube defects Congenital anomalies that involve incomplete development of the brain, spinal cord, and/or their protective coverings.

Neuralgia Pain caused by chronic nerve damage.

Neuroeffector junction Interface between a neuron and its target tissue.

Neurogenic shock Shock with hypotension caused by a sudden loss of control over the sympathetic nervous system. Loss can be caused by a variety of mechanisms from traumatic injury to disease and infection.

Neuroglia Supporting cells of nervous tissue; functions include nourishment, protection, and insulation.

Neurons Conducting cells of nervous tissue; composed of a cell body, dendrites, and axon.

Neuropeptide A protein that may interact with a receptor after circulation through the blood.

Neuroses Mental diseases related to upbringing and personality in which the person remains "out of touch" with reality.

Neurotransmitters A chemical released from one nerve that crosses the synaptic cleft to reach a receptor.

Neutralizing agent A substance that counteracts the effects of acids or bases; brings the pH of a solution back to 7.0.

Neutron radiation Penetrating radiation that can result in whole-body irradiation.

Neutrophils A form of granulocyte that is short lived but often first to arrive at the site of injury; capable of phagocytosis.

Newborn asphyxia The inability of a newborn to begin and continue breathing at birth.

Newly born An infant in the first minutes to hours after birth.

Nodule An elevated, solid lesion in the deep skin or subcutaneous tissues.

Noncardiogenic pulmonary edema Fluid collection in the alveoli of the lung that does not result from heart failure.

Nonfeasance Failure to perform a required act or duty.

Nonproprietary name Generic name.

Nonsteroidal antiinflammatory drug (NSAID) Medications used primarily to treat inflammation, mild to moderate pain, and fever.

Nonverbal cues Expressions, motions, gestures, and body language that may be used to communicate other than with words.

Normal flora Nonthreatening bacteria found naturally in the human body that, in some cases, are necessary for normal function.

Nuclear envelope The outer boundary between the nucleus and the rest of the cell to the endoplasmic reticulum for protein synthesis.

Nuclear membrane Membrane in the cell that surrounds the nucleus.

Nucleoplasm Protoplasm of the nucleus as contrasted with that of the cell.

Nucleus Area within a cell where the genetic material is stored.

Nullipara A woman who has not borne a child.

Numerator The number or mathematic expression written above the line in a fraction; the numerator is a portion of the denominator.

Nystagmus Involuntary rapid movement of the eyes in the horizontal, vertical, or rotary planes of the eyeball.

Obesity An excessively high amount of body fat or adipose tissue in relation to lean body mass.

Objective information Verifiable findings, such as information seen, felt, or heard by the paramedic.

Obsessive-compulsive disorder (OCD) An anxiety disorder marked by frequent, intrusive, unwanted, and bothersome thoughts (obsessions) and repetitive rituals (compulsions).

Obstructed lane +1 Blocking with an emergency vehicle to stop the flow of traffic in the lane in which the damaged vehicle is positioned plus one additional lane or the shoulder of the roadway.

Occipital lobe Most rearward portion of the cerebrum; mainly responsible for processing the sense of sight.

Occupational Safety and Health Administration (OSHA) A unit of the U.S. Department of Labor that establishes protective standards, enforces those standards, and reaches out to employers and employees through technical assistance and consultation programs.

Official name A drug's name as listed in the *United States Pharmacopoeia*.

Offline medical direction Prospective and retrospective medical direction.

Oils In medicine, substances extracted from flowers, leaves, stems, roots, seeds, or bark for use therapeutic treatments.

Olfactory Sense of smell.

Olfactory fatigue Desensitization of the sense of smell.

Olfactory tissue Located within the nasopharynx; contains receptors that enable the ability of smell (olfaction).

Omphalocele Protrusion of abdominal organs into the umbilical cord.

Oncotic pressure The net effect of opposing osmotic pressures in the capillary beds.

Online medical direction Direct voice communication by a medical director (or designee) to a prehospital professional while he or she is attending to the patient; also called *direct medical direction*.

Oocyte The female gamete; product of the female reproductive system.

Oogenesis Egg production.

Open-ended questions A form of interview question that allows patients to respond in narrative form so that they may feel free to answer in their own way and provide details and information that they believe to be important.

Open fracture Fracture of the bone tissue that breaks the skin and may or may not still be exposed.

Open pneumothorax Injury to the thoracic cavity in which the cavity is breached, allowing air into the space between the lung and the chest wall.

Operations Carries out the tactical objectives of the incident commander.

Ophthalmic Route of administration in which medications are applied to the eye, such as antibiotic eye drops.

Ophthalmoscope An instrument used to examine the inner parts of the eye; consists of an adjustable light and multiple magnification lenses.

Opioids Powerful pain-relieving drugs derived from the seed pods of the poppy plant or drugs that are similar in molecular structure.

Oral A route of administration in which the medication is placed in the mouth and swallowed; the drug is absorbed through the gastrointestinal tract.

Oral cavity First part of the gastrointestinal tract; includes salivary glands, teeth, and tongue.

Organ A structure composed of two or more kinds of tissues organized to perform a more complex function than any one tissue alone can.

Organ of Corti Organ of hearing located in the cochlea.

Organ systems The coordination of several organs working together.

Organelles Numerous structures within the cell.

Organic An etiology of an illness that stems from a biologic cause, such as a stroke or electrolyte imbalance.

Organism An entity composed of cells and capable of carrying on life functions.

Organophosphate A pesticide that inhibits acetylcholinesterase.

Orogastric (OG) tube A tube placed by way of the mouth into the stomach.

Oropharynx Starts at the uvula; back of the oral cavity that extends down to the epiglottis.

Orphan drugs Products developed for the diagnosis and/or treatment of rare diseases or conditions, such as sickle cell anemia and cystic fibrosis.

Orthopnea Dyspnea relieved by a change in position (either sitting upright or standing).

Orthostatic vital signs Serial measurements of the patient's pulse and blood pressure taken with the patient recumbent, sitting, and standing. Results are used to assess possible volume depletion; also called the *tilt test* or *postural vital signs*.

Osmolarity The number, or concentration, of solute per liter of water.

Osmosis The passive movement of water from a higher to a lower concentration.

Osmotic gradient The difference in the concentration from one side of a membrane to the other in the presence of an imbalance in the ionic concentration.

Osmotic pressure The pressure exerted by the concentration of the solutes in a given space.

Osteoarthritis A disorder in which the cartilaginous covering of the joint surface starts to wear away, resulting in pain and inflammation of a joint; also known as *degenerative joint disease.*

Osteomyelitis An infection of bone.

Osteoporosis Reduction in the amount of bone mass, which leads to fractures after minimal trauma.

Ostomy Hole; usually refers to a surgically made hole in some part of the body (e.g., tracheostomy, gastrostomy, colostomy).

Otic Route of administration in which medications are applied to the ear, such as antibiotic drops.

Otitis externa A condition manifested by redness and irritation of the external auditory canal; also called *swimmer's ear.*

Otosclerosis Abnormal growth of bone that prevents structures in the ear from working properly; thought to be a hereditary disease.

Otoscope An instrument used to examine the inner ear; consists of a light source and magnifying lens; the tip is covered with a disposable cone.

Oval window A membranous structure that separates the middle ear from the inner ear.

Ovarian follicle The ovum and its surrounding cells.

Ovarian medulla Inner portion of the ovary.

Ovarian torsion Twisting of an ovary on its axis such that the venous flow to the ovary is interrupted.

Ovaries Site of egg production in females.

Overdose The accidental or intentional ingestion of an excess of a substance with the potential for toxicity.

Over-the-counter (OTC) Drugs that can be purchased without a prescription.

Overweight State of increased body weight in relation to height.

Ovulation Mid-cycle release of an ovum during the menstrual cycle.

Ovum (oocyte) Human egg that, when fertilized, implants in the lining of the uterus and results in pregnancy.

Oxidation A normal chemical process in the body caused by the release of oxygen atoms created during normal cell metabolism.

Oxidation ability The ability of a substance to readily release oxygen to stimulate combustion.

Oxygen-limiting silo A vertical structure used to store ensiled plant material in an anaerobic environment.

Oxyhemoglobin Hemoglobin that has oxygen molecules bound to it.

P wave First wave in the cardiac cycle; represents atrial depolarization and the spread of the electrical impulse throughout the right and left atria.

Pacemaker Artificial pulse generator that delivers an electrical current to the heart to stimulate depolarization.

Pacemaker cells Specialized cells of the heart's electrical conduction system capable of spontaneously generating and conducting electrical impulses.

Packaging Placing the injured or ill patient in a litter and securing him or her for evacuation.

Painful stimulus Any stimulus that causes discomfort to the patient, triggering some sort of response.

Palliative care Provision of comfort measures (physical, social, psychological, and spiritual) to terminally ill patients.

Pallor Pale, washed-out coloration of skin. Often a result of extreme anemia or chronic illness. A patient with pallor can be referred to as pallid.

Palpation The process of applying pressure against the body with the intent of gathering information.

Palpitations An unpleasant awareness of one's heartbeat.

Pancreatitis Inflammation of the pancreas.

Pandemic A disease that affects the majority of the population of a single region or that is epidemic at the same time in many different regions.

Panic attack A sudden, paralyzing anxiety reaction characterized by an overwhelming sense of fear, anxiety, and impending doom, often with physical symptoms such as chest pain and difficulty breathing.

Papillary dermis Section of the dermis composed of loose connective tissue that contains vasculature that feeds the epidermis.

Papillary muscles Muscles attached to the chordae tendineae of the heart valves and the ventricular muscle of the heart.

Papule An elevated, solid lesion usually less than 0.5 centimeters in diameter; may arise from the epidermis, dermis, or both.

Para The number of pregnancies carried to term.

Paracrine communication Method of intercellular communication in which cells communicate with cells in close proximity through the release of paracrine factors, or cytokines.

Paradoxic motion (of a segment of the chest wall) Part of the chest moves in an opposite direction from the rest during respiration.

Paranoid delusions False perceptions of persecution and the feeling that one is being hunted or conspired against; this is the most common type of delusion.

Paranoid schizophrenia A form of schizophrenia characterized by persistent preoccupation with illogical, absurd, and changeable delusions, usually of a persecutory, grandiose, or jealous nature, accompanied by related hallucinations.

Paraphimosis Tight, constricting band caused by the foreskin when it is retracted behind the glans penis.

Paraplegia Paralysis of the lower limbs and trunk.

Parasites An organism that lives within or on another organism (the host) but does not contribute to the host's survival.

Parasympathetic division A division of the autonomic nervous system; responsible for the relaxed state of the body known as "feed and breed."

Parasympathetic nervous system The subdivision of the autonomic nervous system usually involved in activating vegetative functions, such as digestion, defecation, and urination.

Parasympatholytics Drugs that block or inhibit the function of the parasympathetic receptors.

Parasympathomimetics Drugs that mimic the parasympathetic division of the autonomic nervous system.

Parenteral Administration route used for systemic effects and given by a route other than the digestive tract.

Paresthesia Abnormal sensation described as numbness, tingling, or pins and needles.

Parietal lobe Section of the cerebrum responsible for the integration of most sensory information from the body.

Parietal pleura Lining of the pleural cavity attached tightly to the interior of the chest cage.

Parity The number of pregnancies that have resulted in a viable infant.

Parkinson's disease Progressive movement disorder caused by dysfunction in the cerebellum; rigidity, tremor, bradykinesia, and postural instability are characteristic.

Parkmedic A National Park Service ranger who has undergone additional wilderness medical training and who operates in certain parks under the medical direction of emergency physicians from University of Southern California–Fresno; scope of practice lies between a traditional EMT-Intermediate and EMT-Paramedic, with additional wilderness medical training.

Paroxysmal atrial tachycardia Atrial tachycardia that starts or ends suddenly.

Paroxysmal nocturnal dyspnea (PND) A sudden onset of difficulty breathing that awakens the patient from sleep.

Paroxysmal supraventricular tachycardia (PSVT) A regular, narrow QRS tachycardia that starts or ends suddenly.

Partial agonist A drug that when bound to a receptor may elicit a physiologic response, but it is less than that of an agonist; may also may block the response of a competing agonist.

Partial pressure The pressure exerted by an individual gas in a mixture.

Partial seizure A seizure confined to one area of the brain.

Partial-thickness burn Burns that involve any layer of the dermis. The depth of these burns varies and depends on location, so they're further subcategorized as superficial partial-thickness or deep partial-thickness burns. Also called *second-degree burns*.

Partially sighted Level of vision in persons who have some type of visual problem and may need assistance.

Passive immunity Induced immunity that only lasts as long as the injected immune agents are alive and active (e.g., immunoglobulin injection).

Passive range of motion Degree of movement at a joint determined when the examiner causes the movement with the patient at rest.

Passive transport The ability of a substance to traverse a barrier without any energy input; generally occurs from a higher to a lower concentration.

Past medical history A summary of all past health-related events.

Patch A flat, circumscribed, discolored lesion.

Pathologic fracture Fractures that occur as a result of an underlying disease process that weakens the mechanical properties of the bone.

Pathophysiology Functional changes that accompany a particular syndrome or disease.

Patients with terminal illness Patients with advanced stage of illness or disease with an unfavorable prognosis and no known cure.

Pattern recognition Gathering patient information, relating it to the health care professional's knowledge of pathophysiology and the signs and symptoms of illnesses and injuries, and determining whether the patient's presentation fits a particular pattern.

Pattern response Anticipating the equipment and emergency care interventions needed on the basis of the patient's history and physical examination findings.

Patterned injuries Those that leave a distinctive mark, indicating that an object was used in the assault (e.g., cigarette burns, electrical cord whipping, human bites, glove injuries, attempted strangulation, and slaps).

Peak expiratory flow The greatest rate of airflow that can be achieved during forced expiration beginning with the lungs fully inflated.

Peak flow meter A device used to assess the severity of respiratory distress.

Pediculosis Human infestation with lice.

Pelvic inflammatory disease (PID) An infection of a woman's reproductive organs, usually from a bacterial infection, that spreads from the vagina to the upper parts of the reproductive tract.

Penetrating trauma Any mechanism of injury that causes a cut or piercing of skin.

Penis Male sex organ with three columns of erectile tissue; transfers sperm during copulation.

Percussion A diagnostic technique that uses tapping on the body to differentiate air, solids, and fluids.

Performance-based response system A contractual agreement between the EMS provider and the government authority to provide ambulance response to a particular municipality or region with time requirements for each response and total responses on a monthly basis.

Perfusion Circulation of blood through an organ or a part of the body.

Pericardial cavity The potential space between the two layers of the pericardium.

Pericardial effusion An increase in the volume and/or character of pericardial fluid that surrounds the heart.

Pericardial tamponade Life-threatening injury in which blood collects within the pericardium until the increasing pressure prevents the heart from filling with blood, causing death.

Pericardiocentesis A procedure in which a needle is inserted into the pericardial space and the excess fluid is drawn out (aspirated) through the needle.

Pericarditis Inflammation of the double-walled sac (pericardium) that encloses the heart.

Pericardium Two-layer serous membrane lining the pericardial cavity.

Perinatal From the twenty-eighth week of gestation through the first 7 days after delivery.

Perineal body See *Perineum.*

Perineum The tissue between the mother's vaginal and rectal openings; may be torn during delivery.

Periodontal membrane/ligament Ligamentous attachment between the root of a tooth and the socket of the bone within which it sits.

Periosteum Fibrous connective tissue rich in nerve endings that envelops bone.

Peripheral nervous system All the nerves outside the central nervous system.

Peripheral vein A vein outside the chest or abdomen, such as the veins of the upper and lower extremities.

Peripherally inserted central catheter (PICC) line A thin tube inserted into a peripheral vein (usually the arm) and threaded into the superior vena cava to allow fluid or medication administration.

Peristalsis The wavelike contraction of the smooth muscle of the gastrointestinal tract.

Peritoneal cavity The space between the parietal and visceral peritoneum; also called the *peritoneal space.*

Peritoneum Double-layered serous membrane that lines the abdominal cavity and covers the organs located in it.

Peritonitis Inflammation of the peritoneum, typically caused by infection or in response to contact with blood or digestive fluids.

Peritonsillar abscess (PTA) An infection of tissue between the tonsil and pharynx, usually the result of a significant infection in the tonsils.

Permeability Ability of a membrane channel to allow passage of electrolytes once it is open.

Permissible exposure limit Allowable air concentration of a substance in the workplace as established by the Occupational Safety and Health Administration; these values are legally enforceable.

Permit-required confined space A confined space with one or more of the following characteristics: (1) contains or has a potential to contain a hazardous atmosphere; (2) contains a material with the potential for engulfing an entrant; (3) has an internal configuration such that an entrant could be trapped or asphyxiated by inwardly converging walls or by a floor that slopes downward and tapers to a smaller cross-section; or (4) contains any other recognized serious safety or health hazard.

Personal protective equipment (PPE) Equipment used to protect personnel; includes items such as gloves, eyewear, masks, respirators, and gowns.

Personal space The area around an individual that the person perceives as an extension of himself or herself. In the United States, personal distance is 1.5 to 4 feet.

Personality disorders Patterns of interacting with others and the world that are rigid and harmful, causing social and occupational problems.

Pertinent negative In a patient assessment, the signs and symptoms found not to be present that support a working diagnosis.

Pertinent positive In a patient assessment, the signs and symptoms found to be present that support a working diagnosis.

Pesticide A chemical material used to control a pest (insect, weed, etc.).

Petechiae A tiny pinpoint rash on the upper area of the neck and the face; may indicate near strangulation or suffocation; caused by an occlusion of venous return from the head while arterial pressure remains normal; may be present in mothers after childbirth; reddish-purple nonblanchable discolorations in the skin less than 0.5 cm in diameter.

pH A numeric assignment used to define the hydrogen ion concentration of a given chemical. The lower the pH, the higher the hydrogen ion concentration and the more acidic the solution.

Phagocyte Cells that are part of the body's immune system that play a predominant role in the destruction of invading microorganisms.

Phagocytosis Ingestion and digestion of foreign materials by phagocytes (cells, such as macrophages, designed to perform this function).

Pharmaceutics The science of preparing and dispensing drugs.

Pharmacogenetics The study of inherited differences (variation) in drug metabolism and response.

Pharmacokinetics The process by which a drug is absorbed, distributed, metabolized, and eliminated by the body.

Pharmacologic restraints Agents such as sedatives that can suppress a patient's neurologic and/or motor capabilities so that the threat to the paramedic is reduced; also known as *chemical restraints.*

Pharmacology The study of drugs, including their actions and effects on the host.

Pharmacopeia A book describing drugs, chemicals, and medicinal preparations in a country or specific geographic area, including a description of the drug, its formula, and dosage.

Phases of rescue The training and organizational concept that groups all the activities that take place at a typical vehicle crash with entrapment into four categories, with each known as a phase of rescue.

Phlebitis Inflammation of a vein.

Phobia An intense fear of a particular object or situation.

Phosphate A salt of phosphoric acid that is important in the maintenance of the acid-base balance of the blood.

Phospholipid bilayer A double layer composed of three types of lipid molecules that comprise the plasma membrane.

Photoreceptor cells Rods and cones contained in the sensory part of the retina; they relay impulses to the optic nerve.

Photosensitivity A condition in which the patient's eyes are sensitive or feel pain when exposed to bright light.

Physical abuse Inflicting a nonaccidental physical injury on another person such as punching, kicking, hitting, or biting.

Physical disabilities Disabilities that involve limitation of mobility.

Physical restraints Straps, splints, and other devices that prevent movement of all or part of the patient's body.

Physician advisor A physician responsible for the oversight of the EMS system and the actions of the paramedics; also known as a *medical director.*

Physiology Study of how the body functions.

Pia mater Last meningeal layer; adheres to the central nervous system.

Pierre Robin sequence A congenital anomaly characterized by a very small lower jaw (micrognathia), a tongue that tends to fall back and downward (glossoptosis), and cleft palate.

Pill Dried powder forms of medication in the form of a small pellet; the term "pill" has been replaced with tablet and capsule.

Pinch points A machinery entanglement hazard formed when two machine parts move together and at least one of the parts moves in a circle.

Pinocytosis Absorption or ingestion of nutrients, debris, and fluids by a cell.

Placards Diamond-shaped signs placed on the sides and ends of bulk transport containers (e.g., truck, tank car, freight container) that carry hazardous materials.

Placenta (afterbirth) The organ inside the uterus that exchanges nutrition and waste between mother and fetus.

Placenta previa Placement of the placenta such that it partially or completely covers the cervix.

Placental abruption (abruptio placenta) Separation of part of the placenta away from the wall of the uterus.

Placental barrier Many layers of cells that form between maternal and fetal circulation that protect the fetus from toxins.

Plague An acute infectious disease caused by the anaerobic, gram-negative bacterium *Yersinia pestis;* transmitted naturally from rodents to human beings through flea bites; three common syndromes are bubonic (most likely form of the disease to be seen from naturally occurring infections), pneumonic (most likely form of the disease to result from an act of terrorism), and septicemic plague.

Plaintiff The person who initiates a lawsuit by filing a complaint; also known as a *claimant, petitioner,* or *applicant.*

Planning Supplies past, present, and future information about the incident.

Plaque An elevated, solid lesion usually greater than 0.5 cm in diameter that lacks any deep component.

Plasma Pale, yellow material in the blood; made of approximately 92% water and 8% dissolved molecules.

Plasma level profile The measurement of blood level of a medication versus the dosage administered.

Plasma membrane The outer covering of a cell that contains the cellular cytoplasm; also known as the *cell membrane.*

Platelets One of three formed elements in the blood; also called *thrombocytes.*

Pleura Serous membrane that lines the pleural cavity.

Pleural cavities Areas that contain the lungs.

Pleural effusion Collection of fluid in the pleural space, usually fluid that has seeped through the lung or chest wall tissue.

Pleural friction rub Noise made when the visceral and parietal pleura rub together.

Pleurisy Painful rubbing of the pleural lining.

Plural Amount that refers to more than one person, place, or thing.

Pluripotent Cell line that has the ability to differentiate into multiple different cell lines based on the right physiologic stimulus.

Pneumomediastinum Air entrapped within the mediastinum; a serious medical condition.

Pneumonia An inflammation and infection of the lower airway and lungs caused by a viral, bacterial, parasitic, or fungal organism.

Pneumonia Infection of the lungs.

Pneumothorax A collection of air in the pleural space, usually from either a hole in the lung or a hole in the chest wall.

Pocket mask A clear, semirigid mask designed for mouth-to-mask ventilation of a nonbreathing adult, child, or infant.

Poikilothermic An organism whose temperature matches the ambient temperature.

Point of maximum impulse (PMI) The apical impulse; the site where the heartbeat is most strongly felt.

Poison Any substance that can harm the human body; also known as a *toxin.*

Poisoning Exposure to a substance that is harmful in any dosage.

Poisonous Describes gases, liquids, or other substances of such nature that exposure to a very small amount is dangerous to life or is a hazard to health; also known as *toxic* (e.g., cyanide, arsenic, phosgene, aniline, methyl bromide, insecticides, pesticides).

Polarized state Period after repolarization of a myocardial cell (also called the *resting state*) when the outside of the cell is positive and the interior of the cell is negative.

Poliomyelitis Viral infection that tends to attack the motor roots of the spinal nerves, often leading to physical disability and even paralysis of the diaphragm.

Polydipsia Excessive thirst.

Polymorphic Varying in shape.

Polyphagia Excessive eating.

Polypharmacy The concurrent use of several medications.

Polyuria Excessive urination.

Pons Area of the brainstem that contains the sleep and respiratory centers for the body, which along with the medulla control breathing.

Portable radio Also referred to as a *walkie-talkie.* These radios are carried by emergency personnel and have a lower wattage output than the mobile or base unit. To use these portable radios with a higher watt output, the units can be connected through a repeater system to increase their output, which increases range.

Portal hypertension Increased venous pressure in the portal circulation.

Portal vein A vein composed of a group of vessels that originate from the digestive system.

Positive battery cable Also known as the *hot cable,* this electrical power cable allows a vehicle's electrical system to carry the current or electrical energy from the battery to the electrically powered appliances throughout the vehicle.

Positive end-expiratory pressure (PEEP) The amount of pressure above atmospheric pressure present in the airway at the end of the expiratory cycle. When forcing air into the lungs (positive-pressure ventilation), airway pressure is maintained above atmospheric pressure at the end of exhalation by means of a mechanical device, such as a PEEP valve.

Positive-pressure ventilation Forcing air into the lungs.

Postconcussion syndrome Symptoms of a concussion that persist for weeks to 1 year after an initial injury to the head.

Posterior The back, or dorsal, surface.

Postganglionic neuron The nerve that travels from the ganglia to the desired organ or tissue.

Postictal State that begins at the termination of seizure activity in the brain and ends with the patient returning to a level of normal behavior.

Postnatal The period immediately following the birth of a child and lasting for approximately 6 weeks.

Postpartum Pertaining to the mother after delivery.

Posttraumatic stress disorder (PTSD) An anxiety disorder that occurs after a traumatic, often life-threatening event.

Posture A patient's overall attitude and frame of mind.

Potassium The main intracellular ion (electrolyte), with the chemical designation K+.

Potential difference Difference in electrical charge between two points in a circuit; expressed in volts or millivolts.

Potentiating To augment or increase the action of.

Potentiation A prolongation or increase in the effect of a drug by another drug.

Pounds per square inch (psi) The amount of pressure on an area that is 1 inch square.

Poverty of speech A disorder of thought form characterized by very little spontaneous, voluntary speech and short answers to questions.

Powder Medication ground into a fine substance.

power take-off Element that connects a tractor to an implement; also called a *driveshaft.*

Prearrival instructions Clinically approved instructions provided by telephone by a trained and certified emergency medical dispatcher.

Precapillary sphincters Smooth muscle located at the entrances to the capillaries; responsive to local tissue needs.

Preeclampsia A complication of pregnancy that includes hypertension, swelling of the extremities and, in its most severe form, seizures (see *Eclampsia*).

Preexcitation Term used to describe rhythms that originate from above the ventricles but in which the impulse travels by a pathway other than the atrioventricular node and bundle of His; thus the supraventricular impulse excites the ventricles earlier than normal.

Prefix A sequence of letters that comes before the word root and often describes a variation of the norm.

Preganglionic neuron The nerve that extends from the spinal cord (central nervous system) to the ganglion.

Prehospital care report (PCR) The report written by the paramedic after the call has been completed. The report becomes part of the patient's permanent medical record.

Preload Force exerted by the blood on the walls of the ventricles at the end of diastole.

Premature birth Delivery between the twentieth and thirty-seventh weeks of pregnancy.

Premature complex Early beat occurring before the next expected beat; can be atrial or ventricular.

Premature or preterm infant Infant born before 37 completed weeks of completed gestation.

Prenatal Preceding birth.

Preoccupation A topic or theme that consistently recurs in a person's thought process and conversations.

Prepuce A fold formed by the union of the labia minora over the clitoris.

Presbycusis Age-related hearing loss.

Presbyopia Loss of function of the lens to adjust to close reading; usual onset in middle age.

Presenting part The first part of the infant to appear at the vaginal opening, usually the head.

Pressured speech Rapid, loud, and intense speech that often results from racing thoughts and frequently is seen during manic episodes.

Preterm birth Birth before 37 weeks of gestation.

Preterm delivery Delivery between the twentieth and thirty-seventh weeks of pregnancy.

Prevalence rate The fraction of the population that currently has a certain disease.

Priapism A prolonged and painful erection.

Primary apnea The newly born's initial response to hypoxemia consisting of initial tachypnea, then apnea, bradycardia, and a slight increase in blood pressure; if stimulated, responds with resumption of breathing.

Primary blast injury Injuries caused by an explosive's pressure wave.

Primary cord injury A spinal cord injury caused by a direct traumatic blow.

Primary hypertension High blood pressure for which no cause is identifiable; also called *essential hypertension.*

Primary injury prevention Keeping an injury from occurring.

Primary skin lesion A lesion that has not been altered by scratching, rubbing, scrubbing, or other types of trauma.

Primary triage The initial sorting of patients to determine which are most injured and in need of immediate care.

Primary tumor A collection of cells that grow out of control, far in excess of normal rates. A primary tumor is a tumor that develops in one tissue only (e.g., a liver primary tumor originates in the liver).

Primigravida A woman who is pregnant for the first time.

Primipara A woman who has given birth to her first child.

Primum non nocere Latin for "first, do no harm."

Prions Infectious agents composed of only proteins.

Prodromal An early symptom of a disease.

Prodrome A symptom indication the onset of a disease.

Prodrug A substance that is inactive when it is given and is converted to an active form within the body.

Profession A group of similar jobs or fields of interest that involve a responsibility to serve the public and require mastery of specific knowledge and specialized skills.

Professional A person who has special knowledge and skills and conforms to high standards of conduct and performance.

Professional malpractice A type of tort case addressing whether a professional person failed to act as a reasonably prudent and careful person with similar training would act under similar circumstances.

Professionalism Following the standards of conduct and performance for a profession.

Progesterone A female hormone secreted after ovulation has occurred that causes changes in the lining of the uterus necessary for successful implantation of a fertilized egg.

Prokaryotes One of the kingdoms of cells; simpler in structure and found in lower life forms such as bacteria.

Proliferative phase Portion of the menstrual cycle in which the endometrial lining grows under the influence of estrogen.

Prone Position in which the patient is lying on his or her stomach (face down).

Proprioception Ability to sense the orientation, location, and movement of the body's parts relative to other body parts.

Prospective medical direction Physician participation in the development of EMS protocols, procedures, and participation in the education and testing of EMS professionals; a type of offline medical direction.

Prostaglandins A class of fatty acids that has many of the properties of hormones.

Prostate Glandular tissue that produces prostatic fluid and muscular portion that contracts during ejaculation to prevent urine flow; dorsal to the symphysis pubis and the base of the urinary bladder.

Protein Any one of a number of large molecules composed of amino acids that form the structural components of cells or carry out biochemical functions.

Protocols A set of treatment guidelines written for the paramedic to follow.

Protoxin A substance converted to a toxin through a biochemical process in the body; would be harmless if they were not converted (e.g., methanol and ethylene glycol).

Proximal A position nearer to the attachment of a limb to the trunk.

Pruritus Itching of the skin.

Psoriasis A common chronic skin disorder characterized by erythematous papules and plaques with a silver scale.

Psychological abuse The verbal or psychological misuse of another person, including threatening, name calling, ignoring, shaming unfairly, shouting, and cursing; mind games are another form of psychological abuse.

Psychomotor Pertaining to motor effects of cerebral or psychic activity.

Psychomotor agitation Excessive motor activity that is usually nonproductive and tedious, resulting from inner tensions (pacing, fidgeting, hand wringing, etc.)

Psychoses A group of mental disorders in which the individual loses contact with reality; psychosis is thought to be related to complex biochemical disease that disorders brain function. Examples include schizophrenia, bipolar disease (also known as *manic-depressive illness*), and organic brain disease.

Psychosis An abnormal state of widespread brain dysfunction characterized by bizarre thought content, typically delusions and hallucinations.

Psychosocial development The social and psychological changes human beings undergo as they grow and age.

Psychosocial factors Life events that affect a person's emotional state, such as marriage, divorce, or death of a loved one.

Public health The discipline that studies the overall health of populations and intervenes on behalf of those populations rather than on behalf of individuals.

Public Safety Answering Point (PSAP) A dispatch center set up to receive and dispatch 9-1-1 calls.

Pull-in point Machinery entanglement hazard created when an operator attempts to remove material being pulled into a machine.

Pulmonary abscess A collection of pus within the lung itself.

Pulmonary arteries Left and right pulmonary arteries supplying the lungs.

Pulmonary bleb Cavity in the lung much like a balloon; may rupture to create a pneumothorax.

Pulmonary circulation Blood from the right ventricle is pumped directly to the lungs for oxygenation through the pulmonary trunk; blood becomes oxygenated and is then delivered through the pulmonary arteries for the left atrium.

Pulmonary edema A buildup of fluid in the lungs, usually a complication of left ventricular fibrillation.

Pulmonary embolism Movement of a clot into the pulmonary circulation.

Pulmonary embolus A blood clot that has lodged in the pulmonary artery, causing shortness of breath and hypoxia.

Pulmonary trunk Vessels that deliver blood from the right ventricle of the heart to the lungs for oxygenation.

Pulmonary veins Vessels that return blood to the left atrium of the heart.

Pulmonic valve Right semilunar valve; separates the right ventricle and the pulmonary trunk.

Pulp Center of a tooth that contains nerves, blood vessels, and connective tissue.

Pulse deficit A difference between the apical pulse and the peripheral pulse rates.

Pulse generator Power source that houses the battery and controls for regulating a pacemaker.

Pulse oximetry A noninvasive method of measuring the percentage of oxygen-bound hemoglobin.

Pulse pressure The difference between the systolic and diastolic blood pressures.

Pulseless electrical activity (PEA) Organized electrical activity observed on a cardiac monitor (other than ventricular tachycardia) without the patient having a palpable pulse.

Pulsus alternans A beat-to-beat difference in the strength of a pulse (also called *mechanical alternans*).

Pulsus paradoxus A fall in systolic blood pressure of more than 10 mm Hg during inspiration (also called *paradoxic pulse*).

Pupil Central opening in the iris.

Purkinje fibers Fibers found in both ventricles that conduct an electrical impulse through the heart.

Purpura Reddish-purple nonblanchable discolorations greater than 0.5 cm in diameter; large purpura are called ecchymoses.

Pustule A lesion that contains purulent material.

Pyelonephritis Infection of the kidney.

Pyrogenic Substances, such as endotoxins from certain bacteria, that stimulate the body to produce a fever.

Pyrophorics Substances that form self-ignitable flammable vapors when in contact with air.

QRS complex Several waveforms (Q wave, R wave, and S wave) that represent the spread of an electrical impulse through the ventricles (ventricular depolarization).

Quadriplegia Paralysis affecting all four extremities.

Quality assurance Programs designed to achieve a desired level of care.

Quality improvement Programs designed to improve the level of care; commonly driven by quality assurance.

Quality improvement unit (QIU) Trained and certified quality specialists who have the knowledge and skills to measure dispatcher performance against established standards accurately and consistently.

Quarantine The seclusion of groups of exposed but asymptomatic individuals for monitoring.

Quick response unit A type of responder with paramedic-level skills but no transport capability.

R wave On an EGG, the first positive deflection in the QRS complex, representing ventricular depolarization.

Raccoon eyes Bruising around the orbits of the eyes.

Racing thoughts The subjective feeling that one's thoughts are moving so fast that one cannot keep up; often seen during manic episodes.

415

Radio frequency Channel that allows communication from one specific user to another. For simple communication, both users must be on the same frequency or channel.

Radioactive The ability to emit ionizing radioactive energy.

Radioactive substances Any material or combination of materials that spontaneously emit ionizing radiation and have a specific activity greater than 0.002 mcCi/g (e.g., plutonium, cobalt, uranium 235, radioactive waste).

Radioactivity The spontaneous disintegration of unstable nuclei accompanied by the emission of nuclear radiation.

Range of motion The full and natural range of a joint's movement.

Rapid medical assessment A quick head-to-toe assessment of a medical patient who is unresponsive or has an altered mental status.

Rapid sequence intubation (RSI) The use of medications to sedate and paralyze a patient to achieve endotracheal intubation rapidly.

Rapid trauma assessment A quick head-to-toe assessment of a trauma patient with a significant mechanism of injury.

Rattles (rhonchi) Attributable to inflammation and mucus or fluid in the larger airway passages; descriptive of airway congestion heard on inspiration. Rhonchi are commonly associated with bronchitis or pneumonia.

Red blood cell count The number of red blood cells per liter of blood.

Rebound tenderness Discomfort experienced by the patient that occurs when the pressure from palpation is released.

Receptor A molecule, such as a protein, found inside or on the surface of a cell that binds to a specific substance (such as hormones, antigens, drugs, or neurotransmitters) and causes a specific physiologic effect in the cell.

Reciprocal change Mirror image ECG changes seen in the wall of the heart opposite the location of an infarction.

Reciprocity The ability for an EMS professional to use his or her certification or license to be able to practice in a different state.

Recompression A method used to treat divers with certain diving disorders, such as decompression sickness.

Rectal The drug administration route for suppositories; the drug is placed into the rectum (colon) and is absorbed into the venous circulation.

Rectum End of the sigmoid colon; feces are further compacted into waste here.

Reentry Spread of an impulse through tissue already stimulated by that same impulse.

Referred pain Pain felt at a site distant to the organ of origin.

Reflection Echoing the patient's message using your own words.

Reflection on actions A final step that may involve a personal reflection or a run critique; in certain instances this may be done formally, but in most instances it is accomplished informally.

Refractoriness Period of recovery that cells need after being discharged before they are able to respond to a stimulus.

Refresher education The process of refreshing information and skills previously learned.

Registration The process of entering an individual's name and essential information into a record as a means of verifying initial certification and monitoring recertification.

Regurgitation Backward flow of blood through a valve during ventricular contraction of the heart.

Rejection In terms of organ transplantation, the process by which the body uses its immune system to identify a transplanted organ and kill it; the medical management of posttransplant patients is largely directed at preventing rejection.

Relative refractory period Corresponds with the downslope of the T wave; cardiac cells can be stimulated to depolarize if the stimulus is strong enough.

Relief medic Emergency medical technician who has obtained additional training and certification in disaster and relief medical operations.

Rem Roentgen equivalent man.

Renal calculi Kidney stones formed by substances such as calcium, uric acid, or cystine.

Renal corpuscle Large terminal end of the nephron.

Renal insufficiency A decrease in renal function to approximately 25% of normal.

Renal pyramids Number of divisions in the kidney.

Repeater A system that receives transmissions from a low-wattage radio and rebroadcasts the signal at a higher wattage to the dispatch center.

Reperfusion phenomenon Series of events that result from the reperfusion of tissue damaged in a crush injury or tissue that is profoundly hypoxic; can lead to crush syndrome (rhabdomyolysis).

Repolarization Movement of ions across a cell membrane in which the inside of the cell is restored to its negative charge.

Res ipsa loquitur Latin phrase meaning "the thing speaks for itself." In negligence cases, this doctrine can be imposed when the plaintiff cannot prove all four components of negligence, but the injury itself would not have occurred without negligence (e.g., a sponge left in a patient after surgery).

Rescue The act of delivery from danger or entrapment.

Residual volume After a maximal forced exhalation, the amount of air remaining in the lungs and airway passages not able to be expelled.

Resistance The amount of weight moved or lifted during isotonic exercise. Also the ability of the body to defend itself against disease-causing microorganisms.

Resistance stage The stage of the stress response in which the specific stimulus no longer elicits an alarm reaction.

Respiration The exchange of gases between a living organism and its environment.

respiratory arrest Absence of breathing.

respiratory distress Increased work of breathing (ventilatory effort).

Respiratory failure Failure of the ventilation system of the body to provide sufficient oxygen to the body; does not require apnea.

Respiratory membrane Where gas exchange takes place; oxygen is picked up in the bloodstream and carbon dioxide is eliminated through the lungs.

Respiratory syncytial virus A virus linked to bronchiolitis in infants and children.

Respiratory tract Passages to move air to and from the exchange surfaces.

Respondeat superior Latin phrase meaning "let the master answer." Under this legal doctrine, an employer is liable for the acts of employees within their scope of employment.

Response area The geographic area assigned to an emergency vehicle for responding to the sick and injured.

Response assignment plan An approved, consistent plan for responding to each call type.

Response mode A type of response, either with or without lights and sirens use.

Response time The time from when the call is received until the paramedics arrive at the scene.

Restraint Any mechanism that physically restricts an individual's freedom of movement, physical activity, or normal access to his or her body.

Restraint asphyxia Suffocation of a patient stemming from an inability to expand the chest cavity during inspiration because of restraint and immobilization.

Reticular activating system Group of specialized neurons in the brainstem; involved in sleep and wake cycles; maintains consciousness.

Reticular cells The cells forming the reticular fibers of connective tissue; those forming the framework of lymph nodes, bone marrow, and spleen are part of the reticuloendothelial system and under appropriate stimulation may differentiate into macrophages.

Reticular dermis Section of the dermis composed of larger and denser collagen fibers; provides most of the skin's elasticity and strength. This layer contains most of the skin structures located within the dermis.

Reticular formation A cloud of neurons in the brainstem and midbrain responsible for maintaining consciousness.

Retina Outer pigmented area and inner sensory layer that responds to light.

Retinal detachment A condition in which the retina is lifted or pulled from its normal position, resulting in a loss of vision.

Retractions Sinking in of the soft tissues above the sternum or clavicle or between or below the ribs during inhalation.

Retreat Leaving the scene when danger is observed or when violence or indicators of violence are displayed; requires immediate and decisive action.

Retrograde Moving backward or moving in the opposite direction to that which is considered normal.

Retrograde amnesia The inability to remember events or recall memories from before an event in which the head was struck.

Retroperitoneal Abdominopelvic organs found behind the peritoneum.

Retrospective medical direction Physician review of prehospital care reports and participation in the quality improvement process; a type of offline medical direction.

Reuptake Absorption of neurotransmitters from the synapse into the presynaptic neuron to be reused or destroyed.

Review of systems A review of symptoms for each organ system.

Rhabdomyolysis Complex series of events that occur in patients with severe muscle injury (e.g., crush injuries); destruction of the muscle tissues results in a release of cellular material and acidosis that can lead to acute renal failure.

Rheumatoid arthritis A painful, disabling disease in which the body's immune system attacks the joints.

Rhinitis Runny nose; inflammation of the mucous membranes of the nose, usually accompanied by swelling of the mucosa and a nasal discharge.

Rhinorrhea Persistent discharge of fluid (such as blood or cerebrospinal fluid) from the nose.

Rhonchi Rattling or rumbling in the lungs.

Ribonucleic acid (RNA) Specialized structures within the cell that carry genetic material for reproduction.

Ribosome Substance in organelle where new protein is synthesized; forms the framework for the genetic blueprint.

Right A position toward the right side of the body.

Right block or left block Terms describing a responding vehicle arriving on scene and turning at a right or left angle. In this block position, the emergency vehicle acts as a physical barrier between the crash scene work area and approaching traffic.

Right coronary artery Blood vessel that provides oxygenated blood to the right side of the heart muscle.

Risk factors Traits and lifestyle habits that may increase a person's chance of developing a disease.

Risus sardonicus Distorted grinning expression caused by involuntary contraction of the facial muscles.

Roentgens Denote ionizing radiation passing through air.

Rolling the dash Rescue tasks involving strategic cuts to the firewall structure followed by pushing, spreading, or even pulling equipment to move the dash, firewall, steering wheel, column, and pedals away from front seat occupants.

Rollover protective structure A structure mounted on a tractor designed to support the weight of the tractor if an overturn occurs; if a tractor has this structure and the operator wears a seat belt, the operator will stay in the safety zone if the tractor overturns.

Root word In medical terminology, the part of the word that gives the primary meaning.

Rotor-wing aircraft Helicopter that can be used for hospital-to-hospital and scene-to-hospital transports;

417

usually travels a shorter distance and is used in the prehospital setting for certain types of transport.

Routes of administration Various methods of giving drugs, including oral, enteral, parenteral, and inhalational.

Rovsing's sign Palpation of the abdomen in the left lower quadrant elicits pain in the right lower quadrant.

S1 The sound of the bicuspid and mitral valves closing.

S2 The sound of the closing of the pulmonary and aortic valves.

Sacrum (sacral vertebrae) A heavy, large bone at the base of the spinal cord between the lumbar vertebrae and the coccyx. Roughly triangular in shape, it comprises the back of the pelvis and is made of the five sacral vertebrae fused together.

Safety officer The person responsible for ensuring that no unsafe acts occur during the emergency incident.

Sagittal plane Imaginary straight line that runs vertically through the middle of the body, creating right and left halves.

Saliva Mucus that lubricates material like food that is placed in it; enzymes begin the digestive process of starchy material.

Salivary glands Located in the oral cavity; produce saliva.

Saponification A form of necrosis in which fatty acids combine with certain electrolytes to form soaps.

Sarin A nerve agent.

Saturation of peripheral oxygen The percentage of hemoglobin saturated with oxygen (SpO_2).

Scabies A contagious skin disease of the epidermis marked by itching and small raised red spots caused by the itch mite *(Sarcoptes scabiei)*.

Scale Thick stratum corneum that results from hyper-proliferation or increased cohesion of keratinocytes (can include eczema or psoriasis).

Scar A collection of new connective tissue; may be hypertrophic or atrophic and implies dermoepidermal damage.

Schizophrenia A group of disorders characterized by psychotic symptoms, thought disorder, and negative symptoms (social isolation and withdrawal); types include paranoid, disorganized, and catatonic.

Sciatica Pain in the lumbar back and leg caused by irritation and impingement of the sciatic nerve, usually from a herniated disc.

Sclera Firm, opaque, white outer layer of the eye; helps maintain the shape of the eye.

Scope of practice A predefined set of skills, interventions, or other activities that the paramedic is legally authorized to perform when necessary; usually set by state law or regulation and local medical direction.

Scrotum Loose layer of connective tissue that support the testes.

Sebaceous glands Found in the dermis; secrete oil (sebum) in the shaft of the hair follicle and the skin.

Sebum Oil secreted by the sebaceous glands in the shaft of the hair follicle and the skin; prevents excessive drying of the skin and hair; also protects from some forms of bacteria.

Second messenger A molecule that relays signals from a receptor on the surface of a cell to target molecules in the cell's nucleus or internal fluid where a physiologic action is to take place; also called a *biochemical messenger.*

Secondary apnea When asphyxia is prolonged, a period of deep, gasping respirations with a simultaneous fall in blood pressure and heart rate; gasping becomes weaker and slower and then ceases.

Secondary blast injury Injuries caused by shrapnel from the fragments of an explosive device and from things that have been attached to it.

Secondary contamination The risk of another person or health care provider becoming contaminated with a hazardous material by contact with a contaminated victim.

Secondary cord injury A spinal cord injury that develops over time after a traumatic injury to the spinal column or the blood vessels that supply the spinal cord with blood. Generally caused by ischemia, swelling, or compression.

Secondary device An explosive, chemical, or biologic device hidden at the scene of an emergency and set to detonate or release its agent after emergency response personnel are on scene.

Secondary hypertension High blood pressure that has an identifiable cause, such as medications or an underlying disease or condition.

Secondary injury prevention Preventing further injury from an event that has already occurred.

Secondary skin lesion Any lesion that has been altered by scratching, scrubbing, or other types of trauma.

Secondary triage Conducted after the primary search; determines the order of treatment and transport of the remaining patients.

Secondary tumor A tumor that has spread from its original location (e.g., lung tumor that spreads to brain); also called *metastasis.*

Secretion Release of water, acids, enzymes, and buffers that aid in the breakdown and digestion of food in the digestive tract.

Secretory phase Portion of the menstrual cycle in which the corpus luteum secretes progesterone to maintain the endometrial lining in case of fertilization.

Sedative-hypnotics Prescription central nervous system depressant drugs that cause powerful relaxation and euphoria when abused; typically barbiturates and benzodiazepines.

Segment Line between waveforms; named by the waveform that precedes and follows it.

Seizure A temporary alteration in behavior or consciousness caused by abnormal electrical activity of one or more groups of neurons in the brain.

Self-injury An unhealthy coping mechanism involving intentionally injuring one's own body, often through cutting or burning oneself to relieve emotional tension; also known as *self-mutilation.*

Sellick maneuver Technique used to compress the cricoid cartilage against the cervical vertebrae, causing occlusion of the esophagus, thereby reducing the risk of aspiration; cricoid pressure.

Semicircular canals Three bony fluid-filled loops in the internal ear; involved in balance of the body.

Semilunar (SL) valves Valves shaped like half moons that separate the ventricles from the aorta and pulmonary artery.

Seminal fluid Liquid produced in the seminal vesicles.

Seminal vesicles Ducts that produce seminal fluids.

Sensing Ability of a pacemaker to recognize and respond to intrinsic electrical activity.

Sensorineural hearing loss A type of deafness that occurs when the tiny hair cells in the cochlea are damaged or destroyed. In addition, damage to the auditory nerve prevents sounds from being transmitted from the cochlea to the brain.

Sensory cortex Area of brain tissue on the frontal lobe responsible for receiving sensory information from different parts of the body.

Sepsis Pathologic state, usually accompanied by fever, resulting from the presence of microorganisms or their poisonous products in the bloodstream; commonly called *blood poisoning.*

Septic abortion An abortion associated with intrauterine infection.

Septic arthritis Invasion of microorganisms into a joint space, causing infection of the joint.

Septic shock Sepsis with hypotension, despite adequate fluid resuscitation, along with the presence of perfusion abnormalities that may include lactic acidosis, decreased urine output, and a sudden change in mental status.

Septicemia A serious medical condition characterized by vasodilation that leads to hypotension, tissue hypoxia, and eventually shock; usually caused by gram-negative bacteria; diagnosed by blood tests called cultures.

Septum Tough piece of tissue that divides the left and right halves of the heart.

Serious apnea Cessation of breathing for longer than 20 seconds or any duration if accompanied by cyanosis and sinus bradycardia.

Serosanguineous discharge Blood and fluid discharged from the body.

Serous membrane Membrane that lines the thoracic, abdominal, and pelvic cavities; composed of the parietal membrane, which adheres to the cavity wall, and the visceral membrane, which adheres to the organ.

Serum base deficit Implies that the blood buffer, bicarbonate, is being used to combat a metabolic acidosis. Metabolic acidosis occurs in the setting of numerous shock states, such as burn shock. This number is reported on a standard blood gas assay and is detected in an arterial or venous blood sample.

Serum lactate Measure in the blood; a byproduct of anaerobic metabolism. As such, it is a good measure of end organ and cellular perfusion in shock states. Elevated serum lactate levels, or lactic acidemia, implies that cells, tissues, or organs are not receiving adequate oxygen to carry out their metabolic activities.

Sesamoid bones Specialized bones found within tendons where they cross a joint; designed to protect the joint (e.g., the patella [kneecap]).

Severe sepsis Sepsis associated with organ dysfunction, shock, or hypotension.

Sexual abuse Forced and/or coerced sex, violent sexual acts against the victim's will (rape), or witholding sex from the victim; includes fondling, intercourse, incest, rape, sodomy, exhibitionism, sexual exploitation, or exposure to pornography. According to the National Center on Child Abuse and Neglect, to be considered child abuse these acts must be committed by a person responsible for the care of a child (e.g., a babysitter, parent, or daycare provider) or related to the child. Child sexual abuse includes a range of behaviors such as oral, anal, or genital penile penetration; genital contact with no intrusion; fondling of a child's breasts or buttocks; indecent exposure; inadequate or inappropriate supervision of a child's voluntary sexual activities; and use of a child in prostitution, pornography, Internet crimes, or other sexually exploitative activities. If a stranger commits these acts, it is considered sexual assault and handled solely by the police and criminal courts.

Sexual assault Sexually explicit conduct used as an expression of interpersonal violence against another individual; nonconsenting sexual acts achieved through power and control.

Shaft The length of a needle; the needle shaft connects to the hub. Also called the *cannula.*

Shear points Hazardous machinery locations created when the edges of two objects are moved toward or next to one another closely enough to cut a relatively soft material.

Shingles Infection of a nerve, often by the herpes zoster virus, causing severe pain and a rash along a unilateral dermatome.

Shock Inadequate systemic perfusion.

Short bones Specialized bones of the skeleton designed for compactness and strength, often with limited movement (e.g., bones of the wrist [carpals])

Short haul The transport of one or more people externally suspended below a helicopter.

Shoulder dystocia Impaction of a newborn's anterior shoulder underneath the mother's pubic bone, slowing or preventing delivery.

Shunt Insertion of catheters into an artery and a vein from outside the body. Most shunts are located on the forearm. When not in use to dialyze a patient, the catheters are connected to each other with clear tubing, allowing the continuous flow of blood from artery to vein, then covered with self-adhering roller gauze for protection.

Side effect An effect of a drug other than the one for which it was given; may or may not be harmful.

Side impact airbags Deployable airbags located inside any or all vehicle doors, front and rear outboard seatbacks, as well as along all or a portion of the roof line.

Sighing Involuntary and periodic slow, deep breath followed by a prolonged expiratory phase. Occurring approximately once per minute, the act of sighing is thought to open atelectatic (collapsed) alveoli.

419

Sigmoid colon Part of the large intestine.

Signs and symptoms Signs are a medical or trauma condition of the patient that can be seen, heard, smelled, measured, or felt during an examination. Symptoms are conditions described by the patient, such as shortness of breath, or pieces of information bystanders tell you about the patient's chief complaint.

Silo gas The gases produced from the fermentation of plant material inside a silo.

Simple asphyxiants Inert gases and vapors that displace oxygen in inspired air (e.g., carbon dioxide, nitrogen).

Simple partial seizure A seizure affecting only one part of the brain without an alteration in consciousness.

Simple pneumothorax Injury to the thoracic cavity in which a lung is ruptured, allowing air into the space between the chest wall and the lungs.

Simplex A system that allows only one-at-a-time communication. The transmission cannot be interrupted; both operators use the same frequency.

Singular command Command type involving one agency.

Sinoatrial node Pacemaker site of the heart; where impulse formation begins in the heart.

Sinus block (barosinusitis) A condition of acute or chronic inflammation of one or more of the paranasal sinuses; produced by a negative pressure difference between the air in the sinuses and the surrounding atmospheric air.

Sinus rhythm A normal heart rhythm.

Sinuses Cavities within the bones of the skull that connect to the nasal cavity.

Situational awareness The state of being aware of everything occurring in the surrounding environment and the relative importance of all these events.

Size-up The art of assessing conditions that exist or can potentially exist at an incident scene.

Skeletal muscles Muscles that affect movement of the skeleton, usually by voluntary contractions.

Skin grafting Transplantation of skin, either from the same person or from a cadaver, to the site of a wound, such as a burn.

Skin turgor The elasticity of the skin; good skin turgor returns the skin's natural shape within 2 seconds.

Slander False statements spoken about a person that blacken the person's character or injure his or her reputation.

Slipped capital femoral epiphysis A disease in which a posterior displacement of the growth plate of the femur occurs (the epiphysis).

SLUDGEM Mnemonic for *s*alivation, *l*acrimation, *u*rination, *d*efecation, *g*astrointestinal pain, *e*mesis, and *m*iosis.

Smallpox A disease caused by variola viruses, which are members of the Orthopoxvirus family; eradicated in the 1970s but still remains a threat as a bioterrorism agent.

Sneezing Occurs from nasal irritation and allows clearance of the nose.

Sniffing position Neck flexion at the fifth and sixth cervical vertebrae, with the head extended at the first and second cervical vertebrae. This position aligns the axes of the mouth, pharynx, and trachea, opening the airway and increasing airflow.

Snoring Noisy breathing through the mouth and nose during sleep; caused by air passing through a narrowed upper airway.

Social distance The acceptable distance between strangers used for impersonal business transactions. In the United States, social distance is 4 to 12 feet.

Sodium bicarbonate Neutralizes hydrochloric acid from the stomach.

Solid organ An organ (a part of the body or group of tissues that performs a specific function) without any channel or cavity within it; examples include the kidneys, pancreas, liver, and spleen.

Solubility Pertaining to the ease with which a drug can dissolve.

Solution A medication dissolved in a liquid, often water.

Soman A G nerve agent. The G agents tend to be nonpersistent, volatile agents.

Somatic Portion of the peripheral nervous system that carries impulses to and from the skin and musculature; responsible for voluntary muscle control.

Somatic delusions False perceptions of the appearance or functioning of one's own body.

Somatic nervous system Division of the peripheral nervous system whose motor nerves control movement of voluntary muscles.

Somatic pain Pain that arises from either the cutaneous tissues of the body's surface or deep tissues of the body, such as musculoskeletal tissue or the parietal peritoneum.

Somatoform disorders A group of disorders characterized by the manifestation of psychological problems as physical symptoms; this includes conversion disorder, hypochondriasis, somatization disorder, and body dysmorphic disorder.

Sore throat Any inflammation of the larynx, pharynx, or tonsils.

Space blanket A blanket resembling aluminum foil used to help the patient maintain body temperature.

Space-occupying lesion A mass, such as a tumor or blood collection, within a contained body space, such as the skull.

Spacer A hollow plastic tube that attaches to the metered-dose inhaler on one end and has a mouthpiece on the other; sometimes called a *holding chamber.*

Span of control The amount of resources that one person can effectively manage.

Special needs Conditions with the potential to interfere with usual growth and development; may involve physical disabilities, developmental disabilities, chronic illnesses, and forms of technologic support.

Specialty center A hospital that has met criteria to offer special care as a burn center, level I trauma center, stroke center, or pediatric center.

Specific gravity The ratio of a liquid's weight compared with an equal volume of water (which has a constant value of 1); materials with a specific gravity of less than 1.0 float on water and materials with a specific gravity greater than 1.0 sink.

Sperm Mucus-type secretion made of prostatic fluid and spermatozoa.

Spermatic cord Nerves, blood vessels, and smooth muscle that surround the vas (ductus) deferens.

Spermatocele Benign accumulation of sperm at the epididymis presenting as a firm mass.

Spermatogenesis Spermatozoa formation.

Spermatozoa Product of the male reproductive system.

Sphincters Smooth muscles that regulate flow through the capillary beds.

Spina bifida Malformation of the meninges and spinal cord in utero, often leading to permanent physical disabilities.

Spina bifida occulta Mildest form of spina bifida in which the spinal cord is intact but one or more vertebrae fail to close in the lumbosacral area.

Spinal cord Part of the central nervous system that connects the brain to the periphery of the body; contains the main reflex centers of the body.

Spinal cord injury (SCI) An injury to the spinal cord that results from trauma; usually a permanent injury.

Spinal cord injury without radiological abnormality A spinal cord injury not detected on a standard radiograph.

Spinal nerves Paired nerves that originate from the spinal cord and exit the spine on either side between vertebrae; each has a sensory root and a motor root.

Spinal shock Shock with hypotension caused by an injury to the spinal cord.

Spirit A medication that contains volatile aromatic substances.

Split-thickness skin graft A skin graft in which only a fraction of the thickness of the natural dermis is taken.

Spontaneous abortion See *Miscarriage.*

Spontaneous bacterial peritonitis (SBP) Infection of cirrhotic fluid in the abdominal cavity.

Spontaneous pneumothorax Pneumothorax occurring without trauma, usually by rupture of a pulmonary bleb.

Sprain An injury to a ligament that results when the ligament is overstretched, leading to tearing or complete disruption of the ligament.

Stagnant phase Vascular response in shock when precapillary sphincters open, allowing the capillary beds to engorge with fluid; follows the ischemic phase.

Stair chair A collapsible, portable chair with handles on the front and back used to carry patients in sitting position down stairs.

Standard of care Conduct exercising the degree of care, skill, and judgment that would be expected under like or similar circumstances by a similarly trained, reasonable paramedic in the same scenario.

Standard operating procedures (SOPs) An organized set of guidelines distributed across the organization.

Standing orders Written instructions that authorize EMS personnel to perform certain medical interventions before establishing direct communication with a physician.

Standard precautions Infection control practices in healthcare designed to be observed with every patient and procedure and prevent the exposure to bloodborne pathogens.

Stapes The stirrup-shaped bone that links the middle ear to the inner ear; connects to the malleus and incus.

Status asthmaticus Condition of severe asthma that is minimally responsive to therapy; a serious condition.

Status epilepticus Any prolonged series of similar seizures without return to full consciousness between them.

Statute A law passed by a legislature.

Statute of limitations A law that sets the time limits within which parties must take action to enforce their rights.

Statutory law Statutes and ordinances enacted by Congress, state legislatures, and city councils.

Steady state An evenly distributed concentration of a drug in the plasma.

Stellate laceration A laceration with jagged margins.

Stem cells Formative cells whose daughter cells may give rise to other cell types.

Stenosis Abnormal constriction or narrowing of a structure.

Stereotyping The attribution of some trait or characteristic to one person on the basis of the interviewer's preconceived notions about a general class of people of similar characteristics.

Sterile Free of any living organism.

Sterilization Process that makes an object free of all forms of life (e.g., bacteria) by using extreme heat or certain chemicals.

Sterilize To kill all microorganisms.

Stimuli Anything that excites or incites an organism or part to function, become active, or respond.

Stomach Organ located at the inferior end of the esophagus; large storage vessel surrounded by multiple layers of smooth muscle; cells within it produce acid.

Stored energy Any energy (mechanical, electrical, hydraulic, compressed air, etc.) that has the potential of being released either intentionally or inadvertently, causing further injury or problems.

Strain An injury to a muscle that results when the muscle is overstretched, leading to tearing of the individual muscle fibers.

Strainer A water hazard formed by an object or structure in the current that allows water to flow but that strains out large objects, such as boats and people.

Strangulation Compression of the vessels that carry blood, leading to ischemia.

Stratum corneum Outer layer of the epidermis where skin cells are shed.

Stress Mental, emotional, or physical pressure, strain, or tension resulting from stimuli.

Stressor A stimulus that produces stress.

Stricture A specific form of narrowing, usually from scar tissue formation.

Stridor A harsh, high-pitched sound heard on inspiration associated with upper airway obstruction; often described as a high-pitched crowing or "seal-bark" sound.

Stroke volume Amount of blood ejected by either ventricle during one contraction; can be calculated as cardiac output divided by heart rate.

Struck-by A situation in which a responder, working in or near moving traffic, is struck, injured, or killed by traffic passing the incident scene.

Stye An external hordeolum.

Stylet A relatively stiff but flexible metal rod covered by plastic and inserted into an endotracheal tube; used for maintaining the shape of the relatively pliant tube and "steering" it into position.

Subarachnoid hemorrhage Bleeding from the arteries between the arachnoid membrane and the pia mater that occurs suddenly and often is fatal.

Subcutaneous (Sub-Q) Injection of medication in a liquid form underneath the skin into the subcutaneous tissue.

Subcutaneous emphysema Air entrapped beneath the skin, typically caused by rupture of a structure containing air; feels like crackling when palpated.

Subcutaneous tissue Thick layer of connective tissue found between the layers of the skin; composed of adipose tissue and areolar tissue; insulates, protects, and stores energy (in the form of fat).

Subdural hematoma A collection of blood in the subdural space, which is between the dura mater and arachnoid layer of the meninges.

Subdural space Area below the dura mater; contains large venous vessels, drains, and a small amount of serous fluid.

Subjective information Information told to the paramedic.

Sublingual Medication placed under the tongue.

Sucking chest wound Open thoracic injury characterized by air being pulled into and pushed out of the wound during respiration.

Sudden cardiac death (SCD) An unexpected death from a cardiac cause that either occurs immediately or within 1 hour of the onset of symptoms.

Suffix Added to the end of a root word to change the meaning; usually identifies the condition of the root word.

Suicide The act of ending one's own life.

Sulfur mustard The most well known and commonly used of the vesicants.

Summarization Briefly reviewing the interview and your conclusions.

Summation The combined effects of two or more drugs equaling the sum of each of their effects.

Superficial burn A burn with a pink appearance that does not exhibit blister formation; painful both with and without tactile stimulation (e.g., sunburn); also known as a *first-degree burn.*

Superficial fascia Connective tissue that contains the subcutaneous fat cells.

Superficial partial-thickness burn Burns involving the more superficial dermis. These burns have a moist, pink appearance, and when lightly touched, are painful and sensate. Blood vessels, hair shafts, nerves, and glands may be injured, but not to the extent that regeneration cannot take place.

Superior Situated above or higher than a point of reference in the anatomic position; top.

Superior vena cava Vessel that returns venous blood from the upper part of the body to the right atrium of the heart.

Supernormal period Period during the cardiac cycle when a weaker than normal stimulus can cause cardiac cells to depolarize; extends from the end of phase 3 to the beginning of phase 4 of the cardiac action potential.

Supine Position in which the patient is lying on his or her back (face up).

Supine hypotensive syndrome A fall in the pregnant patient's blood pressure when she is placed supine; caused by the developing fetus and uterus pressing against the inferior vena cava.

Suppository Medications combined to make them a solid at room temperature; when placed in a body opening such as the rectum, vagina, or urethra, they dissolve because of the increase in body temperature and are absorbed through the surrounding mucosa.

Supraglottic Any airway structure above the vocal cords (e.g., the epiglottis).

Suprasternal notch A depression easily felt at the base of the anterior aspect of the neck, just above the angle of Louis.

Supraventricular Originating from a site above the bifurcation of the bundle of His, such as the sinoatrial node, atria, or atrioventricular junction.

Supraventricular dysrhythmias Rhythms that begin in the sinoatrial node, atrial tissue, or the atrioventricular junction.

Surfactant Specialized cells within each alveolus that keep it from collapsing when little or no air is inside.

Surge capacity The ability to expand care based on a sudden mass casualty incident developed in the emergency management plan.

Susceptibility Vulnerability or weakness; the opposite of resistance.

Suspension Medication suspended in a liquid, such as an oral antibiotic.

Sutures Seams between flat bones.

Sweat glands Odor-forming glands in the body; two types are merocrine and apocrine.

Swimmer's ear See *Otitis externa.*

Sympathetic division of the autonomic nervous system Division of the autonomic nervous system that, when stimulated, provides a fight-or-flight response, including increased heart rate, pupil dilation, bronchodilation, and the shunting of blood to the muscles.

Sympathetic nervous system Division of the autonomic nervous system that prepares the body for stress or the classic fight-or-flight response.

Sympatholytics Drugs that block or inhibit adrenergic receptors.

Sympathomimetics Drugs that mimic the sympathetic division of the autonomic nervous system.

Sympathy Sharing the patient's feelings or emotional state in relation to an illness.

Symphysis Cartilaginous joint; unites two bones by means of fibrocartilage.

Synapse Microscopic space at the neuroeffector junction that neurotransmitters cross to stimulate target tissues.

Synaptic communication Method of intercellular communication in which neural cells communicate to adjacent neural cells by using neurotransmitters.

Synaptic junction The open space in which neurotransmitters traverse to reach a receptor.

Synchondroses Cartilaginous joint; unites the bones by means of hyaline cartilage.

Synchronized intermittent mandatory ventilation (SIMV) A ventilator setting.

Syncope A brief loss of consciousness caused by a temporary decrease in blood flow to the brain.

Syndesmosis Joint in which the bones are united by fibrous, connective tissue forming an intraosseous membrane or ligament.

Synergism The interaction of drugs such that the total effect is greater than the sum of the individual effects.

Synonym A root word, prefix, or suffix that has the same or almost the same meaning as another word, prefix, or suffix.

Synovial fluid Fluid located within the joint capsules of synovial joints; provides lubrication and cushioning during manipulation of the joint.

Synovial joint Freely movable; enclosed by a capsule and synovial membrane.

Synovium Soft tissue that lines the noncartilaginous surfaces of a joint.

Synthetic drugs Drugs chemically developed in a laboratory; also called *manufactured drugs.*

Syrup A medication dissolved in water with sugar or a sugar substitute to disguise taste.

System At least two kinds of organs organized to perform a more complex task than can a single organ.

System Status Management The dynamic process of staffing, stationing, and moving ambulances based on projected call volumes; also called *flexible deployment.*

Systemic damage Damage remote to the site of exposure or absorption.

Systemic effect Drug action throughout the body.

Systemic inflammatory response syndrome A response to infection manifested by a change in two or more of the following: temperature, heart rate, respiratory rate, and white blood cell count.

Systole Contraction of the heart (usually referring to ventricular contraction) during which blood is propelled into the pulmonary artery and aorta; when the term is used without reference to a specific chamber of the heart, the term implies ventricular systole.

Systolic blood pressure The pressure exerted against the walls of the large arteries at the peak of ventricular contraction.

T lymphocytes Cells present in the lymphatic system that mediate cell-mediated immunity (also known as *T cells*).

Tablets Medications that have been pressed into a small form that is easy to swallow. They are a specific shape, color, and may have engraving for identification.

Tachycardia A heart rate grater than 100 beats/min.

Tachyphylaxis The rapidly decreasing response to a drug or physiologically active agent after administration of a few doses; rapid cross-tolerance.

Tachypnea A respiratory rate persistently faster than normal for age; in adults, a rate faster than 20 breaths/min.

Tactical EMS EMS personnel specially trained and equipped to provide prehospital emergency care in tactical environments.

Tactical patient care Patient care activities that occur inside the scene perimeter or hot zone.

Tangential thinking A progression of thoughts related to each other but that become less and less related to the original topic.

Tardive dyskinesia A neurologic syndrome caused by the long-term or high-dose use of dopamine antagonists, usually antipsychotic medications, characterized by repetitive, involuntary, and purposeless movements. The patient may appear to be grimacing. Rapid movements of the face, tongue, and extremities occur. Lip smacking, puckering, and rapid eye blinking may also be seen. No standard treatment is available. Symptoms may last for a significant period after removal of the offending agent.

Teachable moment The time just after an injury has occurred when the patient and observers remain acutely aware of what has happened and may be more receptive to learning how the event or illness could have been prevented.

Teamwork The ability to work with others to achieve a common goal.

Teeth Provide mastication of food products in preparation for entry into the stomach.

Telemetric A system set up as mayday call reporting, such as On-Star and Tele-aid. This system can send information from an automobile that has been involved in an accident directly to an emergency dispatch center with the exact location and the amount of damage that may have occurred.

Telephone aid Ad-libbed instructions most often used in emergency dispatch centers by dispatchers who have had previous training as paramedics, EMTs, or cardiopulmonary resuscitation providers; strictly relies on the dispatcher's experience and prior knowledge of a particular situation or medical condition and is considered an ineffective form of telephone treatment.

423

Telson Venom-containing portion of a scorpion's abdomen that is capable of venomous injection into human beings.

Temporal demand Measurement of call demand by hour of the day.

Temporal lobe Section of the cerebrum that receives and evaluates smell and auditory input; plays a key role in memories.

Temporal modeling Predicting the times when calls occur.

Tendonitis Inflammation of a tendon, often caused by overuse.

Tendons Tough, fibrous bands of connective tissue that connect muscle to muscle and muscle to bones.

Tension-building phase Period when tension in the relationship is high and heightened anger, blaming, and arguing may occur between the victim and the abuser.

Tension pneumothorax Life-threatening injury in which air enters the space between the lungs and the chest wall but cannot exit. With each breath, the pressure increases until it prevents ventilation and causes death.

Teratogen A drug or agent that is harmful to the development of an embryo or fetus.

Term gestation A gestation equal to or longer than 37 weeks.

Terminal drop A theory that holds that mental and physical functioning decline drastically only in the few years immediately preceding death.

Terminal illness Advanced stage of illness or disease with an unfavorable prognosis and no known cure.

Tertiary blast injury Injuries caused by the patient being thrown like a projectile.

Testes Male reproductive organs suspended within the scrotum.

Testicular torsion Twisting of the spermatic cord inside the scrotum that cuts off the blood supply to the testis.

Testosterone Male hormone secreted within the testes.

Tetany Repeated, prolonged contraction of muscles, especially of the face and limbs.

Tetraplegia Paralysis to all four extremities as a result of a spinal cord injury high in the spine. The injury can either be complete (a complete loss of muscle control and sensation below the injury site) or incomplete (a partial loss of muscle control or sensation below the injury site).

Thalamus Structure located within the limbic system that is the switchboard of the brain, through which almost all signals travel on their way in or out of the brain.

Therapeutic abortion Planned surgical or medical evacuation of the uterus.

Therapeutic dose The dose required to produce a beneficial effect in 50% of the drug-tested population; also called *effective dose.*

Therapeutic index The ratio between the amount of drug required to produce a therapeutic dose and a lethal dose of the same drug. A narrow therapeutic index is dangerous because the possibility of underdosing or overdosing is higher.

Therapeutic threshold The level of a drug that elicits a beneficial physiologic response.

Thermogenesis The process of heat generation.

Thermolysis A chemical process by which heat is dissipated from the body; sometimes results in chemical decomposition.

Thermoreceptor A sensory receptor that responds to heat and cold.

Third space Extravascular and extracellular milieu; also known as the *interstitium.*

Thirst mechanism Sensation activated by cells in the hypothalamus when cells called osmoreceptors detect an imbalance in body water; as the body is replenished by drinking fluid, the osmoreceptors sense a return to baseline and turn off this mechanism.

Thoracic vertebrae A group of 12 vertebrae in the middle of the spinal column that connect to ribs.

Thought blocking A symptom of thought disorder in which a patient is speaking and then stops mid-sentence, unable to remember what he or she was saying and unable to continue.

Thought content The dominant themes and ideas of a patient; may include delusions, hallucinations, and preoccupations.

Threatened abortion Vaginal bleeding or uterine cramping during the first half of pregnancy without cervical dilation.

Threshold limit value The airborne concentrations of a substance; represents conditions under which nearly all workers are believed to be repeatedly exposed day after day without adverse effects.

Thrombocytes One of three formed elements in the blood; also known as *platelets.*

Thrombocytopenia A lower than normal number of platelets circulating in the blood.

Thromboembolism Movement of a clot within the vascular system.

Thrombophlebitis Development of a clot in a vein in which inflammation is present.

Thromboplastin Blood coagulation factor.

Thrombus Blood clot.

Thrush A fungal infection of the mouth.

Thyroid storm Severe form of hyperthyroidism characterized by tachypnea, tachycardia, shock, hyperthermia, and delirium.

Thyrotoxicosis A condition in which the thyroid gland produces excess thyroid hormone; also called *hyperthyroidism* or *Graves' disease.*

Tidal volume The volume of air moved into or out of the lungs during a normal breath; can be indirectly evaluated by observing the rise and fall of the patient's chest and abodmen.

Time on task The average time a unit is committed to manage an incident.

Tincture A medicine consisting of an extract in an alcohol solution (e.g., tincture of iodine, tincture of mercurochrome).

Tinea capitis Located on the head and scalp; appears as a round, scaly area where no hair is growing; diffuse scaling.

Tinea corporis Located on the body; appears annular (e.g. ringworm).

Tinea cruris Located on the groin and genitalia; appears as a sharply demarcated area with elevated scaling, geographic borders.

Tinea manuum Located on the hands; appears as dry, diffuse scaling, usually on the palm.

Tinea pedis Located on the feet; appears as maceration between the toes, scaling on soles or sides of the foot, sometimes vesicles and/or pustules.

Tinea unguium Located on or under fingernails or toenails; appears as dark debris under the nails.

Tinea versicolor Located on the trunk; appears as pink, tan, or white patches with fine, desquamating scale.

Tinnitus A ringing, roaring sound or hissing in the ears that is usually caused by certain medicines or exposure to loud noise.

Tissue A group of cells that are similar in structure and function.

Tocolytic A medication used to slow uterine contractions.

Tolerance Decreasing responsiveness to the effects of a drug; increasingly larger doses are necessary to achieve the effect originally obtained by a smaller dose.

Tongue Muscular organ that provides for the sensation of taste; also directs food material toward the esophagus.

Tonic-clonic seizure Form of generalized seizure with a tonic phase (muscle rigidity) and a clonic phase (muscle tremors).

Topical Medication administered by applying it directly to the skin or mucous membrane.

Tort A wrong committed on the person or property of another.

Total body surface area burned (TBSAB) Used to describe the amount of the body injured by a burn and expressed as a percentage of the entire body surface area.

Total body water (TBW) The total amount of fluid in the body at any given time.

Totally blind Description of someone who has no vision and uses nonvisual media or reads Braille.

Toxic organic dust syndrome A flulike illness caused by the inhalation of grain dust, with symptoms including fever, chest tightness, cough, and muscle aches; inhalation may occur in an agricultural setting or from covering a floor with straw.

Toxicology The study of poisons.

Toxidrome A classification system of toxic syndromes by signs and symptoms.

Toxin A poisonous substance of plant or animal origin.

TP segment Interval on the ECG between two successive PQRST complexes during which electrical activity of the heart is absent; begins with the end of the T wave through the onset of the following P wave and represents the period from the end of ventricular repolarization to the onset of atrial depolarization.

Trachea Air passage that connects the larynx to the lungs.

Tracheal stoma A surgical opening in the anterior neck that extends from the skin surface into the trachea, opening the trachea to the atmosphere.

Tracheitis Inflammation of the mucous membranes of the trachea.

Tracheostomy The surgical creation of an opening into the trachea.

Trade name The name given a chemical compound by the company that makes it; also called the *brand name* or *proprietary name.*

Transcellular compartment Compartment classified as extracellular but distinct because it is formed from the transport activities of cells; cerebrospinal fluid, bladder urine, the aqueous humor, and the synovial fluid of the joints are considered transcellular.

Transdermal Through the skin.

Transection A complete cutting (severing) across the spinal cord.

Transient ischemic attack (TIA) Neurologic dysfunction caused by a temporary blockage in blood flow; by definition the symptoms resolve within 24 hours but usually within 1 or 2 hours.

Transient synovitis A nonspecific inflammation of a joint, usually the hip, that affects the synovium and synovial fluid in children.

Transverse colon Part of the large intestine.

Transverse plane Imaginary straight line that divides the body into top (superior) and bottom (inferior) sections; also known as the *horizontal plane.*

Traumatic asphyxia Life-threatening injury in which the thorax is severely crushed, preventing ventilation; typically results in death.

Traumatic iritis An inflammation of the iris caused by blunt trauma to the eye.

Triage Classifying patients based on the severity of illness or injury.

Tricuspid valve Right atrioventricular valve of the heart.

Trigeminal neuralgia Irritation of the seventh cranial nerve (trigeminal nerve), causing episodes of severe, stabbing pain in the face.

Trip audit The review of a prehospital care report written by a paramedic to a peer or a third party.

Tripod position Position used to maintain an open airway that involves sitting upright and learning forward with the neck slightly extended, chin projected, and mouth open and supported by the arms.

Trismus Spasm of the muscles used for chewing, resulting in limited movement of the mouth because of pain.

Trunking system A system that uses multiple repeaters (five or more) so that the computer can search for an open channel to transmit by.

Tube trailers Trailers that carry multiple cylinders of pressurized gases.

Tuberculosis (TB) A highly contagious bacterial infection known for causing pneumonia and infecting other parts of the body.

Tularemia A disease resulting from infection of *Francisella tularensis;* normally transmitted through

425

handling infected small mammals such as rabbits or rodents or through the bites of ticks, deerflies, or mosquitoes that have fed on infected animals; also known as *rabbit fever* or *deer fly fever.*

Tumor, benign A cancer that is not malignant (i.e., is not known for spreading and growing aggressively).

Tumor, malignant A cancer that is known for being aggressive and spreading to other parts of the body.

Tumor necrosis factor-alpha An inflammatory cytokine released in response to a variety of physical trauma, including burns. In burn injuries, massive quantities are produced by the liver; has been implicated as the causative agent in myocardial depression seen in burns.

Tumor, primary A tumor in the location where it originates (e.g., a primary lung tumor is in the lung).

Tumor, secondary A tumor that has spread from its original location (e.g., lung tumor that spreads to the brain); also called *metastasis.*

Tunica adventitia Outermost layer of the blood vessel; made of mainly elastic connective tissue; allows the vessel to expand to great pressure or volume.

Tunica intima Innermost layer of the blood vessel; composed of a single layer of epithelial cells; provides almost no resistance to blood flow.

Tunica media Middle layer of the blood vessel; mainly composed of smooth muscle; functions to alter the diameter of the lumen of the vessel and is under autonomic control, which enables the body to adjust blood flow quickly to meet immediate needs.

Tunics Layers of an elastic tissue and smooth muscle in the blood vessels.

Tunnel vision Focusing on or considering only one aspect of a situation without first taking into account all possibilities.

Turbinates Large folds found in the nasal cavity; highly vascular area in the nose that warms and humidifies inhaled air.

Turgor Normal tension of a cell or tissue.

Tympanic membrane A thin, translucent, pearly gray oval disk that protects the middle and conducts sound vibrations; eardrum.

Type and crossmatch Mixing a sample of a recipient's and donor's blood to evaluate for incompatibility.

Type I ambulance Regular truck cab and frame with a modular ambulance box mounted on the back.

Type II ambulance Van-style ambulance.

Type III ambulance A van chassis with a modified modular back.

Type IV (quaternary) blast injuries All other miscellaneous injuries caused by an explosive device.

Ulcer A full-thickness crater that involves the dermis and epidermis, with loss of the surface epithelium; this lesion is depressed and may bleed; it usually heals with scarring.

Umbilical An administration route that may be used on a newborn infant; because the umbilical cord was the primary source of nutrient and waster exchange, it provides an immediate source of drug exchange.

Umbilical cord The cord, containing two arteries and a vein, that connects the fetus to the placenta.

Umbilical cord prolapse Appearance of the umbilical cord in front of the presenting part, usually with compression of the cord and interruption of blood supply to the fetus.

Umbilical vein route Route of administration that achieves access through the one umbilical vein set between the two umbilical arteries.

Unethical Conduct that does not conform to moral standards of social or professional behavior.

Unified command Command type involving multiple agencies.

Unintentional injury Injuries and deaths not self-inflicted or perpetrated by another person (accidents).

Unintentional tort A wrong that the defendant did not mean to commit; a case in which a bad outcome occurred because of the failure to exercise reasonable care.

Unipolar lead Lead that consists of a single positive electrode and a reference point; a pacing lead with a single electrical pole at the distal tip of the pacing lead (negative pole) through which the stimulating pulse is delivered. In a permanent pacemaker with a unipolar lead, the positive pole is the pulse generator case.

Unit hour utilization (UhU) A measure of ambulance service productivity and staff workload.

United Nations (UN) number The four-digit number assigned to chemicals during transit by the U.S. Department of Transportation; the *2004 Emergency Guidebook* lists useful information about these chemicals.

Upper airway Portion of the respiratory tract above the glottis.

Upper flammable limit The concentration of fuel in the air above which the vapors cannot be ignited; above this point too much fuel and not enough oxygen are present to burn (too rich); also called the *upper explosive limit.*

Upper respiratory tract infection (URI) Viral syndrome causing nasal congestion, coughing, fever, and runny nose.

Upregulation The process by which a cell increases the number of receptors exposed to a given substance to improve its sensitivity to that substance.

Upstream A term describing the approaching traffic side of the damaged vehicles and the crash scene.

Uremia A term used to describe the signs and symptoms that accompany chronic renal failure.

Uremic frost Dried crystals of urea excreted through the skin that appear to be a frosting on the patient's body.

Ureter Tube that drains urine from the kidney to the bladder.

Urethra Passageway for both urine and male reproductive fluids; opening at the end of the bladder.

Urethral meatus Opening of the urethra between the clitoris and vagina.

Urinary bladder Hollow organ that stores urine; surrounded by smooth muscle.

Urinary retention The inability to empty the bladder or completely empty the bladder when urinating.

Urinary system Eliminates dissolved organic waste products by urine production and elimination.

Urticaria Also known as *hives;* a skin condition in which a wheal on the skin forms from edema; often caused by a reaction to a drug or through contact with substances (skin contact or even inhaled), causing hypersensitivity in the patient.

Uterine cavity Innermost region of the uterus.

Uterine prolapse Protrusion of part or all of the uterus out of the vagina.

Uterine tubes Tubular structures that extend from each side of the superior end of the body of the uterus to the lateral pelvic wall; they pick up the egg released by the ovary and transport it to the uterus; also known as *fallopian tubes.*

Uterus Muscular organ approximately the size of a pear; grows with the developing fetus.

Uvula Fleshy tissue resembling a grape that hangs down from the soft palate.

Vagina Female organ of copulation, the lower part of the birth canal, extending from the uterus to the outside of the body; extends from the cervix to the outside of the body.

Vaginal orifice Opening of the vagina.

Vaginitis An inflammation of the vaginal tissues.

Vallecula The depression or pocket between the base of the tongue and the epiglottis.

Vancomycin-resistant *Enterococcus* Bacteria resistant to vancomycin (a potent antibiotic); commonly acquired by patients in the hospital or patients who have indwelling catheters.

Vapor density The weight of a volume of pure gas compared with the weight of an equal volume of pure dry air (which has a constant value of 1); materials with a vapor density less than 1.0 are lighter than air and rise when released; materials with a vapor density greater than 1.0 are heavier than air and sink when released.

Vapor pressure The pressure exerted by a vapor against the sides of a closed container; a measure of volatility — high vapor pressure means it is a volatile substance.

Varicella An acute contagious vesicular skin eruption caused by the varicella zoster virus (chickenpox).

Varices Distended veins.

Varicocele Dilation of the venous plexus and internal spermatic vein, presenting as a lump in the scrotum.

Variola major A member of the *orthopoxvirus* family that causes the most common form of smallpox; the most likely form of the organism to be used as a weapon.

Vas deferens Tubes that extend from the end of the epididymis and through the seminal vesicles; also known as the *ductus deferens.*

Vascular access device Type of intravenous device used to deliver fluids, medications, blood, or nutritional therapy; usually inserted in patients who require long-term intravenous therapy.

Vascular headaches Headaches that involve changes in the diameter or size and chemistry of blood vessels that supply the brain.

Vascular resistance Amount of opposition that the blood vessels give to the flow of blood.

Vascular tunic Layer of the eye that contains most of the vasculature of the eye.

Vector A mode of transmission of a disease, typically from an insect or animal.

Vegetative functions Autonomic functions the body requires to survive.

Vehicle hazards Hazards directly related to the vehicle itself, including undeployed airbags; fuel system concerns; electrical system and battery electricity; stability of the vehicle; sharp glass and metal; leaking hot antifreeze; and engine oil, transmission oil, or antifreeze spills. Even the contents inside a vehicle's trunk or cargo area are typical vehicle hazards that can be encountered.

Vehicle stabilization Immediate action taken to prevent any unwanted movement of a crash-damaged vehicle.

Vena cava One of two large veins returning blood from the peripheral circulation to the right atrium of the heart.

Venipuncture Piercing of a vein.

Venom The poison injected by venomous animals such as snakes, insects, and marine creatures.

Venous return Amount of blood flowing into the right atrium each minute from the systemic circulation.

Ventilation The mechanical process of moving air into and out of the lungs.

Ventral Referring to the front of the body; anterior.

Ventricles Two pumping chambers in the heart.

Ventricular fibrillation Disorganized electrical activity of the ventricular conduction system of the heart, resulting in inefficient contractile force. This is the main cause of sudden cardiac death in electrical injuries.

Venules Small venous vessels that return blood to the capillaries.

Verbal apraxia Speech disorder in which the person has difficulty saying what he or she wants to say in a correct and consistent manner.

Verbal stimulus Any noise that elicits some sort of response from the patient.

Vertebrae Specialized bones comprising the spinal column.

Vertebral foramen Open space in the middle of vertebra.

Vertigo An out-of-control spinning sensation not relieved by lying down that may get worse when the eyes are closed.

Very high frequency A type of radio signal used to make two-way radio contact between the communications center and the responders. Now considered old technology compared with more contemporary 800-MHz radio systems.

427

Vesicants Agents named from the most obvious injury they inflict on a person; will burn and blister the skin or any other part of the body they touch; also known as *blister agents* or *mustard agents.*

Vesicles The shipping containers of the cell. They are very simple in structure, consisting of a single membrane filled with liquid; they transport a wide variety of substances both inside and outside the cell.

Vestibule Space or cavity that serves as the entrance to the inner ear.

Veterinary medical assistance team Teams designed to provide animal care and assistance during disasters.

Vials Glass containers with rubber stoppers at the top.

Viral hemorrhagic fevers A group of viral diseases of diverse etiology (arenaviruses, filoviruses, bunyaviruses, and flaviviruses) having many similar characteristics, including increased capillary permeability, leukopenia, and thrombocytopenia, resulting in a severe multisystem syndrome.

Viral shedding Release of viruses from an infected host through some vector (e.g., sneezing, coughing, bleeding).

Virions Small particles of viruses.

Virulence A term to describe the relative pathogenicity or the relative ability to do damage to the host of an infectious agent.

Virus Microorganism that invades cells and uses their machinery to live and replicate; cannot survive without a host, does not have a cell wall of its own, and consists of a strand of DNA or RNA surrounded by a capsid.

Visceral Portion of the peripheral nervous system that processes motor and sensory information from the internal organs, includes the autonomic nervous system.

Visceral pain Deep pain that arises from internal areas of the body that are enclosed within a cavity.

Visceral pleura Lining of the pleural cavity that adheres tightly to the lung surface.

Viscosity The thickness of a liquid; a high-viscosity liquid does not flow easily (e.g., oils and tar); a low-viscosity liquid flows easily (e.g., gasoline) and poses a greater risk for aspiration and consequent pulmonary damage.

Visual acuity card A standardized board used to test vision.

Vitreous chamber The most posterior chamber of the eyeball.

Vitreous humor Thick, jellylike substance that fills the vitreous chamber of the eyeball.

Voice over Internet protocol Telephone technology that gives Internet users the ability to make voice telephone calls.

Volatility A measure of how quickly a material passes into the vapor or gas state; the greater the volatility, the greater its rate of evaporation.

Volkmann contracture A deformity of the hand, fingers, and wrist caused by injury to the muscles of the forearm; also known as *ischemic contracture.*

Voltage Difference in electrical charge between two points.

Voluntary guarding Conscious contraction of the abdominal muscles in an attempt to prevent painful palpation.

Volvulus Intestinal obstruction caused by a knotting and twisting of the bowel.

Vomiting Forceful ejection of stomach contents through the mouth.

Vowel The letters *a, e, i, o, u,* and sometimes *y.*

Vulva External female genitalia.

Vulvovaginitis Inflammation of the external female genitalia and vagina.

VX Most toxic of the nerve agent class of military warfare agents.

Warm zone Area surrounding the hot zone that functions as a safety buffer area, decontamination area, and as an access and egress point to and from the hot zone; also called the *contamination reduction zone.*

Warts Benign lesions caused by the papillomavirus.

Washout phase Vascular response in shock when postcapillary sphincters open, allowing fluid in the capillary beds to be pushed into systemic circulation; follows the stagnant phase.

Water solubility The degree to which a material or its vapors are soluble in water.

Water-reactive materials Materials that violently decompose and/or burn vigorously when they come in contact with moisture.

Waveform Movement away from the baseline in either a positive or negative direction.

Wernicke-Korsakoff syndrome Neurologic disorder caused by a thiamine deficiency; most often seen in chronic alcoholics; characterized by ataxia, nystagmus, weakness, and mental derangement in the early stages. In later stages, the condition is much more likely to become permanent and is characterized by amnesia, disorientation, delirium, and hallucinations.

Wheal A firm, rounded, flat-topped elevation of skin that is evanescent and pruritic (itches); also known as a *hive.*

Wheeze A musical, whistling sound heard on inspiration and/or expiration resulting from constriction or obstruction of the pharynx, trachea, or bronchi. Wheezing is commonly associated with asthma.

Wilderness command physician A physician who has received additional training by a Wilderness Emergency Medical Services Institute–endorsed course in wilderness medical care and medical direction of wilderness EMS providers and operations.

Wilderness emergency medical technician An emergency medical technician who has obtained EMT certification by Department of Transportation criteria and has completed additional modules in wilderness care; sometimes abbreviated as WEMT, W-EMT, or EMT-W.

Wilderness EMS An individual or group that preplans to administer care in an austere environment and then is called on to perform these duties when needed.

Wilderness EMS system A formally structured organization integrated into or part of the standard EMS system and configured to provide wilderness medical care to a discrete region.

Wilderness first aid A level of certification indicating a provider has been trained in traditional first aid with added training in wilderness care and first aid administration in austere environments.

Wilderness first responder A first responder who has obtained certification by Department of Transportation criteria and has completed additional modules in wilderness care.

Wilderness medicine Medical management in situations where care and prevention are limited by environmental considerations, prolonged extrication, or resource availability.

Window phase The period after infection during which the antigen is present but no antibody is detectable.

Withdrawal Physical and/or psychological signs and symptoms that result from discontinuing regular administration of a drug; effects are usually the opposite of the effects of the drug itself because the body has changed itself to maintain homeostasis.

Wolff-Parkinson-White syndrome Type of preexcitation syndrome characterized by a slurred upstroke of the QRS complex (delta wave) and wide QRS.

Word root The foundation of a word; establishes the basic meaning of a word.

Word salad The most severe form of looseness of associations in which the topic shifts so rapidly that it interrupts the flow of sentences themselves, producing a jumble of words.

Workload management Planning resources and support services around demand.

Wrap point A machinery entanglement hazard formed when any machine component rotates.

Xenografting Transplanting tissue from a member of a different species (e.g., porcine heart valves harvested from pigs).

Years of potential life lost (YPLL) A method that assumes that, on average, most people will live a productive life until the age of 65 years.

Yeast A unicellular type of fungus that reproduces by budding.

Yersinia pestis The anaerobic, gram-negative bacterium that causes plague disease in human beings and rodents.

Zone of coagulation In a full-thickness burn wound, the central area of the burn devoid of blood flow. This tissue is not salvageable and becomes visibly necrotic days after the injury.

Zone of stasis or ischemia Outside the zone of coagulation, where blood supply is tenuous. The capillaries may be damaged but oxygenated blood can still pass through them to perfuse the surrounding tissues.

Illustration Credits

CHAPTER 7

Brain, Hearts, Lymphatic system

Drake, R., Vogl, W., & Mitchell, A. (2005). *Gray's anatomy for students*. New York: Churchill Livingstone.
Herlihy, B. (2007). *The human body in health and illness* (3rd ed.). Philadelphia: Saunders.

CHAPTER 22

Aehlert, B. (2006). *ECGs made easy* (3rd ed.). St Louis: Mosby.

CHAPTER 23

Aehlert, B. (2006). *ECGs made easy* (3rd ed.). St Louis: Mosby.

CHAPTER 27

Aehlert, B. (2006). *ECGs made easy* (3rd ed.). St Louis: Mosby